Complementary and Alternative Medicine for Health Professionals

Complementary and Alternative Medicine for Health Professionals

Edited by Penelope Higgins

hayle
medical

New York

Hayle Medical,
750 Third Avenue, 9th Floor,
New York, NY 10017, USA

Visit us on the World Wide Web at:
www.haylemedical.com

ISBN: 978-1-63241-816-6

Trademark Notice: Registered trademark of products or corporate names are used only for explanation and identification without intent to infringe.

Cataloging-in-Publication Data

Complementary and alternative medicine for health professionals / edited by Penelope Higgins.
    p. cm.
Includes bibliographical references and index.
ISBN 978-1-63241-816-6
1. Alternative medicine. 2. Medicine. 3. Alternative medicine specialists--Guidebooks. I. Higgins, Penelope.
R733 .C66 2019
615.5--dc23

Table of Contents

Preface

Integrative health care is the approach to health and wellness that combines the benefits of conventional and complementary health practices in a holistic and patient-focused manner. Alternative medicine approaches include mind and body practices along with the use of natural products. Yoga, meditation, and chiropractic and osteopathic manipulation are some of the popular mind and body practices. Hypnotherapy, acupuncture, tai chi, qi gong, Trager psychophysical integration, etc. are other such practices. Natural products include a variety of products, such as probiotics, herbs, vitamins and minerals. Complementary and alternative medicine (CAM) uses conventional medical treatment with alternative medicinal practices for improved results. Integrative medicine can help people by reducing pain, fatigue and anxiety. Some of the clinical conditions treated under integrative medicine include musculoskeletal and joint pain, gastrointestinal conditions, cancer, women's health issues, stress management, etc. This book covers in detail some existing theories and innovative concepts revolving around complementary and alternative medicine. It aims to shed light on some of the unexplored aspects of integrative health care and the recent researches in this field. It will help new researchers by foregrounding their knowledge in this field.

After months of intensive research and writing, this book is the end result of all who devoted their time and efforts in the initiation and progress of this book. It will surely be a source of reference in enhancing the required knowledge of the new developments in the area. During the course of developing this book, certain measures such as accuracy, authenticity and research focused analytical studies were given preference in order to produce a comprehensive book in the area of study.

This book would not have been possible without the efforts of the authors and the publisher. I extend my sincere thanks to them. Secondly, I express my gratitude to my family and well-wishers. And most importantly, I thank my students for constantly expressing their willingness and curiosity in enhancing their knowledge in the field, which encourages me to take up further research projects for the advancement of the area.

Editor

Coconut water vinegar ameliorates recovery of acetaminophen induced liver damage in mice

Nurul Elyani Mohamad[1], Swee Keong Yeap[2], Boon-Kee Beh[3,4], Huynh Ky[5], Kian Lam Lim[6], Wan Yong Ho[7], Shaiful Adzni Sharifuddin[4], Kamariah Long[4*] and Noorjahan Banu Alitheen[1,3*] (iD)

Abstract

Background: Coconut water has been commonly consumed as a beverage for its multiple health benefits while vinegar has been used as common seasoning and a traditional Chinese medicine. The present study investigates the potential of coconut water vinegar in promoting recovery on acetaminophen induced liver damage.

Methods: Mice were injected with 250 mg/kg body weight acetaminophen for 7 days and were treated with distilled water (untreated), Silybin (positive control) and coconut water vinegar (0.08 mL/kg and 2 mL/kg body weight). Level of oxidation stress and inflammation among treated and untreated mice were compared.

Results: Untreated mice oral administrated with acetaminophen were observed with elevation of serum liver profiles, liver histological changes, high level of cytochrome P450 2E1, reduced level of liver antioxidant and increased level of inflammatory related markers indicating liver damage. On the other hand, acetaminophen challenged mice treated with 14 days of coconut water vinegar were recorded with reduction of serum liver profiles, improved liver histology, restored liver antioxidant, reduction of liver inflammation and decreased level of liver cytochrome P450 2E1 in dosage dependent level.

Conclusion: Coconut water vinegar has helped to attenuate acetaminophen-induced liver damage by restoring antioxidant activity and suppression of inflammation.

Keywords: *Cocos nucifera*, Paracetamol, Phenolic, Acetification, Inflammation

Background

Acetaminophen or more commonly known as paracetamol is among the most commonly used mild analgesic drug worldwide [1]. Although acetaminophen is generally considered safe, unintentional or deliberate overdoses have resulted in acute liver failure especially in United States [2]. Acetaminophen is metabolized by cytochrome P450 2E1 (CYP2E1) in the liver into the reactive metabolite N-acetyl-p-benzoquinone imine (NAPQI). When consumed in safe dosage, NAPQI can be easily detoxified by glutathione (GSH) into acetaminophen-glutathione conjugate.

When acetaminophen was consumed in overdose, metabolism by CYP2E1enzyme produced excessive NAPQI that depletes the liver GSH and caused mitochondrial oxidative stress. Subsequently, mitochondrial oxidative stress promotes hepatocyte cell death and release of hepatocyte contents such as ALT. Massive release of liver enzymes such as ALT also results in formation of pro-inflammatory mediators and chronic inflammation [3].

Bioactive food ingredients and herbal medicine have been widely used to alleviate chronic liver disease. The hepatoprotective effect from these food ingredients and herbal medicine was contributed by the active metabolites such as curcumin from turmeric and silymarin from milk thistle seeds [4]. Although these food or herbal ingredients have been widely consumed and generally believed as safe, their efficacy and safety will still need further validation [4]. Coconut (*Cocos nucifera* L.) water

* Correspondence: amai@mardi.gov.my; noorjahan@upm.edu.my
[4]Biotechnology Research Centre, Malaysian Agricultural Research and Development Institute (MARDI), 43400 Serdang, Selangor, Malaysia
[1]Department of Cell and Molecular Biology, Faculty of Biotechnology and Biomolecular Science, Universiti Putra Malaysia, 43400 Serdang, Selangor, Malaysia
Full list of author information is available at the end of the article

is a delicious and refreshing drink in coconut producing countries. In addition, coconut water is also consumed for various health benefits. Previous study has reported that coconut water is rich in antioxidant and lack of anti-nutritional factors. Antioxidants in the coconut water have contributed to prevent lipid peroxidation in the animal that fed with fish oil diet [5]. In addition, normal animals fed with coconut water were recorded with reduction of liver enzymes and thus proposed as potential hepatoprotective agent [6]. Moreover, coconut water has also been reported with hepatoprotection activity on carbon tetrachloride (CCl_4) induced liver damaged [7−9] and alloxan induced diabetic [10] rat models by restoring the liver antioxidant level. However, in the coconut industry, coconut water particularly from the mature coconut was commonly handled as waste by-product due to the cost and processing flow [11]. As coconut water contained substantial amount of sugar [12], thus it is suitable as starting material to be converted as fermented end product such as vinegar.

Vinegar is widely used as food seasoning and traditional Chinese medicine [13]. It has been reported with various bioactivities including anti-diabetic, anti-hypertension, anti-microbe, liver protection and anti-tumor effects [14]. However, vinegar produced using different source of carbohydrate and strains of microbes may possess different level of bioactivities particularly on the antioxidant activity [15]. Previously, nipa water vinegar and roselle vinegar were reported with higher antioxidant level than the unfermented fruit [16, 17]. As coconut water was reported to exhibit hepatoprotective effect on CCl4 induced liver inflammation, the fermentation of this fruit water may enhance the effect. Our recent finding on hepatoprotective effect of nipa vinegar also has demonstrated a significant restoration of liver inflammation in mice treated with nipa vinegar sample [16]. Nonetheless, acetification of some fruits was reported with reduction of antioxidant activity due to decrease of total phenolics [18]. Thus, although coconut water has been reported as potential hepatoprotective agent [7−9] and coconut water vinegar has been commonly consumed to treat various disease including liver disorders and inflammation in coconut producing countries, the hepato-recovery effect of coconut water vinegar was still unclear. Thus, this study was performed to evaluate the effect of coconut water vinegar in promoting recovery of acetaminophen induced liver damage.

Methods

Organic acid and antioxidant level of coconut water vinegar

Coconut water vinegar (batch no:2, 9th May 2014) was obtained from Malaysian Agricultural Research and Development Institute (MARDI) (Selangor, Malaysia) in year 2013. Details of preparation method were described in Beh et al. [16]. The coconut water vinegar was standardized to 5% acetic acid and confirmed by reversed phase chromatography with eternal calibration graph (Result not shown). Organic acids in the sample were separated on an Extrasil ODS column (250 mm × 4.6 mm, 5 μm) and the detector was set at $\lambda = 210$ nm and $\lambda = 245$ nm. Determination of acetic acid was carried out at isocratic conditions at 45 °C, using a mobile phase of 50 mM phosphate solution (6.8 g potassium dihydrogen phosphate in 900 ml water, pH 2.8). The flow rate of the mobile phase was set at 0.7 ml/min. Total phenolic content and total antioxidant capacity were profiled using Folin-Ciocalteu and FRAP assays [14].

Animals

The study was performed according to international rules and approved by Universiti Putra Malaysia Animal Care and Use Committee (IACUC) (UPM/FPV/PS/3.2.1. 551/AUP-R168). In brief, a total of 35 BALB/c mice (male, 5−6 weeks old) were purchased from Animal House of the Faculty of Veterinary Sciences, Universiti Putra Malaysia and were placed in plastic cages at 22 ± 1 °C with 12 h of dark/light cycle and relative humidity approximately 60%.. The mice were maintained on a basal diet (22% crude protein, 5% crude fiber, 3% fat, 13% moisture, 8% ash, 0.85−1.2% calcium, 0.6−1% phosphorus and 49% nitrogen free extract) (Mouse pellet 702-P from Gold Coin Co, Limited, Malaysia) and were given distilled water *ad libitum*. The mice were divided into 5 groups and all mice were pre-treated with acetaminophen (250 mg/kg BW) for 7 days via stomach gavage to induce liver inflammation except for normal control group (N). The post-treatment with coconut vinegar begin after 7 days of acetaminophen induction where distilled water was given to the untreated group (UT), 50 mg/kg BW silybin was given to positive control group (S), 0.08 mL/kg BW coconut vinegar was given to low concentration treatment group (CL) and 2 mL/kg BW was given to high concentration treatment group (CH). All samples were prepared freshly prior to usage. At the end of the treatment, the mice were euthanized under ketamine-xylazine anesthesia (100 mg ketamine and 10 mg xylazine per kg body weight). Blood samples were collected from their hearts by cardiac puncture and liver was harvested for further analysis.

Serum biochemical analysis

Serum samples were analyzed for liver marker (ALT, AST and ALP) and lipid profile (cholesterol, triglyceride, LDL and HDL) using ELISA assay kits (Roche, Germany).

Liver tissue histological analysis

Histology of liver tissues was performed as reported previously [14]. The liver was rinsed with PBS and fixed in buffered formalin for 24 h. Then, the liver was embedded in paraffin, sectioned, deparaffinized and rehydrated using the standard techniques before further stained with hematoxylin and eosin. The morphology of the liver was then observed using bright field optic under a Nikon Eclipse 90imicroscope (New York, USA) at 40 times magnification.

Liver antioxidant level

Excised liver was weighted and meshed in phosphate buffer saline (PBS) at a ratio of 1 g of liver to 10 mL of PBS. The supernatant was centrifuged at 10000 rpm for 10 min and the upper clear part of the supernatant was collected and kept in -20 °C prior to the antioxidant analyses. The antioxidant activity in this study was evaluated through superoxide dismutase (SOD) assay, lipid peroxidation (MDA) and glutathione reductase activity (GSH). MDA and SOD was done according to the previous study [14] while GSH was done using Glutathione assay kit according to the manufacturer's protocol (Sigma, USA).

Liver cytochrome P450 2E1 level

Cytochrome P450 (Abcam, USA) protein expression level was determined using Western blot technique as reported previously [14]. In brief, fresh liver tissue was weighed and meshed in liquid nitrogen before lysed in Radio Immuno Precipitation Assay (RIPA) buffer (150 mM sodium chloride, 1.0% NP-40 or Triton X-100 0.5% sodium deoxycholate, 0.1% SDS (sodium dodecyl sulphate) and 50 mM Tris, pH 8.0) added with protease inhibitor cocktail (Pierce, Thermo Fisher Scientific, USA). Protein was measured using the standard Bradford protein assay with Bradford reagent (Bio-Rad, USA). Using SDS page, an equal amount of protein was separated and transferred to nitrocellulose membrane (PALL, USA). Then, the membrane was then blocked with 5% non-fat milk (Biobasic, USA) overnight. The next day, the membrane was washed with TBST (10 mM Tris, 140 mM NaCl, 0.1% Tween-20, pH 7.6) and further incubated in primary antibody for 1 h at 4 °C followed by washing with TBST before incubated with appropriate 2° antibody for another 1 h. Then, it was washed again and incubated with HRP substrate for 10 min before viewed using a Chemidoc imager (UVP, USA). The density results obtained were analyzed using Vision Work LS Analysis software, UVP, USA.

Liver iNOS and NF-kB mRNA expression analysis

Total RNA from liver tissue was isolated using the RNeasy kit (Qiagen, Germany). Then, first-strand cDNA was synthesized using 1 μg of total RNA in a 20 μL reverse transcriptase reaction mixture using Bio-rad iScript cDNA synthesis kit following the manufacturer's protocol. PCR amplification was performed in a 96-well plate with a 20 μL reaction mixture containing cDNA template and 1 μM of forward and reverse primers. Quantitative real-time PCR assays iNOS and NF-kB were carried out using iQ5 (Bio-Rad, USA). The differences in CT values and the relative fold change in gene expression between groups of control and treated groups was analyzed using Bio-Rad software.

Liver nitric oxide level

The NO activity was determined using Griess reagent kit protocol given by the manufacturer (Invitrogen, USA). Hundred and fifty μL of liver homogenate was mixed with 20 μL of Griess Reagent and 130 μL of distilled water in a 96-well plate and incubated for 30 min at room temperature. The absorbance was read at 540 nm using an ELISA Reader (Bio-tek Instrument, USA).

Statistical analysis

Data are reported as mean ± SD and were analyzed using SPSS 16 software by one-way analysis of variance (ANOVA). K-S (with Lilliefors correction) tests in SPSS was used to test for the normality of the results in this study. Normal distribution was obtained for results in all subgroups in all tested assays. Duncan's multiple range tests was performed as post-hoc analysis. P values less than 0.05 were considered significant.

Results

Total antioxidant and organic acids content

Comparing between fresh coconut water (total phenolic acid 167.24 ± 0.35 μg GAE/ml; FRAP: 222.87 ± 1.11 μg TE/ml) with coconut water vinegar (total phenolic acid 106.45 ± 0.01 μg GAE/ml; FRAP: 176.65 ± 0.01 μg TE/ml), total phenolic content (TPC) was recorded with ~ 36% of reduction, which has contributed to ~ 20% reduction of Ferric reducing ability of plasma (FRAP) antioxidant content. Acetic acid was not detected in fresh coconut water but the concentration of acetic acid in coconut water vinegar was 4.95% (Result not shown).

Serum liver enzyme and lipid levels

Acetaminophen induced a remarkable increase in serum liver enzyme ALT, ALP and AST comparing to the normal healthy mice. In addition, serum cholesterol and triglyceride level were raised while HDL/LDL ratio was reduced in the untreated acetaminophen challenged mice. Silymarin and coconut water vinegar treatment were able to significantly reduced both serum liver enzymes and lipid profiles. In addition, improvement of serum liver and lipid profiles by coconut vinegar treatment in the acetaminophen challenged mice were in dosage dependent manner (Table 1).

Histologic analysis of liver

Histologic analysis of the livers in each group is shown in Fig. 1. Dilated sinusoids (SC) and pyknotic nuclei (black rectangle) were present in the liver of untreated acetaminophen challenged mice (UT). On the other hand, mice treated with both silymarin (S) and coconut water vinegar (CL and CH) were observed with less incident of dilated sinusoids and binuclear hepatocytes (BN) indicating recovery of liver cell from the damage caused by acetaminophen. Comparing between low and high dose of coconut water vinegar, higher amount of binuclear hepatocytes and absence of pyknotic nuclei in the CH indicated that high dose of coconut water vinegar promotes better recovery.

SOD, GSH and lipid peroxidation level in the liver

Drastic reduction of SOD enzyme (Fig. 2a) and GSH peptide (Fig. 2b) level associated with increase of lipid peroxidation (Fig. 2c) was observed in the liver of untreated acetaminophen challenged mice. On the contrary, Silymarin and coconut water vinegar treatment helped to restore the SOD enzyme and GSH peptide level in the liver (Fig. 2a and b). More interestingly, GSH peptide level in both CL and CH treated mice was higher than normal healthy mice indicating that coconut water vinegar promotes antioxidant level in the mice by stimulating production of GSH in mice (Fig. 2b). Enhancement of liver antioxidant by both silymarin and coconut water vinegar were observed with significant ($p < 0.01$) reduction of lipid peroxidation in the liver as indicated by the level of malondialdehyde (MDA) (Fig. 2c).

CYP2E1 level in the liver

Normal healthy mice were recorded with lowest level of cytochrome P450 2E1 (CYP2E1) level comparing to the other groups. In terms of silymarin, CL and CH treated mice, -1.45, -1.05 and -2 folds down-regulation of CYP2E1 level in the liver compared to the untreated acetaminophen challenged mice, respectively (Fig. 3).

mRNA expression of iNOS and NF-kB in the liver

The liver mRNA expression levels of iNOS and NF-kB are shown in Fig. 4. Down-regulation of iNOS and NF-kb mRNA expression were observed in the liver of normal, silymarin treated and coconut water vinegar treated mice compared to the untreated acetaminophen challenged mice (Fig. 4).

Nitric oxide (NO) level in the liver

Nitric oxide (NO) level in the liver of mice untreated acetaminophen challenged mice was significantly higher compared to other groups. Silymarin and CH treatments have reduced the liver NO level close to the normal healthy mice (Fig. 5).

Discussion

Unlike other types of vinegars [16, 17], coconut water vinegar was recorded with reduced total antioxidant activity contributed by reduction of total phenolic content as described in section 2.1. This phenomenon was common as previous study has shown that acetification of fruit that is rich in phenolic acid has slight reduction of antioxidant [18]. Previous studies have proposed that antioxidant in the coconut water contributes to the hepatoprotective effect [7–9]. Although comparatively coconut vinegar is slightly less effective than fruit vinegar, previous study has reported that even synthetic vinegar that only contained acetic acid also possessed substantial hepatoprotective and anti-inflammatory effects [14]. Thus, it is important to evaluate the hepatoprotective, antioxidant and anti-inflammatory effect of coconut water vinegar in the acetaminophen challenged mice.

In this study, acetaminophen treatment was found to cause liver damage as indicated by the high level of serum liver enzymes profile and liver histology changes [1]. In addition, elevation of serum lipid profile as shown in Table 2 also indirectly indicates mild liver function failure as liver is the major organ of fat metabolism [19]. Coconut water vinegar treatment was able to reduce serum liver enzymes level and serum lipid profiles (Table 2) indicating that liver damage caused by acetaminophen was

Table 1 Primer sequences of inducible nitric oxide synthase (iNOS) and nuclear factor kappa-light-chain-enhancer of activated B cells (NF-kB) used in the quantitative real time PCR (qRT-PCR) assay. Beta-actin (β-actin), hypoxanthine phosphoribosyltransferase (HPRT) and glyceraldehyde 3-phosphate dehydrogenase (GAPDH) were used as housekeeping genes for normalization of the iNOS and NF-kB gene expression

	Forward primer (5'-3')	Reverse primer (3'-5')
iNOS	5'-GCACCGAGATTGGAGTTC-3'	3'-GAGCACAGCCACATTGAT-5'
NF-κB	5'-CATTCTGACCTTGCCTATCT-3'	3'-CTGCTGTTCTGTCCATTCT-5'
β-actin	5'-TTCCAGCCTTCCTTCTTG-3'	3'-GGAGCCAGAGCAGTAATC-5'
GAPDH	5'-GAAGGTGGTGAAGCAGGCATC-3'	3'-GAAGGTGGAAGAGTGGGAGTT-5'
HPRT	5'-CGTGATTAGCGATGATGAAC-3'	3'-AATGTAATCCAGCAGGTCAG-5'

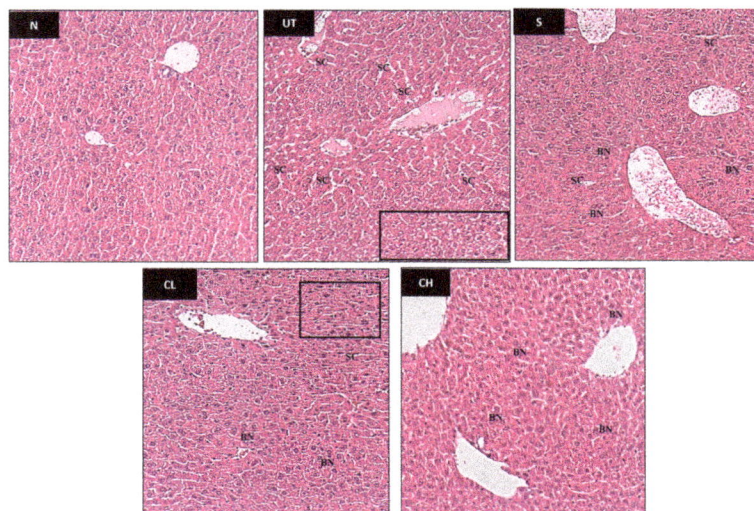

Fig. 1 Effect of coconut water vinegar against acetaminophen-induced liver histopathological changes in mice (magnification 200×). N: Liver from normal control mice with normal histological appearance. UT: Untreated acetaminophen challenged mice with pyknotic nuclei (rectangle), and dilated sinusoidal (SC). S: Silybin treated acetaminophen challenged mice and CL: 0.08 ml/kg BW coconut vinegar treated acetaminophen challenged mice showed reduced number of dilated sinusoidal (SC) and increasing binuclear hepatocyte (BN) comparing to UT. CH: 2 ml/kg BW coconut vinegar treated acetaminophen challenged mice histological appearance similar to normal control mice with higher incidence of binuclear hepatocyte (BN)

improving after 2 weeks of treatment with coconut water vinegar. These results were supported by the higher event of binuclear hepatocytes observed in the histological study indicating liver cells underwent regeneration [20].

The liver damage induced by over-dosage of acetaminophen was reported due to the development of oxidative stress in the liver [1, 3]. Cytochrome P450 2E1 (CYP2E1) is the main enzyme involved in metabolism of toxic substrates such as alcohol, acetaminophen and

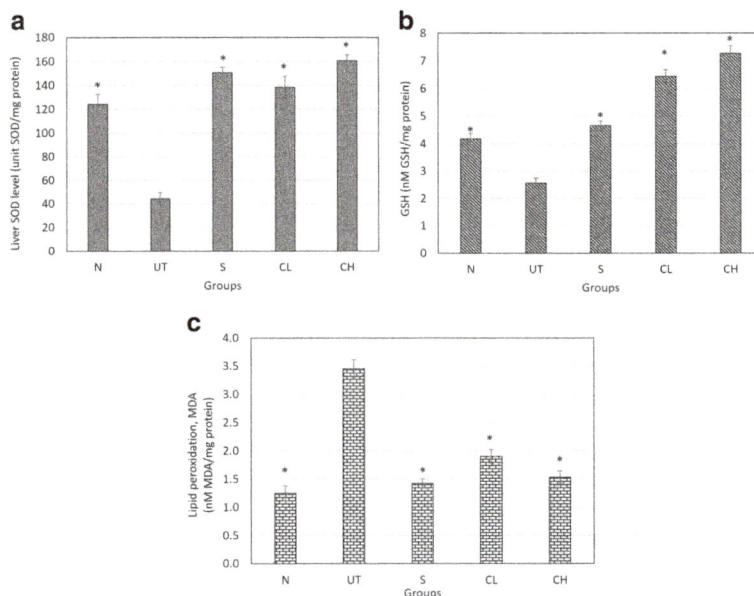

Fig. 2 Effect of coconut water vinegar on liver **a** SOD **b** GSH and **c** MDA levels in the liver of acetaminophen-challenged mice. All values are expressed as means mean ± SD of 6 mice in each group. *$P < 0.01$ as compared with the untreated control group. N: normal healthy control; UT: untreated acetaminophen-induced control; S: acetaminophen-induced treated with 50 mg/kg silybin; CL: acetaminophen-induced treated with 0.08 ml/kg coconut water vinegar; CH: acetaminophen-induced treated with 2 ml/kg coconut water vinegar

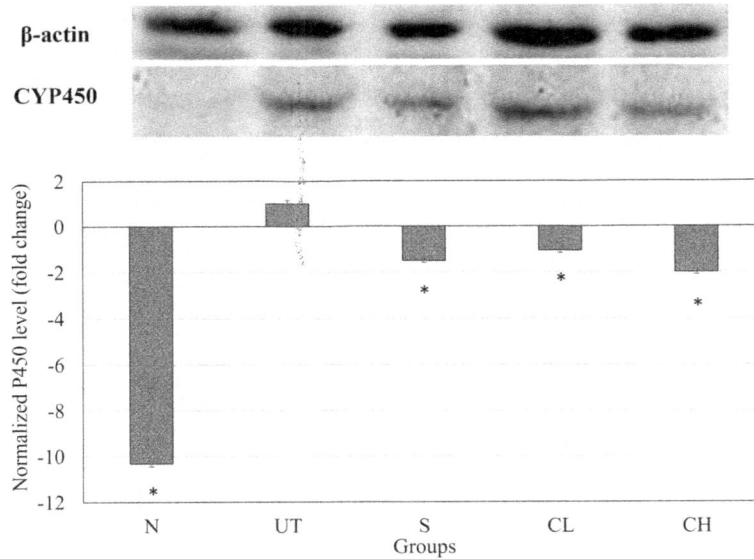

Fig. 3 Western blot analyses of CYP2E1 and β-actin proteins in the liver. All values are expressed as means mean ± SD of 6 mice in each group. *P < 0.01 as compared with the untreated control group. N: normal healthy control; UT: untreated acetaminophen-induced control; S: acetaminophen-induced treated with 50 mg/kg silybin; CL: acetaminophen-induced treated with 0.08 ml/kg coconut water vinegar; CH: acetaminophen-induced treated with 2 ml/kg coconut water vinegar

CCl_4. Overexpression of CYP2E1, which is commonly associated with hepatotoxicity was correlated with the increase susceptibility of apoptosis-induced liver injury [21]. During metabolism of acetaminophen by CYP2E1 enzyme in the liver, reactive N-acetyl-p-benzo-quinone imine (NAPQI), which is toxic, was formed. NAPQI can be neutralized by glutathione peptide to form non-toxic cysteine and mercapturic acid conjugates. However, over-dosage of acetaminophen can effectively deplete the GSH peptide thus caused oxidative stress in the liver [3].

Lipid peroxidation, which is normally measured by quantifying malondialdehyde, was the consequence of oxidative stress caused by acetaminophen [22]. Up regulation of lipid peroxidation contributes directly but not solely to acetaminophen overdose liver injury [23]. In this study, coconut water vinegar treatment was found to effectively restore the GSH peptide level in the liver associated with lower level of CYP2E1 and lipid peroxidation. These results have shown that although coconut water vinegar was detected with slightly lower total

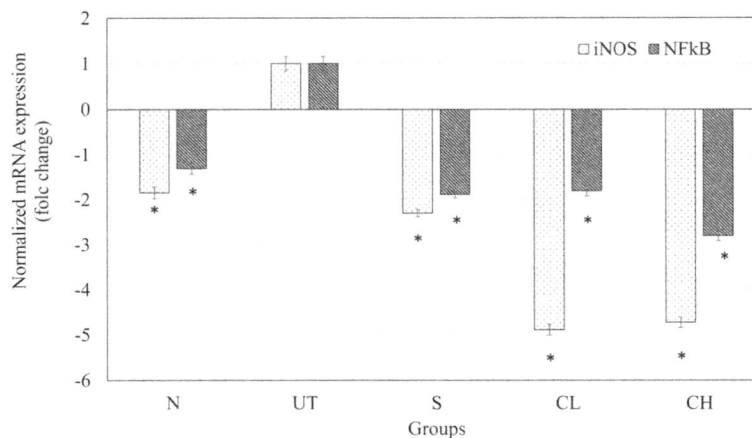

Fig. 4 Effect of coconut water vinegar on normalized mRNA expression of iNOS and NF-kB in liver of acetaminophenchallenged mice. All values are expressed as means mean ± SD of 6 mice in each group. *P < 0.01 as compared with the untreated control group. N: normal healthy control; UT: untreated acetaminophen-induced control; S: acetaminophen-induced treated with 50 mg/kg silybin; CL: acetaminophen-induced treated with 0.08 ml/kg coconut water vinegar; CH: acetaminophen-induced treated with 2 ml/kg coconut water vinegar

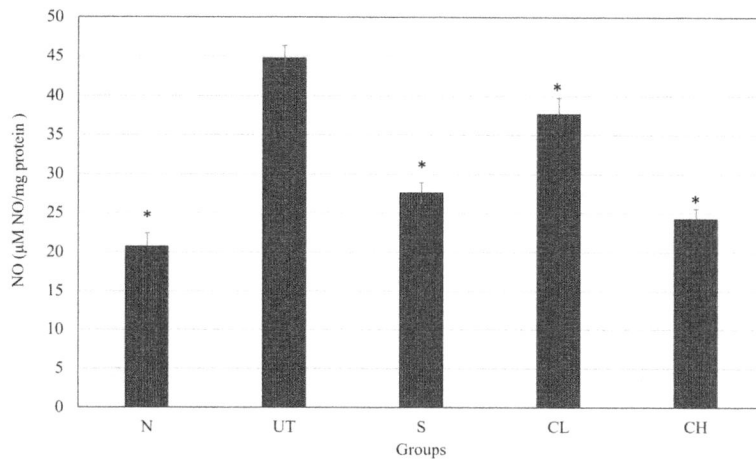

Fig. 5 Effect of coconut water vinegar on liver nitric oxide (NO) level in the liver of acetaminophen challenged mice. All values are expressed as means mean ± SD of 6 mice in each group. *$P < 0.01$ as compared with the untreated control group. N: normal healthy control; UT: untreated acetaminophen-induced control; S: acetaminophen-induced treated with 50 mg/kg silybin; CL: acetaminophen-induced treated with 0.08 ml/kg coconut water vinegar; CH: acetaminophen-induced treated with 2 ml/kg coconut water vinegar

antioxidant capacity and total phenolic content, the in vivo antioxidant effect was not compromised. Gallic and vanillic acids were the two major phenolic acids detected in the coconut water vinegar [24]. These phenolic acids were previously reported as hepatoprotective agents [20, 25]. They may have contributed to the hepato-recovery effect of coconut water vinegar as previous studies have proposed that phenolic acids reduced the CYP2E1 expression and prevent GSH depletion via inhibiting transportation of acetaminophen into the hepatocytes via the hepatic organic anion-transporting polypeptide [26, 27].

Based on this study, overdose of acetaminophen was observed with reduction of Superoxide dismutase (SOD) enzyme (Fig. 2a). In the absence of nitric oxide (NO), superoxide that accumulates in the liver promoted lipid peroxidation mediated toxicity. However, acetaminophen overdose was also commonly observed with NO accumulation produced by pro-inflammatory reaction indicated by overexpression of inflammatory mediators including iNOS and NF-kB [1, 3] as observed in this study. Accumulated superoxide contributed by depletion

of SOD enzyme preferentially react with NO to produce toxic peroxynitrite [28], which is another main agent that contributed to the hepatocyte cell death besides lipid peroxidation [23]. Coconut water vinegar was observed with anti-inflammatory effect where it suppressed the expression of inflammatory mediators' iNOS and NF-kB, associated with lower level of NO in the liver. Concurrently, coconut water vinegar also improved the SOD activity (Fig. 2a). Thus, coconut water vinegar may have the potential to prevent peroxynitrite mediated hepatocyte damage.

Conclusion

In summary, we concluded that acetification of coconut water to produce vinegar has significantly reduced antioxidant capacity of the coconut water vinegar due to the reduction of total phenolic content compared to the fresh coconut water. However, this phenomenon did not compensate the hepato-recovery effect of coconut water vinegar against acetaminophen induced hepatotoxicity. Coconut water vinegar promoted the recovery of liver

Table 2 Serum liver and lipid profiles of normal (N), acetaminophen untreated (UT), acetaminophen 50 mg/kg BW silymarin (S) treated, acetaminophen 0.08 ml/kg BW coconut vinegar (CL) treated and acetaminophen 2 ml/kg BW coconut vinegar (CH) treated mice

Group	ALT (U/L)	ALP (U/L)	AST (U/L)	Cholesterol (mmol/L)	Triglyceride (mmol/L)	HDL/LDL
N	61.23 ± 5.57*	85.67 ± 2.32*	145.20 ± 15.15*	3.30 ± 0.36*	2.33 ± 0.64*	15.93 ± 0.21*
UT	123.94 ± 7.25	104.44 ± 2.31	368.76 ± 9.83	3.75 ± 0.23	3.44 ± 0.56	13.33 ± 0.17
S	72.44 ± 8.23*	81.75 ± 1.51*	250.46 ± 11.14*	3.10 ± 0.21*	2.11 ± 0.24*	20.46 ± 0.23*
CL	39.80 ± 3.77*	75.17 ± 2.39*	163.33 ± 15.26*	2.94 ± 0.29*	2.20 ± 0.61*	18.43 ± 0.18*
CH	38.03 ± 3.35*	73.33 ± 1.52*	119.51 ± 15.49*	2.97 ± 0.36*	1.54 ± 0.37*	19.31 ± 0.23*

The data presented were representative as mean ± SD of biological replicated of mice from the same treatment group. Significant values were calculated against untreated group (*$P < 0.05$)

damage induced by acetaminophen by improving the hepatic antioxidant level and suppressing the liver inflammation in dosage dependent manner. Future studies including detailed mechanisms of the coconut water vinegar hepatoprotective effect and clinical trials shall be carried out to validate the potential of coconut vinegar as a potential food supplement to ameliorate chemical induced liver damage.

Abbreviations
ALP: Alkaline phosphatase; ALT: Alanine transaminase; ANOVA: one-way analysis of variance; AST: Aspartate aminotransferase; BN: Binuclear hepatocytes; CCl_4: Carbon tetrachloride; CH: Acetaminophen-induced treated with 2 ml/kg coconut water vinegar; CL: Acetaminophen-induced treated with 0.08 ml/kg coconut water vinegar; CYP2E1: Cytochrome P450 2E1; FRAP: Ferric reducing ability of plasma; GAPDH: Glyceraldehyde 3-phosphate dehydrogenase; GSH: Glutathione; HPRT: Hypoxanthine phosphoribosyltransferase; iNOS: inducible nitric oxide synthase; MDA: Malondialdehyde; N: healthy normal control group; NAPQI: N-acetyl-p-benzoquinone imine; NF-kB: Nuclear factor kappa-light-chain-enhancer of activated B cells; NO: Nitric oxide; qRT-PCR: quantitative real time PCR; S: acetaminophen-induced treated with 50 mg/kg silybin; SC: Dilated sinusoids; SDS: Sodium dodecyl sulphate; SOD: Superoxide dismutase; TPC: Total phenolic content; UT: Untreated acetaminophen-induced control; β-actin: Beta-actin

Funding
This study was supported by Grant Pembangunan RMK10, Mardi from Ministry of Agriculture, Malaysia. The authors have no conflicts of interest to report.

Authors' contributions
SKY, KL and NBA designed the experiment; KL and SAS performed HPLC and prepared coconut water vinegar; NEM, SKY and BKB performed the experiment; HK and WYH performed qRT-PCR; KLL performed Western blot analysis; NEM and SKY prepared the manuscript; all authors have gone through and approved the manuscript.

Competing interests
The authors declare that they have no competing interests.

Author details
[1]Department of Cell and Molecular Biology, Faculty of Biotechnology and Biomolecular Science, Universiti Putra Malaysia, 43400 Serdang, Selangor, Malaysia. [2]China-ASEAN College of Marine Sciences, Xiamen University Malaysia, Jalan Sunsuria, Bandar Sunsuria, 43900 Sepang, Selangor, Malaysia. [3]Institute of Bioscience, Universiti Putra Malaysia, Serdang, Selangor, Malaysia. [4]Biotechnology Research Centre, Malaysian Agricultural Research and Development Institute (MARDI), 43400 Serdang, Selangor, Malaysia. [5]Department of Genetics and Plant Breeding, College of Agriculture and Applied Biology, Cantho University, 3/2 Street, CanTho City, Vietnam. [6]Faculty of Medicine and Health Sciences, Universiti Tunku Abdul Rahman, Sungai Long Campus, Jalan Sungai Long, Bandar Sungai Long, Cheras, 43000 Kajang, Selangor, Malaysia. [7]School of Biomedical Sciences, the University of Nottingham Malaysia Campus, Jalan Broga, 43500 Semenyih, Selangor, Malaysia.

References
1. Fontana RJ. Acute liver failure including acetaminophen overdose. Med Clin N Am. 2008;92:761–94.
2. Nourjah P, Ahmad SR, Karwoski C, Willy M. Estimates of acetaminophen (paracetomal)-associated overdoses in the United States. Pharmacoepidemiol Drug Saf. 2006;15:398–405.
3. McGill MR, Sharpe MR, Williams CD, Taha M, Curry SC, Jaeschke H. The mechanism underlying acetaminophen-induced hepatotoxicity in humans and mice involves mitochondrial damage and nuclear DNA fragmentation. J Clin Invest. 2012;122:1574–83.
4. Hong M, Li S, Tan HY, Wang N, Tsao SW, Feng Y. Current status of herbal medicines in chronic liver disease therapy: the biological effects, molecular targets and future prospects. Int J Mol Sci. 2015;16:28705–45.
5. Santoso U, Kubo K, Ota T, Tadakoro T, Maekawa A. Antioxidative effect of coconut (Cocos nucifera L.) water extract on TBARS value in liver of rats fed fish oil diet. Indo Food Nutri Prog. 1996;3:42–50.
6. Offor C, Adetarami O, Nwali B, Igwenyi I, Afiukwa C. Effect of Cocos nuciferawater on liver enzymes. Middle-East J Sci Res. 2014;21:844–7.
7. Loki AL, Rajamohan T. Hepatoprotective and antioxidant effect of tender coconut water on carbon tetrachloride induced liver injury in rats. Indian J Biochem Biophys. 2003;40:354–7.
8. Ndubuka GI, Okafor WC, Jervas E, Chidi IS, Oh U, Illiams OI. Protective effect of immature coconut water on hepatocytes against carbontetrachloride-induced liver damage in Wister rats. Int J Sci Res. 2014;4:1427–31.
9. Okafor WC, Ndubuka GI, Jervas E, Chidi IS, Udoka OC, Osuchukwu IW. Effects of immature coconut water on the hepatocytoarchitecture against Carbontetrachloride-induced Liver damaging wistar rats. IOSR J Den Med Sci. 2014;1:60–5.
10. Preetha P, Girija Devi V, Rajamohan T. Comparative effects of mature coconut water (Cocos nucifera) and glibenclamide on some biochemical parameters in alloxan induced diabetic rats. Rev Bras Farmacogn Braz J Pharmacogn. 2013;23:481–7.
11. Satheesh N, Prasad N. Production of fermented coconut water beverages. J Food Ag-Ind. 2013;6:281–9.
12. Yong JW, Ge L, Ng YF, Tan SN. The chemical composition and biological properties of coconut (Cocos nucifera L.) water. Molecules. 2009;14:5144–64.
13. Li J, Yu G, Fan J. Alditols and monosaccharides from sorghum vinegar can attenuate platelet aggregation by inhibiting cyclooxygenase-1 and thromboxane-A2 synthase. J Ethnopharmacol. 2014;155:285–92.
14. Mohamad NE, Yeap SK, Lim KL, Yusof HM, Beh BK, Tan SW, Ho WY, Sharifuddin SA, Jamluddin A, Long K, Rahman NMANA, Alitheen NB. Antioxidant effects of pineapple vinegar in reversing of paracetamol-induced liver damage in mice. Chin Med. 2015;10:1–14.
15. Nishidai S, Nakamura Y, Torikai K, Yamamoto M, Ishihara N, Mori H, Ohigashi H. Kurosu, a traditional vinegar produced from unpolished rice, suppresses lipid peroxidation in vitro and in mouse skin. Biosci Biotechnol Biochem. 2000;64:1909–14.
16. Beh BK, Mohamad NE, Yeap SK, Lim KL, Ho WY, Yusof HM, Sharifuddin SA, Jamaluddin A, Long K, Alitheen NB. Polyphenolic profiles and the in vivo antioxidant effect of nipa vinegar on paracetamol induced liver damage. RSC Adv. 2016;6:63304–13.
17. Kongkiattikajorn J. Antioxidant properties of roselle vinegar production by mixed culture of Acetobacter Acetiand Acetobacter cerevisiae. Kasetsart J (Nat Sci). 2014;48:980–8.
18. Cunha MAA, Lima KP, Santos VAQ, Heinz OL, Schmidt CAP. Blackberry vinegar produced by successive acetification cycles: Production, characterization and bioactivity parameters. Braz Arch Biol Techn. 2016;59:1–10.
19. Basu S, Haldar N, Bhattacharya Sanji BS, Biswas M. Hepatoprotective activity of Litchi chinensis leaves against paracetamol-induced liver damage in rats. Am-Eur J Sci Res. 2012;7:77–81.
20. Rasool MK, Sabina EP, Ramya SR, Preety P, Patel S, Mandal N, Mishra PP, Samuel J. Hepatoprotective and antioxidant effects of gallic acid in paracetamol-induced liver damage in mice. J Pharm Pharmacol. 2010;62: 638–43.
21. Wang X, Lu Y, Cederbaum AI. Induction of cytochrome P450 2E1 increases hepatotoxicity caused by Fas agonistic Jo2 antibody in mice. Hepatology. 2005;42:400–10.
22. Dusan M, Milica N, Danijela V, Miodrag C, Marjan M, Vera T, Milena S, Tatjana R. The effects of ethanol on paracetamol-induced oxidative stress in mice liver. J Serb Chem Soc. 2013;78:179–95.
23. Knight TR, Fariss MW, Farhood A, Jaeschke H. Role of lipid peroxidation as a mechanism of liver injury after acetaminophen overdose in mice. Toxicol Sci. 2003;76:229–36.
24. Mohamad NE, Yeap SK, Ky H, Ho WY, Boo SY, Chua J, Beh BK, Sharifuddin SA, Long K, Alitheen NB. Dietary coconut water vinegar for improvement of obesity-associated inflammation in high-fat-diet treated mice. Food Nutr Res. 2017;61:1368322.

25. Itoh A, Isoda K, Kondoh M, Kawase M, Watari A, Kobayashi M, Tamesada M, Yagi K. Hepatoprotective effect of syringic acid and vanillic acid on CCl4-induced liver injury. Biol Pharm Bull. 2010;33:983–7.

26. Mandery K, Bujok K, Schmidt I, Keiser M, Siegmund W, Balk B, Konig J, Fromm MF, Glaeser H. Influence of the flavonoids apigenin, kaempferol, and quercetin on the function of organic anion transporting polypeptides 1A2 and 2B1. Biochem Pharmacol. 2010;80:1746–53.

27. Priyadarsini RV, Nagini S. Quercetin suppresses cytochrome P450 mediated ROS generation and NFκB activation to inhibit the development of 7, 12-dimethylbenz [a] anthracene (DMBA) induced hamster buccal pouch carcinomas. Free Radic Res. 2012;46:41–9.

28. James LP, Mayeux PR, Hinson JA. Acetaminophen-induced hepatotoxicity. Drug Metab Dispos. 2003;31:1499–506.

2

Patterns of conventional and complementary non-pharmacological health practice use by US military veterans

Melvin T. Donaldson[1,2]* (iD), Melissa A. Polusny[1,4], Rich F. MacLehose[3], Elizabeth S. Goldsmith[1,3], Emily M. Hagel Campbell[1], Lynsey R. Miron[1], Paul D. Thuras[1] and Erin E. Krebs[1,4]

Abstract

Background: Non-pharmacological therapies and practices are commonly used for both health maintenance and management of chronic disease. Patterns and reasons for use of health practices may identify clinically meaningful subgroups of users. The objectives of this study were to identify classes of self-reported use of conventional and complementary non-pharmacological health practices using latent class analysis and estimate associations of participant characteristics with class membership.

Methods: A mailed survey (October 2015 to September 2016) of Minnesota National Guard Veterans from a longitudinal cohort ($n = 1850$) assessed current pain, self-reported overall health, mental health, substance use, personality traits, and health practice use. We developed the Health Practices Inventory, a self-report instrument assessing use of 19 common conventional and complementary non-pharmacological health-related practices. Latent class analysis was used to identify subgroups of health practice users, based on responses to the HPI. Participants were assigned to their maximum-likelihood class, which was used as the outcome in multinomial logistic regression to examine associations of participant characteristics with latent class membership.

Results: Half of the sample used non-pharmacological health practices. Six classes of users were identified. "Low use" (50%) had low rates of health practice use. "Exercise" (23%) had high exercise use. "Psychotherapy" (6%) had high use of psychotherapy and support groups. "Manual therapies" (12%) had high use of chiropractic, physical therapy, and massage. "Mindfulness" (5%) had high use of mindfulness and relaxation practice. "Multimodal" (4%) had high use of most practices. Use of manual therapies (chiropractic, acupuncture, physical therapy, massage) was associated with chronic pain and female sex. Characteristics that predict use patterns varied by class. Use of self-directed practices (e.g., aerobic exercise, yoga) was associated with the personality trait of absorption (openness to experience). Use of psychotherapy was associated with higher rates of psychological distress.

Conclusions: These observed patterns of use of non-pharmacological health practices show that functionally similar practices are being used together and suggest a meaningful classification of health practices based on self-directed/active and practitioner-delivered. Notably, there is considerable overlap in users of complementary and conventional practices.

Keywords: Complementary integrative health, Alternative medicine, Non-pharmacological therapies, Latent class analysis, Veterans

---

* Correspondence: donax007@umn.edu
[1]Minneapolis VA Health Care System, One Veterans Drive, Minneapolis, MN 55417, USA
[2]University of Minnesota Medical Scientist Training Program, Minneapolis, MN 55455, USA
Full list of author information is available at the end of the article

Background

Non-pharmacological therapies and self-management practices include approaches considered "conventional," such as exercise and manual physical therapy, and those considered "complementary," such as yoga and chiropractic manipulation. These health practices are commonly used by American adults [1, 2] and are recommended for prevention and management of a wide variety of illnesses, including, for example, hypertension [3], chronic musculoskeletal pain [4–6] and depression [7].

Prior studies have characterized users of individual practices [8] and types of practices [9], typically by examining practices categorized according to expert opinion [10] or researchers' interests. Categorization of non-pharmacological health practices can vary widely between studies. Although most studies distinguish between complementary and conventional practices, the utility of this distinction is unclear. Evidence suggests people do not use individual complementary practices in isolation, but rather in combination with other complementary and conventional modalities [11, 12]. Certain health practices may cluster in meaningful ways that could define functionally meaningful categories of non-pharmacological health practices. Understanding factors associated with these patterns could help tailor care for patients and increase uptake of evidence-based practices.

The aims of this study were 1) to identify distinct patterns and categories of health practice use through latent class analysis; and 2) to estimate associations between latent class membership and sociodemographic, psychological, behavioral, and pain characteristics of users. We also describe development of a self-report tool for assessing health practice use.

Methods

Development of Health Practices Inventory

We developed the Health Practices Inventory (HPI) to facilitate valid self-report assessment of non-pharmacological therapies and health-related practices, including complementary and conventional approaches. Our primary goal was to evaluate use of therapies and practices for management of chronic pain; however, the inventory was designed to be broadly applicable beyond pain treatments. An initial list of 28 therapies and practices with brief definitions was developed after review of the National Health Interview Survey Complementary and Alternative Medicine (CAM) supplement, questionnaires used by prior studies, and chronic pain management guidelines. Definitions of complementary practices were based on descriptions provided in the National Health Interview Survey [13] and the National Center for Complementary and Integrative Health website [14]. Key informant interviews with 4 expert clinicians were used to refine health practice definitions.

One author (MAP) conducted cognitive interviews using a preliminary version of the HPI with 5 participants.

Participants were mailed a questionnaire and instructed to complete it in one sitting, marking any items that were confusing or raised questions. Subsequently, semi-structured cognitive interviews were conducted to gather in-depth information about participants' responses, following published recommendations [15, 16]. To assess whether they answered questions as intended by the developers, participants were instructed to "think aloud" as they completed the inventory. The cognitive interviewing process largely confirmed comprehension and clarity of items. Only minor changes were made after the cognitive interviews.

The final HPI covers 19 distinct health practices, each accompanied by a brief description (Additional file 1: Figure S1, for full text of the HPI including descriptions of practices). Questions ask about use of each practice in the past year. For each endorsed practice, follow-up questions ask about reasons for use (improve well-being/general health, manage pain, or manage a condition other than pain) and frequency of use in the past month (not at all, several days, more than half the days, nearly every day).

Procedures and participants

Study participants were members of the Readiness and Resilience in National Guard Soldiers (RINGS) [17] longitudinal cohort study, which was originally designed to identify predictors of post-deployment health outcomes. Eligible cohort participants included 3890 Army National Guard Soldiers who were deployed to Iraq, Afghanistan, or Kuwait between 2006 and 2011, completed a baseline assessment before or during deployment, and completed at least 1 follow-up assessment post-deployment.

Data were collected from October 2015 to September 2016 using standard multiple-contact mailed survey methodology [18]. A questionnaire, cover letter, and $20 incentive were mailed to 3833 participants (52 others had untrackable addresses, 1 was incarcerated, and 4 were deceased). A postcard reminder and 2 additional survey mailings were sent to non-responders at 2-week intervals, with the final mailing delivered by priority mail. The overall response rate was 48.3% ($n = 1850$). The non-responders were slightly younger than responders and less likely to be female, but otherwise similar (see Additional file 2: Table S1, for characteristics of responders and non-responders). All study procedures were approved by the institutional review boards of the Minneapolis VA Health Care System and University of Minnesota. A waiver of documentation of informed consent was approved by both IRBs.

Measures

Data for this study are cross-sectional and obtained from the 2015–2016 RINGS cohort follow-up survey described above. The mailed questionnaire included the HPI described above and measures assessing deployment experiences, pain, quality of life, mental health, substance use, and personality characteristics. For this analysis, variables were selected based on previously-demonstrated or hypothesized associations with non-pharmacological or complementary health practice use.

Demographics

Age at time of survey mailing was recorded from administrative records. Participants self-reported gender, race, ethnicity, educational attainment, employment, and length of military service.

Pain

Pain is a common reason for use of both complementary and conventional non-pharmacological therapies. The National Pain Strategy population health [19] pain persistence item (5 response version) was used to define chronic pain as the presence of pain on at least half the days in the previous 6 months. Pain severity was measured with the 3-item Pain, Enjoyment of life, General Activity (PEG) scale [20]. The 3 items ask participants to rate on a 0 to 10 scale over the past week their average pain severity, pain interference with enjoyment of life, and pain interference with general activity. The PEG has good responsiveness [21] and concurrent validity [20].

Military deployment experiences

To assess past combat exposure, participants were asked, "During any deployment, were you ever a participant or observer in direct combat operations?" They could respond, "Yes, participated in direct combat operation(s)"; "yes, observed or witnessed combat operation(s) but not participated"; "no." To assess deployment injuries, participants were asked, "Were you wounded or injured during any deployment?" (response options, yes or no).

Self-reported health

Overall health was self-reported using the single-item global heath and 1-year retrospective global health questions from the Veterans RAND 12 Item Health Survey (VR-12) [22, 23]. Participants were asked, "In general would you say your health is: excellent, very good, good, fair or poor?" Overall health was dichotomized as excellent/very good versus good/fair/poor. For the retrospective questions, participants were asked, "Compared to one year ago, how would you rate your... Physical health in general now?" and "Emotional problems (such as feeling anxious, depressed or irritable) now?" Participants could respond, "much worse", "slightly worse", "about the same", "slightly better", or "much better." These items were dichotomized as slightly worse/much worse versus much better/slightly better/about the same.

Mental health

Anxiety, depression, and poor self-rated health may be more prevalent in people who use complementary approaches than those who do not. [10, 24] Anxiety symptoms were measured using the Patient Reported Outcomes Measurement Information System (PROMIS) short form 8a anxiety scale [25]. The scale was dichotomized at 22 (corresponding to a T-score > 60) [26], consistent with moderate or severe anxiety. Depressive symptoms were measured with the 8-item Patient Health Questionnaire depression scale (PHQ-8) [27]. The PHQ-8 was dichotomized at 10 [27], consistent with moderate or severe depression. Posttraumatic stress symptoms were measured with the PTSD Checklist-5 (PCL-5) [28]. The PCL-5 was dichotomized at 33, consistent with probable PTSD [28].

Substance use

Alcohol use was measured with the Alcohol Use Disorders Identification Test (AUDIT) [29]. The AUDIT score was dichotomized above 7, consistent with problem alcohol use [29]. Illicit drug use was measured with the Drug Abuse Screening Test (DAST) [30]. A score above 0 represents any illicit drug use in the previous year.

Personality

Absorption (the tendency to be open to experiences and mindful states), is 1 of 11 primary traits measured by the Multidimensional Personality Questionnaire [31, 32]. Absorption has been shown to be positively associated with use of complementary non-pharmacological therapies [33]. Absorption was measured using the 12-item absorption subscale from the Multidimensional Personality Questionnaire-Brief Form [31, 32].

Statistical analyses

We used latent class analysis (LCA) to identify distinct subgroups of users of health practices. LCA is an exploratory data reduction technique that categorizes participants into multiple discrete, non-overlapping classes based on similar patterns of observed data. Because the classes are latent, they cannot be directly observed and can only be estimated using observed response patterns. The purpose of the LCA in this study was to combine the HPI responses to the 19 practices into a small number of substantively meaningful classes about which inferences could be made. For an LCA with binary data, as in this study, the model estimates the probability that a member of each class endorses each item (i.e. each health practice). Estimates from the latent class model were used to calculate the probability an individual was in a class as a function of their actual response pattern.

Frequency of health practice use was dichotomized as any use versus no use in the previous 12 months. Fewer than 2% of participants reported using biofeedback, Tai

Chi/Qi Gong, Healing Touch/Reiki, homeopathy, and hypnotherapy; including these rare approaches led to estimability problems, so they were excluded from the LCA. The latent class model used only self-report of individual health practices to predict class membership. Separate models were fit with 1 to 11 latent classes. The fit of these models was compared using the Bayesian Information Criterion and Akaike's Information Criterion to determine the best fitting number of classes. Participants were assigned to classes based on maximum posterior probability.

To examine associations of participant characteristics with latent class membership, selected variables (described above) were used as predictors in a multinomial regression model with the latent classes as outcomes. Marginal effects (i.e. difference in class membership probabilities) were calculated from the regression results by standardizing to the distribution of covariates in the total sample and calculating the difference in probability of class membership between levels of the covariate [34]. All analyses were performed in Stata 15 [35].

Missing data

Approximately 14% of participants had missing data for at least 1 predictor variable in the multinomial regression model. To address the concern that this missingness could bias results, we imputed 20 datasets by chained multiple imputation to allow all participants to be included [36–38]. Continuous measures and ordered scales were imputed by predictive mean matching with 5 nearest neighbors and imputed values were drawn from 20 independent bootstrap samples [39, 40]. Continuous measures were dichotomized after imputation. Binary and factor variables were imputed by logistic regression or multinomial logistic regression. All imputed variables were included in the chained equations and maximum probability latent class was included as a fixed (not imputed) variable. The scales that were not included in the multinomial logistic regression were still included in the chained imputation equations to improve performance of the imputation.

Results

Table 1 presents demographic characteristics of participants and mean scores on self-report scales. Participants were mostly male and white, with a mean age of 39 years (SD = 9); 41% had chronic pain and over 20% screened positive for mental health problems (e.g., depression, anxiety, PTSD).

Table 2 summarizes HPI responses of all participants. Complete data about past-year use of all 19 health practices were available for 1817 participants (98%). Twenty-five participants (1%) completely skipped HPI past-year use items; 6 (< 1%) skipped past-year use for 1 of the modalities; and 2

Table 1 Characteristics of Minnesota National Guard Veterans who responded to the mailed survey conducted from October 2015 to September 2016 (N = 1850)

Characteristic	Mean (SD) or % (N)
Male, % (N)	90.3% (1668)
Age, Mean (SD)	38.7 (9.2)
White, % (N)	90.1% (1656)
Obtained 4-year degree, % (N)	42.6% (772)
Injured on deployment, % (N)	27.0% (493)
Pain	
Chronic pain, % (N)	41.2% (749)
Intensity and interference (PEG), Mean (SD)	2.4 (2.4)
Self-rated health	
Current health excellent/very good[a], % (N)	43.1% (796)
Mental health	
Anxiety at least moderate (PROMIS-Anxiety 8a ≥ 22), % (N)	21.8% (400)
Depression (PHQ-8 ≥ 10), % (N)	21.7% (392)
Probable PTSD (PCL-5 ≥ 33), % (N)	19.5% (339)
Problem alcohol use (AUDIT ≥8), % (N)	21.6% (394)
Past year illicit drug use (DAST > 0), % (N)	10.3% (184)
Absorption (MPQ-BF Absorption, T-scores), Mean (SD)	47.6 (10.8)

Abbreviations: PEG 3-item PEG scale, *VR-12* Veterans RAND 12-Item Health Survey
[a]Current health excellent/very good vs good/fair/poor; VR-12 overall health item

(< 1%) skipped several of the past-year items. Practices commonly used for pain tended to be practitioner-delivered, including acupuncture, chiropractic, massage and manual physical therapy. Practices used for well-being or general health tended to be active, self-directed practices, including yoga, meditation/mindfulness, aerobic exercise and strengthening/stretching exercise.

Classes of health practice users

The best-fitting latent class model had 6 distinct and substantively meaningful classes (see Additional file 3: Table S2, for model fit statistics; see Additional file 4: Table S3, for characteristics of class members). Table 3 presents the prevalence of use of the HPI modalities within the 6 latent classes, which were labeled to reflect the distinguishing prevalence of modalities between classes. One "low use" class represented very low rates of health practice use (50% of participants, n = 923). Five classes represented greater use of health practices compared to the low use class. The "exercise" class (23%, n = 426) had high rates of aerobic exercise (used by 86% of class members) and strength/stretching exercise (86%) and lower use of other health practices compared to the total sample. The

Table 2 Self-reported past-year use of Health Practices Inventory approaches by Minnesota National Guard Veterans ($N = 1825$), who participated in the mailed survey conducted from October 2015 to September 2016

Health practice[a]	%	n	Reason for use[b]						Past month frequency of use[c]					
			Well-being/ general health		Treat pain		Treat another condition		None		Several days		More	
			%	n	%	n	%	n	%	n	%	n	%	n
Acupuncture	5%	86	37%	32	72%	62	22%	19	69%	59	28%	24	0%	0
Biofeedback	2%	30	70%	21	13%	4	17%	5	47%	14	33%	10	13%	4
Chiropractic	32%	578	31%	179	83%	477	8%	47	46%	268	46%	266	2%	14
Massage	24%	431	52%	226	63%	272	8%	35	56%	242	33%	144	2%	9
Manual physical therapy	13%	242	15%	37	80%	193	12%	30	41%	100	43%	105	8%	20
Healing Touch/Reiki	1%	21	52%	11	52%	11	38%	8	48%	10	43%	9	5%	1
Hypnotherapy	1%	9	33%	3	22%	2	44%	4	67%	6	0%	0	22%	2
Psychotherapy	13%	233	54%	125	9%	22	50%	116	39%	91	46%	107	5%	12
Support groups	4%	79	62%	49	8%	6	39%	31	30%	24	46%	36	13%	10
Spiritual/traditional healing system	6%	115	78%	90	14%	16	29%	33	10%	11	39%	45	44%	51
Relaxation	18%	335	63%	212	19%	65	37%	125	13%	42	54%	182	25%	84
Meditation/Mindfulness	10%	190	74%	140	12%	22	32%	60	10%	19	52%	99	25%	47
Yoga	10%	174	85%	148	33%	58	14%	24	31%	54	50%	87	8%	14
Tai Chi/Qi Gong	1%	15	87%	13	33%	5	7%	1	27%	4	33%	5	13%	2
Strength/stretch exercise	44%	799	76%	604	34%	269	10%	78	9%	69	37%	296	45%	360
Aerobic exercise	36%	661	88%	580	12%	80	9%	56	4%	28	42%	278	45%	300
Diet	7%	120	77%	92	21%	25	19%	23	9%	11	18%	21	63%	76
Herbal supplement	10%	175	80%	140	15%	27	19%	34	5%	8	26%	46	60%	105
Homeopathy	1%	25	60%	15	44%	11	40%	10	36%	9	32%	8	28%	7

The practices are listed in the order they appear in the survey (Additional file 1: Figure S1, for full text of the Health Practices Inventory)

[a]The Health Practices Inventory approaches are grouped based on the a priori categorization described in the text; a summary variable was created for each of the groupings indicating use of any of the modalities in that group

[b]Participants who reported using a Health Practices Inventory modality were asked to identify their reason(s) for using it; the reasons are not mutually exclusive and they could pick any combination of the 3 reasons listed or none at all

[c]Participants who reported using a Health Practices Inventory modality were asked to identify the frequency they used it in the past month; these frequencies are mutually exclusive but do not always add up to 100% because of missingness

"psychotherapy" class (6%, $n = 112$) was the only class with high use of psychotherapy and of support groups, and also had high use of mindfulness and relaxation. The "manual therapies" class (12%, $n = 213$) had high use of practitioner-delivered manual therapies, including chiropractic, massage, and acupuncture, and moderate use of exercise practices. The "mindfulness" class (5%, $n = 101$) had high use of relaxation practices, mindfulness and yoga, and moderate use of exercise. The "multimodal" class (4%, $n = 75$) was the smallest class and had high use of every modality except psychotherapy and support groups. The 6 classes identified in the best-fit latent class model were robust across other latent class model solutions with different numbers of classes. Notably, the low use, exercise and psychotherapy classes were easy to identify in the next best-fit models (5 and 7 classes). Major distinctions between latent class models related to differential use of specific complementary health practices between classes. With 7 classes, the manual

therapies class was split into 2 classes, a class with high rates of strengthening/stretching and aerobic exercise and a class with low rates of exercise. With 5 classes, the mindfulness and multimodal classes merged into one class.

Use of complementary approaches varied among the classes in the final model, as measured by the number of different complementary practices endorsed (range: 0 to 12). Compared with 31% of members of the low use class, 100% of members of the manual therapies, mindfulness, and multimodal classes reported use of at least 1 complementary health practice. The distributions were highly skewed. The multimodal class had the highest overall use of complementary approaches (median = 5; SE: 0.1). The manual therapies class (median = 2; SE: 0.06), mindfulness (median = 2; SE: 0.1) and psychotherapy (median = 2; SE: 0.1) classes had similar moderate use of complementary approaches. The exercise (median = 1; SE: 0.04) and low use (median = 0; SE: 0.02) classes had the least.

Table 3 Probability of use of Health Practices Inventory approaches within latent classes of 1850 Minnesota National Guard Veterans who participated in a mailed survey conducted from October 2015 to September 2016.

Latent class, (% sample in class by maximum probability classification)							
	Low use (50%, n=923)	Exercise (23%, n=426)	Psychotherapy (6%, n=112)	Manual therapies (12%, n=213)	Mindfulness (5%, n=101)	Multimodal (4%, n=75)	Total use† (100%, n=1850)
Health practice, Probability of class member endorsing use of particular health practice							
Acupuncture	**1%***	**0%**	11%	**21%**	**0%**	**20%**	4.7%
Manual physical therapy	6%	9%	25%	35%	4%	**49%**	13%
Chiropractic	22%	23%	26%	**78%**	10%	**70%**	32%
Massage	7%	22%	32%	**64%**	28%	**76%**	24%
Strength/stretch exercise	**11%**	**86%**	28%	61%	74%	**97%**	44%
Aerobic exercise	**5%**	**86%**	18%	40%	69%	**78%**	36%
Relaxation	**4%**	13%	**65%**	13%	**83%**	**89%**	18%
Mindfulness/ Meditation	**1%**	**0%**	**42%**	4%	**100%**	**52%**	10%
Yoga	**1%**	12%	4%	15%	**34%**	**47%**	9.5%
Herbal supplements	**1%**	14%	**1%**	17%	22%	**49%**	9.6%
Diet	**0%**	12%	2%	8%	12%	**41%**	6.6%
Spiritual Healing	**1%**	9%	18%	4%	13%	**39%**	6.3%
Psychotherapy	6%	9%	**79%**	11%	14%	28%	13%
Support groups	1%	2%	**49%**	**0%**	2%	12%	4.3%

Lower use				Higher Use

Health practices were listed in an order that maximized the visual clustering of modalities with similar use within classes
Bolding** added to highlight proportions that distinguish classes; all proportions that represent an odds ratio greater than 5 compared to use among all responders were considered much higher use than in the total sample and were **bolded**; all proportions that represent an odd ratio less than 0.2 compared to use among all responders were considered much lower use than in the total sample and were ***bolded and italicized
†Total use represents the proportion of use of modalities in the total sample. This is not a latent class

Associations of participant characteristics with health practice class

Figure 1 presents estimates of the effect of each covariate on probability of membership in each of the latent classes, compared with low use. A positive value means that the covariate increases the probability of membership in that latent class compared to the low use class. For example, being female was associated with a 0.25 greater prevalence of the multimodal class relative to the low use class. Also, a positive screen for problem alcohol use instead of a negative screen was associated with a 0.08 decrease in the prevalence of the manual therapies class compared to the low use class. Female sex was positively associated with membership in the multimodal class and problem alcohol use was negatively associated with membership in the manual therapies class, compared to the low use class. (see Additional file 5: Table S4, for effects with confidence intervals in tabular form.)

Some demographic characteristics predicted higher rates of health practice use in general, while others distinguished between specific classes. Higher absorption and higher education were associated with higher prevalence of the 5 health practice use classes (compared to the low use class). Depression was not associated with any of the HPI-use classes. PTSD was only associated with the psychotherapy class. Problem alcohol use was only (negatively) associated with the manual therapies users class.

Each class had a unique set of covariates that were associated with a difference in prevalence compared to the low use class. For example, higher anxiety was associated with the psychotherapy class and the multimodal class, but higher anxiety and higher PTSD distinguished the psychotherapy class from the multimodal class. Chronic pain was associated with the manual therapies class and the multimodal class; however, chronic pain

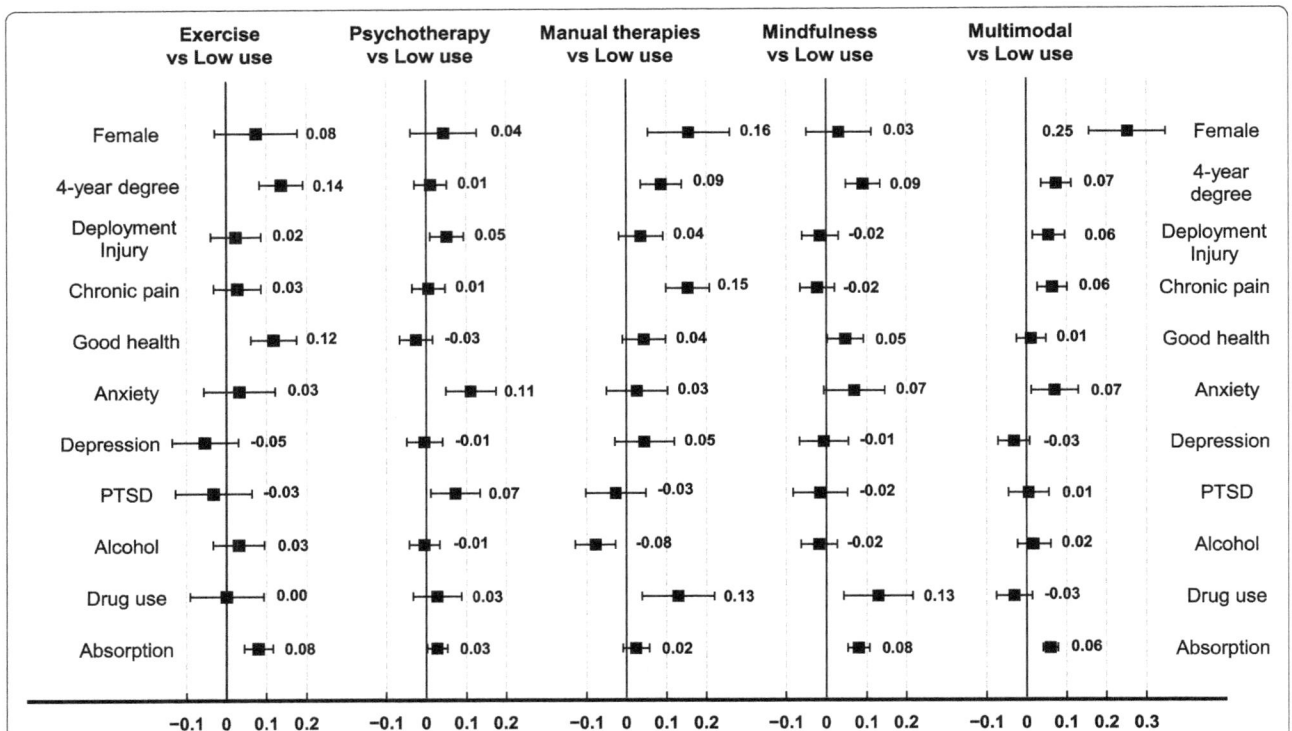

Fig. 1 Prevalence differences of class membership due to covariates; results of multinomial logistic regression from Minnesota National Guard Veterans who participated in the mailed survey conducted from October 2015 to September 2016. Interpreted as the difference in risk (probability) of membership in this latent class between levels of the covariate where a negative value means lower probability of membership in this class compared to probability at the reference level of the covariate; other covariates are standardized to their distribution among all responder. All covariates are dichotomous except for absorption, which is continuous. For absorption, a one-unit change represents a 2-point change on the absorption scale, equivalently a 7-point change on the T-score

with higher absorption distinguished the multimodal class from the manual therapies class. Both the manual therapies and the mindfulness classes were associated with higher education and higher illicit drug use; however, the manual therapies class was distinguished by being female and having chronic pain, whereas the mindfulness users class was distinguished by higher absorption and better self-rated health.

Discussion

This study found that integrated patterns of complementary and conventional approaches identify unique classes of health practice users. These classes had unique sets of predictors. For example, the exercise class was characterized by better self-rated health, higher educational attainment, and more open and mindful personality (absorption), while the psychotherapy class was characterized by higher psychological distress compared to the low use class. These data were collected using a novel instrument, the HPI. The HPI is an efficient way to collect self-report data on individuals' use of multiple complementary and conventional non-pharmacological therapies with minimal missing data.

Results from this study, which used LCA to explore data-driven patterns of use of health approaches, are broadly consistent with prior classifications based on qualitative research and expert opinion. In this study, active approaches, such as exercise, yoga, and mindfulness, tended to cluster together (Table 3). Similarly, practitioner-delivered approaches, such as chiropractic, massage, or manual physical therapy, tended to cluster together. Authors of the National Health Interview Survey CAM supplement previously noticed a distinction between active and practitioner-delivered practices [41]. Through qualitative interviews, they found participants experienced active practices differently than practitioner-delivered practices [41]. This distinction has persisted in the CAM supplement questions. In other instances, practices are classified based on expert opinion. Categorizations differ between experts. The National Center for Complementary and Integrative Health (NCCIH) has broadly classified practices as Mind and Body, Natural Products, and Others [42]. On the other hand, authors from the National Center for Health Statistics (NCHS) have classified approaches as Natural Products, Practitioner-based, Mind and Body, or Whole Medical Systems [43]. Even the categories that share the same name do not contain the same list of practices (e.g. chiropractic and acupuncture are "Mind and Body" in the NCCIH taxonomy but chiropractic is "Practitioner-based" and acupuncture is "Whole Medical Systems" in the NCHS taxonomy).

Classifying practices based on practitioner-delivered versus active/self-directed emerged in the patterns we observed in the present study. Our categorization were based on real-world patterns of use, instead of expert opinion or practitioner experience. These 3 different approaches to classifying nonpharmacological health practices (i.e. categorization by expert opinion, categorization based on experiences of health practice users informed by qualitative interview, and latent class statistical categorization based on observed patterns of use) all triangulate towards similar, meaningful categories of health practices. Convergence of findings using several different approaches adds external validity to the emergent classes of the present analysis.

The distinction between active and practitioner-delivered practices appears to be functionally important. This study found differences in the reported reasons for using practices from these 2 categories. Participants were more likely to report using practitioner-delivered approaches for pain rather than well-being, and far more likely to report using active approaches for well-being rather than pain. In fact, the practices most-often used for wellness were aerobic exercise, yoga, and tai chi/qi gong, and the practices most-often used for pain were manual physical therapy, chiropractic, and acupuncture. Despite this difference in reason for use, practitioner-delivered practices have not been shown to be superior to active practices for pain [44–46].

Prior studies have found that use of complementary health approaches is greater among women, middle age groups, people with more education and higher income, and people reporting a musculoskeletal pain disorder [2, 43]. Our results are largely consistent with prior studies; higher use of non-pharmacological practices generally was predicted by female sex and higher educational attainment. Higher absorption has been shown to be associated with higher use of complementary approaches [33], although our results suggest this may apply more to active than practitioner-delivered practices. We observed that the predictors of use are quite variable within classes.

This study has several limitations. First, although the HPI allows collection of detailed data about how often and why participants use non-pharmacological therapies, we dichotomized health practice use as any versus no use in the past year, which statistically equates daily use and one-time use. We did this because when we included frequency in our LCA the groups seemed to be defined by frequency of use of the exercise practices, which did not suit the purposes of this study. Frequency of exercise practices may have dominated because they were the most common practices and variability in

exercise frequency was large. A second limitation is the small prevalence of some classes (e.g., multimodal). Although there is no consensus on adequate class size, estimability problems due to small class prevalence are diminished in large total sample sizes (500 or 1000) [47]. Furthermore, model fit statistics supported the model we chose as best fit for these data. Third, the overall response rate was 48.3% for the follow-up survey; however, non-responders were not substantially different from responders, and the response rate is reasonable considering some cohort members have been followed for 10 years already. Fourth, there was a small amount of item missingness. We used multiple imputation to address this and results were consistent with complete case analysis. Fifth, participants were National Guard veterans, whose characteristics and health practice behaviors likely differ from the general population; therefore, it is important these findings be replicated in other samples.

Conclusions

The practical categorization of health practices as active or practitioner-delivered emerged in the distinct patterns of use identified in this sample of recently deployed veterans. Our analyses show the value of considering integrated use of health practices. There are important similarities among individuals within latent classes of use that would be obscured by collapsing all users of individual practices or collapsing all users of complementary practices. Because individuals use multiple health practices that may have overlapping effects, it may be important to consider overlapping effects in studies of individual health practices. Our findings should be investigated in other contexts and with other samples. In particular, latent class analyses with new samples could provide evidence for or against these 6 classes.

Abbreviations
AUDIT: Alcohol Use Disorders Identification Test; CAM: Complementary and Alternative Medicine; DAST: Drug Abuse Screening Test; HPI: Health Practices Inventory; LCA: Latent class analysis; NCCIH: National Center for Complementary and Integrative Health; NCHS: National Center for Health Statistics; PCL-5: PTSD Checklist, DSM-V criteria; PEG: Pain, Enjoyment of life, General Activity [pain scale]; PHQ-8: 8-item Patient Health Questionnaire [depression scale]; PROMIS: Patient Reported Outcomes Measurement Information System; RINGS: Readiness and Resilience in National Guard Soldiers [study]; VA: [Department of] Veterans Affairs; VR-12: Veterans RAND 12-item Health Survey

Acknowledgments
We thank Dr. Barbara Stussman, who provided valuable feedback on development of the Health Practices Inventory. We would like to thank the other members of the RINGS-CAM study team: Christopher Erbes, Paul Arbisi, Shannon Kehle-Forbes, Siamak Noorbaloochi, Shelly Hubbling, Ann Bangerter, Erin Amundson, Andrea Cutting, Erin Koffel, and David Leverty.

Funding
This research was supported by the National Institutes of Health National Center for Complementary Integrative Health (R01AT008387; Polusny & Krebs, Co-PIs). M. Donaldson was supported by an individual fellowship from National Center for Complementary and Integrative Health (F30AT009162), and the University of Minnesota Medical Scientist Training Program (T32GM00824). This material is the result of work supported with resources and the use of facilities at the Minneapolis VA Health Care System, Minneapolis, MN.

Disclosures
M. Donaldson presented data from this manuscript as a poster at the 2018 International Congress on Integrative Medicine and Health, Baltimore, MD, USA, May 8, 2018.

Authors' contributions
MD designed and performed statistical analyses and drafted the manuscript. MAP and EEK designed and conducted the study and developed main conceptual ideas. EMHG contributed to data management and analysis. All authors contributed to analytical design and interpretation. All authors have been involved in critically revising the manuscript and have approved the final version.

Competing interests
None of the authors report current or future competing interests or disclosures of financial interests and relationships. The views expressed in this article are those of the authors and do not reflect the official policy or position of the Department of Veterans Affairs, Department of the Army, or Department of Defense. The authors declare that they have no competing interests.

Author details
[1]Minneapolis VA Health Care System, One Veterans Drive, Minneapolis, MN 55417, USA. [2]University of Minnesota Medical Scientist Training Program, Minneapolis, MN 55455, USA. [3]Division of Epidemiology and Community Health, University of Minnesota School of Public Health, Minneapolis, MN 55454, USA. [4]University of Minnesota Medical School, Minneapolis, MN 55455, USA.

References
1. Clarke TC, Norris T, Schiller JS. Early release of selected estimates based on data from the 2016 National Health Interview Survey: Lesiure-time physical activity. 2017; https://www.cdc.gov/nchs/data/nhis/earlyrelease/Earlyrelease201705_07.pdf .
2. Clarke TC, Black LI, Stussman BJ, Barnes PM, Nahin RL. Trends in the use of complementary health approaches among adults: United States, 2002–2012. Natl Health Stat Report. 2015;(79):1–16.
3. Whelton PK, Carey RM, Aronow WS, Casey DE, Collins KJ, Dennison Himmelfarb C, et al. 2017 ACC/AHA/AAPA/ABC/ACPM/AGS/APhA/ASH/ASPC/NMA/PCNA guideline for the prevention, detection, evaluation, and Management of High Blood Pressure in adults. Hypertension. 2017;:HYP.0000000000000065 doi:https://doi.org/10.1161/HYP.0000000000000065.
4. Chou R, Deyo R, Friedly J, Skelly A, Hashimoto R, Weimer M, et al. Nonpharmacologic therapies for low back pain: a systematic review for an American college of physicians clinical practice guideline. Ann Intern Med. 2017;166:493–505.
5. Kligler B, Bair MJ, Banerjea R, DeBar L, Ezeji-Okoye S, Lisi A, et al. Clinical Policy Recommendations from the VHA State-of-the-Art Conference on Non-Pharmacological Approaches to Chronic Musculoskeletal Pain. J Gen Intern Med. 2018; https://doi.org/10.1007/s11606-018-4323-z.
6. Tick H, Nielsen A, Pelletier KR, Bonakdar R, Simmons S, Glick R, et al. Evidence-based nonpharmacologic strategies for comprehensive pain care. EXPLORE. 2018; https://doi.org/10.1016/j.explore.2018.02.001.
7. Gartlehner G, Gaynes BN, Amick HR, et al. Nonpharmacological Versus Pharmacological Treatments for Adult Patients With Major Depressive Disorder [Internet]. Rockville (MD): Agency for Healthcare Research and Quality (US); 2015 Dec. (Comparative Effectiveness Reviews, No. 161.) Available from: https://www.ncbi.nlm.nih.gov/books/NBK338245/.
8. Park CL, Finkelstein-Fox L, Barnes DM, Mazure CM, Hoff R. CAM use in recently-returned OEF/OIF/OND US veterans: demographic and psychosocial predictors. Complement Ther Med. 2016;28:50–6.
9. Edmond SN, Becker WC, Driscoll MA, Decker SE, Higgins DM, Mattocks KM, et al. Use of non-pharmacological pain treatment modalities among veterans with chronic pain: results from a cross-sectional survey. J Gen Intern Med. 2018;33:54–60. https://doi.org/10.1007/s11606-018-4322-0.
10. Park C, Mind-Body CAM. Interventions: current status and considerations for integration into clinical Health Psychology. J Clin Psychol. 2013;69:45–63.
11. Eisenberg DM, Kessler RC, Foster C, Norlock FE, Calkins DR, Delbanco TL. Unconventional medicine in the United States -- prevalence, costs, and patterns of use. N Engl J Med. 1993;328:246–52. https://doi.org/10.1056/NEJM199301283280406.
12. Eisenberg DM, Kaptchuk TJ, Post DE, Hrbek AL, O'Connor BB, Osypiuk K, et al. Establishing an integrative medicine program within an academic health center. Acad Med. 2016;91:1223–30. https://doi.org/10.1097/ACM.0000000000001173.
13. 2012 NHIS Questionnaire - Adult CAM: Adult Alternative Health/Complementary And Alternative Medicine. ftp://ftp.cdc.gov/pub/Health_Statistics/NCHS/Survey_Questionnaires/NHIS/2012/English/qalthealt.pdf. Accessed 26 Mar 2018.
14. National Center for Complementary and Integrative Health. Use of Complementary Health Approaches in the U.S.: National Health Interview Survey (NHIS). 2017. https://nccih.nih.gov/research/statistics/NHIS/2012/key-findings. Accessed 1 Feb 2018.
15. Willis GB. Cognitive Interviewing: A "how to" guide. In: 1999 Meeting of the American Statistical Association. http://www.chime.ucla.edu/publications/docs/cognitive interviewing guide.pdf. Accessed 1 Feb 2018.
16. Willis G. Cognitive interviewing. Thousand Oaks: SAGE Publications, Inc.; 2005. https://doi.org/10.4135/9781412983655.
17. Polusny MA, Erbes CR, Murdoch M, Arbisi PA, Thuras P, Rath MB. Prospective risk factors for new-onset post-traumatic stress disorder in National Guard soldiers deployed to Iraq. Psychol Med. 2011;41:687–98. https://doi.org/10.1017/S0033291710002047.
18. Dillman DA, Smyth JD, Christian LM. Internet, phone, mail, and mixed-mode surveys: the tailored design method. 4th ed. Hoboken: Wiley; 2014.
19. Von Korff M, Scher AI, Helmick C, Carter-Pokras O, Dodick DW, Goulet J, et al. United States National Pain Strategy for population research: concepts, definitions, and pilot data. J Pain. 2016;17:1068–80. https://doi.org/10.1016/j.jpain.2016.06.009.
20. Krebs EE, Lorenz KA, Bair MJ, Damush TM, Wu J, Sutherland JM, et al. Development and initial validation of the PEG, a three-item scale assessing pain intensity and interference. J Gen Intern Med. 2009;24:733–8.
21. Kean J, Monahan PO, Kroenke K, Wu J, Yu Z, Stump TE, et al. Comparative responsiveness of the PROMIS pain interference short forms, brief pain inventory, PEG, and SF-36 bodily pain subscale. Med Care. 2016;54:414–21. https://doi.org/10.1097/MLR.0000000000000497.
22. Selim AJ, Rogers W, Fleishman JA, Qian SX, Fincke BG, Rothendler JA, et al. Updated U.S. population standard for the veterans RAND 12-item health survey (VR-12). Qual Life Res. 2009;18:43–52. https://doi.org/10.1007/s11136-008-9418-2.
23. Jones D, Kazis L, Lee A, Rogers W, Skinner K, Cassar L, et al. Health status assessments using the veterans SF-12 and SF-36: methods for evaluating otucomes in the veterans health administration. J Ambul Care Manag. 2001;24:68–86. https://doi.org/10.1097/00004479-200107000-00011.
24. Bishop FL, Lewith GT. Who uses CAM a narrative review of demographic characteristics and health factors associated with CAM use. Evidence-Based Complement Altern Med. 2010;7:11–28.
25. Pilkonis PA, Choi SW, Reise SP, Stover AM, Riley WT, Cella D, et al. Item banks for measuring emotional distress from the patient-reported outcomes measurement information system (PROMIS®): depression, anxiety, and anger. Assessment. 2011;18:263–83. https://doi.org/10.1177/1073191111411667.
26. Patient-Reported Outcomes Measurement Information System. PROMIS Scoring Guide: Version 1.0 short forms. 2011. https://www.assessmentcenter.net/documents/PROMIS%20Scoring%20Manual-%20CATs,%20Profiles,%20Short%20Forms.pdf.
27. Kroenke K, Strine TW, Spitzer RL, Williams JBW, Berry JT, Mokdad AH. The PHQ-8 as a measure of current depression in the general population. J Affect Disord. 2009;114:163–73. https://doi.org/10.1016/j.jad.2008.06.026.
28. Wortmann JH, Jordan AH, Weathers FW, Resick PA, Dondanville KA, Hall-Clark B, et al. Psychometric analysis of the PTSD Checklist-5 (PCL-5) among treatment-seeking military service members. Psychol Assess. 2016;28(11): 1392–1403.

29. Saunders JB, Aasland OG, Babor TF, De La Fuente JR, Grant M. Development of the alcohol use disorders identification test (AUDIT): WHO collaborative project on early detection of persons with harmful alcohol consumption--II. Addiction. 1993;88:791–804. https://doi.org/10.1111/j.1360-0443.1993.tb02093.x.

30. Skinner HA. The drug abuse screening test. Addict Behav. 1982;7:363–71. https://doi.org/10.1016/0306-4603(82)90005-3.

31. Tellegen A, Atkinson G. Openness to absorbing and self-altering experiences ("absorption"), a trait related to hypnotic susceptibility. J Abnorm Psychol. 1974;83:268–77.

32. Patrick CJ, Curtin JJ, Tellegen A. Development and validation of a brief form of the multidimensional personality questionnaire. Psychol Assess. 2002;14: 150–63. https://doi.org/10.1037/1040-3590.14.2.150.

33. Galbraith N, Moss T, Galbraith V, Purewal S. A systematic review of the traits and cognitions associated with use of and belief in complementary and alternative medicine (CAM) [published online ahead of print (February 22, 2018)]. Psychol Health Med. 2018; https://doi.org/10.1080/13548506.2018.1442010.

34. Muller CJ, Maclehose RF. Estimating predicted probabilities from logistic regression: different methods correspond to different target populations. Int J Epidemiol. 2014;43:962–70.

35. StataCorp. Stata Statistical Software: Release 15. 2017.

36. Raghunathan TE, Lepkowski JM, Van Hoewyk J, Solenberger P. A multivariate technique for multiply imputing missing values using a sequence of regression models. Surv Methodol. 2001;27:85–95.

37. Van Buuren S, Brand JPL, Groothuis-Oudshoorn CGM, Rubin DB. Fully conditional specification in multivariate imputation. J Stat Comput Simul. 2006;76:1049–64. https://doi.org/10.1080/10629360600810434.

38. Rubin DB. Inference and missing data. Biometrika. 1976;63:581–92. https://doi.org/10.1093/biomet/63.3.581.

39. Morris TP, White IR, Royston P. Tuning multiple imputation by predictive mean matching and local residual draws. BMC Med Res Methodol. 2014;14:75.

40. Little RJA. Missing-data adjustments in large surveys. J Bus Econ Stat. 1988;6: 287–96. https://doi.org/10.2307/1391881.

41. Stussman BJ, Bethell CD, Gray C, Nahin RL. Development of the adult and child complementary medicine questionnaires fielded on the National Health Interview Survey. BMC Complement Altern Med. 2013;13:328. https://doi.org/10.1186/1472-6882-13-328.

42. National Center for Complementary and Integrative Health. 2016 Strategic Plan: Exploring the Science of Complementary and Integrative Health. NIH Publication No. 16-AT-7643. 2016. https://nccih. nih.gov/sites/nccam.nih.gov/files/NCCIH_2016_Strategic_Plan.pdf. Accessed 7 Feb 2018.

43. Clarke TC, Nahin RL. Use of Complementary Health Approaches for Musculoskeletal Pain Disorders Among Adults: United States, 2012. Natl Heal Stat Rep. 2016;98:1–8. https://www.cdc.gov/nchs/data/nhsr/nhsr098.pdf

44. Chou R, Qaseem A, Snow V, Casey D, Cross JTJ, Shekelle P, et al. Diagnosis and treatment of low back pain: A joint clinical practice guideline from the American College of Physicians and the American Pain Society. Ann Intern Med. 2007;147:478–91. https://doi.org/10.7326/0003-4819-147-7-200710020-00006.

45. Qaseem A, Wilt TJ, McLean RM, Forciea MA. Noninvasive treatments for acute, subacute, and chronic low back pain: a clinical practice guideline from the American College of Physicians. Ann Intern Med. 2017;166:514–30.

46. Crawford C, Lee C, Freilich D. Effectiveness of active self-care complementary and integrative medicine therapies: options for the Management of Chronic Pain Symptoms. Pain Med. 2014;15:S86–95. https://doi.org/10.1111/pme.12407.

47. Nylund KL, Asparouhov T, Muthén BO. Deciding on the number of classes in latent class analysis and growth mixture modeling: a Monte Carlo simulation study. Struct Equ Model. 2007;14:535–69.

3

Oleanolic acid attenuates TGF-β1-induced epithelial-mesenchymal transition in NRK-52E cells

Wei-ming He[1†], Jia-qi Yin[2†], Xu-dong Cheng[3†], Xun Lu[4], Li Ni[2], Yi Xi[2], Gui-dong Yin[2], Guo-yuan Lu[2], Wei Sun[1] and Ming-gang Wei[2*]

Abstract

Background: Epithelial-to-mesenchymal transition (EMT) plays an important role in the progression of renal interstitial fibrosis, which finally leads to renal failure. Oleanolic acid (OA), an activator of NF-E2-related factor 2 (Nrf2), is reported to attenuate renal fibrosis in mice with unilateral ureteral obstruction. However, the role of OA in the regulation of EMT and the underlying mechanisms remain to be investigated. This study aimed to evaluate the effects of OA on EMT of renal proximal tubular epithelial cell line (NRK-52E) induced by TGF-β1, and to elucidate its underlying mechanism.

Methods: Cells were incubated with TGF-β1 in the presence or absence of OA. The epithelial marker E-cadherin, the mesenchymal markers, α-smooth muscle actin (α-SMA), fibronectin, Nrf2, klotho, the signal transducer (p-Smad2/3), EMT initiator (Snail), and ILK were assayed by western blotting.

Results: Our results showed that the NRK-52E cells incubated with TGF-β1 induced EMT with transition to the spindle-like morphology, down-regulated the expression of E-cadherin but up-regulated the expression of α-SMA and fibronectin. However, the treatment with OA reversed all EMT markers in a dose-dependent manner. OA also restored the expression of Nrf2 and klotho, decreased the phosphorylation of Smad2/3, ILK, and Snail in cells which was initiated by TGF-β1.

Conclusion: OA can attenuate TGF-β1 mediate EMT in renal tubular epithelial cells and may be a promising therapeutic agent in the treatment of renal fibrosis.

Keywords: Oleanolic acid, EMT, TGF-β1, Nrf2, Klotho

Background

The epithelial-mesenchymal transition (EMT) is a highly conserved process in which polarized, immobile epithelial cells are converted into motile mesenchymal cells with motile mesenchymal phenotypes [1–3]. The EMT is involved in various pathological processes, such as inflammation, fibrosis and tumorigenesis. Accumulating evidences show that EMT occurred in kidney plays an important role in the progression of renal interstitial fibrosis [4–7]. It is important to understand the mechanism to reverse EMT which is valuable establishing therapeutic strategies preventing progressive renal failure. Among many fibrogenic factors regulating renal fibrotic process, transforming growth factor-β1 (TGF-β1) is the key mediators that play critical roles in inducing EMT and renal fibrosis through the TGF-β1/Smads signal pathway [8–11]. The EMT process is characterized by the loss of epithelial markers such as E-cadherin and acquiring mesenchymal features, including α-smooth muscle actin (α-SMA) and fibronectin concomitantly with the increase in the expression of Snail protein [12–14], which is a zinc finger protein and functions as a core EMT transcription factors that plays critical roles in fibrosis via the down regulation of E-cadherin expression [15–17]. ILK plays critical role in renal tubular EMT process mainly by upregulating the expression of Snail [18–21]. In concert, the inhibition of

* Correspondence: weiminggang@suda.edu.cn
†Wei-ming He, Jia-qi Yin and Xu-Dong Cheng contributed equally to this work.
²The First Affiliated Hospital of Soochow University, Suzhou 215006, Jiangsu, China
Full list of author information is available at the end of the article

TGF-β1 signaling has been included in several therapeutic approaches for preventing renal fibrosis [22, 23].

OA is a natural triterpenoid compounds that exist widely in food, medicinal herbs and other plants, which has recently attracted considerable attention for its anti-oxidant properties through the induction of Nrf2 activation [24–28]. Recently studies have also shown that OA is effective in protecting chemically induced liver injury in laboratory animals. Nrf2 is a basic leucine-zipper (bZip) transcription factor that protects cells and tissues from oxidative and electrophilic stress by activating antioxidant and detoxifying enzymes [29–31]. Recently study also shows that Nrf2 can restore the klotho expression and protect against renal fibrosis [32]. Klotho gene, a new anti-aging gene, is predominantly expressed in renal tubular epithelial cells [33]. Previous studies have found that the reduction of renal klotho gene expression is associated with the emergence and development of the pathological process of renal diseases [34]. The klotho protein can directly bind to the type-II TGF-β1 receptor and inhibit TGF-β1 binding to cell surface receptors, thereby inhibiting TGF-β1 signaling and reduced EMT responses [35]. We previously reported that the JiaWeiDangGui decoction, OA is one of the most effective components. OA reduces the accumulation of ECM in the kidneys of rats with Adriamycin-induced nephropathy [36]. However, protective effects of OA, an Nrf2 activator, against renal fibrosis induced by TGF-β1 has not been investigated.

In this study, we investigated the effects of OA on EMT of NRK-52E induced by TGF-β1 in vitro. We found that OA inhibited TGF-β1-induced EMT via upregulation of Nrf2 and klotho, it also inhibits the TGF-β1/Smads pathway.

Methods

Drug and reagents

Oleanolic acid (OA) (Fig. 1) was purchased from Tauto Biotech (Shanghai. China) (Purity higher than 98%). OA was dissolved in DMSO for its administration. Recombinant TGF-β1 was purchased from Peprotech (Cat. No. 100-21C, USA). All other chemicals used in this study were either HPLC or analytical grade.

Cell culture and treatment

NRK-52E cells were purchased from the Institute of Biochemistry and Cell Biology (Shanghai, China) and cultured in DMEM/F12 (Gibco, USA) with 10% fetal bovine serum (FBS) (Gibco, USA) in an atmosphere of 5% CO_2 at 37 °C. To determine the effects of OA treatment on the EMT, NRK-52E cells were incubated into 6-well plates with 50–60% confluence were starved for 24 h by incubation with DMEM/F12 containing 0.5% FBS and then divided into following groups: (1) normal control group incubated in DMEM/F12 containing 0.1% DMSO (i.e., vehicle); (2) TGF-β1 group stimulated with recombinant TGF-β1 (5 ng/mL); and (3) OA-treated groups stimulated with recombinant TGF-β1(5 ng/mL) and simultaneously treated with different concentrations of OA (2, 4, and 8 μM). After 48 h, cells were harvested and processed for western blot analysis.

Western blotting

Western blot assays were used to evaluate the expression of the protein levels. Briefly, cells were lysed in lysis buffer (20 mM Tris, 1 mM EDTA, 1% Triton X-100, 1 mM Na3VO4, 20 mg/ml Aprotinin, 20 mg/ml Leupeptin, 1 mM DTT, and 1 mM PMSF) and the crude protein lysate (40 μg) was resolved by 12% SDS-PAGE. After protein was transferred to a polyvinylidene difluoride (PVDF) membrane, the PVDF membrane was blocked with 5% (w/v) non-fat milk in Tris buffered saline (TBST) for 1 h at 37 °C. The blots were probed with a dilution of primary antibody. Antibodies used were as follows: anti-fibronectin (ab23751, Abcam, Cambridge, UK), anti-E-cadherin (ab133597, Abcam, Cambridge, UK), anti-α-SMA (ab5694, Abcam, Cambridge, UK), anti-Klotho antibody (ab203576), anti-Nrf2 antibody (ab137550), anti-pSmad2/3 (ab63399, Abcam, Cambridge, UK), anti-Smad2/3 (ab63672, Abcam, Cambridge, UK), anti-ILK (ab137912, Abcam, Cambridge, UK), anti-Snail (ab180714, Abcam, Cambridge, UK), and β-actin (Santa Cruz Biotechnology, Inc.). After hybridization, the blots were washed and hybridized with 1:5000 (v/v) dilutions of goat anti-rabbit IgG, horseradish peroxidase-conjugated secondary antibody (Santa Cruz Biotechnology, Inc.). The signal was generated by adding enhanced chemiluminescent reagent, with β-actin used as an internal control.

Statistical analysis

Data are shown as means ± standard deviation The statistical difference between groups was mined by the paired Student's t-test. A P-value les 0.05 was considered significant.

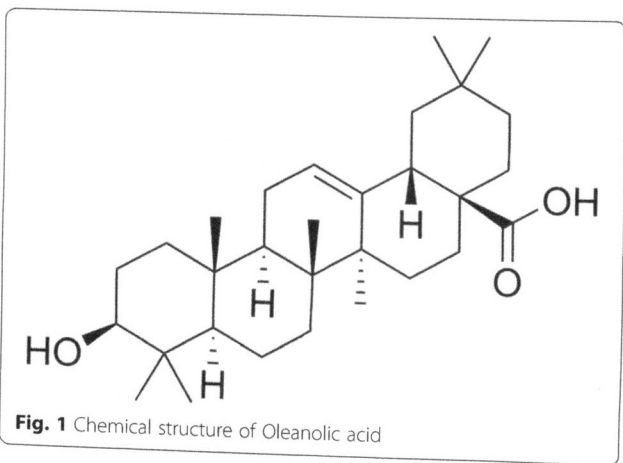

Fig. 1 Chemical structure of Oleanolic acid

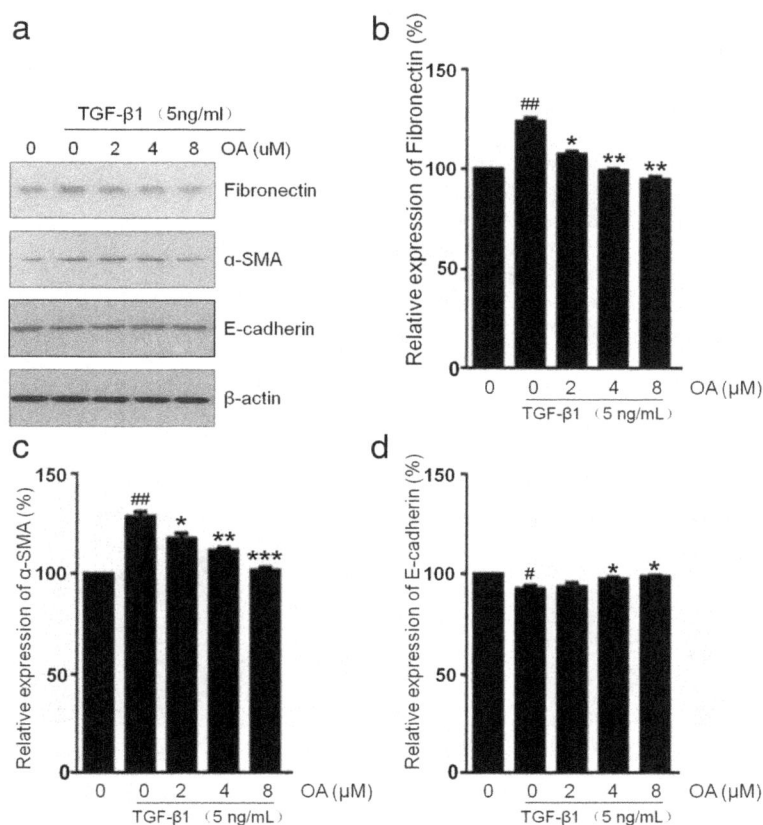

Fig. 3 Effects of OA on TGF-β1-induced EMT in NRK-52E cells. The cells were incubated with 5 ng/mL of TGF-β1 for 48 h with different concentrations of OA (0, 2, 4, 8 μM). **a** The expression of Fibronectin, α-SMA and E-cadherin was determined by Western blotting. **b, c, d** The expression level was quantitatively analyzed with Image J software. The data showing mean ± SD. # $P < 0.05$, ## $P < 0.01$, and ### $P < 0.005$ vs. 0 ng/mL TGF-β1. * $P < 0.05$, ** $P < 0.01$, and *** $P < 0.005$ vs. 0 μM OA in the presence of 5 ng/mL TGF-β1

Effects of OA on the ILK and snail expression in NRK-52E cells

ILK has been shown to be a key intracellular mediator which controls EMT in tubular epithelial cells by inducing key EMT-regulatory gene Snail expression [18, 19]. To examine whether TGF-β1 promotes ILK and Snail expression and whether OA abolish the EMT process via these process, Western blots were performed. Our results showed that the expressions of ILK and Snail in NRK-52E cells were up-regulated by TGF-β1 but suppressed by OA (Fig. 6).

Discussion

EMT defines a physiological process that allows polarized epithelial cells converting into motile mesenchymal cells [1–3]. Recent evidences have indicated that EMT may play an important role in the kidney fibrosis. The inhibition of EMT attenuates renal fibrosis induced by TGF-β1, a well-known profibrotic cytokine in the renal fibrosis [10]. Accumulating evidences suggest that OA has beneficially effects on many cellular processes, but its protective activity against EMT remains largely unclear. The model of EMT induced by TGF-β1 in epithelial cells

(NRK-52E) has been employed widely in studies of renal fibrosis [39–41]. In this study, we evaluated the effects of OA on EMT of renal proximal tubular epithelial cell line (NRK-52E) induced by TGF-β1, and elucidated its underlying mechanism. In agreement with previous reports on the TGF-β1 response, NRK-52E cells loses their classic cobblestone-like morphology and adopts a mesenchymal spindle-like appearance after treated by TGF-β1. Moreover OA alleviated changes in the expression of these markers induced by TGF-β1, indicating that OA could attenuate TGF-β1-induced EMT in NRK-52E cells.

As we known, OA is a nature potent activator of Nrf2 which has antioxidant activity. Previous reports have shown that Nrf2 can protect fibrosis induced by TGF-β1 via reducing EMT [31]. We investigated the expression level of Nrf2 during the EMT process. The results showed that the expression of Nrf2 in the TGF-β1 treatment group decreased compared to the untreated group, but increased by OA treatment in a dose dependent manner. Klotho is an anti-aging protein predominantly expressed in renal tubular epithelial cells. Evidences showed that the upregulation of Klotho could suppress

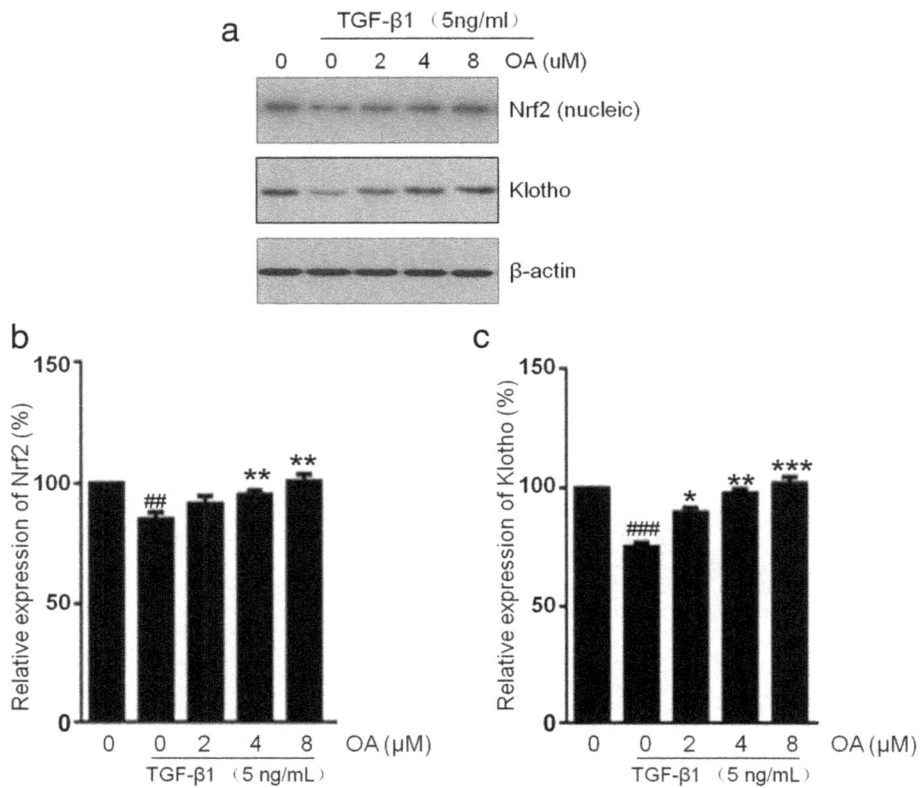

Fig. 4 Effects of OA on the Nrf2 and klotho expression in NRK-52E cells. The cells were incubated with 5 ng/mL of TGF-β1 for 48 h with different concentrations of OA (0, 2, 4, 8 μM). **a** The expression level of Nrf2 and klotho was determined by Western blotting. **b, c** The expression level was quantitatively analyzed with Image J software. The data showing mean ± SD. # $P < 0.05$, ## $P < 0.01$, and ### $P < 0.005$ vs. 0 ng/mL TGF-β1. * $P < 0.05$, ** $P < 0.01$, and *** $P < 0.005$ vs. 0 μM OA in the presence of 5 ng/mL TGF-β1

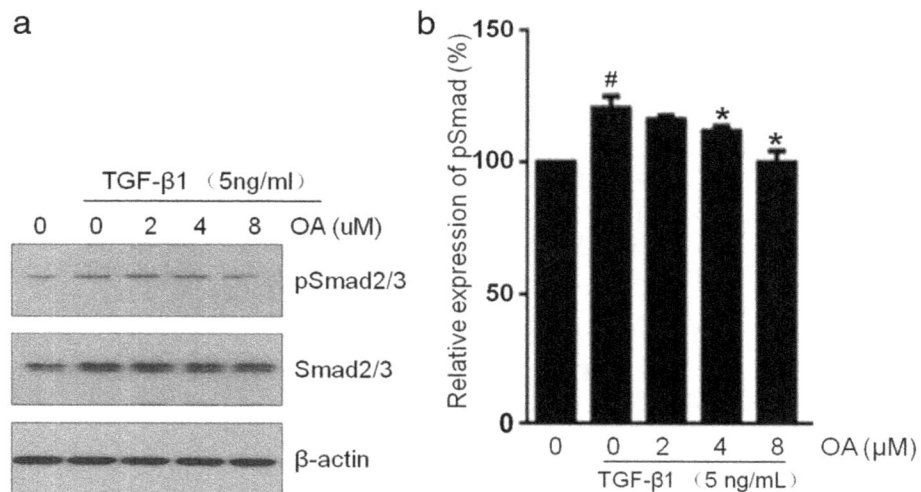

Fig. 5 Effects of OA on the expression of pSmad2/3 in NRK-52E cells. The cells were incubated with 5 ng/mL of TGF-β1 for 48 h with different concentrations of OA (0, 2, 4, 8 μM). **a** The expression level of Smad2/3 and pSmad2/3 was determined by Western blotting. **b** The pSmad2/3 was quantitatively analyzed with Image J software. The data showing mean ± SD. # $P < 0.05$ vs. 0 ng/mL TGF-β1. * $P < 0.05$ vs. 0 μM OA in the presence of 5 ng/mL TGF-β1

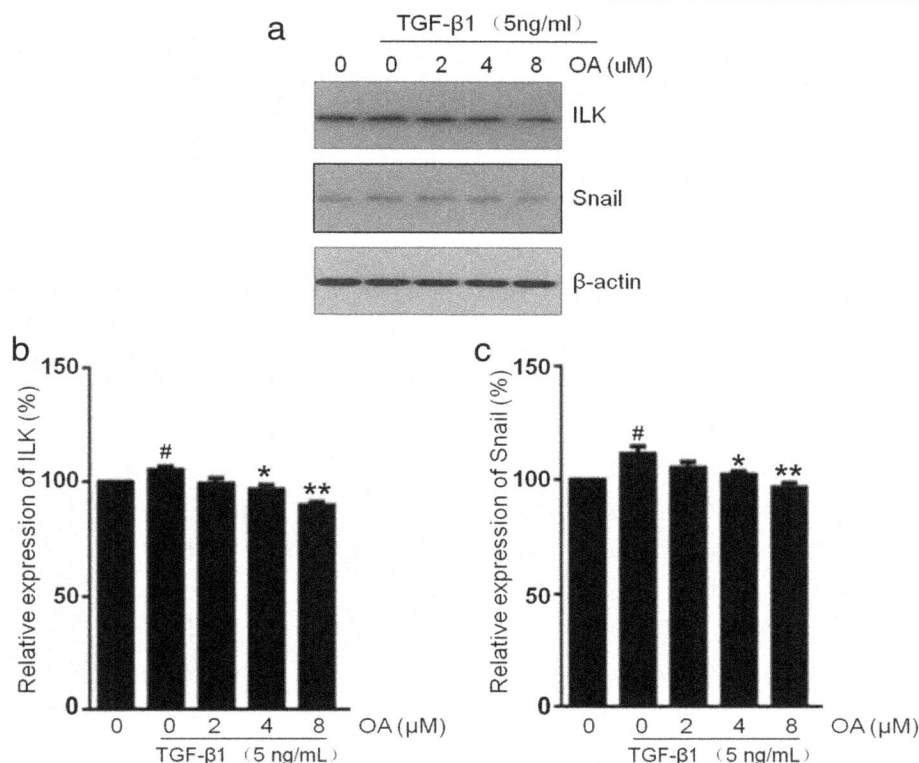

Fig. 6 Effects of OA on the ILK and Snail expression in NRK-52E cells. The cells were incubated with 5 ng/mL of TGF-β1 for 48 h with different concentrations of OA (0, 2, 4, 8 μM). **a** The expression level of ILK and Snail was determined by Western blotting. **b**, **c** The expression level was quantitatively analyzed with Image J software. The data showing mean ± SD. # $P < 0.05$ vs. 0 ng/mL TGF-β1. * $P < 0.05$, and ** $P < 0.01$ vs. 0 μM OA in the presence of 5 ng/mL TGF-β1

the EMT process induced by TGF-β1 [35], and Nrf2 activation can restore the expression of klotho and then attenuates oxidative stress and inflammation in CKD [32]. In our study, treatment with OA could restore the expression of klotho in NRK-52E cells which is down-regulated by TGF-β1. The results showed that OA attenuates renal EMT induced by TGF-β1 in NRK-52E cells may be primarily involved the upregulation of Nrf2 and klotho expression.

To further address the mechanism by which OA inhibits EMT in NRK-52E cells induced by TGF-β1, we focused on components downstream of TGF-β1 signaling. TGF-β1/Smads pathway plays a critical role in TGF-β1-induced EMT in epithelial cells. It has been demonstrated that activation of TGF-β1 signaling triggers a dramatic induction of Smad2/3 phosphorylation. Previous reports showed that Nrf2 is involved in the inhibition of smad activation pathway by TGF-β1. Moreover, many reports have shown that klotho suppresses TGF-β1-induced EMT responses in cultured cells, including decreased epithelial marker expression, increased mesenchymal marker expression, and/or increased cell migration by inhibiting TGF-β1/Smads pathway [35]. The results in this study suggests that OA attenuates TGF-β1-induced EMT in NRK-52E cells associated with the modulation of the TGF-β1/Smads pathway. Snail,

a key EMT-regulatory gene, downregulates E-cadherin expression and upregulates fibronectin expression, leading to a full EMT phenotype induced primarily by TGF-β1. ILK is well documented as a key intracellular mediator that promotes EMT in tubular epithelial cells by inducing Snail expression [18–21]. Our study demonstrated that ILK and Snail were down-regulated in response to OA during TGF-β1-induced EMT.

The above observation demonstrated that OA attenuates renal EMT processes induced by TGF-β1 in NRK-52E cells. The possible mechanisms involve the upregulation of Nrf2 and klotho expression, suppression of the TGF-β1/Smads pathway and the subsequent inhibition of ILK and Snail expression, and the inhibition of EMT processes. Thus, the anti-fibrotic effect of OA requires further study for future clinical usage.

Conclusion

In conclusion, we demonstrated that OA, an activator of Nrf2, could dose-dependently attenuate TGF-β1-induced EMT in NRK-52E cells. Therefore, OA may be a potential therapeutic agent which can prevent or attenuate EMT process.

Abbreviations

bZip: basic leucine-zipper; CKD: Chronic kidney disease; DMEM/F-12: Dulbecco's Modified Eagle Medium/Nutrient Mixture F-12; DMSO: Dimethyl sulfoxide; DTT: dithiothreitol; EMT: Epithelial-to-mesenchymal transition; FBS: fetal bovine serum; HPLC: High-performance liquid chromatography; Nrf2: NF-E2-related factor 2; OA: Oleanolic acid; PBS: Phosphate buffer saline; PMSF: Phenylmethylsulfonyl fluoride; PVDF: polyvinylidene difluoride; SD: Standard deviation; TBST: Tris buffered saline; TGF-β1: transforming growth factor-β1; α-SMA: α-smooth muscle actin

Funding

This work was supported by the grant from the Natural Science Foundation of China (No. 81273723, No. 81473633, No. 81673896, No. 81774269), Research Project for Practice Development of National TCM Clinical Research Bases (No. JDZX2015096), Suzhou Science and Technology Program (SYS201602, SYSD2016186).

Authors' contributions

JQY, XDC, XL, LN, YX, and GDY carried out experiment studies. MGW and WMH drafted the manuscript. MGW, WS and GYL participated in the design of the study and performed the statistical analysis. All authors read and approved the final manuscript.

Competing interests

The authors declare that they have no competing interests.

Author details

[1]Affiliated Hospital of Nanjing University of Chinese Medicine, Nanjing 210029, Jiangsu, China. [2]The First Affiliated Hospital of Soochow University, Suzhou 215006, Jiangsu, China. [3]Suzhou Hospital of Traditional Chinese Medicine, Suzhou 215006, Jiangsu, China. [4]Suzhou Municipal Hospital, Affiliated Hospital of Nanjing Medical University, Suzhou 215006, Jiangsu, China.

References

1. Kalluri R, Neilson EG. Epithelial-mesenchymal transition and its implications for fibrosis. J Clin Invest. 2003;112:1776–84.
2. Lee JM, Dedhar S, Kalluri R, Thompson EW. The epithelial-mesenchymal transition: new insights in signaling, development, and disease. J Cell Biol. 2006;172:973–81.
3. Kalluri R, Weinberg RA. The basics of epithelial-mesenchymal transition. J Clin Invest. 2009;119:1420–8.
4. Liu Y. Epithelial to mesenchymal transition in renal fibrogenesis: pathologic significance, molecular mechanism, and therapeutic intervention. J Am Soc Nephrol. 2004;15:1–12.
5. Hewitson TD. Renal tubulointerstitial fibrosis: common but never simple. Am J Physiol Renal Physiol. 2009;296:1239–44.
6. Liu Y. New insights into epithelial-mesenchymal transition in kidney fibrosis. J Am Soc Nephrol. 2010;21:2–22.
7. Inoue T, Umezawa A, Takenaka T, Suzuki H, Okada H. The contribution of epithelial-mesenchymal transition to renal fibrosis differs among kidney disease models. Kidney Int. 2015;87:233–8.
8. Border WA, Noble NA. Transforming growth factor beta in tissue fibrosis. N Engl J Med. 1994;331:1286–92.
9. Kasai H, Allen JT, Mason RM, Kamimura T, Zhang Z. TGF-β1 induces human alveolar epithelial to mesenchymal cell transition (EMT). Respir Res. 2005;6:56.
10. Xu J, Lamouille S, Derynck R. TGF-beta-induced epithelial to mesenchymal transition. Cell Res. 2009;19:156–72.
11. Sutariya B, Jhonsa D, Saraf MN. TGF-β: the connecting link between nephropathy and fibrosis. Immunopharmacol Immunotoxicol. 2016;38:39–49.
12. Yang J, Liu Y. Dissection of key events in tubular epithelial to myofibroblast transition and its implications in renal interstitial fibrosis. Am J Pathol. 2001; 159:1465–75.
13. Zeisberg M, Neilson EG. Biomarkers for epithelial-mesenchymal transitions. J Clin Invest. 2009;119:1429–37.
14. Veerasamy M, Nguyen TQ, Motazed R, Pearson AL, Goldschmeding R, Dockrell ME. Differential regulation of E-cadherin and α-smooth muscle actin by BMP 7 in human renal proximal tubule epithelial cells and its implication in renal fibrosis. Am J Physiol Renal Physiol. 2009;297:1238–48.
15. Jiao W, Miyazaki K, Kitajima Y. Inverse correlation between E-cadherin and snail expression in hepatocellular carcinoma cell lines in vitro and in vivo. Br J Cancer. 2002;86:98–101.
16. Barrallo-Gimeno A, Nieto MA. The snail genes as inducers of cell movement and survival: implications in development and cancer. Development. 2005; 132:3151–61.
17. Yoshino J, Monkawa T, Tsuji M, Inukai M, Itoh H, Hayashi M. Snail1 is involved in the renal epithelial-mesenchymal transition. Biochem Biophys Res Commun. 2007;362:63–8.
18. Li Y, Yang J, Dai C, Wu C, Liu Y. Role for integrin-linked kinase in mediating tubular epithelial to mesenchymal transition and renal interstitial fibrogenesis. J Clin Invest. 2003;112:503–16.
19. Li Y, Tan X, Dai C, Stolz DB, Wang D, Liu Y. Inhibition of integrin-linked kinase attenuates renal interstitial fibrosis. J Am Soc Nephrol. 2009;20:1907–18.
20. Kang YS, Li Y, Dai C, Kiss LP, Wu C, Liu Y. Inhibition of integrin-linked kinase blocks podocyte epithelial-mesenchymal transition and ameliorates proteinuria. Kidney Int. 2010;78:363–73.
21. Serrano I, McDonald PC, Lock FE, Dedhar S. Role of the integrin-linked kinase (ILK)/Rictor complex in TGFβ-1-induced epithelial-mesenchymal transition (EMT). Oncogene. 2013;32:50–60.
22. Böttinger EP. TGF-beta in renal injury and disease. Semin Nephrol. 2007; 27:309–20.
23. Qin W, Chung AC, Huang XR, Meng XM, Hui DS, Yu CM, al e. TGF-β/Smad3 signaling promotes renal fibrosis by inhibiting miR-29. J Am Soc Nephrol. 2011;22:1462–74.
24. Reisman SA, Aleksunes LM, Klaassen CD. Oleanolic acid activates Nrf2 and protects from acetaminophen hepatotoxicity via Nrf2-dependent and Nrf2-independent processes. Biochem Pharmacol. 2009;77:1273–82.
25. Shin S, Wakabayashi J, Yates MS, Wakabayashi N, Dolan PM, Aja S, et al. Role of Nrf2 in prevention of high-fat diet-induced obesity by synthetic triterpenoid CDDO-imidazolide. Eur J Pharmacol. 2009;620:138–44.
26. Martín R, Carvalho-Tavares J, Hernández M, Arnés M, Ruiz-Gutiérrez V, Nieto ML. Beneficial actions of oleanolic acid in an experimental model of multiple sclerosis: a potential therapeutic role. Biochem Pharmacol. 2010;79:198–208.
27. Santos RS, Silva PL, Oliveira GP, Cruz FF, Ornellas DS, Morales MM, et al. Effects of oleanolic acid on pulmonary morphofunctional and biochemical variables in experimental acute lung injury. Respir Physiol Neurobiol. 2011;179:129–36.
28. Bachhav SS, Patil SD, Bhutada MS, Surana SJ. Oleanolic acid prevents glucocorticoid-induced hypertension in rats. Phytother Res. 2011;25:1435–9.
29. Kay HY, Kim YW, Ryu DH, Sung SH, Hwang SJ, Kim SG. Nrf2-mediated liver protection by sauchinone, an antioxidant lignan, from acetaminophen toxicity through the PKCδ-GSK3β pathway. Br J Pharmacol. 2011;163:1653–65.
30. Ma Q. Role of nrf2 in oxidative stress and toxicity. Annu Rev Pharmacol Toxicol. 2013;53:401–26.
31. Zhou W, Mo X, Cui W, Zhang Z, Li D, Li L, et al. Nrf2 inhibits epithelial-mesenchymal transition by suppressing snail expression during pulmonary fibrosis. Sci Rep. 2016;6:38646.
32. Son YK, Liu SM, Farzaneh SH, Nazertehrani S, Khazaeli M, Vaziri ND. Activation of Nrf2 restores klotho expression and attenuates oxidative stress and inflammation in CKD. J Appl Life Sci Int. 2015;2:22–34.
33. Kuro-o M, Matsumura Y, Aizawa H, Kawaguchi H, Suga T, Utsugi T, et al. Mutation of the mouse klotho gene leads to a syndrome resembling ageing. Nature. 1997;390:45–51.
34. Zhou Q, Lin S, Tang R, Veeraragoo P, Peng W, Wu R. Role of Fosinopril and valsartan on klotho gene expression induced by angiotensin II in rat renal tubular epithelial cells. Kidney Blood Press Res. 2010;33:186–92.
35. Doi S, Zou Y, Togao O, Pastor JV, John GB, Wang L, et al. Klotho inhibits transforming growth factor-beta1 (TGF-beta1) signaling and suppresses renal fibrosis and cancer metastasis in mice. J Biol Chem. 2011;286:8655–65.

36. Wei MG, He WM, Lu X, Ni L, Yang YY, Chen L, et al. JiaWeiDangGui decoction ameliorates proteinuria and kidney injury in Adriamycin-induced rat by blockade of TGF-β/Smad signaling. Evid Based Complement Alternat Med. 2016;2016:5031890.

37. Ryoo IG, Ha H, Kwak MK. Inhibitory role of the KEAP1-NRF2 pathway in TGFβ1-stimulated renal epithelial transition to fibroblastic cells: a modulatory effect on SMAD signaling. PLoS One. 2014;9:e93265.

38. Derynck R, Muthusamy BP, Saeteurn KY. Signaling pathway cooperation in TGF-β-induced epithelial-mesenchymal transition. Curr Opin Cell Biol. 2014; 31:56–66.

39. Rhyu DY, Yang Y, Ha H, Lee GT, Song JS, Uh ST, Lee HB. Role of reactive oxygen species in TGF-beta1-induced mitogen-activated protein kinase activation and epithelial-mesenchymal transition in renal tubular epithelial cells. J Am Soc Nephrol. 2005;16:667–75.

40. Xiong M, Jiang L, Zhou Y, Qiu W, Fang L, Tan R, Wen P, Yang J. The miR-200 family regulates TGF-β1-induced renal tubular epithelial to mesenchymal transition through Smad pathway by targeting ZEB1 and ZEB2 expression. Am J Physiol Renal Physiol. 2012;302:F369–79.

41. Zhang W, S S, F L, Y L, Zhang Y. Beta-casomorphin-7 prevents epithelial-mesenchymal transdifferentiation of NRK-52E cells at high glucose level: involvement of AngII-TGF-β1 pathway. Peptides. 2015;70:37–44.

4

Ginkgolide B inhibits platelet and monocyte adhesion in TNFα-treated HUVECs under laminar shear stress

Ming Zhang[1,2†], Jie Sun[1†], Beidong Chen[1], Yanyang Zhao[1], Huan Gong[1], Yun You[3] and Ruomei Qi[1,2*] (iD)

Abstract

Background: Endothelial cells are sensitive to changes in both blood components and mechanical stimuli. Endothelial cells may undergo phenotypic changes, such as changes in adhesion protein expression, under different shear stress conditions. Such changes may impact platelet and monocyte adhesion to endothelial cells. This phenomenon is linked to chronic vascular inflammation and the development of atherosclerosis. In the present study, we investigated the effects of ginkgolide B on platelet and monocyte adhesion to human umbilical vein endothelial cells (HUVECs) under different conditions of laminar shear stress.

Methods: Platelet and monocyte adhesion to endothelial cells was determined by the Bioflux 1000. HUVECs were incubated with ginkgolide B or aspirin for 12 h, and then TNFα was added for 2 h to induce the inflammatory response under conditions of 1 and 9 dyn/cm^2 laminar shear stress. The protein expression was analyzed by Western blot.

Results: The number of platelets that adhered was greater under conditions of 1 dyn/cm^2 than under conditions of 9 dyn/cm^2 of laminar shear stress (74.8 ± 19.2 and 59.5 ± 15.1, respectively). Ginkgolide B reduced the tumor necrosis factor α (TNFα)-induced increase in platelet and monocyte adhesion to HUVECs at 1 and 9 dyn/cm^2 of laminar shear stress. In TNFα-treated HUVECs, the number of monocytes that adhered was greater under conditions of 1 dyn/cm^2 of laminar shear stress compared with 9 dyn/cm^2 (29.1 ± 4.9 and 22.7 ± 3.7, respectively). Ginkgolide B inhibited the TNFα-induced expression of vascular cell adhesion molecule-1(VCAM-1), VE-cadherin, and Cx43 in HUVECs at 1 and 9 dyn/cm^2. The expression of these proteins was not different between 1 and 9 dyn/cm^2.

Conclusions: Ginkgolide B suppressed platelet and monocyte adhesion under different conditions of laminar shear stress. Moreover, ginkgolide B reduced VCAM-1, VE-cadherin and Cx43 expression in TNFα-treated HUVECs under laminar shear stress. This suggested that ginkgolide B might shed light on the treatment of inflammation in atherosclerosis.

Keywords: Ginkgolide B, Endothelial cells, Platelets, VCAM-1, VE-cadherin, Shear stress

Background

Endothelial cells are the initial barriers on the vessel wall. Endothelial cell dysfunction is a primary cause of cardiovascular disease. Endothelial cells are sensitive to changes in both blood components and mechanical

* Correspondence: ruomeiqi@163.com
†Ming Zhang and Jie Sun contributed equally to this work.
[1]MOH Key Laboratory of Geriatrics, Beijing Hospital, National Center of Gerontology, Beijing, China
[2]Graduate School of Peking Union Medical College, Chinese Academy of Medical Sciences, Beijing, China
Full list of author information is available at the end of the article

stimuli [1–3]. In humans, normal physiological flow ranges from 10 to 50 dyn/cm^2 and is highly pulsatile in arteries and ~ 10-fold less with minimal pulsation in veins [4]. High shear stress that results from laminar flow promotes endothelial cell survival and quiescence, alignment in the direction of the flow, and the secretion of substances that promote vasodilation and anticoagulation [5, 6]. Low shear stress or changes in the direction of shear stress, as found in turbulent flow, promotes vasoconstriction, coagulation, and platelet aggregation [7, 8]. The precise mechanisms by which endothelial cells sense shear stress to affect cell-cell interactions are still not completely understood. Endothelial cells may undergo phenotypic changes, such as changes in adhesion protein expression, under different shear stress conditions. Such changes may impact platelet and monocyte adhesion to endothelial cells. This phenomenon is linked to chronic vascular inflammation and the development of atherosclerosis [9–11].

In the physiological state, endothelial cells maintain vessel integrity through junction proteins. VE-cadherin is a calcium-dependent cell-cell adhesion protein that is composed of five extracellular cadherin repeats and a transmembrane region [12]. VE-cadherin antibodies were shown to increase monolayer permeability in cultured cells [13]. We recently reported that VE-cadherin was involved in monocyte translocation in oxidized low-density lipoprotein (ox-LDL)-treated endothelial cells. Treatment with VE-cadherin siRNA reduced monocyte translocation in ox-LDL-treated endothelial cells [14]. Cx43 is also a junction protein that belongs to the gap junction protein family. Gap junctions play a role in intercellular communication between cells to regulate cell death, proliferation, and differentiation [15]. Gap junctions are involved in connecting adjacent cells to permit the exchange of low-molecular-weight molecules, such as ions and secondary messengers, to maintain homeostasis [16, 17].

Tumor necrosis factor α (TNFα) is a member of the cytokine family and involved in various inflammatory processes. TNFα is implicated in several human diseases, including atherosclerosis and cardiovascular disease. It is a potent inducer of nuclear factor κB (NF-κB) signaling, which is involved in the transcription of many inflammatory proteins. TNFα is also involved in endothelial cell injury under pathological conditions, such as atherosclerosis [18].

Ginkgolide B is a *Ginkgo biloba* leaf extract that can completely bind platelet-activating factor receptor (PAFR) and inhibit platelet activation [19]. Our recent studies showed that ginkgolide B inhibited inflammatory protein expression that was induced by ox-LDL in human umbilical vein endothelial cells (HUVECs) [20, 21]. However, remaining unknown is whether ginkgolide B inhibits platelet and monocyte adhesion to endothelial cells under different shear stress conditions. In the present study, we investigated the effects of ginkgolide B on platelet and monocytes adhesion to endothelial cells and phenotypic changes under different laminar shear stress conditions.

Methods

Materials

Ginkgolide B (95% purity) was purchased from Daguanyuan Company (Xuzhou, Jiangsu, China). Mouse tail type I collagen were purchased from Sigma-Aldrich (St. Louis, MO, USA). Monoclonal anti-connexin 43 antibody, polyclonal anti-VCAM-1 antibody and monoclonal anti-actin antibody were purchased from Santa Cruz Biotechnology (Santa Cruz, CA, USA). Monoclonal anti-VE-cadherin antibody was purchased from Abcam (Boston, MA, USA). Bioflux 48-well plates (1–20 dyn/cm^{-2}; 910–0047) were purchased from Fluxion Biosciences (South San Francisco, CA, USA).

Preparation of platelets

Fresh citrate anti-coagulated venous blood was obtained from human donors who had not taken any medication for a minimum of 2 weeks before blood collection. The blood was centrifuged at 400 × g for 15 min to obtain platelet-rich plasma (PRP). The PRP was washed twice in Tyrode's/HEPES buffer with 2 mM ethylene glycol tetraacetic acid (EGTA). Platelets were suspended in Tyrode's/HEPES buffer at a concentration of 2 × 108 cells/ml [22].

Preparation of monocytes

The THP-1 human monocytic cell line was obtained from the American Type Culture Collection (Manassas, VA, USA). The cells were maintained at 37 °C in RPMI 1640 medium supplemented with 10% fetal calf serum (FCS), 100 IU penicillin, 100 μg/ml streptomycin, and 2 mM L-glutamine in a humidified 5% carbon dioxide atmosphere [23].

Preparation and culture of human umbilical vein endothelial cells

HUVECs were purchased from ScienCell Research Laboratories (Carlsbad, CA, USA). HUVECs were redissolved in a 37 °C constant temperature water bath. The cells were cultured in M199 medium that contained 10% fetal bovine serum (Gibco, NY, USA), 2 mM glutamine, 100 U/ml penicillin, 100 μg/ml streptomycin, and 20 ng/ml endothelial growth factor (R&D, Minneapolis, MN, USA) in an incubator at 37 °C and 5% CO_2. Cells up to passage 4 were used in the experiments [24].

Platelet and monocyte adhesion to HUVECs assay

The Bioflux 1000 system (Fluxion Biosciences Inc., CA, USA) was used in the present study. The flow experiments were performed as previously described [25]. Briefly, the microfluidic channel was coated with type I collagen (20 μg/ml) that was dissolved in 0.02 M acetic acid. HUVECs (3×10^7) were seeded in microfluidic well plates until > 90% of the cells covered the well plate that was used for the experiments. HUVECs were treated with ginkgolide B (0.6 mg/ml) or aspirin (1 mM) for 12 h, and then TNFα was added for another 2 h under conditions of 1 and 9 dyn/cm^2 laminar shear stress. The platelet suspension (300 μl, 2×10^8) or monocyte suspension (300 μl, 5×10^6) was added to the input channel for 45 min for cell adhesion under condition of 0.2 dyn/cm^2. Images were captured by a Nikon Ti100 CCD camera in five locations in the flow chamber and analyzed using Bioflux Montage software.

Western blot

HUVECs were incubated with ginkgolide B (0.6 mg/ml) or aspirin (1 mM) for 12 h, and then TNFα (20 ng/ml) was added for 2 h under conditions of 1 and 9 dyn/cm^2 laminar shear stress. The platelet or monocyte suspension was perfused for 45 min under condition of 0.2 dyn/cm^2 for adhesion. After that the microfluidic channel was washed with PBS to remove unadhered platelets or monocytes for 5 min under condition of 2 dyn/cm^2, and then lysis buffer (1% Triton X-100, 100 mM Tris/HCl [pH 7.2], 50 mM NaCl, 5 mM ethylenediaminetetraacetic acid [EDTA], 5 mM EGTA, 1 μM phenylmethylsulfonyl fluoride [PMSF], and 100 μg/ml leupeptin) was added. Lysates were centrifuged at 12000 × g at 4 °C for 5 min. To obtain sufficient protein, three parallel microfluidic flow channels were used in each group. The cell lysates were separated by 10% sodium dodecyl sulfatepolyacrylamide gel electrophoresis (SDS-PAGE), and transferred to a polyvinylidene difluoride membrane (Millipore, Billerica, MA, USA. Primary antibody incubations were performed overnight at 4 °C. Horseradish peroxidase-conjugated secondary antibody was applied for 1 h at room temperature and developed using Super Signal developing reagent (Pierce, Thermo Scientific). Blot densitometry was then performed, and the bands were analyzed using the Gene Genius Bio Imaging System.

Statistical analysis

Quantitative data are presented as mean ± SEM. Significant differences between two groups were analyzed by two-tail unpaired Student's t-test. All of the calculations were performed using SPSS 18.0 software (Armonk, NY, USA). Values of $p < 0.05$ were considered statistically significant.

Results

Ginkgolide B decreases platelet adhesion to TNFα-treated HUVECs under conditions of laminar shear stress

To investigate the interaction between platelets and HUVECs, platelet adhesion was determined in TNFα-treated HUVECs under conditions of 1 and 9 dyn/cm^2 of shear stress. Our previous studies showed that 0.6 mg/ml ginkgolide B and 1 mM aspirin significantly inhibited the inflammatory response of endothelial cells. Therefore, we applied the same doses of ginkgolide B and aspirin in the present study. As shown

in Fig. 1, at 1 dyn/cm^2, the number of platelets that adhered was 74.8 ± 19.2 and 36.1 ± 4.4 in TNFα-treated and -untreated HUVECs, respectively. The number of platelets that adhered was 39.5 ± 12.3 in ginkgolide B-treated HUVECs. We used aspirin (1 mM) as a control. Aspirin treatment also reduced the number of platelets that adhered (35.8 ± 10.1) in TNFα-treated HUVECs. At 9 dyn/cm^2, the number of platelets that adhered was 59.5 ± 15.1 and 28.8 ± 3.7 in TNFα-treated and -untreated HUVECs. The number of platelets that adhered was 31.5 ± 4.9 and 32.1 ± 4.3 in the ginkgolide B- and aspirin-treated groups, respectively.

Ginkgolide B suppresses VCAM-1, VE-cadherin, and Cx43 expression in TNFα-treated HUVECs that present platelet adhesion under conditions of laminar shear stress

We first investigated the effects of ginkgolide B on VCAM-1 expression under laminar shear stress. As shown in Fig. 2a, at 1 dyn/cm^2, VCAM-1 expression increased by 31.7% ± 2.9% in TNFα-treated HUVECs compared with the control. Ginkgolide B and aspirin completely inhibited TNFα-induced VCAM-1 expression. VCAM-1 expression increased by 46.9% ± 10.1% in TNFα-treated HUVECs under conditions of 9 dyn/cm^2 of laminar shear stress. Ginkgolide B (0.6 mg/ml) almost completely attenuated TNFα-induced VCAM-1 expression. Similar results were found in the aspirin-treated group.

We next evaluated the effects of ginkgolide B on the expression of the tight junction proteins VE-cadherin and Cx43 under different conditions of laminar shear stress. As shown in Fig. 2b and c, TNFα treatment increased VE-cadherin expression by 31.8% ± 2.2% and 38.9% ± 9.1% under conditions of 1 and 9 dyn/cm^2 of laminar shear stress, respectively. Ginkgolide B (0.6 mg/ml) and aspirin (1 mM) completely abolished TNFα-induced VE-cadherin expression at 1 and 9 dyn/cm^2. Cx43 expression increased by 37.7% ± 9.8 and 30.5% ± 6.1% in TNFα-treated HUVECs that presented platelet adhesion at 1 and 9 dyn/cm^2, respectively. Ginkgolide B (0.6 mg/ml) and aspirin (1 mM) significantly inhibited TNFα-induced Cx43 expression at both 1 and 9 dyn/cm^2.

Ginkgolide B decreases monocyte adhesion to TNFα-treated HUVECs under conditions of laminar shear stress

Furthermore, monocyte adhesion to endothelial cells was evaluated under conditions of laminar shear stress. As shown in Fig. 3a, at 1 dyn/cm^2, the number of monocytes that adhered was 29.1 ± 4.9 in TNFα-treated HUVECs. The number of monocytes that adhered was 11.3 ± 1.9 in the control group. At 9 dyn/cm^2, the number of monocytes that adhered was 22.7 ± 3.7 in TNFα-treated HUVECs. The number of monocytes that adhered was 14.3 ± 4.5 in the

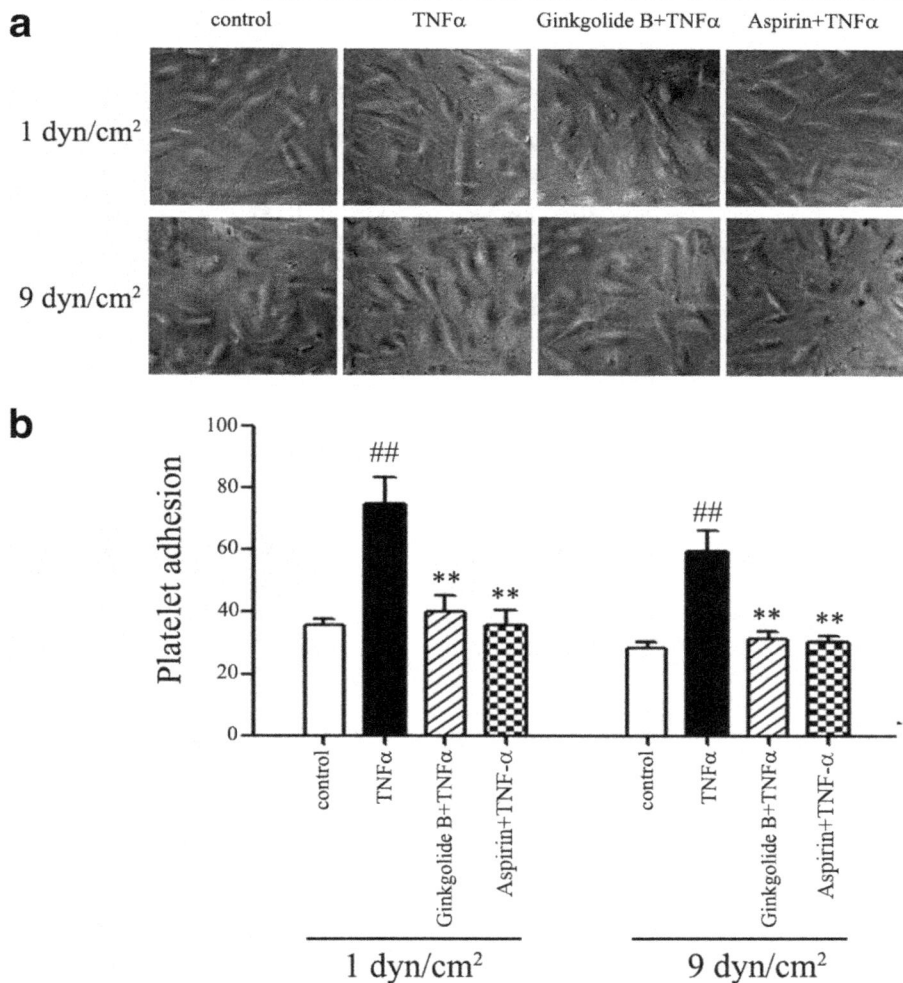

Fig. 1 Ginkgolide B reduced platelet adhesion in TNFα-treated HUVECs under different conditions of laminar shear stress. HUVECs were incubated with ginkgolide B (0.6 mg/ml) or aspirin (1 mM) for 12 h, and then TNFα (20 ng/ml) was added for another 2 h. The platelet suspension was then added to the input well under conditions of 1 and 9 dyn/cm^2 of laminar shear stress for 45 min. The data were obtained from three independent experiments. **a** Ginkgolide B decreased the number of platelets that adhered to TNFα-treated HUVECs at 1 and 9 dyn/cm^2. **b** Platelet adhesion to HUVECs. $^{\#\#}p < 0.01$, significant difference between TNFα-treated and -untreated HUVECs. $^{**}p < 0.01$, significant difference between TNFα-treated cells and ginkgolide B- and aspirin-treated cells

control group. Ginkgolide B (0.6 mg/ml) inhibited monocyte adhesion to TNFα-treated HUVECs. The number of monocytes that adhered was 17.0 ± 2.8 at 1 dyn/cm^2 and 15.7 ± 4.8 at 9 dyn/cm^2. In the aspirin-treated group, the number of monocytes that adhered was 20.7 ± 1.8 and 14.7 ± 5.4 at 1 and 9 dyn/cm^2, respectively. Significant differences were found between TNFα-treated cells and ginkgolide B- and aspirin-treated cells.

Ginkgolide B suppresses VCAM-1, VE-cadherin, and Cx43 expression in TNFα-treated HUVECs that present monocyte adhesion under conditions of laminar shear stress

We also evaluated the effects of ginkgolide B on adhesion proteins and tight junction proteins under conditions of laminar shear stress and monocyte adhesion in HUVECs. As shown in Fig. 4a-c, VCAM-1 expression increased by $29.8\% \pm 2.9\%$ at 1 dyn/cm^2 and by $48.6\% \pm 10.1\%$ at 9 dyn/cm^2 in TNFα-treated HUVECs. Ginkgolide B inhibited TNFα-induced VCAM-1 expression at both 1 and 9 dyn/cm^2. Similar results were found in aspirin-treated HUVECs.

TNFα treatment increased VE-cadherin expression by $36.9\% \pm 6.6$ and $28.2\% \pm 6.0\%$ at 1 and 9 dyn/cm^2, respectively. Ginkgolide B and aspirin reduced TNFα-induced VE-cadherin expression at 1 and 9 dyn/cm^2. Cx43 expression increased by $20.9\% \pm 7.1$ and $21.8\% \pm 5.4\%$ at 1 and 9 dyn/cm^2 in TNFα-treated HUVECs, respectively. Both ginkgolide B and aspirin completely suppressed TNFα-induced Cx43 expression at 1 and 9 dyn/cm^2.

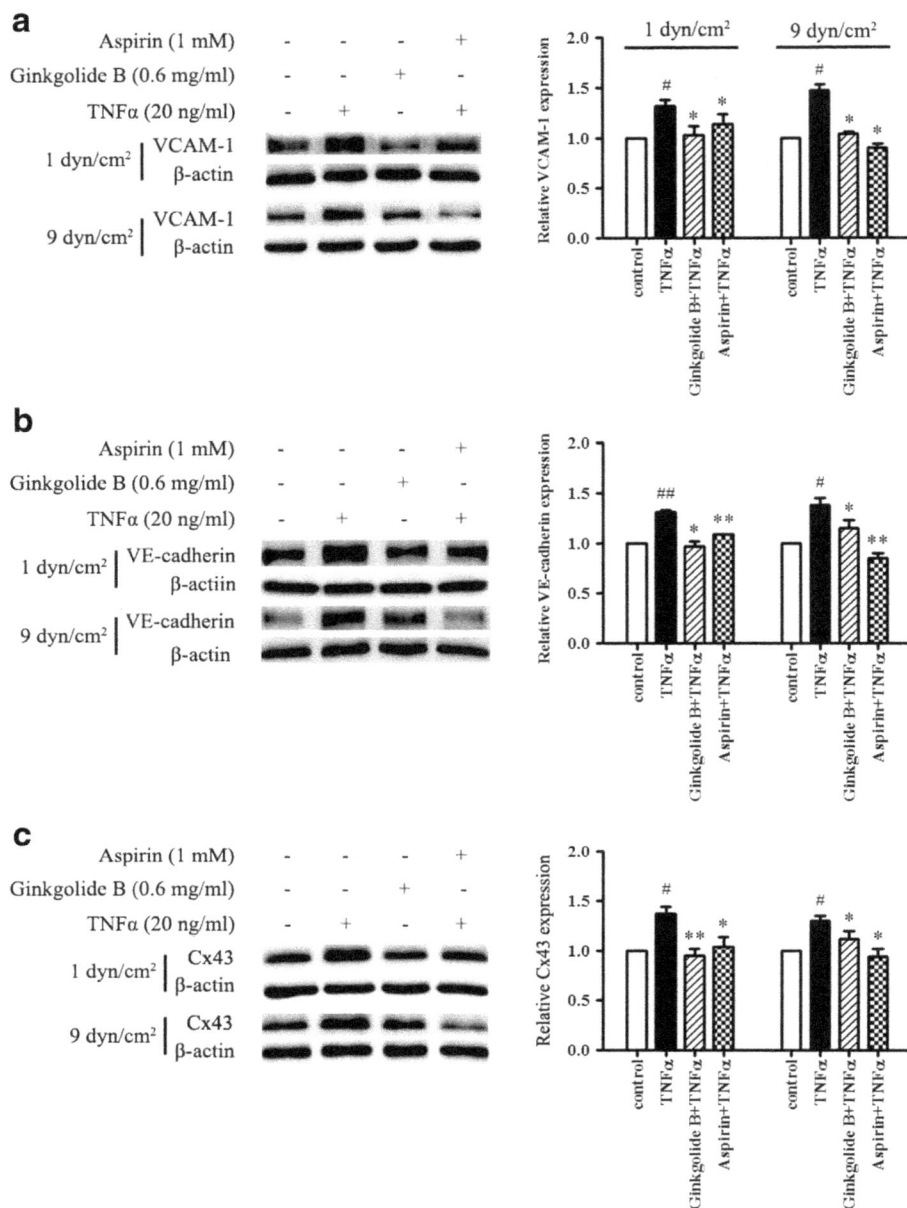

Fig. 2 Ginkgolide B suppressed VCAM-1, VE-cadherin, and Cx43 expression in TNFα-treated HUVECs that presented platelet adhesion under different conditions of laminar shear stress. HUVECs were incubated with ginkgolide B (0.6 mg/ml) or aspirin (1 mM) for 12 h, and then TNFα (20 ng/ml) was added for another 2 h. The platelet suspension was then added to the input well at 1 and 9 dyn/cm^2 of laminar shear stress for 45 min. Unadhered platelets were removed by the addition of PBS buffer for 2 min. Lysates were then collected by the addition of lysis buffer. Protein expression was analyzed by Western blot. The data were obtained from three independent experiments. **a** Ginkgolide B inhibited TNFα-induced VCAM-1 expression at 1 and 9 dyn/cm^2. **b** Ginkgolide B decreased TNFα-induced VE-cadherin expression at 1 and 9 dyn/cm^2. **c** Ginkgolide B reduced TNFα-induced Cx43 expression at 1 and 9 dyn/cm^2. $^\#p < 0.05$, significant difference between TNFα-treated and -untreated HUVECs. $^{**}p < 0.01$, significant difference between TNFα-treated cells and ginkgolide B- and aspirin-treated cells

Discussion

Platelets, monocytes, and endothelial cells interact in pathological states. Platelets release several inflammatory mediators, such as platelet factor 4 (PF4), regulated on activation, normal T-cell expressed and secreted chemokine (RANTES), P-selectin, and CD40 ligand, to recruit

monocytes to the site of damaged endothelial cells [26–28]. The adhesion of platelets through the expression of adhesion proteins can also elicit an inflammatory response in endothelial cells [29]. Monocyte adhesion to endothelial cells and enter intima where phagocytosis lipids and transform into macrophage and foam cells

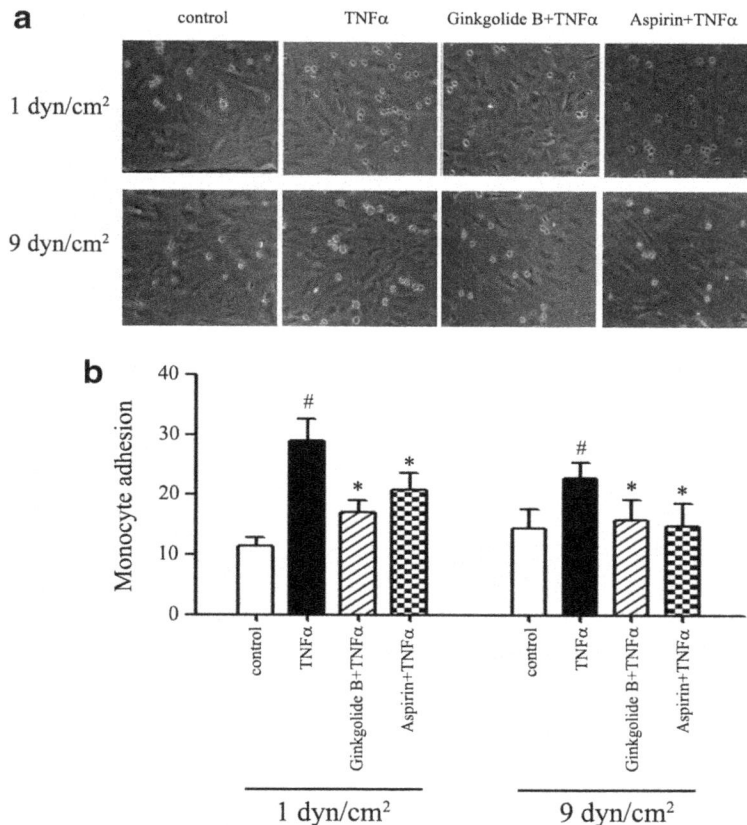

Fig. 3 Ginkgolide B reduced monocyte adhesion to TNFα-treated HUVECs under different conditions of laminar shear stress. HUVECs were incubated with ginkgolide B (0.6 mg/ml) or aspirin (1 mM) for 12 h, and then TNFα (20 ng/ml) was added for another 2 h. The monocyte suspension was then added to the input well at 1 and 9 dyn/cm² of laminar shear stress for 45 min. The data were obtained from three independent experiments. **a** Ginkgolide B reduced TNFα-induced monocyte adhesion to HUVECs at 1 and 9 dyn/cm². **b** Monocyte adhesion to HUVECs. #$p < 0.05$, significant difference between TNFα-treated and -untreated HUVECs. *$p < 0.01$, significant difference between TNFα-treated cells and ginkgolide B- and aspirin-treated cells

[30–32]. This process is involved in plaque formation in atherosclerosis. Therefore, the inhibition of platelet and monocyte adhesion to endothelial cells might be a strategy for preventing atherosclerosis.

In the present study, we used the Bioflux 1000 microfluidic device to investigate platelet and monocyte adhesion to endothelial cells under different conditions of laminar shear stress. High shear stress in the laminar flow promotes endothelial cell survival and anticoagulation. Low shear stress in the laminar flow promotes endothelial cell proliferation, apoptosis, and coagulation [33]. However, the precise mechanisms by which these processes occur are still unknown. To determine the effects of different conditions of shear stress on the interaction between platelets/monocytes and endothelial cells, two conditions of shear stress were used (1 and 9 dyn/cm²). Laminar shear stress at 1 dyn/cm² reflects a pathological state, and 9 dyn/cm² reflects a physiological state [34]. Areas of low shear stress in vessels may be linked to endothelial cell dysfunction, reflected by lower

nitric oxide and prostacyclin production. The present results showed that the number of platelets that adhered to HUVECs at 1 dyn/cm² was greater than the number that adhered at 9 dyn/cm². Monocyte adhesion presented a similar trend. The number of monocytes that adhered to HUVECs at 1 dyn/cm² was greater than the number that adhered at 9 dyn/cm². These results support the hypothesis that platelets and monocytes under conditions of low shear stress easily adhere to endothelial cells. We also observed phenotypic changes in endothelial cells under conditions of low and high shear stress. The expression of VCAM-1, VE-cadherin, and Cx43 was not different between 1 and 9 dyn/cm². This implies that 9 dyn/cm² of laminar shear stress does not impact TNFα-induced VCAM-1, VE-cadherin, or Cx43 expression. Both ginkgolide B and aspirin exerted protective actions against the expression of these proteins that was induced by TNFα under conditions of laminar shear stress. This is consistent with our previous study, in which increases in VE-cadherin and Cx43 expression

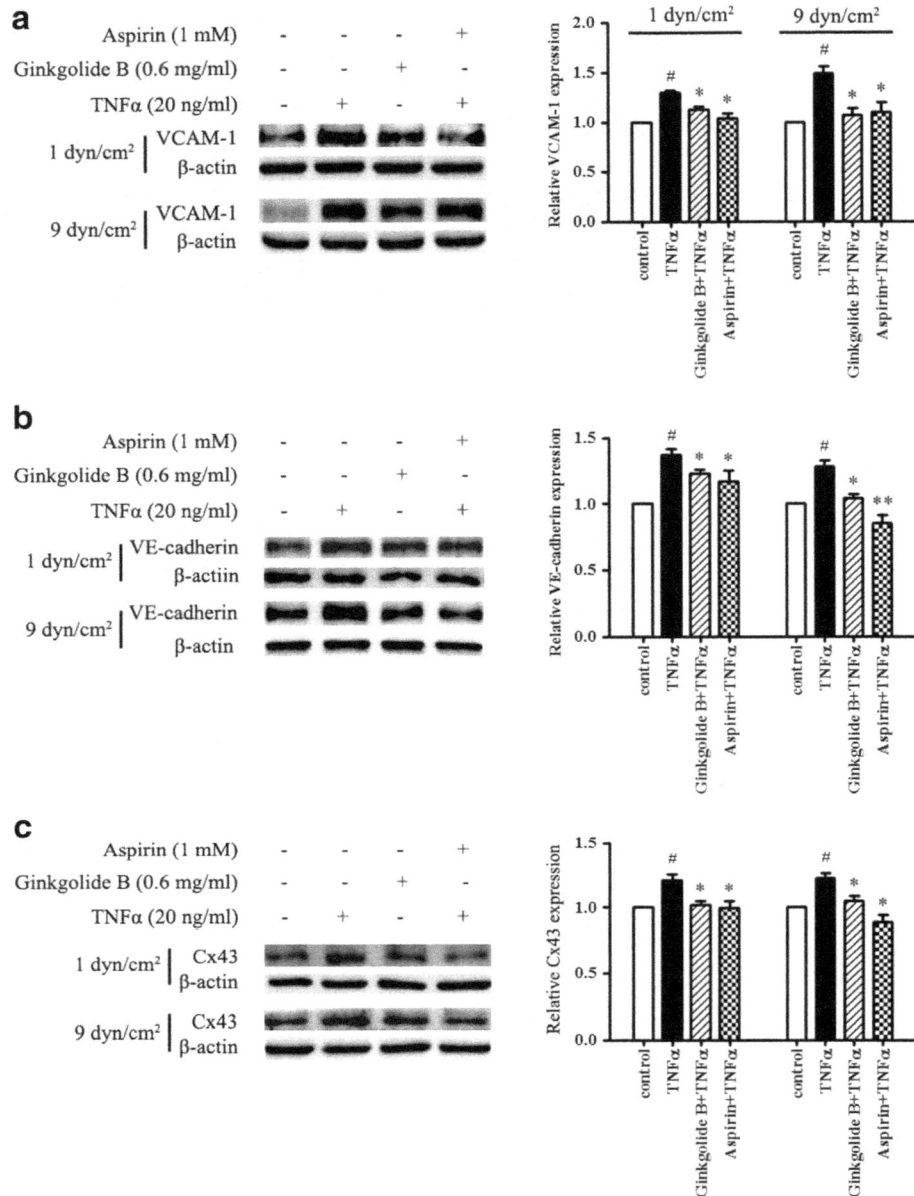

Fig. 4 Ginkgolide B suppressed VCAM-1, VE-cadherin, and Cx43 expression in TNFα-treated HUVECs that presented monocyte adhesion under different conditions of laminar shear stress. HUVECs were incubated with ginkgolide B (0.6 mg/ml) or aspirin (1 mM) for 12 h, and then TNFα (20 ng/ml) was added for another 2 h. The monocyte suspension was then added to the input well at 1 and 9 dyn/cm^2 of laminar shear stress for 45 min. Unadhered monocytes were removed by the addition of PBS buffer for 2 min. Lysates were then collected by the addition of lysis buffer. Protein expression was analyzed by Western blot. **a** Ginkgolide B inhibited TNFα-induced VCAM-1 expression at 1 and 9 dyn/cm^2. **b** Ginkgolide B decreased TNFα-induced VE-cadherin expression at 1 and 9 dyn/cm^2. **c** Ginkgolide B reduced TNFα-induced Cx43 expression at 1 and 9 dyn/cm^2. $^#p < 0.05$, significant difference between TNFα-treated and -untreated HUVECs. $^*p < 0.05$, $^{**}p < 0.01$, significant difference between TNFα-treated cells and ginkgolide B- and aspirin-treated cells

were linked to monocyte migration that was induced by ox-LDL. Furthermore, the knockdown of VE-cadherin and Cx43 gene expression by siRNA decreased the number of monocytes that migrated in ox-LDL-treated HUVECs [14]. This suggests VE-cadherin and Cx43 mediate monocyte migration, and this phenomenon might occur independently of their function at cell junctions. In the present study, platelet and monocyte adhesion decreased under conditions of high shear stress, but the underlying mechanism needs clarification.

Growing evidence has shown the protective action of ginkgolide B on cardiovascular and nervous system diseases. Our previous studies showed that ginkgolide B inhibited platelet aggregation and reduced CD40L, RANTES and PF4 secretion induced by thrombin and collagen. Moreover, ginkgolide B treatment decreased platelet adhesion on aortic plaque in Apo E gene defective mice [20]. Recent a study reported that ginkgolide B promoted microglia/macrophage transferring from inflammatory M1 phenotype to anti-inflammatory phenotype M2 in vivo and in vitro [35]. In recent years *Ginkgo biloba* extracts have been widely used as a phytomedicine in Europe and in the United States. These studies demonstrated that ginkgolide B might be a promising drug in clinic application.

Conclusion

In conclusion, we found that platelet and monocyte adhesion was stronger under conditions of 1 dyn/cm^2 of laminar shear stress compared with 9 dyn/cm^2. Ginkgolide B inhibited TNFα-induced platelet and monocyte adhesion to endothelial cells and attenuated VCAM-1, VE-cadherin, and Cx43 expression under conditions of laminar shear stress. No differences in the expression of these proteins were found between 1 and 9 dyn/cm^2. These findings suggest that ginkgolide B might shed light on the treatment of inflammation in atherosclerosis.

Acknowledgements
We thank Dr. Yun You and Dr. Fulong Liao provides Bioflux 1000 facility for the present study. We would like to thank all the participants in the present study. We also thank the funding NSFC for the financial support.

Funding
This study was funded by National Natural Science Foundation of China (NSFC) (grant numbers 80471051, 81270379, 81070231, and 91649110). The funding agency had no role in the design of the study; in the collection, analyses, or interpretation of data; in the writing of the manuscript; or in the decision to publish the results.

Authors' contributions
Conceived and designed the experiments: RMQ and YY. Performed the experiments: JS, MZ, YYZ, BDC, and HG. Analyzed the data: MZ and JS. Wrote the paper: RMQ. All author reviewed and approved the manuscript.

Competing interests
The authors declare that they have no competing interests.

Author details
[1]MOH Key Laboratory of Geriatrics, Beijing Hospital, National Center of Gerontology, Beijing, China. [2]Graduate School of Peking Union Medical College, Chinese Academy of Medical Sciences, Beijing, China. [3]Institute of Chinese Materia Medica, China Academy of Chinese Medical Sciences, Beijing, China.

References
1. Nakajima H, Yamamoto K, Agarwala S, Terai K, Fukui H, Fukuhara S, et al. Flow-dependent endothelial YAP regulation contributes to vessel maintenance. Dev Cell 2017;40:523–536.
2. Urschel K, Garlichs CD, Daniel WG, Cicha I. VEGFR2 signalling contributes to increased endothelial susceptibility to TNF-alpha under chronic non-uniform shear stress. Atherosclerosis. 2011;219:499–509.
3. Johnson BD, Mather KJ, Wallace JP. Mechanotransduction of shear in the endothelium: basic studies and clinical implications. Vasc Med. 2011;16:365–77.
4. Paszkowiak JJ, Dardik A. Arterial wall shear stress: observations from the bench to the bedside. Vasc Endovasc Surg. 2003;37:47–57.
5. Schuler D, Sansone R, Freudenberger T, Rodriguez-Mateos A, Weber G, Momma TY, et al. Measurement of endothelium-dependent vasodilation in mice–brief report. Arterioscler Thromb Vasc Biol. 2014;34:2651–2657.
6. Inaba H, Takeshita K, Uchida Y, Hayashi M, Okumura T, Hirashiki A, et al. Recovery of flow-mediated vasodilatation after repetitive measurements is involved in early vascular impairment: comparison with indices of vascular tone. PLoS One 2014;9:e83977.
7. Verbeke FH, Pannier B, Guérin AP, Boutouyrie P, Laurent S, London GM. Flow-mediated vasodilation in end-stage renal disease. Clin J Am Soc Nephrol. 2011;6:2009–15.
8. Okorie UM, Denney WS, Chatterjee MS, Neeves KB, Diamond SL. Determination of surface tissue factor thresholds that trigger coagulation at venous and arterial shear rates: amplification of 100 fM circulating tissue factor requires flow. Blood. 2008;111:3507–13.
9. Ahmadsei M, Lievens D, Weber C, Von HP, Gerdes N. Immune-mediated and lipid-mediated platelet function in atherosclerosis. Curr Opin Lipidol. 2015; 26:438–48.
10. Soehnlein O. Monocytes chat with atherosclerotic lesions. Arterioscler Thromb Vasc Biol. 2016;36:1720–1.
11. Badimon L, Suades R, Fuentes E, Palomo I, Padró T. Role of platelet-derived microvesicles as crosstalk mediators in Atherothrombosis and future pharmacology targets: a link between inflammation, atherosclerosis, and thrombosis. Front Pharmacol. 2016;7:293.
12. Gavard J. Endothelial permeability and VE-cadherin: a wacky comradeship. Cell Adhes Migr. 2013;7:455–61.
13. Corada M, Liao F, Lindgren M, Lampugnani MG, Breviario F, Frank R, et al. Monoclonal antibodies directed to different regions of vascular endothelial cadherin extracellular domain affect adhesion and clustering of the protein and modulate endothelial permeability. Blood 2001;97:1679–1684.
14. Liu X, Sun W, Zhao Y, Chen B, Wu W, Li B, et al. Ginkgolide B inhibits JAM-A, Cx43, and VE-cadherin expression and reduces monocyte transmigration in oxidized LDL-stimulated human umbilical vein endothelial cells. Oxidative Med Cell Longev 2015;2015:907926.
15. Cheng JC, Chang HM, Fang L, Sun YP, Leung PC. TGF-β1 up-regulates connexin43 expression: a potential mechanism for human trophoblast cell differentiation. J Cell Physiol. 2015;230:1558–66.
16. Laird DW. Syndromic and non-syndromic disease-linked Cx43 mutations. FEBS Lett. 2014;588:1339–48.
17. Ghosh S, Kumar A, Chandna S. Connexin-43 downregulation in G2/M phase enriched tumour cells causes extensive low-dose hyper-radiosensitivity (HRS) associated with mitochondrial apoptotic events. Cancer Lett. 2015;363:46–59.
18. Chin-Feng H, Hsia-Fen H, Wei-Kung T, Thung-Lip L, Yu-Feng W, Kwan-Lih H, et al. Glossogyne tenuifolia extract inhibits TNF-α-induced expression of adhesion molecules in human umbilical vein endothelial cells via blocking the NF-kB signaling pathway. Molecules 2015;20:16908–16923.
19. Hu L, Chen Z, Xie Y, Jiang Y, Zhen H. New products from alkali fusion of Ginkgolides a and B. J Asian Nat Prod Res. 2000;2:103–10.
20. Liu X, Zhao G, Yan Y, Bao L, Chen B, Qi R. Ginkgolide B reduces atherogenesis and vascular inflammation in ApoE(−/−) mice. PLoS One. 2012;7:e36237.
21. Zhang S, Chen B, Wu W, Bao L, Qi R. Ginkgolide B reduces inflammatory protein expression in oxidized low-density lipoprotein-stimulated human vascular endothelial cells. J Cardiovasc Pharmacol. 2011;57:721–7.
22. Reiss C, Mindukshev I, Bischoff V, Subramanian H, Kehrer L, Friebe A, et al. The sGC stimulator riociguat inhibits platelet function in washed platelets but not in whole blood. Br J Pharmacol 2015; 172:5199–5210.
23. Scipione CA, Sayegh SE, Romagnuolo R, Tsimikas S, Marcovina SM, Boffa MB, et al. Mechanistic insights into Lp(a)-induced IL-8 expression: a role for oxidized phospholipid modification of apo(a). J Lipid Res 2015;56:2273–2285.
24. Qin WD, Mi SH, Li C, Wang GX, Zhang JN, Wang H, et al. Low shear stress induced HMGB1 translocation and release via PECAM-1/PARP-1 pathway to induce inflammation response. PLoS One 2015;10:e0120586.
25. Sato M, Levesque MJ, Nerem RM. Micropipette aspiration of cultured bovine aortic endothelial cells exposed to shear stress. Arteriosclerosis. 1987;7:276–86.

26. Woller G, Brandt E, Mittelstädt J, Rybakowski C, Petersen F. Platelet factor 4/CXCL4-stimulated human monocytes induce apoptosis in endothelial cells by the release of oxygen radicals. J Leukoc Biol. 2008;83:936–45.

27. Von HP, Weber KS, Huo Y, Proudfoot AE, Nelson PJ, Ley K, et al. RANTES deposition by platelets triggers monocyte arrest on inflamed and atherosclerotic endothelium. Circulation 2001;103:1772–1777.

28. Lievens D, Zernecke A, Seijkens T, Soehnlein O, Beckers L, Munnix IC, et al. Platelet CD40L mediates thrombotic and inflammatory processes in atherosclerosis. Blood 2010;116:4317–4327.

29. Blann AD, Nadar SK, Lip GY. The adhesion molecule P-selectin and cardiovascular disease. Eur Heart J. 2003;24:2166–79.

30. Hilgendorf I, Swirski FK, Robbins CS. Monocyte fate in atherosclerosis. Arterioscler Thromb Vasc Biol. 2015;35:272–9.

31. Plotkin JD, Elias MG, Dellinger AL, Kepley CL. NF-κB inhibitors that prevent foam cell formation and atherosclerotic plaque accumulation. Nanomedicine. 2017;13:2037–48.

32. Fong GH. Potential contributions of intimal and plaque hypoxia to atherosclerosis. Curr Atheroscler Rep. 2015;17:1–10.

33. Cunningham KS, Gotlieb AI. The role of shear stress in the pathogenesis of atherosclerosis. Lab Investig. 2005;85:9–23.

34. Stepp DW, Nishikawa Y, Chilian WM. Regulation of shear stress in the canine coronary microcirculation. Circulation. 1999;100:1555–61.

35. Shu ZM, Shu XD, Li HQ, Sun Y, Shan H, Sun XY, et al: Ginkgolide B protects against ischemic stroke via modulating microglia polarization in mice. CNS Neurosci Ther 2016;22:729–739.

5

Sotetsuflavone inhibits proliferation and induces apoptosis of A549 cells through ROS-mediated mitochondrial-dependent pathway

Shaohui Wang[1] ⓘ, Yanlan Hu[1], Yu Yan[1], Zhekang Cheng[1] and Tongxiang Liu[2]*

Abstract

Background: Sotetsuflavone is isolated from *Cycas revoluta* Thunb., which has biological activity against tumors. However, the anti-proliferative effects of sotetsuflavone on A549 cells and its mechanism are not fully elucidated.

Methods: This study investigated the mechanisms of growth inhibition, cell cycle arrest and apoptosis in non-small cell lung cancer A549 cells induced by sotetsuflavone and evaluated whether sotetsuflavone can be safely utilized by humans as therapeutic agent.

Results: We found that sotetsuflavone had significant antiproliferative activity against A549 cells. At the same time, the reactive oxygen species (ROS) content increased while the mitochondrial membrane potential and the ratio of Bcl-2/Bax decreased. Cleaved caspase-3, cleaved caspase-9, cytochrome C and Bax expression increased, and Cyclin D1, CDK4, cleaved caspase-8 and Bcl-2 expression decreased. Interestingly, we demonstrated that sotetsuflavone could effectively inhibit the G0/G1 cycle progression, and then induce the endogenous apoptosis pathway. Our results show that sotetsuflavone could inhibit the growth of A549 cells by up-regulating intracellular ROS levels and causing the mitochondrial membrane potential to collapse, inducing G0/G1 phase arrest and endogenous apoptosis.

Conclusions: In short, we confirm that sotetsuflavone had an inhibitory effect on A549 cells and discovered that it causes apoptosis of A549 lung cancer cells. Sotetsuflavone may be used as a novel candidate for anti-tumor therapy in patients with lung cancer.

Keywords: Sotetsuflavone, Reactive oxygen species (ROS), Apoptosis, Mitochondria-dependent pathway, Cycle arrest

Background

Lung cancer, also known as Primary Bronchogenic Carcinoma, is a serious threat to human health and quality of life, ranking first among malignant tumors in morbidity and mortality [1–3]. The morbidity and mortality of lung cancer all over the world has increased rapidly within the last 10 years, and more significantly in developed countries [4]. The cancers are mainly divided into small cell lung cancer (SCLC) and non-small cell lung cancer (NSCLC), and NSCLC accounts for 80–85% [5]. The main counter measures are chemotherapy and radiotherapy, targeted therapy, and immune therapy. Although the existing methods of chemotherapy based on Cisplatin can have some effect, the five years survival rate of lung cancer patients is still only about 17%, while it causes a serious economic burden to the patients [6].

Apoptosis or programmed cell death is important for the stability and growth of cells, as well as is controlled at molecular level [7]. It is associated with several diseases, especially cancer [8]. Many anticancer agents mediate their effects on apoptosis induction [9]. Apoptosis is an active and highly ordered process involving a series of enzymes involved in gene regulation. There are three

---

* Correspondence: tongxliu123@hotmail.com
[2]School of Pharmacy, Minzu University of China, Key Laboratory of Ethnomedicine (Minzu University of China), Minority of Education, No. 27 Zhongguancun South Street, Haidian District, Beijing 100081, China
Full list of author information is available at the end of the article

apoptosis signaling pathways: the mitochondrial pathway, the death receptor pathway and the endoplasmic reticulum pathway, in which the mitochondrial pathway is the major one [10]. Mitochondria release cytochrome c and apoptosis inducing factors, thereby activating downstream apoptotic executors [11]. The mitochondrial apoptosis signaling pathway is regulated by the Bcl-2 protein family [11]. The protein family is divided according to different functions, including the inhibitory subfamily (such as Bcl-2, Bcl-x etc.) and the promoter subfamily (such as Bax, Bak, Bad, Bid). The anti-apoptotic members of the Bcl-2 family are usually up-regulated, while pro-apoptotic members are down-regulated in many cancers [12]. The cysteinyl aspartate specific proteinase family (Caspases) is an important factor in the molecular mechanism of apoptosis and occupies a central role in the process of apoptosis, and its members are directly involved in apoptosis initiation, signal transduction and apoptosis. Among them, cysteinyl aspartate specific proteinase-3 (Caspase-3) is the most critical protease in the apoptosis pathway. Activated Caspase-3 can initiate a Caspase cascade, inducing apoptosis after important protein degradation in cells, caspase 8 is a key factor in the death receptor pathway, and caspase 9 is an important factor in mitochondrial pathway [13]. The cell cycle is precisely ordered and regulated with cyclin and cyclin-dependent kinase (CDK) as key elements [14]. Cyclin D1 is an important cell cycle regulatory protein. By combining with cyclin-dependent kinase 4 (CDK 4), phosphorylation and the deactivation of retinoblastoma protein (pRb), it plays an important role in the G1 to S transition in the cell cycle progression [15]. Reactive oxygen species (ROS) play a key role in cell growth in many cellular signaling pathways [16]. Increased ROS in cancer cells is associated with a variety of changes in cell function, such as cell proliferation, migration, differentiation and apoptosis [8].

Cycas revolute Thunb. is an evergreen palm woody plant with ornamental, medicinal and edible value. Its main components are double flavonoid compounds, amino acids and sugars. Ancient records report that it is sweet, flat, astringent, and slightly toxic, with fever-reducing and coagulant abilities, dispersing congestion [17]. We first studied the activity of total flavonoids from *Cycas revolute* Thunb. in vivo, and found it can regulate the expression of interleukin-2 and interleukin-10 in immune cells and inhibit the growth and metastasis of tumor cells in lewis lung cancer model mice [18]. To tap its medicinal and edible value, and ensure its safety, we isolated the chemical constituents from *Cycas revolute* Thunb. and carried out anti-tumor activity screening. Sotetsuflavone had the strongest inhibitory effect on A549 cells. Thus, in order to clarify the effect of Sotetsuflavone on A549 cells, we studied its potential molecular mechanism, and evaluated whether Sotetsuflavone can be safely utilized by humans as therapeutic agent.

Methods

Plant material, chemicals, reagents, and antibodies

Sotetsuflavone was isolated from *Cycas Revolute* Thunb. in our laboratory (purity: > 98%, HPLC) (Fig. 1d). The isolation of sotetsuflavone was done using the protocol described by Zhouyan et al. [19]. The leaf of *Cycas Revolute* Thunb. was collected from AnGuo herbal medicine market in HeBei Province of China in May 2015, and was identified by Prof. Tong-Xiang Liu at Minzu University of China. A voucher specimen (No. GRT2015–05) was deposited in the 404 laboratory of Pharmaceutical Research Institute, School of Pharmacy, Minzu University of China, Beijing, China. A549 cells (AS6011), 3-(4,5-Dimethylthiazol-2-yl)-2,5-diphenyltetrazoliunbromide (MTT) assay kit (AS1035), crystalline violet dye (AS1086), Hoechst dye (AS1041) were purchased from Wuhan Aspen Biotechnology Co., Ltd. (Wuhan, China). Dulbecco's modified eagle medium (DMEM) high glucose medium (SH30022) was purchased from HyClone. (Los Angeles, USA). Cell cycle detection kit (CY2001-O), Annexin-FITC cell apoptosis detection kit (AO2001-02P-G), N-acetyl-L-cysteine (NAC) were obtained from Tianjin three arrows Biotechnology Co., Ltd. (Tianjin, China). JC-1 test kit (C2006), ROS active oxygen kit (S0033), anti-bodies against Cyclin D1, CDK4, Caspase-3, Caspase-9, Caspase-8, cytochrome C, Bcl-2, Bax, and GAPDH were purchased from Beyotime Biotechnology Co., Ltd. (Shanghai, China). DR-200Bs ELISA detection microplate reader was purchased from Wuxi Hiwell Diatek Instruments Co., Ltd. (Wuxi, China). MicroPublisher imaging system (QImaging) was purchased from Shanghai puch Biotechnology Co. Ltd. (Shanghai, China). FACScalibur flow cytometry was obtained from Medical devices Co., Ltd. (BD). (Shanghai, China). CX-21 Ordinary Optical Microscope was purchased from OLYMPUS. (Shanghai, China). All other chemicals made in China were of analytical grade.

Cell culture

In our previous experiments, we found that sotetsuflavone had a significant growth inhibiting effect on human lung cancer cells (A549) (IC_{50} = 71.12 μmol / L), human colon adenocarcinoma cells (Caco-2) (IC_{50} = 79.70 μmol / L), Human esophageal cancer cells (EC-109) (IC_{50} = 76.68 μmol / L), Human prostate cancer cells (PC-3)(IC_{50} = 106.31 μmol / L) and human hepatoma cells (HepG2) (IC_{50} = 87.14 μmol / L). A549 cells were much more sensitive than the other cell lines. Moreover, sotetsuflavone showed better anti-proliferative activity on A549 than CDDP (Cisplatin) [20]. Based on this results, we used A549 cells to continue the follow-up experiments. A549 cells were cultured in dulbecco's modified eagle medium (DMEM) medium containing 10% fetal bovine serum, penicillin and streptomycin 100 U/ml, and cultured under

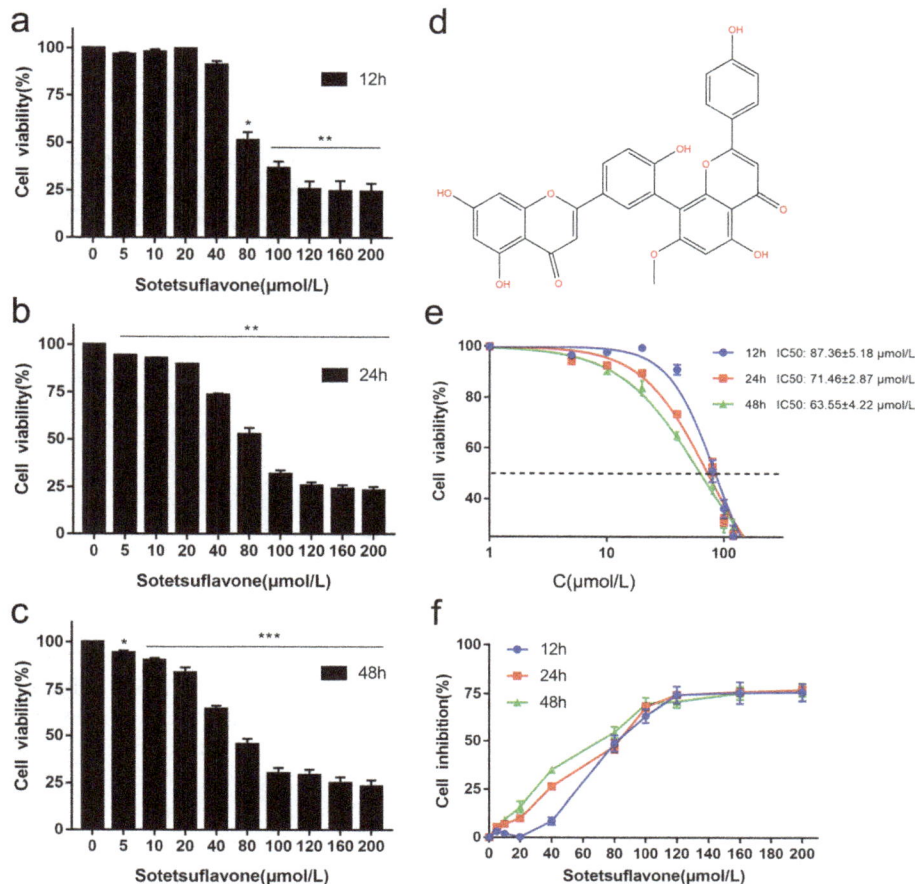

Fig. 1 Effects of sotetsuflavone on A549 cells survival. **a**, **b**, **c** show changes of cell viability of A549 cells treated with different concentrations of sotetsuflavone for 12 h, 24 h and 48 h respectively. The viability of A549 cells were significantly different after 12 h, 24 h and 48 h compared with that of control groups ($P < 0.05$, ** $P < 0.01$, *** $P < 0.001$). **d** Molecular structure of sotetsuflavone. **e** The cytotoxicity of sotetsuflavone in A549 cells, there was no significant difference in IC50 values between 24 h and 48 h after drug treatment ($P > 0.05$). **f** The inhibition rate of sotetsuflavone at 12, 24 and 48 h. When the drug concentration was more than 80 µmol/L, the inhibitory effect of the three times gradients was not different ($P > 0.05$). Combined with Fig. 1a, b, c, e, f, the final selection of 24 h as the follow-up experimental treatment time, and the subsequent experimental concentration adjusted to 0, 64, 128 µmol/L. The results from three independent experiments were expressed as mean ± SD compared with the control group, *$P < 0.01$, **$P < 0.01$, ***$P < 0.001$

constant temperature at 37 °C and 5%CO_2. Cells were taken during the logarithmic growth phase.

MTT assay

A549 cells from the logarithmic growth phase were adjusted to 5×10^4 cells/mL, seeded in 96 well plates, 100 µL/well, incubated for 24 h in adherent cells change medium, adding 100 µL in DMEM culture medium with varying concentrations of Sotetsuflavone (0(control), 5, 10, 20, 40, 80, 100, 120, 160, 200 µmol/L). After incubation for 12 h, 24 h, and 48 h, 20 µl of 5 mg/mL MTT working fluid was added to all wells and incubated for 4 h. The supernatant was carefully removed and replaced with 200 µL of dimethyl sulfoxide per well. Plate was then placed on a micro-vibrator for 10 min, and the absorbance at 490 nm was measured [8].

Cell apoptosis analysis

A549 cells were treated with 0 µmol/L(control), 64 µmol/L, 128 µmol/L sotetsuflavone for 24 h, washed once with precooled PBS and resuspended in 300 µl of a binding buffer diluted with phosphate-buffered saline (PBS). 5 µL Annexin V-FITC was added after incubation for 10 min, then 5 µL PI was added and mixed well, and then incubated for 5 min, detected within one hour by flow cytometry [9].

Cell cycle analysis

The same method was used to collect A549 cells, washed twice with pre-cooled PBS, and then 70% pre-cooled ethanol was added slowly, gently blowed and resuspended overnight at 4 °C. The cells were collected again before the test, washed twice with pre-cooled PBS, and 500 μL RNase / PI added to resuspend and stained the cells for 20 min, detected within one hour by flow cytometry [14].

Hoechst 33,258 staining

The cells in the six-well plate were treated as described in the part of cell apoptosis analysis experiment. The cells were washed three times with pre-cooled PBS and then fixed with 4% paraformaldehyde for 30 min, the appropriate amount of Hoechst was added dropwise to the plate after washing with PBS for three times and incubated at room temperature for 15 min, PBS washed three times, then, observed under a fluorescence microscope and photographed [21].

ROS detection

The cells in in the six-well plate were treated as described in the part of cell apoptosis analysis experiment, collected the cells and added 10 μM DCFH-DA working solution diluted with serum-free liquid. Cells were incubated at 37 °C for 30 min. Reversed the mixture every 3–5 min so that the probe and the cells were in full contact. The cells were subsequently washed 1 to 2 times with serum-free cell culture medium and detected by Flow Cytometry [8].

Mitochondrial membrane potential detection

The cells in the six-well plate were treated as described above. Cells were collected in 0.5 ml DMEM, and 0.5 mL of JC-1 staining solution was added. The solution was mixed several times and incubated at 37 °C for 20 min. After incubation, cells were centrifuged 5 min, and the supernatant was discarded. The pellet was washed with JC-1 staining buffer (1×) two times, then cells were resuspended in 0.5 mL JC-1 staining buffer (1×) and detected by flow cytometry analysis [9].

Western blot assay

After the cells were treated with each concentration (0(control), 64, 128 μmol/L), the total protein was extracted with RIPA lysis buffer. The protein samples were subjected to SDS-PAGE and then transferred onto the PVDF membrane. The cells were blocked with Tris-buffered saline tween (TBST) solution containing 5% skimmed milk powder for 1 h. Then the membranes were incubated with primary antibodies of cleaved Caspase-3, cleaved Caspase-9, cleaved Caspase-8, cytochrome C, Bax, Bcl-2, Cyclin D1 and CDK 4 at 4 °C overnight. The membranes were washed with TBST buffer three times and then incubated with a horse radish peroxidase coupled secondary antibodies. Subsequently, the membranes were washed with TBST buffer three times again, and finally detected by the chemiluminescent

substrate system and the results were analyzed with the AlphaEase FC software [20].

Statistical analysis

The experimental data were processed by SPSS 20.0 statistical software. All experiments were repeated at least three times. The measurement data were expressed as mean ± standard deviation (SD). A one-way ANOVA was used to analyze the variance, when the variance was homogeneous, with a Least Significant Difference, Student-Newman-Keuls test. Conversely, we used the Dunnett T3 test when the variance was not uniform. Differences were considered statistically significant for *$P<0.05$,**$P<0.01$,***$P<0.001$.

Results

Growth inhibition of A549 cells by sotetsuflavone

A549 cells treated with 0(control), 5, 10, 20, 40, 80, 100, 120, 160, and 200 μmol/L sotetsuflavone for 12, 24 and 48 h, MTT assay showed a time and dose-dependent inhibition of the growth of A549 cells (Fig. 1a, b, c, f). The IC_{50} values were (87.36 ± 5.18) μmol / L, (71.46 ± 2.87) μmol / L, (63.55 ± 4.22) μmol / L, respectively (Fig. 1e).

Sotetsuflavone induces apoptosis of A549 cells

Annexin V-FITC and PI double staining was performed to determine the apoptosis in A549 cells. Untreated cells were primarily Annexin V-FITC and PI-negative, indicating that they were viable and not undergoing apoptosis. After treatment with different concentrations of sotetsuflavone (0 μmol/L(control), 64 μmol/L, 128 μmol/L), intense FITC green in the membrane and PI red in the nucleus were observed (Fig. 2a). Sotetsuflavone induced and accelerated apoptosis of A549 cells, with the increase in drug concentration (Fig. 2b, c). Hoechst 33,258 is a dye that stains the nucleus, which can reflect the number of apoptotic cells, and the even distribution of chromatin, the nuclear-stained uniform blue cells are considered normal but when the nucleus was condensed and fragmented bright blue cells were counted as apoptotic cells. The results of the Hoechst 33,258 staining showed that the A549 cells gradually increased with the increase in of concentration of sotetsuflavone (0 μmol/L(control), 64 μmol/L, 128 μmol/L) (Fig. 3b). And the apoptosis rate increased with increasing drug concentration. We also found that the apoptotic rate of A549 cells is inconsistent with the results of cell viability assay, and this probably because sotetsuflavone promote cell death, not only by inducing cell apoptosis, but also by other types of cell death, such as autophagy. Etc. which requires further research.

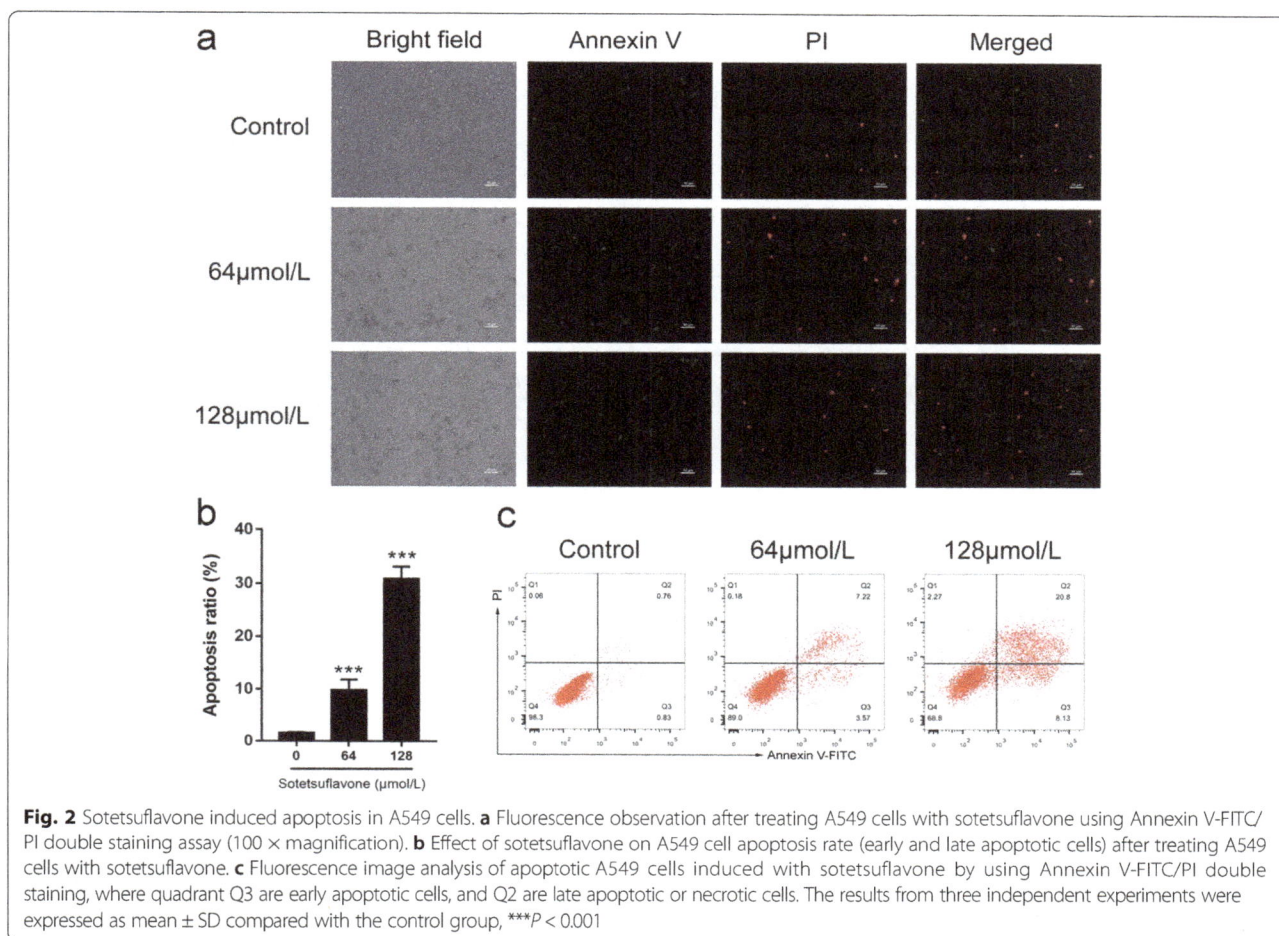

Fig. 2 Sotetsuflavone induced apoptosis in A549 cells. **a** Fluorescence observation after treating A549 cells with sotetsuflavone using Annexin V-FITC/PI double staining assay (100 × magnification). **b** Effect of sotetsuflavone on A549 cell apoptosis rate (early and late apoptotic cells) after treating A549 cells with sotetsuflavone. **c** Fluorescence image analysis of apoptotic A549 cells induced with sotetsuflavone by using Annexin V-FITC/PI double staining, where quadrant Q3 are early apoptotic cells, and Q2 are late apoptotic or necrotic cells. The results from three independent experiments were expressed as mean ± SD compared with the control group, ***$P < 0.001$

Sotetsuflavone on A549 cell cycle arrest in the G0 / G1 phase

After 24 h, with increasing concentrations of sotetsuflavone (0 μmol/L(control), 64 μmol/L, 128 μmol/L), A549 cells cycle arrest in G0/G1 phase gradually increased (Fig. 3a, c): (55.28 ± 0.94)%,(57.10 ± 2.56)%, and(83.53 ± 3.24)%.

Sotetsuflavone increases the ROS expression in A549 cells

Reactive oxygen species as an inevitable product of cell metabolism, can play an anti-tumor role by promoting a variety of signaling pathways, such as cell apoptosis, cell necrosis and autophagic cell death. Increased ROS levels can activate ROS-mediated signaling pathways, then causing changes in cell cycle-associated protein levels. The DCFH-DA probe can be hydrolyzed by esterase to form DCFH across the cell membrane, and the reactive oxygen species in the cell can convert the non-fluorescent DCFH into a fluorescent DCF.

The intracellular reactive oxygen species can convert non-fluorescent DCFH into fluorescent DCF [22]. Therefore, the fluorescence intensity of DCF can reflect the level of ROS [23]. It was found that the control group had no green fluorescence and the ROS level was low in the control group, but higher in the treated groups.

With increasing drug concentration, the ROS levels in A549 cells increased gradually (Fig. 4a, b, c). The premise of oxidative stress-induced cell apoptosis is the imbalance between oxidation and oxidation resistance in cells. Therefore, we added antioxidant NAC in the experiment. By comparing the changes of each index before and after using NAC, we found that the activity of A549 cells and the number of apoptotic cells were decreased significantly (Fig. 4d, e, f). it was further explained that sotetsuflavone induced apoptosis of A549 cells through the ROS mediated mitochondrial pathway.

Sotetsuflavone reduces mitochondrial membrane potential of A549 cells

After cells are damaged, the membrane potential drops, and JC-1 will appear in the form of green fluorescence. Mitochondrial membrane potential (mitochondrial membrane potential, MMP) collapse is one of the signs of early cell apoptosis. We found that with the increase of sotetsuflavone (0 μmol/L(control), 64 μmol/L, 128 μmol/L), the green fluorescence gradually increased and the mitochondrial membrane potential decreased (Fig. 5a). Consistent with this, flow cytometry results showed that the

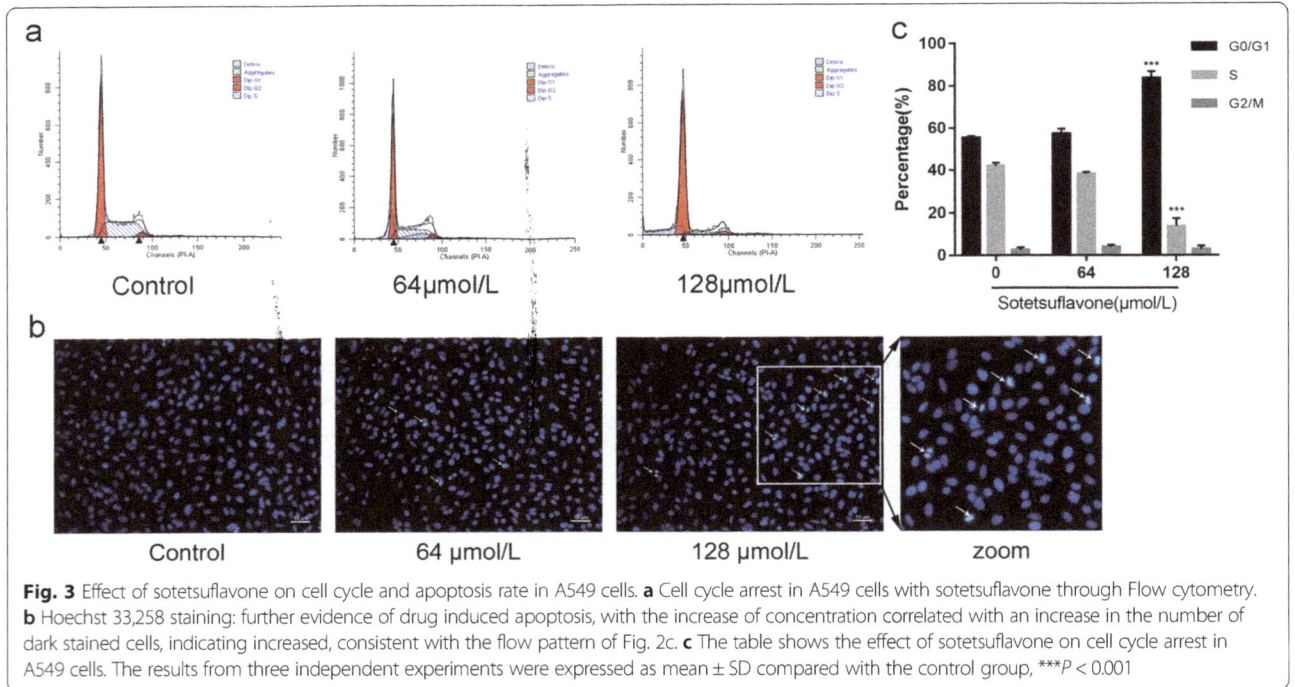

Fig. 3 Effect of sotetsuflavone on cell cycle and apoptosis rate in A549 cells. **a** Cell cycle arrest in A549 cells with sotetsuflavone through Flow cytometry. **b** Hoechst 33,258 staining: further evidence of drug induced apoptosis, with the increase of concentration correlated with an increase in the number of dark stained cells, indicating increased, consistent with the flow pattern of Fig. 2c. **c** The table shows the effect of sotetsuflavone on cell cycle arrest in A549 cells. The results from three independent experiments were expressed as mean ± SD compared with the control group, ***$P < 0.001$

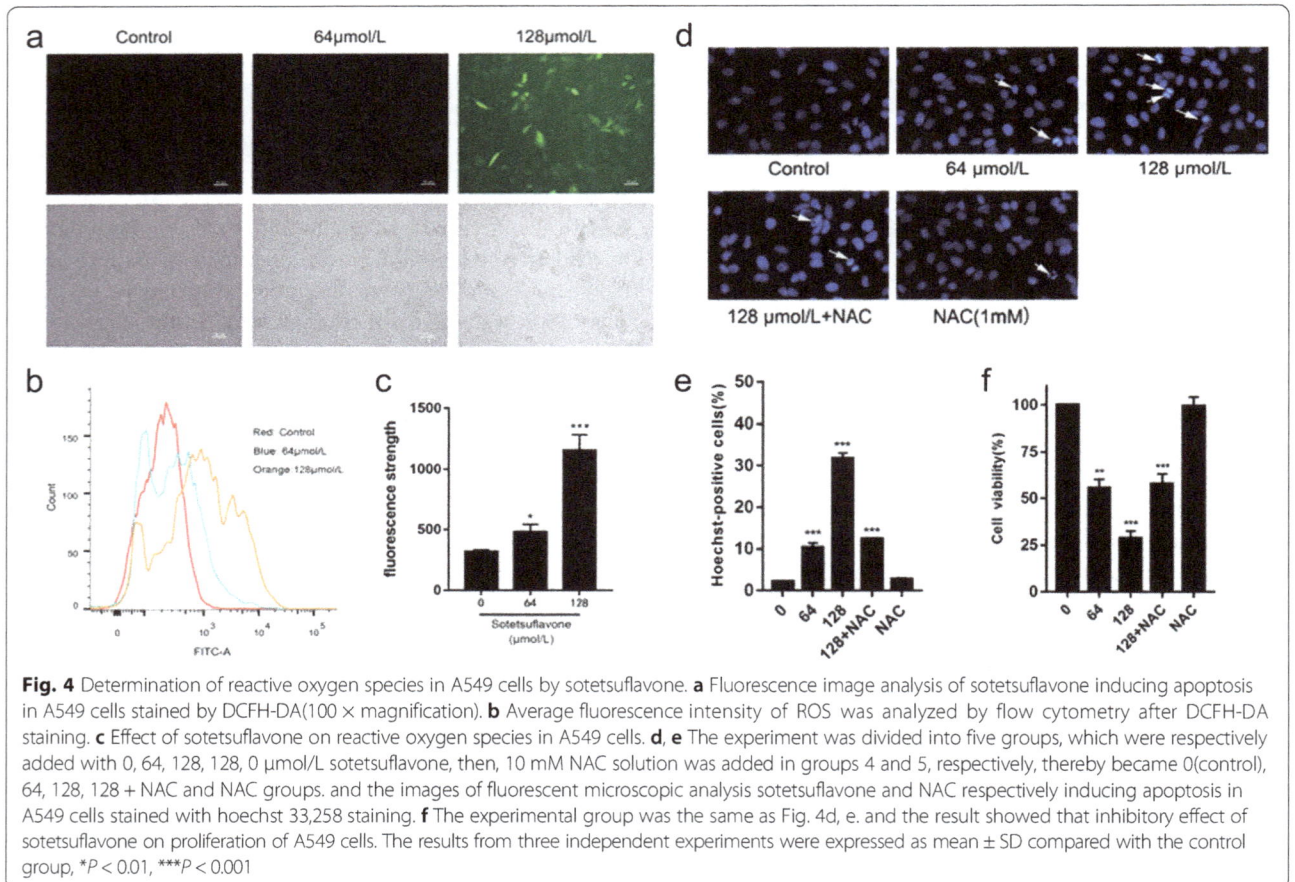

Fig. 4 Determination of reactive oxygen species in A549 cells by sotetsuflavone. **a** Fluorescence image analysis of sotetsuflavone inducing apoptosis in A549 cells stained by DCFH-DA(100 × magnification). **b** Average fluorescence intensity of ROS was analyzed by flow cytometry after DCFH-DA staining. **c** Effect of sotetsuflavone on reactive oxygen species in A549 cells. **d**, **e** The experiment was divided into five groups, which were respectively added with 0, 64, 128, 128, 0 μmol/L sotetsuflavone, then, 10 mM NAC solution was added in groups 4 and 5, respectively, thereby became 0(control), 64, 128, 128 + NAC and NAC groups. and the images of fluorescent microscopic analysis sotetsuflavone and NAC respectively inducing apoptosis in A549 cells stained with hoechst 33,258 staining. **f** The experimental group was the same as Fig. 4d, e. and the result showed that inhibitory effect of sotetsuflavone on proliferation of A549 cells. The results from three independent experiments were expressed as mean ± SD compared with the control group, *$P < 0.01$, ***$P < 0.001$

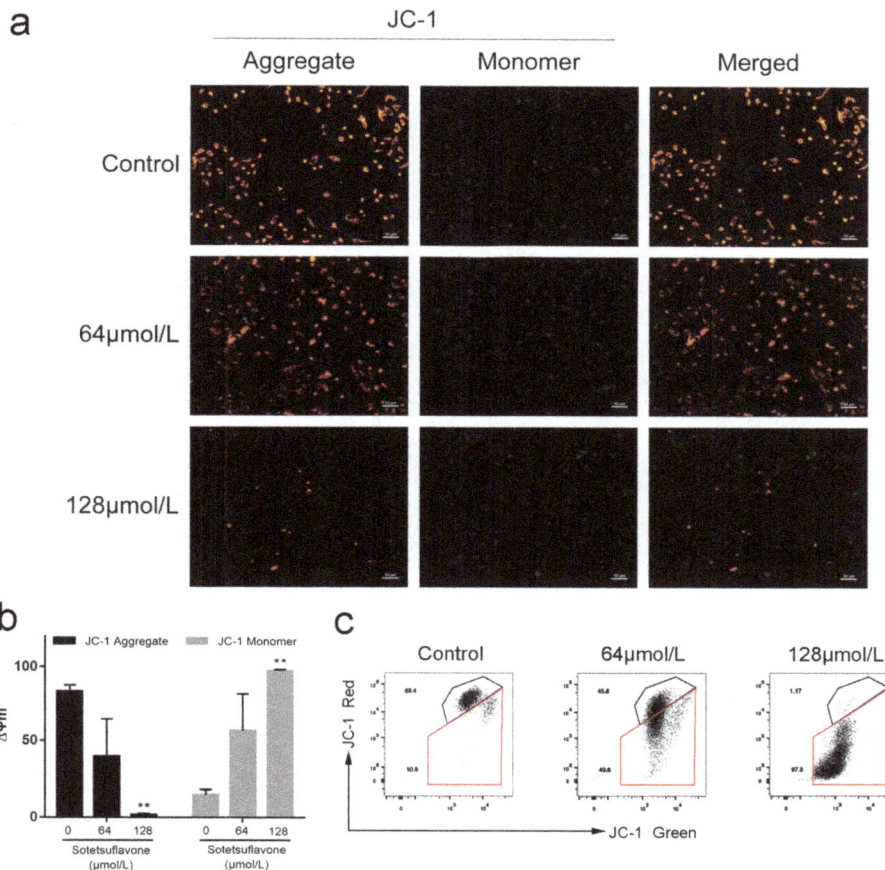

Fig. 5 Sotetsuflavone reduces mitochondrial membrane potential of A549 cells. **a** JC-1 fluorescence. **b** Changes of mitochondrial membrane potential after drug treatment. JC-1 Red channel; normal membrane potential cells. JC-1 Green channel; membrane potential collapse of cells. **c** Change of mitochondrial membrane potential after drug treatment. The results from three independent experiments were expressed as mean ± SD compared with the control group, **$P < 0.01$

proportion of cells corresponding to green fluorescence intensity increased from 10.8 to 97.3% with the increase of drug concentration, and the number of cells corresponding to red fluorescence intensity decreased (Fig. 5b, c).

Sotetsuflavone changes the expression level of apoptosis and cycle-related proteins

Apoptosis signaling is regulated by various proteins. Bcl-2, Bax, cleaved-caspase9, cleaved-caspase3, cleaved-caspase 8 and cytochrome C are important apoptosis-related proteins. Compared with the control group (0 μmol/L), sotetsuflavone (64 μmol/L, 128 μmol/L) down-regulated the expression of Bcl-2 protein and up-regulated the expression of Bax protein, which significantly increased Bax/Bcl-2, and it is suggested that sotetsuflavone has a significant induction effect on apoptotic related proteins. The increase of Bax/Bcl-2 can make mitochondrial membrane permeability changes, and cause caspase waterfall activation, which leads to apoptosis. The expression of Cyclin

D1 and CDK4 protein was seen to be decreased by detecting cell cycle related proteins, and the progression of G0/G1 phase was inhibited. The expression of cleaved-caspase9, cleaved-caspase3, and cytochrome C were increased, and the expression of cleaved-caspase 8 was decreased, it indicated that sotetsuflavone could not induce apoptosis of A549 cells through death receptor pathway but the mitochondrial pathway (Fig. 6a, b).

Discussion

Traditional Chinese medicines are convenient, inexpensive, and generally exhibit low side effects. More importantly, traditional medicines can relieve clinical symptoms, and improve the quality of life. Some may even be effective in treating cancer, and here we explore one such possibility.

Apoptosis is an important self-regulating mechanism for multicellular organisms to maintain a stable internal environment. Inducing apoptosis has become a common methodology in tumor therapy and an important index

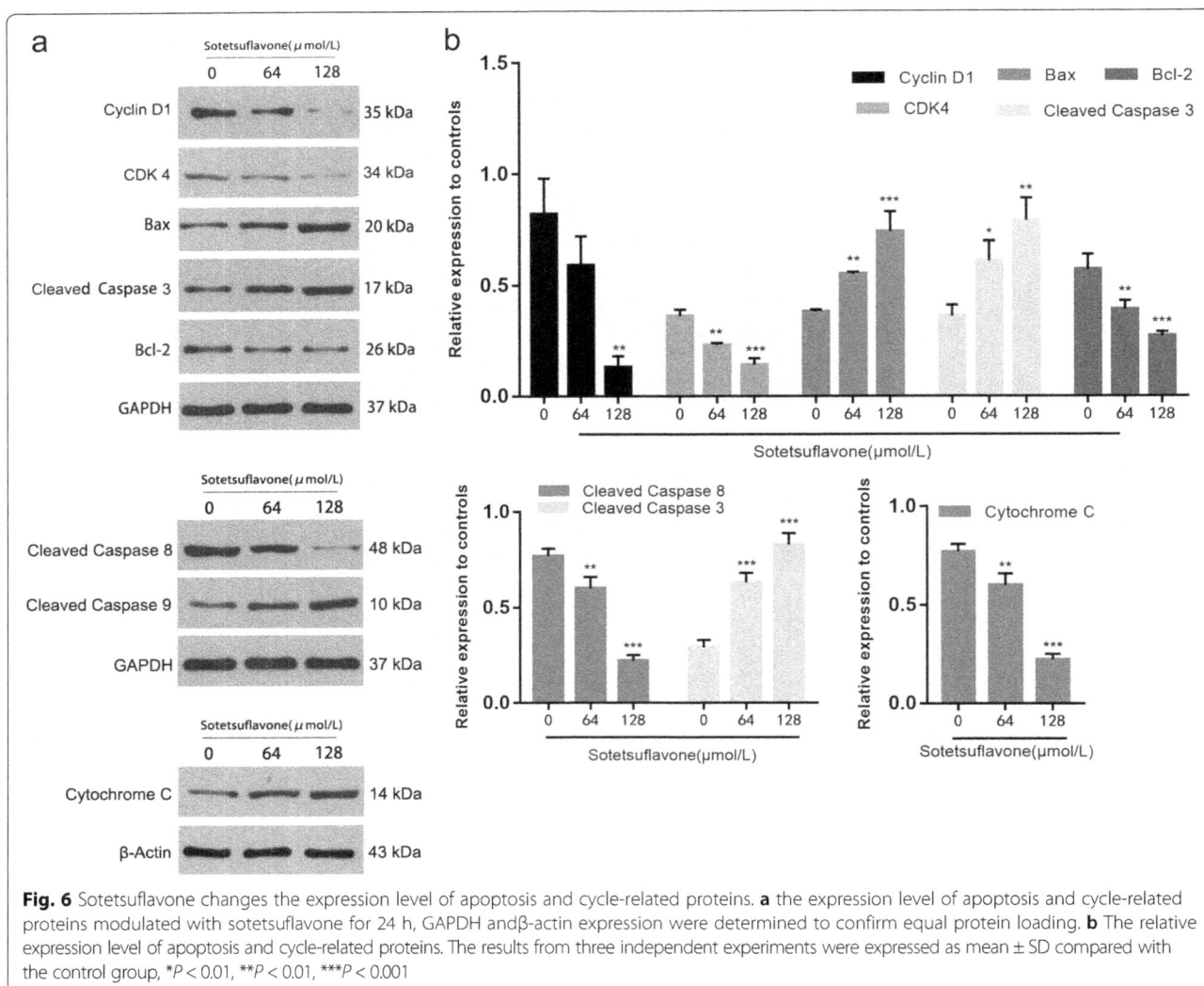

Fig. 6 Sotetsuflavone changes the expression level of apoptosis and cycle-related proteins. **a** the expression level of apoptosis and cycle-related proteins modulated with sotetsuflavone for 24 h, GAPDH andβ-actin expression were determined to confirm equal protein loading. **b** The relative expression level of apoptosis and cycle-related proteins. The results from three independent experiments were expressed as mean ± SD compared with the control group, *$P < 0.01$, **$P < 0.01$, ***$P < 0.001$

to evaluate the efficacy of anticancer drugs [24, 25]. We showed that sotetsuflavone inhibited the proliferation of A549 cells and showed a dose and time-dependent manner markedly (Fig. 1f). A flow cytometry assay showed that treatment with sotetsuflavone for 24 h resulted apoptosis in A549 cells. Moreover, the proportion of apoptotic cells was significantly increased with elevating levels of drug concentrations (Figs. 2 and 3b). In addition, the study found that anti-apoptosis protein of Bcl-2 expression was down-regulated. On the contrary, the pro-apoptosis protein of Bax was up-regulated (Fig. 6). The Bcl-2 protein family is a special family, some members promote apoptosis, such as Bad, Bid, Bax, and some members block apoptosis, such as Bcl-2, Bcl-w. Bcl-2 can inhibit cytochrome C release from the mitochondria into the cytoplasm, thereby inhibiting apoptosis [26]. Bcl-2 protein is an endometrial protein, mainly localized in mitochondria, endoplasmic reticulum membrane and the nuclear membrane, and is present in

a variety of tumor cells. It can increase the mitochondrial membrane potential, inhibit the release of calcium ions, prevent the activation of endonuclease, and then play an anti-apoptotic effect. Bax protein can directly activates the death effect factor caspase or changes the permeability of cell membrane, causing cytochrome C to release ions and small molecules through the cell membrane, thereby promoting cell apoptosis. The Bcl-2/Bax change can regulate apoptosis, when Bcl-2 is dominant, cell have anti-apoptotic effects, Conversely, when Bax is overexpressed, cells are prone to apoptosis [27].

The decline of mitochondrial membrane potential is an early phenomenon of apoptosis. The opening of mitochondrial permeability transition pore (MPTP) decreases mitochondrial membrane potential, and sotetsuflavone reduces the mitochondrial membrane potential of A549 cells in a concentration dependent manner (Fig. 5). Caspase-3 is the most critical enzyme in the pathways of apoptosis. The mitochondrial-dependent pathway of apoptosis is activated

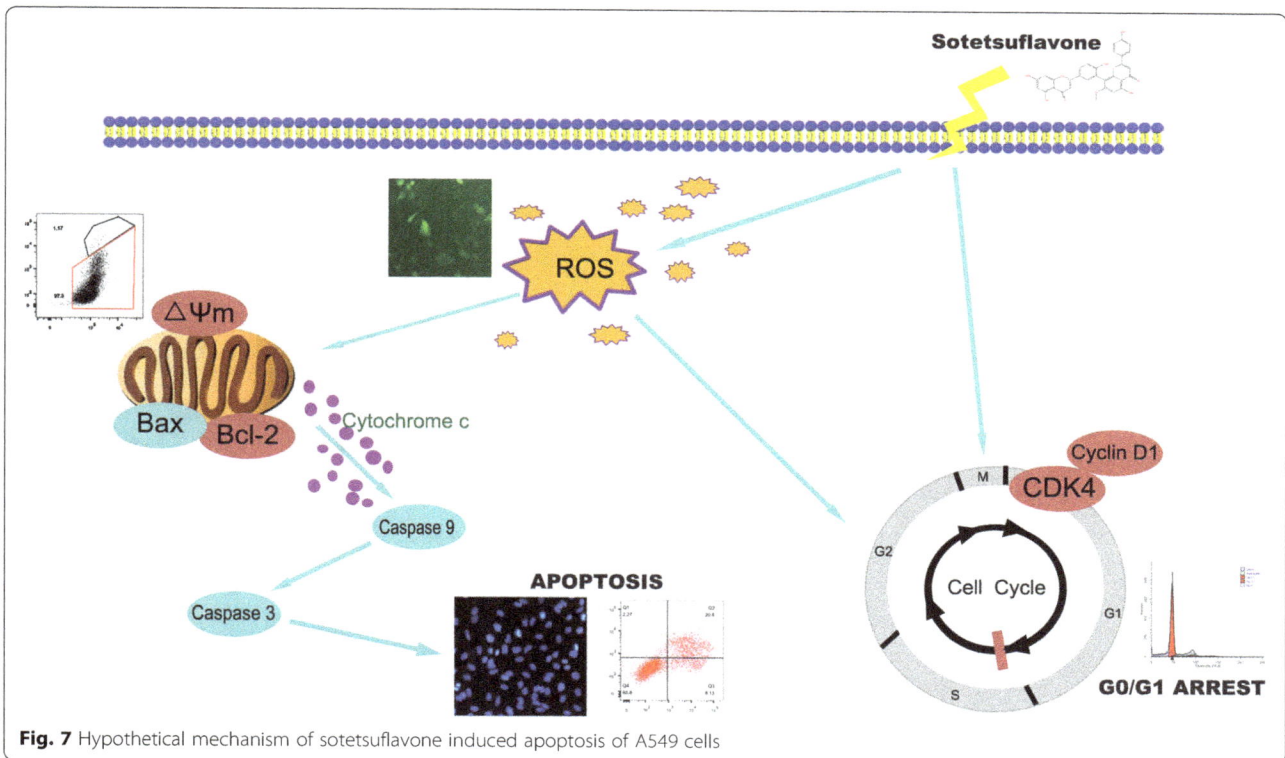

Fig. 7 Hypothetical mechanism of sotetsuflavone induced apoptosis of A549 cells

as a result of intracellular stress or damage, which engages the Bcl-2 family of pro-apoptosis proteins, including Bcl-2, Bak and Bax [28]. Western blot results showed that the proportion of Bcl-2/Bax protein expression was decreased while Cleaved-Caspase 3 was increased significantly (Fig. 6a). It demonstrated that sotetsuflavone induced apoptosis in A549 cells through mitochondrial-dependent pathway.

Studies have shown that increased intracellular ROS can cause cell membrane potential collapse and thus block the cell cycle, ROS entering the cytoplasm can re-enter the cell nucleus to cause DNA damage, further stimulate endogenous pathway apoptosis, and ultimately lead to cell death [29, 30]. ROS is a key molecule in apoptosis, and Bcl-2 plays a role in the relationship between ROS and apoptosis, regulating and maintaining the activity of intracellular antioxidants. Intracellular ROS produced in apoptotic cells is also associated with changes in Bax protein expressions, generation of ROS in the cells by causing increased expression of Bax and decreased Bcl-2 are considered as indicators of activation of mitochondrial cell death pathway [31]. ROS content increased after 24 h of drug action (Fig. 4a). to confirm whether induction of apoptosis on A549 cells was via ROS-mediated mitochondria-dependent pathway or not, we added antioxidant NAC in the experiment, by detecting the cell viability and apoptosis ratio, we found that after the treatment of NAC, the activity of A549

cells and the number of apoptotic cells were decreased significantly (Fig. 4d, e, f). It is indicated that sotetsuflavone induced A549 cells to apoptosis through the ROS-mediated mitochondrial pathway. The accumulation of ROS disrupts the redox control of cell cycle progression via cell cycle regulatory proteins such as Cyclins and CDKs, leading to aberrant cell proliferation and apoptosis [32]. Cyclin D1 and CDK 4 play an important role in the regulation of cell cycle progression. The expression levels of Cyclin D1 and CDK 4 were significantly reduced by western blotting (Fig. 6a). Flow Cytometry assay showed that the number of apoptotic cells in G0/G1 phase increased with the increase of drug concentration (Fig. 3a, c), which indicated that sotetsuflavone could block A549 cells in G0/G1 phase.

Conclusions

In summary, sotetsuflavone can inhibit the proliferation of A549 cells. The cell cycle is mainly blocked in the G0/G1 phase by increasing intracellular ROS levels, and the enhanced ROS generation resulted in increased oxidative stress, thereby Bcl-2/Bax reduction resulted in an increase in Cleaved-caspase3 expression, subsequently, inducing A549 cells apoptosis (Fig. 7). Taken together, sotetsuflavone induced apoptosis on A549 cells via ROS-mediated mitochondria-dependent pathway. In conclusion, sotetsuflavone may be used as a novel candidate for anti-tumor therapy in patients with lung cancer.

Abbreviations

Bax: Bcl-2 Associated X Protein; Bcl-2: B cell lymphoma 2; Caspase-3: Cysteinyl aspartate specific proteinase-3; CDK 4: Cyclin-dependent kinase 4; DCFH-DA: 2-(2,7-dichloro-3,6-diacetyloxy-9H-xanthen-9-yl)-benzoic acid; DMEM: Dulbecco's modified eagle medium; GAPDH: Glyceraldehyde-3-phosphate dehydrogenase; MTT: 3-(4,5-dimethyl-2-thiazolyl)-2,5-diphenyl-2-H-tetrazolium bromide; NAC: N-acetyl-L-cysteine; NSCLC: Non-small cell lung cancer; PBS: Phosphate-buffered saline; ROS: Reactive oxygen species

Funding

This study was supported by the Creative Item of Innovative Team of Ministry of Education (No. IRT-13R63); National Training Programs of Innovation and Entrepreneurship for Undergraduates (No. GCYS2016110001) and Training Programs of Innovation and Entrepreneurship for Undergraduates of of Minzu University of China (No. MCYS2017110007).

Authors' contributions

All authors have made substantial contributions in the research, preparation and revision of manuscript. The principal contributor for the design, data acquisition, analysis and interpretation of the experiment as well as manuscript writing was WSH. HYL, YY, CZK and LTX involved in the design of the study, revising the manuscript critically for important intellectual content. Each author has participated in the work and has given final approval of the version to be published.

Competing interests

The authors declare that they have no competing interests.

Author details

[1]School of Pharmacy, Minzu University of China, No. 27 Zhongguancun South Street, Haidian District, Beijing 100081, China. [2]School of Pharmacy, Minzu University of China, Key Laboratory of Ethnomedicine (Minzu University of China), Minority of Education, No. 27 Zhongguancun South Street, Haidian District, Beijing 100081, China.

References

1. Couzin-Frankel J. Clinical trials. Experimental cancer therapies move to the front line. Science. 2012;335:282–3.
2. Underwood JM, Townsend JS, Tai E, Davis SP, Stewart SL, White A, Momin B, Fairley TL. Racial and regional disparities in lung cancer incidence. Cancer. 2012;118:1910–8.
3. Choi YJ, Uehara Y, Ji YP, Chung KW, Ha YM, Ji MK, Yu MS, Chun P, Park JW, Moon HR. Suppression of melanogenesis by a newly synthesized compound, MHY966 via the nitric oxide/protein kinase G signaling pathway in murine skin. J Dermatol Sci. 2012;68:164–71.
4. Tariq N, Jiang W, Ralph S, Nagla AK. Thyroid metastasis from non-small cell lung cancer. Case Rep Oncol Med. 2013;20:208–13.
5. Siegel R, Ma J, Zou Z, Jemal A. Cancer statistics, 2014. CA Cancer J Clin. 2014;64:9–29.
6. Keith RL, Miller YE. Lung cancer chemoprevention: current status and future prospects. Nat Rev Clin Oncol. 2013;10:334–43.
7. Yuko E, Katsuhiko Y, Yuichi K, Michiko Y, Takashi Y, Airo T. Green tea extract atten-uates MNU-induced photoreceptor cell apoptosis via suppression of heme oxygenase-1. J Toxicol Pathol. 2016;29:61–5.
8. Kao SJ, Lee WJ, Chang JH, Chow JM, Chung CL, Hung WY, Chien MH. Suppression of reactive oxygen species-mediated ERK and JNK activation sensitizes dihydromyricetin-induced mitochondrial apoptosis in human non-small cell lung cancer. Environ Toxicol. 2017;32:1426–38.
9. Ahmed K, V Lakshma N, Chandrakant B, Vishnuvardhan MVPS, Adla M. Investigation of the mechanism and apoptotic pathway induced by 4β cinnamido linked podophyllotoxins against human lung cancer cells A549. Apoptosis. 2015;20:1518–29.
10. Norberg E, Orrenius S, Zhivotovsky B. Mitochondrial regulation of cell death: processing of apoptosis-inducing factor (AIF). Biochem Biophys Res Commun. 2010;396:95–100.
11. Brasacchio D, Alsop AE, Noori T, Lufti M, Iyer S, Simpson KJ, Bird PI, Kluck RM, Johnstone RW, Trapani JA. Epigenetic control of mitochondrial cell death through PACS1-mediated regulation of BAX/BAK oligomerization. Cell Death Differ. 2017;4:961–70.
12. Moghtaderi H, Sepehri H, Attari F. Combination of arabinogalactan and curcumin induces apoptosis in breast cancer cells in vitro and inhibits tumor growth via overexpression of p53 level in vivo. Biomed Pharmacother. 2017;88:582–94.
13. Zhou XL, Shi T, Yang L, Guo J, Peng SF, Shi ZH. Research on the effect and mechanism of total ginkgo flavones-glycoides on hepatocyte apoptosis in rats weih nonalcoholic fatty liver diserse. Chin J Intergr Trad West Med Dig. 2017;25:439–48.
14. Shu W, Ma QJ, Ye X. CyclinE-CDK2 and its Related Proteins in the Cell Cycle. Lett Biotechnol. 2008;19:97–100.
15. Fang Y, Hou Q, Lu Y. Effects of isorhapontigenin on cell cycle arrest and downregulation of cyclin D1 expression in bladder cancer cells. Chin J Pathophysiol. 2013;29:442–8.
16. Wei B, Huang Q, Huang S, Mai W, Zhong X. Trichosanthin-induced autophagy in gastric cancer cell MKN-45 is dependent on reactive oxygen species (ROS) and NF-κB/p53 pathway. J Pharmacol Sci. 2016;131:77–83.
17. Kowalska MT, Itzhak Y, Puett D. Presence of aromatase inhibitors in cycads. J Ethnopharmacol. 1995;28:113–6.
18. Wang SH, Liu TX. Effects of total flavonoids from Cycas revolute on inhibition and immune function of model mice with Lewis lung cancer. Chin J Immun. 2016;32:1598–602.
19. Zhou Y, Zang XR, Jiang SY, CL LI, Peng SL. Chemical constituents of *cycas panzhihuaensis*. Chin J Appl Environ Biol. 1999;5:367–70.
20. Wang S, Yan Y, Cheng Z, Hu Y, Liu T. Sotetsuflavone suppresses invasion and metastasis in non-small-cell lung cancer A549 cells by reversing EMT via the TNF-α/NF-κB and PI3K/AKT signaling pathway. Cell Death Disco. 2018;4:26.
21. Xu H, Gong Z, Zhou S, Yang S, Wang D, Chen X, Wu J, Liu L, Zhong S, Zhao J, Tang J. Liposomal curcumin targeting endometrial Cancer through the NF-κB pathway. Cell Physiol Biochem. 2018;48:569–82.
22. Lebel CP, Ischiropoulos H, Bondy SC. Evaluation of the probe 2',7'-dichlorofluorescin as an indicator of reactive oxygen species formation and oxidative stress. Chem Res Toxicol. 1992;5:227–31.
23. Xiong Q, Kadota S, Tani T, Namba T. Anti-oxidative effects of phenylethanoids from Cistanche deserticola. Biol Pharm Bull. 1996;19:1580–5.
24. Koff JL, Ramachandiran S, Bernal-Mizrachi L. A time to kill: targeting apoptosis in cancer. Int J Mol Sci. 2015;16:2942–55.
25. Renault TT, Chipuk JE. Death upon a kiss: mitochondrial outer membrane composition and organelle communication govern sensitivity to BAK/BAX-dependent apoptosis. Chem Biol. 2014;21:114–23.
26. Zhang Q, An R, Tian X, Yang M, Li M, Lou J, Xu L, Dong Z. β-Caryophyllene pretreatment alleviates focal cerebral ischemia-reperfusion injury by activating PI3K/Akt signaling pathway. Neurochem Res. 2017;42:1459–69.
27. Chen HC, Kanai M, Inoue-Yamauchi A, Tu HC, Huang Y, Ren D, Kim H, Takeda S, Reyna DE, Chan PM. An interconnected hierarchical model of cell death regulation by the BCL-2 family. Nat Cell Biol. 2015;17:1270–81.
28. Trotta AP, Chipuk JE. Mitochondrial dynamics as regulators of cancer biology. Cell Mol Life Sci. 2017;74:1999–2017.
29. Pant K, Gupta P, Damania P, Yadav AK, Gupta A, Ashraf A, Venugopal SK. Mineral pitch induces apoptosis and inhibits proliferation via modulating reactive oxygen species in hepatic cancer cells. BMC Complement Altern Med. 2016;16:148.
30. Yang J, Wu LJ, Tashino S, Onodera S, Ikejima T. Protein tyrosine kinase pathway-derived ROS/NO productions contribute to G2/M cell cycle arrest in evodiamine-treated human cervix carcinoma HeLa cells. Free Radic Res. 2010;44:792–802.
31. Mondal A, Bennett LL. Resveratrol enhances the efficacy of sorafenib mediated apoptosis in human breast cancer MCF7 cells through ROS, cell cycle inhibition, caspase 3 and PARP cleavage. Biomed Pharmacother. 2016;84:1906–14.
32. Shi H, Li Y, Ren X, Zhang Y, Yang Z, Qi C. A novel quinazoline-based analog induces G2/M cell cycle arrest and apoptosis in human A549 lung cancer cells via a ROS-dependent mechanism. Biochem Biophys Res Commun. 2017;486:314–20.

6

Antimicrobial and antioxidant activities of triterpenoid and phenolic derivatives from two Cameroonian Melastomataceae plants: *Dissotis senegambiensis* and *Amphiblemma monticola*

Raissa Tioyem Nzogong[1†], Fabrice Sterling Tchantchou Ndjateu[1,4†], Steve Endeguele Ekom[2],
Jules-Arnaud Mboutchom Fosso[2], Maurice Ducret Awouafack[1,3], Mathieu Tene[1*], Pierre Tane[1], Hiroyuki Morita[3],
Muhammad Iqbal Choudhary[4] and Jean-de-Dieu Tamokou[2*] ⓘ

Abstract

Background: Antimicrobial resistance is a serious threat against humankind and the search for new therapeutics is needed. This study aims to investigate the antimicrobial and antioxidant activities of ethanol extracts and compounds isolated from *Dissotis senegambiensis* and *Amphiblemma monticola*, two Cameroonian Melastomataceae species traditionally used for the treatment of fever, malaria and infectious diseases.

Methods: The plant extracts were prepared by maceration in ethanol. Standard chromatographic and spectroscopic methods were used to isolate and identify fourteen compounds from the two plant species [1–6 (from *D. senegambiensis*), 3, 4 and 7–14 (from *A. monticola*)]. A two-fold serial micro-dilution method was used to determine the minimum inhibitory concentration (MIC) against four bacterial strains including two resistant bacterial strains, methicillin resistant *S. aureus* (MRSA3) and methicillin resistant *S. aureus* (MRSA4) and three yeast strains.

Results: The fractionation of EtOH extracts afforded fourteen compounds belonging to triterpenoid and phenolic derivatives. The ethanol extracts, compounds 3, 5–8, 10 and the mixture of 10 + 12 were active against all the tested bacterial and fungal species. Compound 7 (MIC = 16–32 μg/mL) and 10 (MIC = 8–16 μg/mL) displayed the largest antibacterial and antifungal activities, respectively. Compounds 7, 10 and the mixture of 10 + 12 showed prominent antibacterial activity against methicillin- resistant *S. aureus* (MRSA) which is in some cases equal to that of ciprofloxacin used as reference antibacterial drug. Compound 8 also showed high radical-scavenging activities and ferric reducing power when compared with vitamin C and butylated hydroxytoluene used as reference antioxidants. The tested samples were non-toxic to normal cells highlighting their good selectivity.

Conclusions: The result of this investigation reveals the potential of *D. senegambiensis* and *A. monticola* as well as the most active compounds in the search for new antimicrobial and antioxidant agents. So, further investigations are needed.

Keywords: *Dissotis senegambiensis*, *Amphiblemma monticola*, Melastomataceae, Triterpenoids, Phenolics, Antibacterial, Antifungal, Methicillin-resistant *S. aureus*

* Correspondence: mtene2001@yahoo.fr; jtamokou@yahoo.fr
†Equal contributors
[1]Laboratory of Natural Products Chemistry, Department of Chemistry, Faculty of Science, University of Dschang, P.O. Box 67, Dschang, Cameroon
[2]Laboratory of Microbiology and Antimicrobial substances, Department of Biochemistry, Faculty of Science, University of Dschang, P.O. Box 67, Dschang, Cameroon
Full list of author information is available at the end of the article

Background

Infectious diseases are among the leading causes of death accounting for approximately one-half of all deaths in developing countries [1]. Despite the successes of the Millennium Development Goals era, the inhabitants of low-income countries still suffer an enormous burden of disease owing to diarrhoea, pneumonia, HIV/AIDS, tuberculosis, malaria and other infectious diseases. Increase in infections as a result of emergence of drug-resistant microorganisms and hitherto unknown pathogenic microbes pose enormous public health concerns [1]. These therefore, necessitate continued search for compounds with antimicrobial activities. Historically, plants have provided a good source of anti-infective agents in the fight against microbial infections [2–5]. The genus *Dissotis* which belongs to the Melastomataceae family comprises about 140 species in Africa [6]. They are climbing shrubs, shrubs or small trees found in some African countries such as Ivory Cost, Benin, Democratic Republic of Congo, Nigeria and Cameroon [7]. Several species are used in folk medicine as antidiarrheic, antimicrobial, antioxidant, antitumoral, antirheumatic, and anti-inflammatory agents, and also in the treatment of skin diseases, fever, malaria, and to lower blood cholesterol [8]. *Dissotis senegambiensis* (Guill. & Perr.) Triana (Syn. *Dissotis irvingiana* Hook) belonging to the Melastomataceae family, is a shrub reaching 120 cm in height. The flowers are purple. In Africa, this plant species is found in tropical areas of Cameroon, Senegal, Ethiopia and Mozambique [7]. This species is used in traditional medicine for the treatment of the kwashiorkor, anemia, marasmus, avitaminose, drepanocytose, cutaneous eruptions and diarrhea [9]. To the best of our knowledge, no phytochemical work has yet been done on *D. senegambiensis*. The genus *Amphiblemma* belonging also to the Melastomataceae family, extends from tropical West Africa to Ethiopia and Cabinda. It contains at least 14 species distributed in Africa [10]. They are herbaceous plants or shrubs that grow in evergreen forests [10]. *Amphiblemma monticola* Jacq.-Fél. is a prostrate herb or sub-shrub reaching 100 cm in height that generally grows in West and South-West Regions of Cameroon [10–12]. This plant species is used by the Bamena populations in West Region of Cameroon against fever and stomach disorders [13]. Previous phytochemical studies of some species of the Melastomataceae family reported the isolation of terpenoids, steroids, simple phenolics, flavonoids and a vast range of polyphenols [14–18]. According to some traditional healers found in the Western region of Cameroon, maceration of the studied plants in raffia wine (a traditional alcoholic beverage produced in several African countries) is used for the treatment of different diseases. Traditional uses of *D. senegambiensis* and *A. monticola* motivated our effort to investigate the phytochemistry and pharmacological activity. Fourteen compounds [β-amyrin palmitate (**1**), α-amyrin

acetate (**2**), ursolic acid (**3**), sitosterol-3-O-β-D-glucopyranoside (**4**), vitexin (**5**) and *trans*-tiliroside (**6**) (from *D. senegambiensis*), ursolic acid (**3**), sitosterol-3-O-β-D-glucopyranoside (**4**), 3,4′-di-O-methylellagic acid (**7**), dimethyl 4,4′,5,5′,6,6′-hexahydroxybiphenyl-2,2′-dicarboxylate (**8**), lupeol (**9**), ellagic acid (**10**), 3-hydroxy-4,5-dimethoxybenzoic acid (**11**), 3-O-methylellagic acid 4′-O-β-D-xylopyranoside (**12**), oleanolic acid (**13**) and amphiblemmone A (**14**) (from *A. monticola*)] were isolated and characterized. This is the first report on the isolation of compounds **1–6** from *D. senegambiensis*. Compounds **3**, **4** and **7–14** were previously isolated from the same source (*A. monticola*) [13]. Antimicrobial and antioxidant activities of ethanol extracts of *D. senegambiensis* and *A. monticola* and some compounds (**3–10**, a mixture of **3** and **13**, and a mixture of **10** and **12**) isolated in sufficient quantities are reported here for the first time.

Methods

General experimental procedures

MS data were measured on JEOL MS Station JMS-700 spectrometer or JEOL 600 MS Route spectrometer. ^{1}H NMR (500 and 400 MHz) and ^{13}C NMR (125 and 100 MHz) were recorded using JEOL spectrometers or Bruker Avance AV-400 spectrometer. The chemical shifts were reported in parts per million (ppm) with TMS as internal standard. Deuterated solvents, methanol (CD$_3$OD), dimethyl sulfoxide (DMSO-d_6), pyridine (C$_5$D$_5$N) and chloroform (CDCl$_3$) were used as solvents for the NMR experiments. CC was performed on silica gel 60 F$_{254}$ (70–230 mesh; Merck) and gel permeation on Sephadex LH-20. TLC was carried out on precoated silica gel Kieselgel 60 F$_{254}$ plates (0.25 mm thick), and spots weredetected with UV lights (254 and 365 nm) and further sprayedwith 20% H$_2$SO$_4$ reagent followed by heating to 100 °C.

Sample collections

Plant materials were collected in two locations of the Western Region of Cameroon: the whole plant of *Dissotis senegambiensis* (Guill. & Perr.) Triana in Bansoa (January 2013) and the roots of *Amphiblemma monticola* Jacq.-Fél. in Bamena (May 2016). Their identification was done by Mr. Fulbert Tadjouteu, a botanist of the Cameroon National Herbarium in Yaoundé, where voucher specimens, N° 24736/SRF/Cam (*D. senegambiensis*) and N° 45094/HNC (*A. monticola*), were deposited.

Extraction

The powdered material of *D. senegambiensis* (1.8 kg) was extracted three times (72 h for each time) by maceration with ethanol (8 L) at room temperature. Evaporation of solvent under vacuum afforded 78 g of crude extract. A portion of this extract (76 g) was successively triturated with *n*-hexane, EtOAc and *n*-butanol. TLC analysis showed that the *n*-hexane and EtOAc extracts (19.5 and 20.5 g, respectively) were qualitatively the same. They were thus combined to afford 40 g of extract called "EtOAc extract".

Dried and pulverized roots (1.5 kg) and aerial part (0.08 kg) of *A. monticola* were respectively macerated with ethanol (5 L with roots and 1 L with aerial part) for 24 h (3 times) at room temperature. Evaporation of solvent under reduced pressure afforded 49 g and 4.28 g of crude extracts, respectively.

Phytochemical analysis

The extracts were screened for secondary metabolites using standard procedures as previously described [19–22]. The plant extracts were screened for the presence of different classes of compounds including triterpenoids, steroids, flavonoids, phenols, glycosides, tannins and alkaloids.

Isolation of constituents

A portion (38 g) of "EtOAc extract" of *D. senegambiensis* was subjected to silica gel (70 to 230 mesh) column chromatography (CC) eluted with gradient of *n*-hexane-EtOAc (100:0, 9:1, 4:1, 7:3, 3:2, 1:1 and 0:100) followed by gradient of EtOAc-MeOH (19:1, 9:1, 4:1, 7:3, 1:1 and 0:100). Fifty-five fractions of 300 mL each were collected and combined into six major fractions on the basis of their TLC profiles: A (1–6; 4.0 g), B (7–12; 4.5 g), C (13–17; 3.6 g), D (18–26; 4.7 g), E (27–36; 5.5 g), and F (37–55; 9.1 g). Fraction A crystallized to afford a mixture of two compounds. This mixture was subjected to silica gel CC and eluted with *n*-hexane- EtOAc (49:1) to yield β-amyrin palmitate (4.2 mg; **1**) and α-amyrin acetate (3. 5 mg; **2**). Fraction C crystallized to afford ursolic acid (15.0 mg; **3**). Fraction E was subjected to silica gel CC and eluted with CH_2Cl_2 –MeOH mixture of increasing polarity to yield sitosterol-3-*O*-β-D-glucopyranoside (35. 1 mg; **4**) and vitexin (28.5 mg; **5**). Similarly as with fraction E, fraction F afforded *trans*-tiliroside (25.0 mg; **6**). A portion (18 g) of the *n*-BuOH extract was also subjected to silica gel CC eluted with gradient of CH_2Cl_2-MeOH (100:0, 19:1, 9:1, 4:1and 0:100). Twenty-two fractions of 300 mL each were collected and combined into four major fractions on the basis of their TLC profiles: G (1–7; 2.7 g), H (8–12; 3.5 g), I (13–18; 3.6 g) and J (19–22; 3.7 g). Fraction G was subjected to silica gel CC and eluted with CH_2Cl_2 –MeOH mixture of increasing polarity to yield vitexin (15.1 mg; **5**) and *trans*-tiliroside (13.1 mg; **6**). An attempt to purify fractions B, D, H, I and J failed.

A portion (47 g) of EtOH extract of the roots of *A. monticola* was fractionated on silica gel CC eluted with CH_2Cl_2-MeOH of increasing polarity to give 25 fractions

of 300 mL each. After comparative TLC, they were combined into 4 major fractions: A (1–8; 7.6 g), B (9–16; 11 g), C (17–21; 5.1 g) and D (22–25; 5.8 g). Fraction A was chromatographed on a silica gel column eluted with a continuous gradient of *n*-hexane-EtOAc to afford lupeol (**9**, 120.8 mg) and a mixture of sterols. Similarly, fractions B and C were eluted with CH_2Cl_2-MeOH of increasing polarity yielding four (B1-B4) and three (C1-C3) sub-fractions, respectively. B2 (1.9 g), B3 (2.3 g), C2 (1.9 g) and C3 (1.2 g) were passed separately on LH-20 Sephadex CC eluted with CH_2Cl_2-MeOH (1:1) to give 3,4′-di-*O*-methylellagic acid (20.0 mg; **7**) from B2, dimethyl 4,4′,5,5′,6,6′-hexahydroxybiphenyl-2,2′-dicarboxylate (15.0 mg; **8**) from B3, ellagic acid (23.0 mg; **10**), 3-hydroxy-4,5-dimethoxybenzoic acid (4.0 mg; **11**) and a mixture of **10** and **12** (7.0 mg) from C2, and 3-*O*-methylellagic acid 4′-*O*-β-D-xylopyranoside (2.3 mg; **12**) from C3. Re-crystallization of B4 (0.7 g) in EtOAc afforded a mixture (31.9 mg) of ursolic acid (**3**) and oleanolic acid (**13**). Fraction D was subjected to silica gel CC eluted with a gradient mixture of CH_2Cl_2-MeOH to afford four sub-fractions (D1-D4). Repeated silica gel CC of D2 (0.8 g), eluted with CH_2Cl_2-MeOH (from 49:1 to 9:1) gave sitosterol-3-O-β-D-glucopyranoside (45.0 mg; **4**) and amphiblemmone A (9.7 mg; **14**).

Due to the small quantity of plant material, the aerial part of *A. monticola* (4.28 g of crude EtOH extract), compared to the roots (same collection in the field), was not further studied in this work.

Antimicrobial activity of extracts and compounds
Tested microorganisms

The microorganisms used in this study include four bacterial (*Staphylococcus aureus* ATCC25923, methicillin sensitive *S. aureus* MSSA1, methicillin resistant *S. aureus* MRSA3 and methicillin resistant *S. aureus* MRSA4) and three yeast strains (*Candida albicans* ATCC10231, *Candida tropicalis* PK233 and *Cryptococcus neoformans* H99). These microorganisms were taken from our laboratory collection. The fungal and bacterial strains were grown at 37 °C and maintained on Sabouraud Dextrose Agar (SDA, Conda, Madrid, Spain) and nutrient agar (NA, Conda) slants respectively.

Inocula preparation

The inocula of bacteria and yeasts were prepared from overnight cultures as previously described [23]. Absorbance was read spectrophotometrically at 530 nm and 600 nm for yeasts and bacteria respectively. The final concentrations of microbial suspensions were 2.5×10^5 cells/mL for yeasts and 10^6 CFU/mL for bacteria.

Antimicrobial assay

The antimicrobial activity was evaluated by determining the minimum inhibitory concentrations (MICs). MICs of extracts and compounds were determined by broth micro dilution [24]. Each test sample was dissolved in 10% v/v aqueous dimethylsulfoxide (DMSO) to give a stock solution. This was serially diluted two-fold in Mueller-Hinton Broth (MHB) for bacteria and Sabouraud Dextrose Broth (SDB) for fungi to obtain a concentration range of 4096 to 0.25 µg/mL. Then, 100 µL of each sample concentration was added to respective wells (96-well micro plate) containing 90 µL of SDB/ MHB and 10 µL of inoculum to give final concentration ranges of 2048 to 4 µg/mL (for extracts) and 256 to 0.125 µg/mL (for compounds). Dilutions of nystatin (Sigma-Aldrich, Steinheim, Germany) and ciprofloxacin (Sigma-Aldrich, Steinheim, Germany) were used as positive controls for yeasts and bacteria respectively. Broth with 10 µL of DMSO was used as negative control. The cultured micro plates were covered; then, the contents of each well were mixed thoroughly using a plate shaker (Flow Laboratory, Germany) and incubated at 37 °C for 24 h (bacteria) and 48 h (yeasts) under shaking. After the incubation period, MICs were assessed visually and were taken as the lowest sample concentration at which there was no growth or virtually no growth. The lowest concentration that yielded no growth after the subculturing was considered as the minimum microbicidal concentrations (MMCs). All the tests were performed in triplicate.

Antioxidant assay
Ferric reducing antioxidant power (FRAP) assay
The FRAP was determined by the Fe^{3+}-Fe^{2+} transformation in the presence of extracts and compounds as previously described [25]. The Fe^{2+} was monitored by measuring the formation of Perl's Prussian blue at 700 nm. Butylated hydroxytoluene (BHT) was used as a positive control. All the tests were performed in triplicate.

Diphenyl-1-picrylhydrazyl (DPPH) free radical scavenging assay
The free radical scavenging activity of extracts and compounds was evaluated according to described methods [26]. The EC_{50} (µg/ml), which is the amount of sample necessary to inhibit by 50% the absorbance of free radical DPPH was calculated [26]. Vitamin C was used as a standard control. All the analyses were carried out in triplicate.

Hemolytic assay
Whole blood (10 mL) from albino rats was collected by cardiac puncture into a conical tube containing EDTA as an anticoagulant. The study was conducted according to the ethical guidelines of the Committee for Control and Supervision of Experiments on Animals (Registration no. 173/CPCSEA, dated 28 January,

2000), Government of India, on the use of animals for scientific research. Erythrocytes were harvested by centrifugation at room temperature for 10 min at 1000 x g and were washed three times in PBS buffer [27]. The cytotoxicity was evaluated as previously described [27].

Statistical analysis
Data were analyzed by one-way analysis of variance followed by Waller-Duncan Post Hoc test. The experimental results were expressed as the mean ± Standard Deviation (SD). Differences between groups were considered significant when $p < 0.05$. All analyses were performed using the Statistical Package for Social Sciences (SPSS, version 12.0) software.

Results
Chemical analysis
The phytochemical screening revealed the presence of steroids, phenols, glycosides and tannins in all the plant extracts (Table 1). Triterpenoids and flavonoids are selectively distributed in the extracts whereas alkaloids were absent in all the extracts (Table 1). The EtOAc and n-BuOH extracts from D. senegambiensis and EtOH extract from the roots of A. monticola were fractionated by silica gel column chromatography to afford fourteen compounds (1–14) (Fig. 1). Compounds obtained from D. senegambiensis were identified as β-amyrin palmitate (1) [28], α-amyrin acetate (2) [29], ursolic acid (3) [30], sitosterol-3-O-β-D-glucopyranoside (4) [31]; vitexin (5) [32] and trans-tiliroside (6) [33]. From A. monticola, compounds were identified as 3,4′-di-O-methylellagic acid (7) [34], dimethyl 4,4′,5,5′,6,6′-hexahydroxybiphenyl-2,2′-dicarboxylate (8) [35], lupeol (9) [36], ellagic acid (10) [16], 3-hydroxy-4,5-dimethoxybenzoic acid (11) [37], 3-O-methylellagic acid 4′-O-β-D-xylopyranoside (12) [38], oleanolic acid (13) [16], and amphiblemmone A (14) [13]. The structures of the compounds

Table 1 Secondary metabolites identified in the studied plant extracts

Metabolites	D. senegambiensis			A. monticola	
	Whole plant			Roots	Aerial part
	Crude EtOH extract	EtOAc extract	n-BuOH extract	Crude EtOH extract	Crude EtOH extract
Triterpenoids	+	+	–	+	+
Steroids	+	+	+	+	+
Flavonoids	+	+	+	+	–
phenols	+	+	+	+	+
Tannins	+	+	+	+	+
Glycosides	+	+	+	+	+
Alkaloids	–	–	–	–	–

(+): presence; (–): absence

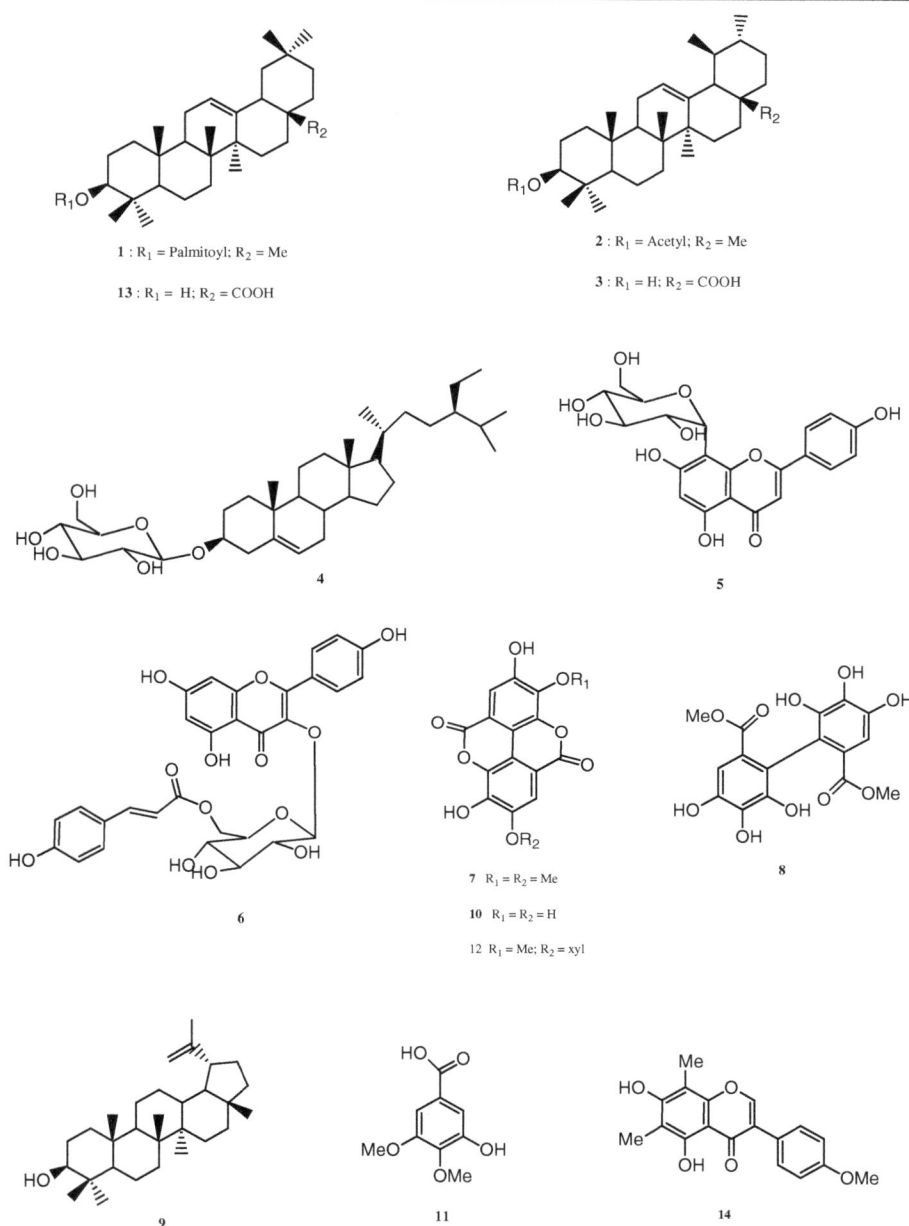

Fig. 1 Chemical structures of compounds isolated from *D. senegambiensis* (**1–6**) and *A. monticola* (**3, 4, 7–14**). **1**: *β*-amyrin palmitate; **2**: *α*-amyrin acetate; **3**: ursolic acid; **4**: sitosterol 3-*O*-*β*-D-glucopyranoside; **5**: vitexin; **6**: *trans*-tilliroside; **7**: 3,4′-di-*O*-methylellagic acid; **8**: dimethyl 4,4′,5,5′,6,6′-hexahydroxybiphenyl-2,2′-dicarboxylate; **9**: lupeol; **10**: ellagic acid; **11**: 3-hydroxy-4,5-dimethoxybenzoic acid; **12**: 3-*O*-methylellagic acid 4′-*O*-*β*-D-xylopyranoside; **13**: oleanolic acid; **14**: amphiblemmone A

(Fig. 1) were determined by analysis of their NMR data and comparison with those reported in the literature (Additional file 1).

Antimicrobial activity

The antimicrobial activity of EtOH extracts from *D. senegambiensis* and *A. monticola* as well as their isolated compounds was performed against four bacterial strains including two resistant bacterial strains, methicillin resistant *S. aureus* (MRSA3) and methicillin resistant *S. aureus* (MRSA4) and three yeast strains (Table 2). The EtOH, EtOAc and *n*-BuOH extracts, as well as compounds **3, 5–8, 10** and the mixture of **10 + 12** were active against all the tested bacterial and fungal species. Among the extracts, the EtOH extract from *D. senegambiensis* (MIC = 64–256 μg/mL) was the most active against *S. aureus* strains whereas

Table 2 Antimicrobial activity (in μg/ml) of extracts and isolated compounds from *D. senegambiensis* and *A. monticola* against bacterial and yeast strains

Crude extracts/ compounds	Inhibition parameters	S. aureus ATCC25923	S. aureus MSSA1	S. aureus MRSA3	S. aureus MRSA4	C. albicans ATCC10231	C. tropicalis PK233	C. neoformans H99
DSEtOH	MIC	128	64	256	128	2048	1024	512
	MMC	256	128	512	256	2048	2048	1024
	MMC/MIC	2	2	2	2	1	2	2
DSEtOAc	MIC	256	128	256	256	2048	1024	512
	MMC	256	256	512	512	> 2048	> 2048	> 2048
	MMC/MIC	1	2	2	1	nd	nd	nd
DSBuOH	MIC	256	64	256	128	2048	1024	1024
	MMC	512	128	512	256	2048	> 2048	> 2048
	MMC/MIC	2	2	2	2	1	nd	nd
AMEtOH	MIC	256	128	256	256	256	128	256
	MMC	256	128	512	512	512	256	256
	MMC/MIC	1	1	2	2	2	2	1
AMEtOAc	MIC	512	256	512	512	512	2048	2048
	MMC	512	512	512	512	1024	> 2048	> 2048
	MMC/MIC	1	2	1	1	2	nd	nd
3	MIC	256	128	128	128	256	256	128
	MMC	> 256	> 256	> 256	> 256	> 256	> 256	> 256
	MMC/MIC	nd	nd	Nd	nd	nd	nd	nd
4	MIC	> 256	> 256	> 256	> 256	256	256	128
	MMC	> 256	> 256	> 256	> 256	> 256	> 256	> 256
	MMC/MIC	nd	nd	Nd	nd	nd	nd	nd
5	MIC	64	64	64	128	128	64	128
	MMC	128	128	128	256	256	128	128
	MMC/MIC	2	2	2	2	2	2	1
6	MIC	32	64	64	128	64	64	64
	MMC	64	64	128	128	64	64	128
	MMC/MIC	2	1	2	1	1	1	2
7	MIC	32	16	16	32	32	32	32
	MMC	32	16	32	64	64	64	32
	MMC/MIC	1	1	2	2	2	2	1
8	MIC	32	32	64	128	128	16	32
	MMC	64	32	128	256	> 256	16	32
	MMC/MIC	2	1	2	2	nd	1	1
9	MIC	256	256	> 256	> 256	> 256	256	256
	MMC	> 256	> 256	> 256	> 256	nd	> 256	> 256
	MMC/MIC	nd	nd	Nd	nd	nd	nd	nd
10	MIC	8	16	32	32	16	8	16
	MMC	16	16	64	32	16	8	16
	MMC/MIC	2	1	2	1	1	1	1
10 + 12	MIC	32	16	32	32	64	64	64
	MMC	64	64	64	64	128	128	64
	MMC/MIC	2	4	2	2	2	2	1
3 + 13	MIC	128	64	> 256	128	> 256	> 256	128

Table 2 Antimicrobial activity (in µg/ml) of extracts and isolated compounds from *D. senegambiensis* and *A. monticola* against bacterial and yeast strains *(Continued)*

Crude extracts/ compounds	Inhibition parameters	*S. aureus* ATCC25923	*S. aureus* MSSA1	*S. aureus* MRSA3	*S. aureus* MRSA4	*C. albicans* ATCC10231	*C. tropicalis* PK233	*C. neoformans* H99
	MMC	256	128	Nd	256	> 256	> 256	256
	MMC/MIC	2	2	nd	2	nd	nd	2
Reference drugs*	MIC	1	1	16	32	2	0.5	1
	MMC	1	1	16	32	2	1	1
	MMC/MIC	1	1	1	1	1	2	1

*: Ciprofloxacin for bacteria and nystatin for fungi; compounds **1–6** and compounds **3, 4, 7–14** were isolated from *D. senegambiensis* and *A. monticola* respectively; compounds **1–2, 11** and **14** were not tested; nd: not determined. MIC: Minimum Inhibitory Concentrations; MMC: Minimum Microbicidal Concentrations; DSEtOH = *D. senegambiensis* EtOH extract; DSEtOAc = *D. senegambiensis* EtOAc extract; DSBuOH = *D. senegambiensis* n-BuOH extract; AMEtOH = *A. monticola* EtOH extract; AMEtOAc = *A. monticola* EtOAc extract; **3**: ursolic acid; **4**: sitosterol 3-O-β-D-glucopyranoside; **5**: vitexin; **6**: *trans*-tilliroside; **7**: 3,4'-di-O-methylellagic acid; **8**: dimethyl 4,4',5,5',6,6'-hexahydroxybiphenyl-2,2'-dicarboxylate; **9**: lupeol; **10**: ellagic acid; **12**: 3-O-methylellagic acid 4'-O-β-D-xylopyranoside; **13**: oleanolic acid

the *A. monticola* EtOH extract (MIC = 128–256 µg/mL) was the most effective against yeast strains. The results also showed that *S. aureus* ATCC25923 and *S. aureus* MSSA1 were the most sensitive bacteria while the most sensitive fungi were *C. tropicalis* and *C. neoformans*. Compound **10** (MIC = 8–16 µg/mL) displayed the largest antifungal activity whereas compound **7** (MIC = 16–32 µg/ml) showed the best anti-staphylococcal activity. Compound **10** (MIC = 8–32 µg/mL) was the most active sample against bacterial and fungal strains following in decreasing order by **7** (MIC = 16–32 µg/mL), **10 + 12** (MIC = 16–64 µg/mL), **8** (MIC = 8–128 µg/mL), **6** (MIC = 32–128 µg/mL), **5** (MIC = 64–128 µg/mL), **3** (MIC = 128–256 µg/mL), **3 + 13** (MIC = 64 - > 256 µg/mL), **9** (MIC = 256 - > 256 µg/mL) and **4** (MIC = 128 - > 256 µg/mL). Compounds **1** and **2**, obtained in small quantities, were not tested against the microorganisms used. The standard drugs used in this study were ciprofloxacin and nystatin for antibacterial and antifungal activity, respectively, and the antibacterial activities of some of the isolated compounds are in some cases equal to those of ciprofloxacin whereas the antifungal activity of the isolated compounds is lesser than that of nystatin.

Ferric reducing antioxidant power (FRAP)

In this study, all the investigated samples showed concentration-dependent reducing power (Fig. 2). The EtOH extracts from *D. senegambiensis* and *A. monticola* displayed the largest reductive abilities when compared with their fractions. Interestingly, compounds **7** and **10 + 12** showed the lowest reducing power whereas compound **8** exhibited the highest reducing power at the different concentrations tested. The antioxidant power of compound **8** is almost equal to that of butylated hydroxytoluene (BHT) used as standard antioxidant.

DPPH free radical scavenging activity

The results of the radical-scavenging activity showed that compounds **7** and **10 + 12** had the highest EC_{50} (i.e. the

lowest activity) while compound **8** had the lowest EC_{50} (i.e. the highest activity) (Fig. 3). Among the extracts, *A. monticola* EtOAc extract (EC_{50} = 40.83 ± 1.57 µg/ml) displayed the lowest activity whereas *D. senegambiensis* and *A. monticola* EtOH extracts had the highest activity (EC_{50} = 22.48 ± 1.62 and 19.74 ± 1.98 µg/ml). The DPPH free radical scavenging activity of compound **8** was comparable to that of the standard antioxidant vitamin C. These results corroborate the FRAP assay, where this compound exhibited the best antioxidant activity.

Hemolytic activity

To investigate the potential use of extracts and compounds **1–14**, the cytotoxicity also has to be evaluated. In this study, none of the tested samples showed hemolytic activities against red blood cells at concentrations up to 256 µg/mL and 2048 µg/mL for isolated compounds and extracts respectively (results not shown). This finding highlights the fact that the observed biological activity is not due to cellular toxicity.

Discussion

The findings of the present study showed that there were differences between the antimicrobial activities of plant extracts. These differences may be due to the different groups of secondary metabolites found in these extracts. Indeed, the antimicrobial activity of medicinal plants is correlated with the presence in their extracts of one or more classes of bioactive secondary metabolites [39]. The results also showed that the fractionation of EtOH extracts of *D. senegambiensis* and *A. monticola* reduced their antimicrobial activity in EtOAc and n-BuOH extracts. This indicates that the active principles might be more concentrated in the EtOH extracts and more diluted in their fractions. The antimicrobial activity of plant extracts is considered to be highly active if the MIC < 100 µg/mL; significantly active when 100 ≤ MIC ≤512 µg/mL; moderately active when 512 < MIC

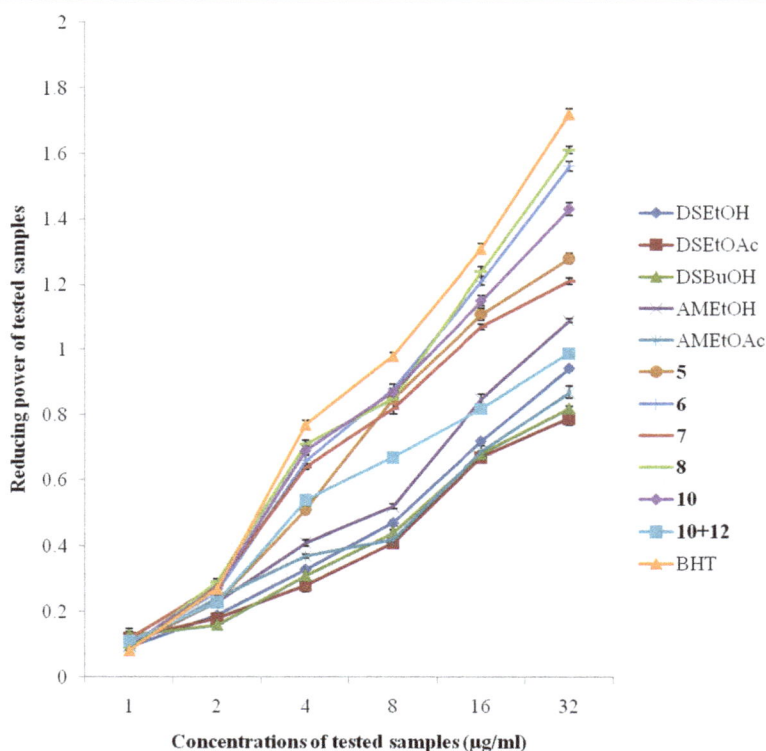

Fig. 2 Reducing power activities of the tested samples as well as butylated hydroxytoluene (BHT). Results represent the mean ± standard deviation of the triplicate reducing power at each concentration. Compounds **1–2**, **11** and **14** were not tested; compounds **3–4**, **9** and **13** were not active; DSEtOH = *D. senegambiensis* EtOH extract; DSEtOAc = *D. senegambiensis* EtOAc extract; DSBuOH = *D. senegambiensis* *n*-BuOH extract; AMEtOH = *A. monticola* EtOH extract; AMEtOAc = *A. monticola* EtOAc extract

≤2048 μg/mL; weakly active if MIC > 2048 μg/mL and not active when MIC > 10 mg/mL [40]. Hence, the EtOH extract of *D. senegambiensis* was highly active (MIC < 100 μg/mL) against *S. aureus* MSSA1; significantly active (100 ≤ MIC ≤512 μg/mL) against *S. aureus* ATCC25923, *S. aureus* MRSA3, *S. aureus* MRSA4 and *C. neoformans*; moderately active (512 < MIC ≤2048 μg/mL) on *C. albicans* and *C. tropicalis*. The antibacterial and antifungal activities of extracts support the use of *D. senegambiensis* and *A. monticola* in traditional medicine for the treatment of microbial infections.

Antimicrobial cutoff points have been defined in the literature to enable the understanding of the potential of pure compounds as follows: highly active: MIC below 1 μg/mL (or 2.5 μM), significantly active: 1 ≤ MIC ≤10 μg/mL (or 2.5 ≤ MIC < 25 μM), moderately active: 10 < MIC ≤100 μg/mL (or 25 < MIC ≤250 μM), low activity: 100 < MIC ≤1000 μg/mL (or 250 < MIC ≤2500 μM and not active: MIC > 1000 μg/mL (or > 2500 μM) [40]. Based on this, most of the antimicrobial activities of the tested triterpenoid and phenolic derivatives could be considered as significant, moderate and weak depending on the sensitive microorganisms.

As mentioned previously, triterpenes are known to display significant antimicrobial properties [41–43]. With this in mind, we examined the inhibitory activity of compounds **3**, **4**, **9** and **13** against *S. aureus* and yeast strains. Although the isolated triterpenoid derivatives did not display any significant antimicrobial activity, these compounds showed some moderate and weak anti-staphylococcal activity as well as weak antifungal activity against *C. albicans*, *C. tropicalis* and *C. neoformans*. Generally, compounds **7**, **10** and the mixture of **10 + 12** showed prominent activity against methicillin-resistant *S. aureus* MRSA3 and MRSA4 and other microbes. Although the test compounds were not as active as the standard drugs, ciprofloxacin and nystatin, these compounds may be employed in situations where there is resistance to anti-staphylococcal drugs. Compounds **7** and **10** are therefore the lead candidates in the search for antimicrobial agents.

From the structure-activity-relationship point of view, compounds **4**, **5** and **6** with the same basic skeleton, have the sugar moieties which should be responsible for the differences in their activity. The difference in the antimicrobial activity of compounds **7** and **10** suggests that the contribution of electron-

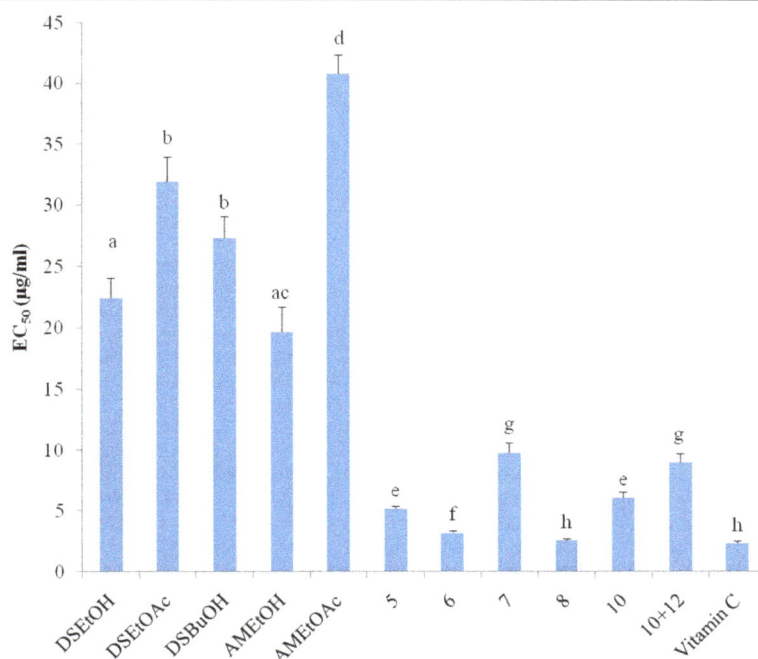

Fig. 3 Equivalent concentrations of tested samples scavenging 50% of DPPH radical (EC_{50}). Results represent the mean ± standard deviation of the triplicate EC_{50} of each sample. Letters a - h indicate significant differences between samples according to one way ANOVA and Waller Duncan test; $p < 0.05$. Compounds **1–2**, **11** and **14** were not tested; compounds **3–4**, **9** and **13** were not active; DSEtOH = *D. senegambiensis* EtOH extract; DSEtOAc = *D. senegambiensis* EtOAc extract; DSBuOH = *D. senegambiensis* n-BuOH extract; AMEtOH = *A. monticola* EtOH extract; AMEtOAc = *A. monticola* EtOAc extract

donating groups (-OH and −OCH$_3$) is remarkable in influencing the activity. The antimicrobial activities of purified phenolic derivatives corroborate with those of the early reports against bacteria and fungi [5, 26, 44]. The antimicrobial inhibitory mechanisms of phenolic compounds found active in this study, may be due to iron deprivation or hydrogen bounding with vital proteins such as microbial enzymes [45]. Lipophilic flavonoids may disrupt microbial membranes whereas terpenes may have the ability to disrupt microbial membrane and this may explain their antimicrobial properties [46].

Reducing power is associated with antioxidant activity and may serve as a significant reflection of the antioxidant activity [47]. In this study, the crude extracts, fractions and isolated compounds from *D. senegambiensis* and *A. monticola* exhibited concentration-dependent reducing power. The reducing capacity of extracts is much related to the presence of biologically active compounds (phenols) with potent donating abilities [48]. The antioxidant potential of each extract/compound was also measured using the change in its absorbance of decolourized DPPH free-radical as it accepts electrons from the antioxidant-rich samples. A free radical is a species capable of independent existence that contains one or more unpaired electrons. Free radicals contribute to the elimination of infected cells, but they can also react with

cellular DNA or other macromolecules, either damaging them directly or setting in motion a chain reaction resulting in extensive damage of cellular structures [49]. The present study showed that the free radical scavenging activity of *D. senegambiensis* and *A. monticola* is due to the presence of antioxidant-rich compounds like phenolic derivatives. Indeed, phenolic compounds are known to be potential antioxidants due to their ability to scavenge free radicals and active oxygen species such as singlet oxygen, superoxide anion and hydroxyl radicals [50]. Hence, the presence of such compounds could explain the antioxidant activity found in the studied plant extracts. The results of the antioxidant study show that extracts from *D. senegambiensis* and *A. monticola* as well as compounds **5–8, 10** and mixture of **10 + 12** may have great relevance in the prevention and therapies of diseases in which oxidants or free radicals are implicated.

Conclusions

The phytochemical study of the EtOH extracts from the studied plant species afforded fourteen triterpenoid and phenolic derivatives. Compounds obtained from *D. senegambiensis* are β-amyrin palmitate (**1**), α-amyrin acetate (**2**), ursolic acid (**3**), sitosterol-3-O-β-D-glucopyranoside (**4**); vitexin (**5**) and *trans*-tiliroside (**6**). Ursolic acid (**3**), sitosterol-3-O-β-D-glucopyranoside (**4**), 3,4′-di-O-methylellagic acid

(7), dimethyl 4,4′,5,5′,6,6′-hexahydroxybiphenyl-2,2′-dicarboxylate (8), lupeol (9), ellagic acid (10), 3-hydroxy-4,5-dimethoxybenzoic acid (11), 3-*O*-methylellagic acid 4′-*O*-β-D-xylopyranoside (12), oleanolic acid (13), and amphiblemmone A (14) were isolated from *A. monticola*. The present study revealed the potential of *D. senegambiensis* and *A. monticola* as well as the most active compounds (7, 8 and 10) in the search for new antimicrobial and antioxidant agents. So, further investigations are needed.

Abbreviations
13C-NMR: Carbon thirteen Nuclear Magnetic Resonance; *1H NMR*: Proton Nuclear Magnetic Resonance; *AMEtOAc*: *A. monticola* EtOAc extract; *AMEtOH*: *A. monticola* EtOH extract; *ATCC*: American Type Culture Collection; *CC*: column chromatography; *DMSO*: Dimethylsulfoxide; *DSBuOH*: *D. senegambiensis* n-BuOH extract; *DSEtOAc*: *D. senegambiensis* EtOAc extract; *DSEtOH*: *D. senegambiensis* EtOH extract; *EtOAc*: Ethyl acetate; *EtOH*: Ethanol; *HNC*: Herbier National du Cameroun; *IR*: Infra-red; *MBC*: Minimum bactericidal concentration; *MFC*: Minimum fungicidal concentration; *MHA*: Mueller Hinton agar; *MHB*: Mueller Hinton broth; *MIC*: Minimum inhibitory concentration; *MMC*: Minimum Microbicidal Concentrations; *MS*: Mass Spectrometry; *NA*: Nutrient agar; *n-BuOH*: n-Butanol; *NMR*: Nuclear Magnetic Resonance; *SDA*: Sabouraud Dextrose Agar; *SDB*: Sabouraud Dextrose Broth; *SRF/CAM*: Section de réserve forestière du Cameroun; *TLC*: Thin Layer Chromatography; *UV*: Ultra-violet

Acknowledgements
Authors are also thankful to the Institute of Medical Mycology, Teikyo University in Japan for providing some clinical bacteria and fungi.

Funding
The authors gratefully acknowledge financial support from the research grant committees of both the University of Dschang and the Cameroonian Ministry of Higher Education. They also thank TWAS-UNESCO for a 6 months research grant at ICCBS, University of Pakistan to one of them (Ndjateu, F.S.T.). We are also grateful to the Japan Society for the promotion of science for postdoctoral fellowship awarded to Dr. M. D. Awouafack as an overseas researcher to work at the Institute of Natural Medicine, University of Toyama.

Authors' contributions
RTN, FSTN and MDA carried out the chemical part; SEE and JAMF did the biological part; MT, PT, HM and MIC contributed to structural elucidation and supervised the chemical part; JDT designed the experiments, supervised the biological part and helped in manuscript writing and editing; all authors read and approved the final manuscript.

Competing interests
The authors declare that they have no competing interests.

Author details
[1]Laboratory of Natural Products Chemistry, Department of Chemistry, Faculty of Science, University of Dschang, P.O. Box 67, Dschang, Cameroon. [2]Laboratory of Microbiology and Antimicrobial substances, Department of Biochemistry, Faculty of Science, University of Dschang, P.O. Box 67, Dschang, Cameroon. [3]Institute of Natural Medicine, University of Toyama, 2630-Sugitani, Toyama 930-0194, Japan. [4]H.E.J Research Institute of Chemistry, University of Karachi, -75270, Karachi, Pakistan.

References
1. Iwu MM, Duncan AR, Okunji CO. New antimicrobials of plant origin. In: Janick J, editor. Perspectives on new crops and new uses. Alexandria: ASHS Press; 1999.
2. Mahady GB, Huang Y, Doyle BJ, Locklear T. Natural products as antibacterial agents. Nat Prod Chem. 2008;35:423–44.
3. Tatsimo NSJ, Tamokou JD, Lamshöft M, Mouafo TF, Lannang MA, Sarkar P, et al. LC-MS guided isolation of antibacterial and cytotoxic constituents from *Clausena anisata*. Med Chem Res. 2015;24(4):1468–79.
4. Pagning NAL, Tamokou JD, Lateef M, Tapondjou AL, Kuiate JR, Ngnokam D, et al. New triterpene and new flavone glucoside from *Rhynchospora corymbosa* (Cyperaceae) with their antimicrobial, tyrosinase and butyrylcholinesterase inhibitory activities. Phytochem Lett. 2016;16(1):121–8.
5. Tebou PLF, Tamokou JD, Ngnokam D, Voutquenne-Nazabadioko L, Kuiate JR, Bag PK. Flavonoids from *Maytenus buchananii* as potential cholera chemotherapeutic agents. South Afri J Bot. 2017;109:58–65.
6. Loigier HA. Descriptive flora of Puerto Rico and adjacent islands, Spermatophyta: Cyrillaceae to Myrtaceae, vol 3. Puerto Rico: University of Puerto Rico Press; 1994, p 462.
7. Maluma V. Les *antherotomadissotis* (inl. *heterotis*), Melastomataceae endémiques d'Afrique Centrale. Revue de Taxonomie et de Nomenclature Botaniques; 2005. p. 1–18.
8. Tchebemou BB, Nganso DYO, Soh D, Zondegoumba NTE, Toghueo KRM, Sidjui SL, et al. Chemical constituents of *Dissotis perkinsiae* (Melastomaceae) and their antimicrobial activity. J Appl Pharm Sci. 2016;6:96–101.
9. Bellakhdar J. La pharmacopée Marocaine traditionnelle: Médecine arabe ancienne et savoirs populaires, vol. 1. Paris-Rabat: Ibis Press-Eds Le Fennec; 1997. p 764.
10. Cheek M, Woodgyer EM. New data on *Amphiblemma monticola* Jacq.-Fél. (Melastomataceae) from western Cameroon. Kew Bull. 2006;61:601–4.
11. Jacques-Félix H. Le genre *Amphiblemma* Naud.(Melastomatacées). Adansonia. 1973;2:429–59.
12. Jacques-Félix H. Un *Amphiblemma* (Melastomataceae) nouveau du Cameroun. Bulletin du Muséum National d'Histoire Naturelle, Section B. Adansonia. 1987;9:125–7.
13. Ndjateu FST, Tene M, Tane P, Choudhary MI. A new C-methyl isoflavone and other compounds from the roots of *Amphiblemma monticola* (Melastomataceae). Nat Prod Commun. 2017;12:1731–2.
14. Calderon AI, Terreaux C, Schenk K, Pattison P, Burdette JE, Pezzuto JM, et al. Isolation and structure elucidation of an isoflavone and a sesterterpenoic acid from *Henriettella fascicularis*. J Nat Prod. 2002;12:1749–53.
15. Zhang Z, Elsohly HN, Li XC, Khan SI, Broedel SE Jr, Raulli RE, et al. Flavanone glycosides from *Miconia trailli*. J Nat Prod. 2003;66:39–41.
16. Ndjateu FST, Tsafack RBN, Nganou BK, Awouafack MD, Wabo HK, Tene M, et al. Antimicrobial and antioxidant activities of extracts and ten compounds from three Cameroonian medicinal plants: *Dissotis perkinsiae* (Melastomataceae), *Adenocarpus mannii* (Fabaceae) and *Barteria fistulosa* (Passifloraceae). South Afri J Bot. 2014;91:37–42.
17. Nono RN, Barboni L, Teponno RB, Quassinti L, Bramucci M, Vitali LA, et al. Antimicrobial, antioxidant, anti-inflammatory activities and phytoconstituents of extracts from the roots of *Dissotis thollonii* Cogn. (Melastomataceae). South Afri J Bot. 2014;93:19–26.
18. Serna DM, Martinez JH. Phenolics and polyphenolics from Melastomataceae species. Molecules. 2015;20:17818–47.
19. Evans WC. Trease and Evans Pharmacognosy. 13th ed. Traiadal, London: Bailere; 1989.
20. Harborne JB. Phytochemical methods: a guide to modern techniques of plant analysis. 2nd ed. London: Chapman and Hall Publishers; 1998.
21. Tiwari P, Kumar B, Kaur M, Kaur G, Kaur H. Phytochemical screening and extraction: a review. Int Pharm Sci. 2011;1:98–106.
22. Banu S, Cathrine L. General techniques involved in phytochemical analysis. Int J Adv Res Chem Sci. 2015;2:25–32.
23. Tsemeugne J, Sopbué FE, Tamokou JD, Tonle I, Kengne IC, Ngongang DA, et al. Electrochemical behavior and *in vitro* antimicrobial screening of some thienylazoaryls dyes. Chem Cent J. 2017;11:119.
24. Tamokou JD, Tala FM, Wabo KH, Kuiate JR, Tane P. Antimicrobial activities of methanol extract and compounds from stem bark of *Vismia rubescens*. J Ethnopharmacol. 2009;124:571–5.
25. Padmaja M, Sravanthi M, Hemalatha KPJ. Evaluation of antioxidant activity of two Indian medicinal plants. J phytol. 2011;3:86–91.
26. Djouossi MG, Tamokou JD, Ngnokam D, Kuiate JR, Tapondjou AL, Harakat D, et al. Antimicrobial and antioxidant flavonoids from the leaves of *Oncoba spinosa* Forssk. (Salicaceae). BMC Compl Altern Med. 2015;15:134.
27. Situ H, Bobek LA. *In vitro* assessment of antifungal therapeutic potential of salivary histatin-5, two variants of histatin-5, and salivary mucin (MUC7) domain 1. Antimicrob Agents Chemother. 2000;44:1485–93.

Antimicrobial and antioxidant activities of triterpenoid and phenolic derivatives from two Cameroonian...

57

28. Marizeth LB, Jorge MD, Pedro Ade PP, Maria LSG, Juceni PD. Fatty acid esters of triterpenes from *Erythroxylum passerinum*. J Braz Chem Soc. 2002; 13:669–73.

29. Nkeoma NO, Daniel LA, Henry NO, Emmanuel EI, Chukwuemeka SN, Festus BCO. Beta-Amyrin and alpha-amyrin acetate isolated from the stem bark of *Alstonia boonei* display profound anti-inflammatory activity. Pharm Biol. 2014;52:1478–86.

30. Seebacher W, Simic N, Weis R, Saf R, Kunert O. Complete assignments of ^{1}H and ^{13}C NMR resonances of oleanolic acid, 18α-oleanolic acid, ursolic acid and their 11- oxo derivatives. Magn Reson Chem. 2003;41:636–8.

31. Tene M, Tane P, Tamokou JD, Kuiate JR, Connolly JD. Degraded diterpenoids from the stem bark of *Neoboutonia mannii*. Phytochem Lett. 2008;1:120–4.

32. Ping W, Huiying H, Ruwei W, Naili W, Xinsheng Y. C glycosylfavones and aromatic glycosides from *Campylotropis hirtella* (Franch.) Schindl. Asian J Trad Med. 2007;2:149–53.

33. Timmers M, Urban S. On-line (HPLC-NMR) and off-line phytochemical profiling of the Australian plant Lasiopetalum macrophyllum. Nat Prod Commun. 2011;7:551–60.

34. Zhang F, Fu T-J, Peng S-L, Liu Z-R, Ding L-S. Two new triterpenoids from the roots of *Sanguisorba officinalis* L. J Integr Plant Biol. 2005;47:251–6.

35. Alam A, Takaguchi Y, Tsuboi S. Synthesis of ellagic acid and its 4,4'-di-O-alkyl derivatives from gallic acid. J Fac environ Sci Technol. Okayama University. 2005;10:111–7.

36. Wang C-M, Chen H-T, Wu Z-Y, Jhan Y-L, Shyu C-L, Chou C-H. Antibacterial and synergistic activity of pentacyclic triterpenoids isolated from *Alstonia scholaris*. Molecules. 2016;21(2):139.

37. Brown BR, Brown PE, Pike WT. The leaf tannin of willow-herb [*Chamaenerion angustifolium* (L.) Scop.]. Biochem J. 1966;100:733–8.

38. Yang X-H, Guo Y-W. Two new ellagic acid glycosides from leaves of *Diplopanax stachyanthus*. J Asian Nat Prod Res. 2004;6:271–6.

39. Reuben KD, Abdulrahman FI, Akan JC, Usman H, Sodipo OA, Egwu GO. Phytochemical screening and *in vitro* antimicrobial investigation of the methanolic extract of *Croton Zambesicus* Muell ARG. Stem bark. Eur J Sci Res. 2008;23(1):134–40.

40. Tamokou JD, Mbaveng TA, Kuete V. Antimicrobial activities of African medicinal spices and vegetables. In: Medicinal spices and vegetables from Africa: therapeutic potential against metabolic, inflammatory, infectious and systemic diseases. 1st ed: Elsevier; 2017, Chapter 8. p. 207–37.

41. Tene M, Ndontsa LB, Tane P, Tamokou JD, Kuiate JR. Antimicrobial diterpenoids and triterpenoids from the stem bark of *Croton macrostachys*. Int J Biol Chem Sci. 2009;3:538–44.

42. Chouna JR, Tamokou JD, Nkeng-Efouet-Alango P, Lenta NB, Sewald N. Antimicrobial triterpenes from the stem bark of *Crossopteryx febrifuga*. Zeitschrift für Naturforschung C. 2015;70(7–8):c:169–73.

43. Catteau L, Zhu L, Van Bambeke F, Quetin-Leclercq J. Natural and hemi-synthetic pentacyclic triterpenes as antimicrobials and resistance modifying agents against *Staphylococcus aureus*: a review. Phytochem Rev 2018. https://doi.org/10.1007/s11101-018-9564-2.

44. Tatsimo NSJ, Tamokou JD, Havyarimana L, Dezso C, Forgo P, Hohmann J, et al. Antimicrobial and antioxidant activity of kaempferol rhamnoside derivatives from Bryophyllum pinnatum. BMC Res Notes. 2012;5:158.

45. Scalbert A. Antimicrobial properties of tannins. Phytochemistry. 1991;30:3875–83.

46. Cowan MM. Plant products as antimicrobial agents. Clin Microbiol Rev. 1999;12:564–82.

47. Olayinka AA, Anthony IO. Preliminary phytochemical screening and *in vitro* antioxidant activities of the aqueous extract of *Helichrysum longifolium* DC. BMC Complement Altern Med. 2010;10:21.

48. Li Y, Guo C, Yang J, Wei J, Xu J, Cheng S. Evaluation of antioxidant properties of pomegranate peel extract in comparison with pomegranate pulp extract. Food Chem. 2006;96(2):254–60.

49. Karou D, Nadembega WMC, Ouattara L, Ilboudo DP, Canini A, Nikiéma JB, et al. African ethnopharmacology and new drug discovery. Med Aromat Plant Sci Biotechnol. 2007;1(1):1–9.

50. Pietta P, Sionetti P, Mauri P. Antioxidant activity of selected medicinal plants. J Agric Food Chem. 1998;46:4487–90.

7

Epigallocatechin gallate inhibits hepatitis B virus infection in human liver chimeric mice

Yu-Heng Lai[1], Cheng-Pu Sun[2], Hsiu-Chen Huang[3], Jui-Chieh Chen[4], Hui-Kang Liu[5,6] and Cheng Huang[7,8*] (iD)

Abstract

Background: Persistent hepatitis B virus (HBV) infection causes liver cirrhosis and hepatocellular carcinoma and constitutes a major worldwide health problem. Currently, anti-HBV drugs are limited to peginterferon and nucleos(t)ide analogs, which are costly and have considerable side effects; the development of novel, effective anti-HBV agents is crucial.

Methods: Catechins are a major group of compounds found in green tea extract and epigallocatechin gallate (EGCG) has been shown to have antiviral properties, including inhibition of cellular entry by HBV. FRG (Fah$^{-/-}$/ Rag2$^{-/-}$/ IL-2Rγ^{-}) mice were used in this study to generate chimeras carrying human primary hepatocytes, to facilitate investigation of the inhibitory effect of EGCG on HBV infection.

Results: Here, we show the inhibitory effect of EGCG on HBV infection and replication in HuS-E/2 cells. The inhibitory effect of EGCG on HBV infection in vivo was confirmed by monitoring HBV DNA and HBsAg in serum and immunostaining the liver tissues of the human liver chimeric mice.

Conclusions: The effects of EGCG suggest a robust strategy for the treatment of HBV infection and EGCG may have therapeutic potential for the treatment of HBV-associated liver diseases.

Keywords: Hepatitis B virus, EGCG, HBsAg, Human liver chimeric mice

Background

Hepatitis B virus (HBV) infection is a major cause of acute and chronic viral hepatitis in humans, with the risk of development of cirrhosis and hepatocellular carcinoma (HCC) [1]. Today, approximately 350 million individuals are chronically infected, despite of the availability of an effective vaccine for more than 25 years [2]. There is an approximately 100-fold greater relative risk of HCC among HBV carriers than non-carriers [2]. However, many HBV-infected patients have not been treated with antiviral drugs, including interferon-alpha and nucleotide analogues that inhibit the viral reverse transcriptase, because of the adverse side effects and

development of drug resistance, as well as the high cost of treatment [3]. Therefore, it is crucial to develop safe and effective, as well as affordable, anti-HBV agents that inhibit viral replication and improve the clinical outcome of HBV patients.

HBV is a small DNA virus with a nucleocapsid that protects the 3.2 kb genome [4]. The nucleocapsid is surrounded by an envelope, which contains three types of hepatitis B surface antigen (HBsAg), the small (S), medium (M) and large (L) forms, with distinct functions [5]. These proteins are encoded by one open reading frame, with three in-phase start codons. The M form of HBsAg (MHBsAg) has a hydrophilic, 55 amino acids (aa) N-terminal extension of the S domain, known as the pre-S2 domain [6]. The L form of HBsAg (LHBsAg) contains the pre-S1 domain, which extends from the pre-S2 domain for another 108 or 119 aa, dependent on the genotype [6]. The LHBsAg protein plays pivotal roles in the viral entry process [7, 8] and, recently, sodium

* Correspondence: chengh@ym.edu.tw
[7]Department of Biotechnology and Laboratory Science in Medicine, National Yang-Ming University, No. 155, Sec. 2, Linong St., Beitou District, Taipei 11221, Taiwan
[8]Department of Earth and Life Sciences, University of Taipei, Taipei 11153, Taiwan
Full list of author information is available at the end of the article

taurocholate cotransporting polypeptide (NTCP) was identified as an HBV receptor [9, 10]. Viral entry begins with binding of the externally exposed region of LHBsAg to NTCP [11] . Entry of HBV into uninfected hepatocytes has long been proposed as a potential target for antiviral intervention [12].

In a previous study, we used immortalized human primary hepatocytes, HuS-E/2 cells, as a model to screen for natural, bioactive compounds against HBV infection [13]. We also found that epigallocatechin gallate (EGCG), a flavonoid that belongs to the subclass of catechins and is present in green tea extract, has antiviral and anti-oncogenic properties [14–16] and is able to inhibit HBV entry and contribute to decreased HBV replication in vitro [17]. In this study, we show that EGCG represses the infection of HBV in HuS-E/2 cells.

Fumacrylacetoacetate (Fah) is an enzyme involved in tyrosine metabolism. Fah-deficient mice develop hypoglycemia and liver dysfunction due to the toxicity of accumulated metabolites [18]. In addition, along with the recombination-activating gene2 and IL-2 receptor knock-out (KO) mice that have disrupted immune development, triple KO mice were generated to engraft human cells in a chimeric model. Previously, FRG (Fah$^{-/-}$/ Rag2$^{-/-}$/ IL-2R$\gamma^{/-}$) mice have been used to generate chimeras carrying human primary hepatocytes. The FRG mouse is well-established and has been used for research into viral liver-associated diseases, providing a solid platform for human hepatic xenorepopulation [19, 20]. These robust primary hepatocytes have replaced the traditional immortal hepatoma cells or hepatoblasts as a research model, with their viability and differentiation status [20]. Therefore, the human chimeric mouse model of HBV infection is crucial for analyzing EGCG dosage and the timing of treatment. To sum up, our study shows potential to predict prognosis in the clinical setting and the accessibility of the therapeutic effects of EGCG in human patients. This suggests a robust strategy for therapeutic intervention in HBV infection in order to treat the associated liver diseases.

Methods
Cell culture
HuS-E/2 [21], and HepG2.2.15 cells (RRID:CVCL_L855), which stably express the HBV genome, were maintained in Dulbecco's modified Eagle's medium supplemented with 10% heat-inactivated fetal calf serum and 100 U/ml of penicillin and 100 µg/ml of streptomycin (Gibco). Both HuS-E/2 and HepG2.2.15 cells were cultured at 37 °C in the presence of 5% CO2.

For HBV infection, HuS-E/2 cells were differentiated by incubation with 2% DMSO for 10 days, as described previously [13].

HBV infection of cell cultures
HBV infection experiments were performed as described previously [13]. Briefly, HBV particles were isolated and concentrated from HepG2.2.15 cells. Differentiated HuS-E/2 cells were incubated for 20 h with purified HBV at a multiplicity of infection (MOI) of 10, in the presence of 0, 10, or 20 µM EGCG or DMSO as control, then the HBV and EGCG were removed and the culture medium was changed every 3 days for 7 days.

DNA and RNA isolation, reverse transcription and real-time PCR
Total DNA was extracted with a Genomic DNA isolation kit (Nexttec Biotechnologie, Germany). Total RNA was isolated from cultured cells using TRIzol® reagent (Invitrogen). Reverse transcription was performed with the RNA templates, AMV reverse transcriptase (Roche), and oligo-dT primer. The products were subjected to real-time PCR with primer sets of specific genes and SYBR Green PCR Master Mix (Bio-Rad). The primer sets used for HBV core, HBsAg, cccDNA and GAPDH were described previously [13]. The results were analyzed with the iCycler iQ real-time PCR detection system (Bio-Rad). Plasmid p1.3HBcl was prepared at 10-fold dilutions ($2*10^4$–$2*10^9$ copies/ml) to generate a standard curve in parallel PCR reactions.

Animals
Eleven 8-week-old female FRG (Fah$^{-/-}$/ Rag2$^{-/-}$/ IL-2Rg$^{/-}$) mice were housed at room temperature with controlled humidity and on a 12 h/12 h light/dark cycle (lights on at 7.00 a.m.) at the Animal Center of the Academia Sinica, Taipei, Taiwan. The weight reached to 25 g in average at 8 weeks old. The food applied was Picolab Rodent Diet 20 (Lab Supply, Inc). Mice were housed in groups using high quality wood pellet hygienic litter bedding (Lignocel HBK 1500–3000, Rettenmaier & Sönne, Germany). Epigallocatechin gallate (EGCE) was injected through the tail vein. Blood was taken from the inferior vena cava during deep anesthesis. The use of animals for this research was approved by the Animal Research Committee of the Academia Sinica and all procedures followed The Guide for the Care and Use of Laboratory Animals (NIH publication, 85–23, revised 1996) and the guidelines of the Animal Welfare Act, Taiwan. On the day of sacrifice, a laparotomy was performed under ketamine and xylazine anesthesia (intramuscular injection of 100 mg/kg body mass and 5 mg/kg body mass, respectively), and whole-blood samples were collected via cardiac puncture.

Generation of human liver chimeric (Hu-FRG) mice
To generate human liver chimeric (Hu-FRG) mice, cryo-preserved human hepatocytes were purchased from

BD Biosciences (San Jose, CA, USA) and CellzDirect/Invitrogen (Durham, NC, USA). FRG (Fah$^{-/-}$/ Rag2$^{-/-}$/ IL-2R$\gamma^{/-}$) mice were transplanted as described previously, except for adopting a protocol of gradually decreasing NTBC in the drinking water [19]. One million viable hepatocytes in 200 μl of William's E medium (Invitrogen Life Technologies, Carlsbad, CA, USA) were injected intrasplenically via a 27-gauge needle. The transplanted mice were given plain water after surgery. To monitor the transplantation rate of human hepatocytes, small amounts of blood were collected monthly from the tail veins of Hu-FRG mice and the serum human albumin (hAlb) levels were determined using a Human Albumin ELISA Quantitation Set (Bethyl Laboratories, Montgomery, TX, USA) according to the manufacturer's protocol. It takes about 4 months to reach human serum albumin concentration of ≥1 mg/mL. Total eleven mice were transplanted and six Hu-FRG mice with human serum albumin concentrations of ≥1 mg/mL were selected for use in the HBV infection studies.

HBV infection of Hu-FRG mice

The Hu-FRG mice were subsequently divided randomly into two groups (HBV, $n = 3$, and HBV + EGCG, $n = 3$). (−)-Eepigallocatechin-3-gallate (EGCG) (≥97.0%, HPLC grade) was purchased from Sigma-Aldrich. An inoculum of $5*10^7$ copies of HBV was injected intraperitoneally on day 1. The mice were injected intravenously with EGCG diluted in sterile saline at a concentration of 10 mg/mL (50 μL/10 g body weight). Injections (50 mg/kg) of EGCG were given twice a day on days 1 to 5 (Fig. 3).

Serological analysis and tissue characterization of Hu-FRG liver chimerism

After HBV infection, mice were sacrificed at week 4 for serological and intrahepatic analyses. Liver specimens were removed during sacrifice and were snap-frozen in liquid nitrogen for further histological and molecular analyses. Serum HBV DNA was quantified by realtime-qPCR at weeks 2 and 4. Serum HBsAg levels were determined by ELISA Quantitation Set (Bio-Rad Laboratories) according to the manufacturer's protocol. To stain human hepatocytes, cryostat sections of chimeric mouse livers were immunostained with human Fah antibodies (Cell Signaling) and polyclonal rabbit anti-HBcAg (Abcam) to detect HBV core antigen (HBcAg). Briefly, the liver sections were incubated with Fah and HBcAg antibodies at 4 °C overnight, then followed by Alexa488-conjugated goat IgG and Alexa594-conjugated goat IgG at 37 °C for 1 h. Hoechst 33258 (Sigma-Aldrich) was used along with the secondary antibody to detect nucleus. The immunostained samples were detected by Leica DM6000B microscope.

Statistical analysis

All values are expressed as mean ± SE. Each value is the mean of at least three animals in each group in vivo experiments. Student's t-test was used for statistical comparison. * indicates that the values are significantly different from the control (*, $p < 0.05$; **, $P < 0.01$; ***, $P ≤ 0.001$.).

Results

Inhibitory effect of EGCG on HBV infection

To evaluate the effects of EGCG on HBV infectivity and replication, HuS-E/2 cells were infected with HBV derived from HepG2.2.15 cells in the presence of EGCG. The replication efficiency was determined by measuring rcDNA and RNA by PCR and RT-PCR, respectively. EGCG treatment during infection resulted in a dose-dependent decrease of HBV rcDNA (Fig. 1a) and HBsAg mRNA (Fig. 1b) in HuS-E/2 cells. In addition, when the cells were treated with 10 μM EGCG, HBV mRNA levels were reduced by 80% compared to control cells. The half-maximal inhibitory concentration (IC$_{50}$) was estimated to be below 10 μM. Taken together, these results suggest that HBV infection is inhibited by EGCG treatment.

EGCG inhibited HBV infection in the Hu-FRG mouse model

To evaluate the EGCG-associated inhibition of HBV infection in vivo, we generated human liver chimeric

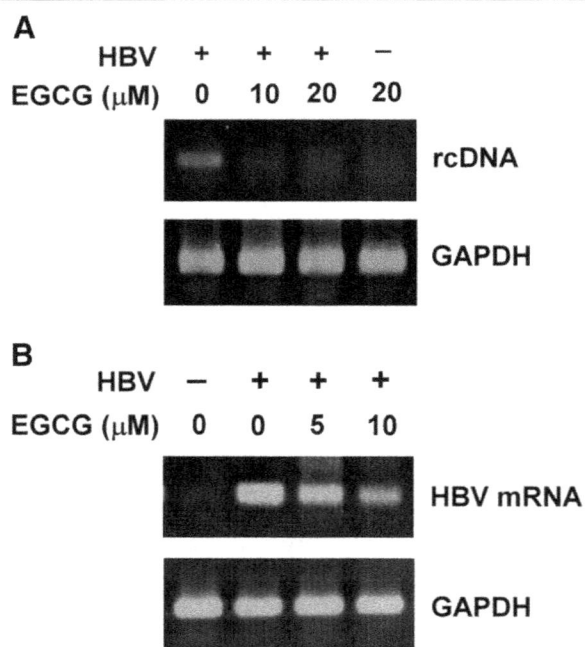

Fig. 1 EGCG inhibited HBV infection. DMSO-differentiated HuS-E/2 cells were infected with HBV for 20 h in the presence of EGCG and incubated for an additional 7 days. Nucleic acids were extracted from the cells and amplified to detect the presence of HBV rcDNA (**a**) and HBsAg mRNA (**b**), to evaluate the infection efficiency

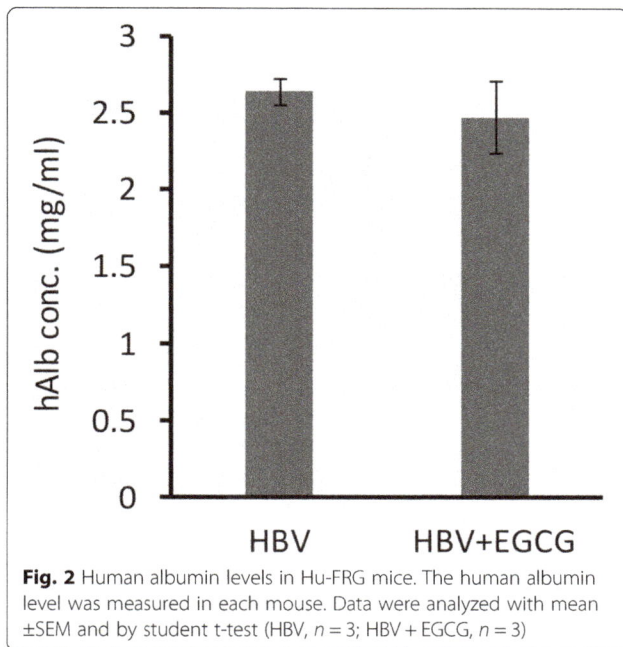

Fig. 2 Human albumin levels in Hu-FRG mice. The human albumin level was measured in each mouse. Data were analyzed with mean ±SEM and by student t-test (HBV, $n = 3$; HBV + EGCG, $n = 3$)

serum. Compared to the control group, the HBV DNA copy number was significantly lower ($p \leq 0.05$) after 4 weeks of treatment with EGCG and challenge with HBV (Fig. 4a). A marked reduction ($p \leq 0.01$) in HBsAg protein level by 70% was detected (Fig. 4b). These data suggest clearly that EGCG inhibits HBV infection in human liver chimeric mice.

EGCG inhibited expression of fah and HBcAg in the livers of human chimeric mice

Liver tissue from Hu-FRG chimeric mice was examined to detect HBV infection with/without EGCG treatment. The human Fah-expressing cells were successfully implanted in the mouse livers (Fig. 5) and the HBV infection was monitored by detecting hepatitis B core antigen (HBcAg) expression. We found that, when the mice were treated with EGCG, the levels of expression of HBcAg in the human cells were lower than in the mice without EGCG treatment. Therefore, based on the immunostaining of the liver tissue of the chimeric mice, we confirmed the inhibitory effect of EGCG on HBV infection.

Discussion

The major components of green tea, polyphenols, which are also known as catechins, have been shown to have a therapeutic effect on a myriad of diseases [22–24]. The catechins in green tea include epicatechin (ECG), epigallocatechin (EGC), epicatechin (EC), catechin (C) and epigallocatechin gallate (EGCG) and EGCG is

(Hu-FRG) mice. We measured the human serum albumin (hAlb) concentrations in the Hu-FRG mice and selected mice with ≥ 1 mg/mL hAlb for the HBV infection studies (Fig. 2). The scheme of EGCG treatment and Hu-FRG mice challenge schedule was shown in Fig. 3. Realtime-qPCR and ELISA assay were used to detect HBV DNA and HBsAg, respectively, in mice

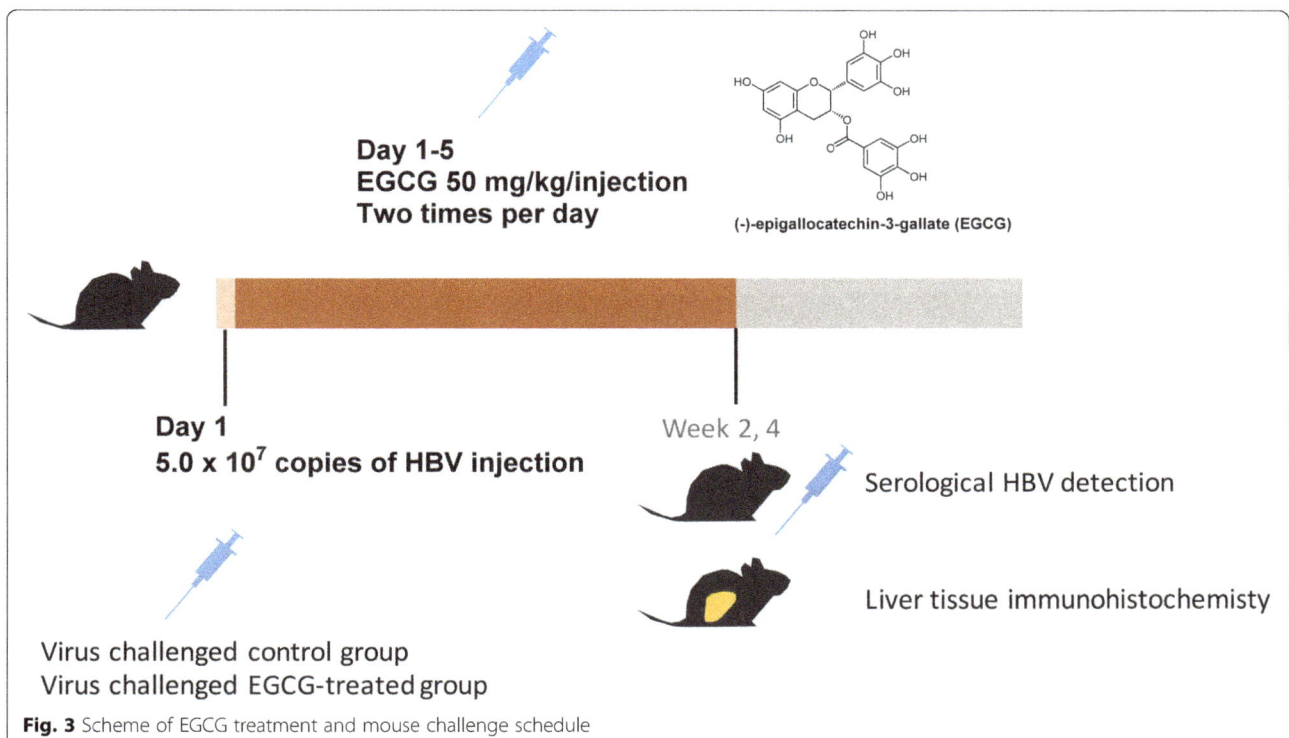

Fig. 3 Scheme of EGCG treatment and mouse challenge schedule

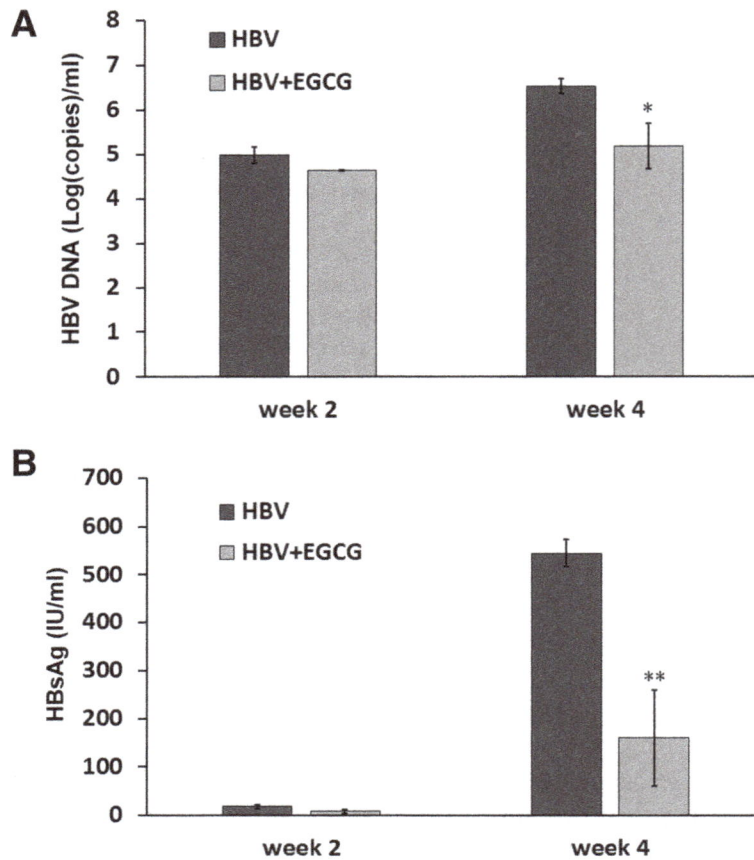

Fig. 4 HBV titers in Hu-FRG mice. HBV titers were determined as HBV DNA copies (**a**), and HBV HBsAg expression levels (**b**). The data are expressed with mean±SEM and were analyzed by student t-test (HBV, n=3; HBV+EGCG, n=3; * p <0.05, ** p <0.01).

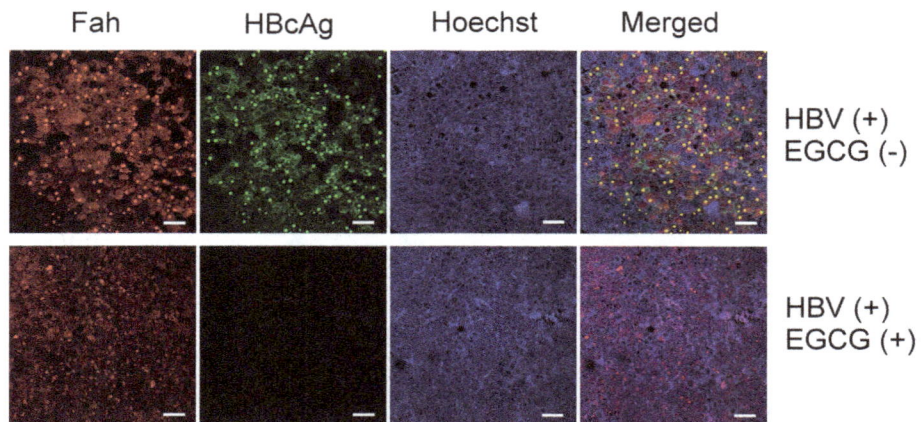

Fig. 5 Expression of Fah and HBcAg in the livers of human chimeric mice. Expression of Fah and HBcAg were examined by immunofluorescence staining with antibodies against Fah and HBcAg, followed by confocal microscopy. The bars on the images represent 100 μm

considered to be the most important in terms of its anti-viral effects through various mechanisms [14, 25]. A previous study by our team showed that EGCG induced clathrin-dependent endocytosis of NTCP and inhibited HBV entry in vitro [17]. In addition, EGCG has been shown to be an inhibitor of the viral serine protease involved in HCV entry [26]. The mechanism of inhibition by EGCG of cellular entry by herpes simplex virus (HSV) may be through disruption of the viral envelope [27]. Several pathways have been reported for the EGCG inhibitory effect on Epstein-Barr virus (EBV) infection, such as interference with the AP-1 pathway [28], reduction of the ability of the virus to bind to host DNA [29], degradation of viral RNA and down-regulation of viral lytic-associated signaling [30].

However, the methods used to elucidate the effects of EGCG were based on cultured cells, including primary human hepatocytes [31]. Therefore, after we confirmed and optimized the EGCG inhibitory efficiency in HuS-E/2 cells, we used a chimeric mouse model to investigate the effect of EGCG on HBV infection in vivo. Previously, an immunodeficient model, based on the urokinase-type plasminogen activator (uPA) mouse, was used for HBV and HCV research [32–34]. To solve the limitation of the uPA mouse model that had high mortality and was difficult to manipulate, the FRG-chimeric mouse model was developed [20]. In our study, we first generated Hu-FRG mice whose livers were repopulated with human hepatocytes. We showed the implantation was efficient by measuring the human albumin level, with no significant difference between the two groups (Fig. 2). Furthermore, we designed an HBV infection strategy and successfully challenged Hu-FRG mice with HBV during EGCG treatment (Fig. 3). Measurement of the HBV DNA copy number and HBsAg titer, as well as immunohistochemical analysis of the liver tissue, provided the solid evidence of inhibition of HBV infection by EGCG (Figs. 4 and 5).

Generally, the HBV DNA copy number exceeded 1.0×10^7 copies/ml 4 weeks after viral challenge in the control group, accompanied by a high titer of HBsAg. We compared the HBV DNA copy number and HBsAg concentration between the untreated and EGCG-treated groups of mice and saw little difference after 2 weeks but, critically, 4 weeks after infection, the HBV titers in the EGCG-treated mice were over 100 fold lower than the control group. To explain the time lag before viral inhibition was apparent, we hypothesized that either the increasing dosage or injection frequency of EGCG blocks HBV entry. We found, despite that the half-life of EGCG is approximately less than 1 h [35], the strategy we applied to boost EGCG was effective and stable enough to block HBV infection. The increasing dosage of EGCG would maintain the EGCG concentration in blood and overcome the degradation of EGCG due to its half-life, which make apparent the effect of EGCG in inhibiting HBV entry into the hepatocytes. Therefore, we may increase the dosage of EGCG in future experiments.

Conclusions

In the present study, the inhibitory effect of EGCG on HBV infection and replication was demonstrated in vitro. Further, it is clear that the use of the Hu-FRG chimeric mouse model to evaluate the inhibitory effect of EGCG was robust and EGCG may have therapeutic potential for the treatment of HBV-associated liver diseases.

Acknowledgments
We thank Dr. K. Shimotohno (Kyoto University, Japan) for providing HuS-E/2 cells, and Dr. Mi-Hua Tao (Academia Sinica, Taiwan) for providing human liver chimeric mice.

Funding
This work was supported by research grant MOST 104–2320-B-077-003- and MOST 106–2320-B-010-038- from the Ministry of Science and Technology, Taiwan.

Authors' contributions
YHL, CPS, and HCH carried out the experiments. JCC and HKL analyzed the data. CH wrote the paper. All authors read and approved the final manuscript.

Competing interests
The authors declare that they have no competing interest.

Author details
[1]Department of Chemistry, Chinese Culture University, Taipei 11114, Taiwan. [2]Institute of Biomedical Sciences, Academia Sinica, Taipei 11529, Taiwan. [3]Department of Applied Science, National Tsing Hua University South Campus, Hsinchu 30014, Taiwan. [4]Department of Biochemical Science and Technology, National Chiayi University, Chiayi 60004, Taiwan. [5]National Research Institute of Chinese Medicine, Ministry of Health and Welfare, Taipei 11221, Taiwan. [6]Program in Clinical Drug Development of Chinese Herbal Medicine, Taipei Medical University, Taipei 11001, Taiwan. [7]Department of Biotechnology and Laboratory Science in Medicine, National Yang-Ming University, No. 155, Sec. 2, Linong St., Beitou District, Taipei 11221, Taiwan. [8]Department of Earth and Life Sciences, University of Taipei, Taipei 11153, Taiwan.

References
1. Arbuthnot P, Kew M. Hepatitis B virus and hepatocellular carcinoma. Int J Exp Pathol. 2001;82(2):77–100.
2. Beasley RP. Hepatitis B virus. The major etiology of hepatocellular carcinoma. Cancer. 1988;61(10):1942–56.
3. Yang JG, et al. Epigallocatechin-3-gallate affects the growth of LNCaP cells via membrane fluidity and distribution of cellular zinc. J Zhejiang Univ Sci B. 2009;10(6):411–21.
4. Chen WN, Oon CJ. Human hepatitis B virus mutants: significance of molecular changes. FEBS Lett. 1999;453(3):237–42.

5. Mehta A, et al. Hepatitis B virus (HBV) envelope glycoproteins vary drastically in their sensitivity to glycan processing: evidence that alteration of a single N-linked glycosylation site can regulate HBV secretion. Proc Natl Acad Sci U S A. 1997;94(5):1822–7.

6. Ni Y, et al. The pre-s2 domain of the hepatitis B virus is dispensable for infectivity but serves a spacer function for L-protein-connected virus assembly. J Virol. 2010;84(8):3879–88.

7. Cooper A, Paran N, Shaul Y. The earliest steps in hepatitis B virus infection. Biochim Biophys Acta. 2003;1614(1):89–96.

8. De Meyer S, et al. Organ and species specificity of hepatitis B virus (HBV) infection: a review of literature with a special reference to preferential attachment of HBV to human hepatocytes. J Viral Hepat. 1997;4(3):145–53.

9. Yan H, et al. Sodium taurocholate cotransporting polypeptide is a functional receptor for human hepatitis B and D virus. Elife. 2012;1:e00049.

10. Watashi K, et al. NTCP and beyond: opening the door to unveil hepatitis B virus entry. Int J Mol Sci. 2014;15(2):2892–905.

11. Yan H, et al. Molecular determinants of hepatitis B and D virus entry restriction in mouse sodium taurocholate cotransporting polypeptide. J Virol. 2013;87(14):7977–91.

12. Gripon P, et al. Infection of a human hepatoma cell line by hepatitis B virus. Proc Natl Acad Sci U S A. 2002;99(24):15655–60.

13. Huang HC, et al. Entry of hepatitis B virus into immortalized human primary hepatocytes by clathrin-dependent endocytosis. J Virol. 2012;86(17):9443–53.

14. Song JM, Lee KH, Seong BL. Antiviral effect of catechins in green tea on influenza virus. Antivir Res. 2005;68(2):66–74.

15. Calland N, et al. (–)-Epigallocatechin-3-gallate is a new inhibitor of hepatitis C virus entry. Hepatology. 2012;55(3):720–9.

16. Isaacs CE, et al. Epigallocatechin gallate inactivates clinical isolates of herpes simplex virus. Antimicrob Agents Chemother. 2008;52(3):962–70.

17. Huang HC, et al. Epigallocatechin-3-gallate inhibits entry of hepatitis B virus into hepatocytes. Antivir Res. 2014;111:100–11.

18. Grompe M, al-Dhalimy M. Mutations of the fumarylacetoacetate hydrolase gene in four patients with tyrosinemia, type I. Hum Mutat. 1993;2(2):85–93.

19. Bissig KD, et al. Repopulation of adult and neonatal mice with human hepatocytes: a chimeric animal model. Proc Natl Acad Sci U S A. 2007; 104(51):20507–11.

20. Azuma H, et al. Robust expansion of human hepatocytes in fah–/–/Rag2 –/–/Il2rg–/– mice. Nat Biotechnol. 2007;25(8):903–10.

21. Aly HH, et al. Serum-derived hepatitis C virus infectivity in interferon regulatory factor-7-suppressed human primary hepatocytes. J Hepatol. 2007; 46(1):26–36.

22. Mak JC. Potential role of green tea catechins in various disease therapies: progress and promise. Clin Exp Pharmacol Physiol. 2012;39(3):265–73.

23. Chen XQ, et al. Preventive effects of Catechins on cardiovascular disease. Molecules. 2016;21(12)

24. Shirakami Y, et al. Catechins and its role in chronic diseases. Adv Exp Med Biol. 2016;929:67–90.

25. Ide K, et al. Anti-influenza virus effects of Catechins: a molecular and clinical review. Curr Med Chem. 2016;23(42):4773–83.

26. Zuo G, et al. Activity of compounds from Chinese herbal medicine Rhodiola kirilowii (regel) maxim against HCV NS3 serine protease. Antivir Res. 2007; 76(1):86–92.

27. Isaacs CE, et al. Digallate dimers of (–)-epigallocatechin gallate inactivate herpes simplex virus. Antimicrob Agents Chemother. 2011;55(12):5646–53.

28. Zhao Y, et al. Epigallocatechin-3-gallate interferes with EBV-encoding AP-1 signal transduction pathway. Zhonghua Zhong Liu Za Zhi. 2004;26(7):393–7.

29. Chen YL, Tsai HL, Peng CW. EGCG debilitates the persistence of EBV latency by reducing the DNA binding potency of nuclear antigen 1. Biochem Biophys Res Commun. 2012;417(3):1093–9.

30. Liu S, et al. (–)-Epigallocatechin-3-gallate inhibition of Epstein-Barr virus spontaneous lytic infection involves ERK1/2 and PI3-K/Akt signaling in EBV-positive cells. Carcinogenesis. 2013;34(3):627–37.

31. Verrier ER, Schuster C, Baumert TF. Advancing hepatitis B virus entry inhibitors. J Hepatol. 2017;66(4):677–9.

32. Heckel JL, et al. Neonatal bleeding in transgenic mice expressing urokinase-type plasminogen activator. Cell. 1990;62(3):447–56.

33. Dandri M, et al. Repopulation of mouse liver with human hepatocytes and in vivo infection with hepatitis B virus. Hepatology. 2001;33(4):981–8.

34. Mercer DF, et al. Hepatitis C virus replication in mice with chimeric human livers. Nat Med. 2001;7(8):927–33.

35. Xifro X, et al. Novel epigallocatechin-3-gallate (EGCG) derivative as a new therapeutic strategy for reducing neuropathic pain after chronic constriction nerve injury in mice. PLoS One. 2015;10(4):e0123122.

8

Astragalus membranaceus (Fisch.) Bunge repairs intestinal mucosal injury induced by LPS in mice

Yizhe Cui[†] [iD], Qiuju Wang[†], Rui Sun, Li Guo, Mengzhu Wang, Junfeng Jia, Chuang Xu[*] and Rui Wu[*]

Abstract

Background: *Astragalus membranaceus (Fisch.) Bunge* is one of the most widely used traditional Chinese herbal medicines. It is used as immune stimulant, tonic, antioxidant, hepatoprotectant, diuretic, antidiabetic, anticancer, and expectorant. The purpose of the study was to investigate the curative effects of the decoction obtained from *Astragalus membranaceus* root in intestinal mucosal injury induced by LPS in mice. An LPS-induced intestinal mucosal injury mice model was applied in the study.

Methods: The mice were post-treated with *Astragalus membranaceus* decoction (AMD) for 4 days after 3 days LPS induction. ELISA kit was used to detect the content of tumor necrosis factor (TNF)-α, interleukin (IL)-1β, IL-4,IL-6 and IL-8 in the serum of each group mice. The morphological changes in intestinal mucosa at the end of the experiments were observed. Both VH (villus height) and CD (crypt depth) were measured using H&E-stained sections.

Results: There were significant differences in IL-1β, IL-4,IL-6, IL-8 and TNF-α levels in AMD-treated group on the 7th day compared to the controls group. The VH was lower in duodenum, jejunum and the ileum in LPS-treated mice compared to the control animals. Similarly, there was also decrease in V/C. Compared to the control mice, for AMD-treated mice, VH and CD had no significantly differences.

Conclusions: *Astragalus membranaceus* reduced intestinal mucosal damage and promoted tissue repair by inhibiting the expression of inflammatory cytokine.

Keywords: *Astragalus membranaceus* (Fisch.) Bunge, Decoction, Mice, Lipopolysaccharide

Background

Intestinal mucosa is a natural barrier against bacteria. It prevents viruses and other harmful bacteria from entering the blood [1]. Endotoxin is the lipopolysaccharide (LPS) in the cell wall of Gram-negative bacteria, which has a variety of biological activity and is decomposed and released in the process of bacterial metabolism or after death. LPS can stimulate the release of inflammatory mediators from macrophages and neutrophils and eventually lead to the imbalance of inflammatory and anti-inflammatory reactions and the occurrence of excessive systemic inflammation [2].

Astragalus membranaceus (Fisch.) Bunge (syn. *Astragalus propinquus* Schischkin) (AM), also known as Huangqi or milk vetch root in China, is an important medicine in traditional Chinese medicine. [3]. This herb possesses many common pharmacological activities, such as multiple organ protection [4, 5], antioxidant [6], hypoglycemic [7], antiviral [8] and so on, and has their own pharmacological properties and mechanisms. Studies have shown that *A. membranaceus* can enhance the contraction of the right ventricular myocardium in rats in a dose-dependent manner [9] and has recently been reported to be a potential promote tissue wound repair. The water extract of *A. membranaceus* is one of the main active preparations obtained from the root of this specie. However, there are not so many reports studies focusing on the decoction of AM. Some studies showed that gastric mucosa and atrophic pathological damage

---

* Correspondence: xuchuang7175@163.com; fuhewu@126.com
[†]Yizhe Cui and Qiuju Wang contributed equally to this work.
College of Animal Science and Veterinary Medicine, Heilongjiang Bayi Agricultural University, 2# Xinyang Road, New Development District, Daqing 163319, Heilongjiang, China

significantly reduced in rats after Huangqi intervention [10]. However, it is still not elucidated whether oral administration of *Astragalus membranaceus* decoction (AMD) could provide a repair effect during intestinal mucosal injury and what is the underlying mechanism. In this study, we explored the repair effect of AMD in LPS induced experimental intestinal mucosal injury in mice.

Methods

Drugs and reagents

LPS (*Escherichia coli* O55:B5) and all other chemicals were obtained from Sigma-Aldrich (St. Louis, MO, USA). Distilled water was filtered through a Milli-Q system from EMD Millipore Corporation (Billerica, MA, USA). LPS was suspended in physiological saline and stored as a 20 mg/ml stock. Dilutions prior to injection were into physiological saline. Animals were weighed prior to injection of LPS and stock LPS was diluted to the appropriate dose for each animal.

Plant material

Astragalus membranaceus was purchased from Fu Rui Bang Chinese Medicine Co., Ltd. (Daqing, China), then it was authenticated by Dr. Pengyu Jia and also deposited in Veterinary drug research and Development Center, Heilongjiang Bayi Agricultural University, Heilongjiang, China) according to Chinese Pharmacopoeia (The Pharmacopoeia Commission of PRC, 2010).

Animals

Male ICR mice weighing 22–25 g were purchased from the Animal Experiment Center of HARBIN MEDICAL UNIVERSITY (DAQING) [Certification no. SYXK (HEI) 2,014,005]. Mice were maintained on a standard light/dark cycle under controlled temperature (22 ± 2 °C) and humidity ($50 \pm 10\%$) with certified standard diet and water adlibitum. Mice were habituated to animal facilities for 1 week before the experiment. All the experimental procedures were approved by, and conducted in accordance with Principles of Laboratory Animal Care and according to the rules and ethics set forth by the Ethical Committee of Heilongjiang Bayi Agricultural University.

Extraction procedure

The general preparation procedure of *Astragalus membranaceus* decoction (AMD) is as follows [11]. Briefly, 100 g the root of *Astragalus membranaceus* was extracted by refluxing with water (1:8, *w/v*) for 1.5 h following sonicating for 30 min, then the extraction solutions were combined to be filtered and concentrated to 100 mL under reduced pressure. The concentrations of the residues were 1 g/mL for *Astragalus membranaceus*. Finally, the concentration be adjusted to the required with distilled water for

intragastrical administration. After being autoclaved at 100 °C for 20 min, the stock solution was stored at 4 °C.

Grouping and treatment

In experiments, animals were randomized into three groups of ten individuals (Fig. 1). The control group, LPS-treated group and AMD-treated group. Mice in the LPS groups and the AMD group, were intraperitoneally injected with LPS (*Escherichia coli* 055:B5, 5 mg/kg; Sigma) for 3 days. The chosen dose of LPS was based on Die Dai's study and preliminary experiments [12]. AMD-treated groups were given *Astragalus membranaceus* decoction by intragastric administration once daily and treatments lasted for 4 days after 3 days LPS induction. Briefly, 1 ml syringe with No. 12 gavage needle was used in intragastric administration. The volume of gavage was usually 0.1 ml/10 g body weight. Mice in control group were received physiological saline for 7 days. After euthanizing the mice by carbon dioxide, blood was obtained by cardiac puncture on the 7th day. On collection, blood samples were centrifuged at 5000 rpm for 10 min, and were subsequently stored at − 80 °C before metabolomics analysis. Survivals were recorded for 72 h.

Determination of inflammatory cytokine levels

Cytokine levels in serum were determined by ELISA by using commercially available kits (Endogen, Cambridge,MA). For each assay, serum was serially diluted to ensure that values obtained were within the linear range of the standards provided with each kit. Each sample was done in duplicate, and data from individual mice were averaged.

Histopathology

Specimens of the intestinal wall of the duodenum, jejunum and ileum were prepared for histological examination by fixing in 4% formalhyde-buffered solution, embedding in paraffin, and sectioning. Paraffin sections were cut into slices of 4 μm and stained with H&E staining solution. Finally, the stained sections were observed and photographed under a light microscope (with 100× magnification). Villous height and the associated crypt depth were evaluated using the Image Pro plus 4 analysis software (Media Cybernetics, Baltimore, MD, USA) processing and analysis system. For each intestinal sample, at least 10 well-oriented were measured and the mean value was calculated. The method was the same as described by Nabuurs et al. [13].

Data analysis

Data were presented as mean and standard deviation (SD). One-way ANOVA showed significant differences among groups. A level of $P < 0.05$ was considered statistically significant. Analysis was performed with the software SPSS version 16.0 (SPSS Inc., USA).

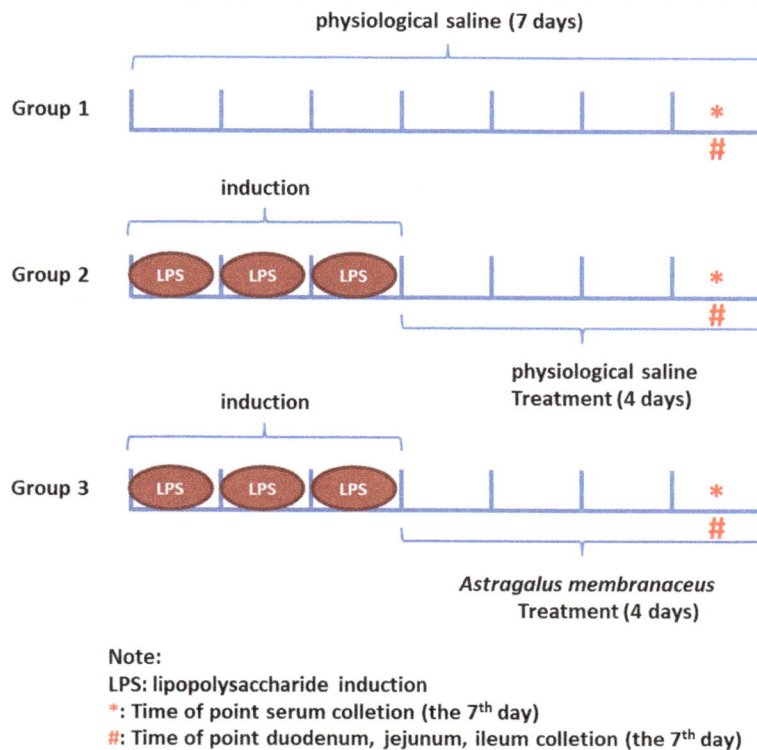

Fig. 1 Experimental design and sampling schedule

Results

Serum concentrations of cytokine

The serum levels of IL-1β, IL-4,IL-6, IL-8 and TNF-α are important biochemical markers for evaluating intestinal mucosal structure and function [14]. In this experiment, the induction of LSP caused significantly higher levels ($P < 0.05$) of IL-1β, IL-4,IL-6, IL-8 and TNF-α in model group on the 7th day compared to the control group (Table 1). Compared with LPS group, the level of inflammatory cytokines decreased significantly ($P < 0.05$) in AMD group. Meanwhile, there were no significant differences of IL-1β, IL-4,IL-6, IL-8 and TNF-α levels in AMD-treated group on the 7th day compared to control group, though the level of IL-4 and IL-1β was higher in AMD group than that in control group, there was no

Table 1 Serum levels of cytokines in LPS- and AMD-treated mice

Parameters	Controls	LPS	AMD
TNF-α (pg/mL)	15.64 ± 1.04	50.30 ± 8.26*	7.29 ± 1.12
IL-1β (pg/mL)	6.21 ± 0.45	9.36 ± 0.71*	7.26 ± 0.45
IL-4 (pg/mL)	3.47 ± 0.33	11.81 ± 0.39*	3.65 ± 0.43
IL-6 (pg/mL)	11.34 ± 0.21	14.25 ± 0.36*	8.96 ± 0.63
IL-8 (pg/mL)	9.51 ± 1.07	11.86 ± 0.66*	7.93 ± 1.13

The data are expressed as the mean ± SD ($n = 10$ per treatment group).
Statistically different from the control group;$P < 0.05$. Tumor necrosis factor (TNF)-α, interleukin (IL) IL-1β, IL-4,IL-6 and IL-8

significant differences. The results suggested that AMD had no effect on the immunity of the body, moreover curative treated AMD was effective in ameliorating LPS-induced intestinal mucosal damage.

Histopathological changes in intestinal tissue

Pathological examinations of the intestinal mucosal injury were carried out and the LPS-treatment and AMD-treatment are shown in Fig. 2. Compared with the control animals, the pathological changes were obvious, LPS-treated groups caused significant mucosal damage, that is, epithelial shedding, villi fracturing, mucosal atrophy, edema and the villus had shortened on the 7th day after LPS injection (Fig. 2). However, as time goes on, the intestinal mucosa damage begins to recover slowly in the AMD-treated groups on the 7th day. These observations showed that AMD has obvious beneficial effects against intestinal mucosal damage.

Histomorphological analyses

The VH and CD, which indicated intestinal villus's absorptive functions, were measured. The experiments showed that the VH was lower in duodenum, jejunum and the ileum in LPS-treated mice compared to the control animals. Similarly, there was decrease in V/C. Compared to the control mice, for AMD-treated mice, VH and CD had no significantly differences (Fig. 3).

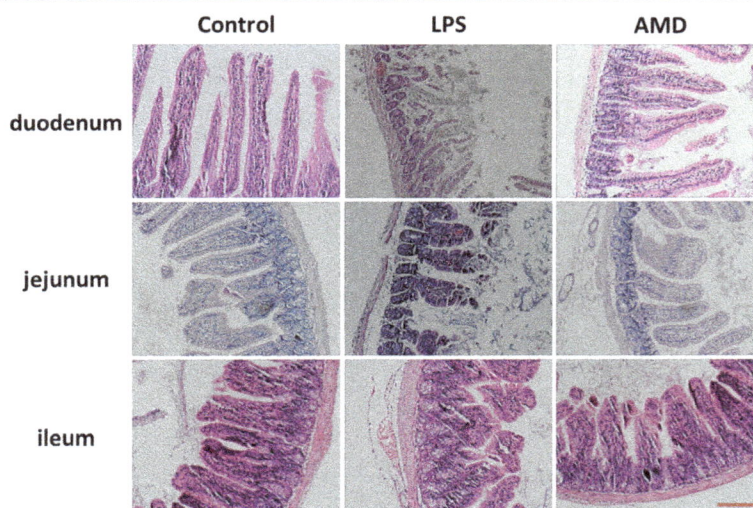

Fig. 2 Histomorphometric analyses of intestinal mucosa time changes. Histological appearance of mice intestinal mucosa after haematoxylin and eosin (H&E) stain (original magnification 100×). Scale bars: 50 μm

Discussion

Intestinal mucosal injury is associated with intestinal inflammation [15]. We investigated whether AMD could ameliorate the inflammatory response in mice induced by LPS. A large number of studies suggest that the intestinal ischemia/reperfusion injury, LPS challenge, and intestinal inflammatory diseases can induce the expression of inflammatory cytokines in humans and animals [16]. Both in vitro and in vivo studies show that over-secretory of inflammatory cytokines can have a negative effects on intestinal mucosal integrity, permeability and epithelial function of the intestinal mucosa [17]. The imbalance of cytokine and chemokine secretion plays an important role in mucosal defense. IL-8 is produced by macrophages and epithelial cells. It can chemotaxis and activate neutrophils, which leads to mucous edema, leukocyte infiltration, increased vascular damage and permeability, resulting in immune inflammatory lesions [18]. IL-4 can play a role in pro-inflammatory factors alone in the gut of mice, which can trigger inflammation [19]. The study showed that LPS was identified by Toll like receptor 4 (TLR4) to release TNF-α, IL-1 beta and IL-6 and other cytokines, which mediate and promote the occurrence of inflammatory bowel disease (IBD) [20]. Intraperitoneal injection of LPS can cause intestinal mucosal inflammation, which is characterized by increased inflammatory and anti-inflammatory cytokines. TNF-α plays a major role in causing intestinal inflammation, and its role is to accumulate inflammatory cells to the local tissues of the inflammation, cause edema, activate coagulation cascade, and form granuloma [21]. The common way to treat IBD in clinic is to inhibit TNF-α by using TNF-α antagonist to improve and alleviate IBD symptoms. In this

experiment, the mice were intraperitoneally injected with LPS to establish a model of intestinal injury in mice. LPS challenge increased the level of TNF-α, IL-1β, IL-4,IL-6 and IL-8 in the serum (Table 1). Importantly, AMD reduced the concentrations of TNF-α, IL-1β, IL-4,IL-6 and IL-8 in the serum, compared to LPS-challenged mice. These findings indicate that the AMD has beneficial effects in reducing intestinal mucosal inflammation. AMD may inhibit intestinal immune damage, reduce intestinal mucosal edema and promote intestinal mucosal repair by downregulating the expression of cytokine.

The structural characteristics of the small intestinal mucosa are circular folds, intestinal villi and microvilli. These characteristics greatly expand the surface area of the small intestine and make the nutrients fully digested and absorbed in the small intestine. The complete structure of the small intestine is the physiological basis of its digestion and absorption function, and its morphological and structural changes directly affect the surface area of villi, thereby affecting the body's ability to absorb nutrients [22]. The integrity and height of the intestinal villi determine the absorption area of the small intestine, the absorption of nutrients and the growth of the animals [23]. Therefore, the increase of the villi height, the ratio of the villi/crypt or the decrease of the depth of the recess is related to the improvement of the digestion and absorption of nutrients [24]. Compared with the LPS group, AMD increased the villus height and villus/crypt ratio of the duodenum, as well as the villus height and chorionic ratio of the jejunum and ileum. Crypt depth was significantly reduced in the duodenum and the jejunum, compared with the LPS group. The expression of inflammatory cytokines was consistent with the

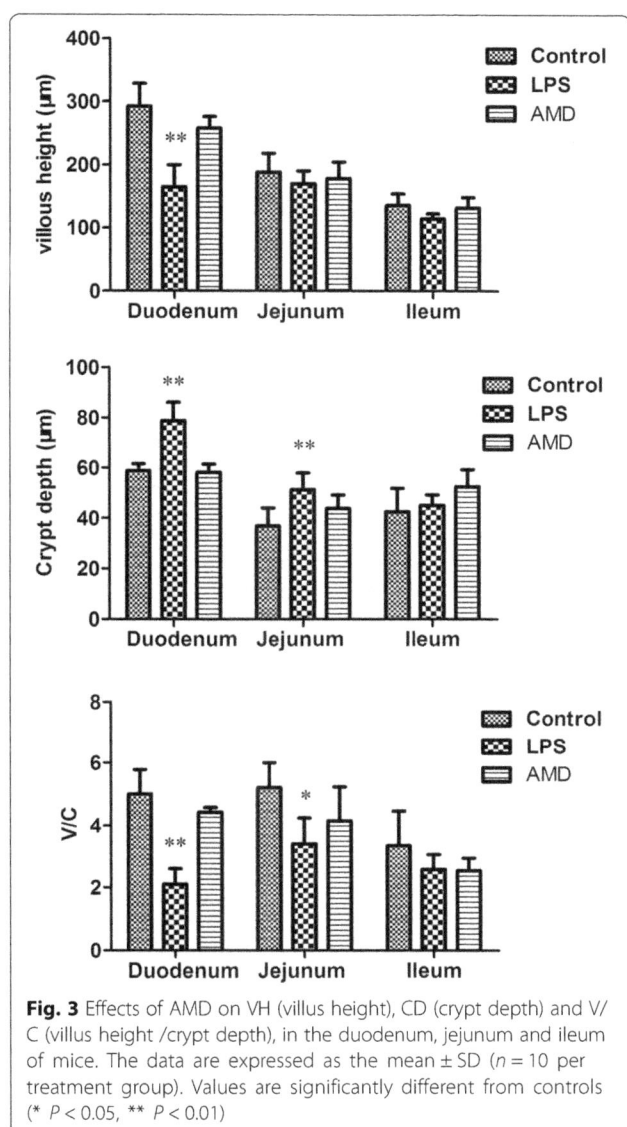

Fig. 3 Effects of AMD on VH (villus height), CD (crypt depth) and V/C (villus height /crypt depth), in the duodenum, jejunum and ileum of mice. The data are expressed as the mean ± SD (n = 10 per treatment group). Values are significantly different from controls (* $P < 0.05$, ** $P < 0.01$)

alteration in the structure of intestinal villi (Table 1). Based on these results, we concluded that AMD protected the intestinal mucosa from the LPS-induced injury.

AM is a well-known medicinal herb for reinforcing Qi (the vital energy) in traditional Chinese medicine [25]. *Astragalus* polysaccharides has the characteristics of antioxidation [26], immunomodulation [27], antiviral, antitumor activities [28] and cardiovascular protection [29]. AM and its active components have been proved to be effective in the treatment of a variety of diseases, such as diabetes mellitus [30] and cardiovascular disorders [31]. In recent years, astragal's polysaccharides effectively reduced the mucosal damage of experimental colitis in mice by shortening colonic length, reducing

colon weight index, and reducing macroscopically and histological scores [32], which is similar to the results of this experiment.

Conclusions

Astragalus membranaceus treatment can protect small intestinal mucosa against LPS injury. Also, *A. membranaceus* promotes tissue repair by inhibiting the expression of inflammatory cytokine. These findings indicate that *A. membranaceus* can partly reduce small intestinal mucosa injury induced by LPS. Further studies of *A. membranaceus* are necessary to develop a new effective plant-derived therapeutic modality for intestinal mucosal injury.

Funding
This work was supported by Natural Science Foundation of Heilongjiang Province (C201444), China Scholarship council (201508230118), Postdoctoral Program Foundation of Heilongjiang Bayi Agricultural University of China (601038), Doctoral Program Foundation of Heilongjiang Bayi Agricultural University of China (XDB-2016-10) and China Postdoctoral Science Foundation (2017 M620124; 2018 T110320).

Authors' contributions
YC and QW contributed equally to this work. YC, QW, CX and RW designed the research; YC, RS, LG, YC performed the research; MW, JJ analyzed the data; and YC and QW wrote the paper. All authors read and approved the final manuscript.

Competing interests
The authors declare that they have no competing interests.

References
1. Vancamelbeke M, Vermeire S. The intestinal barrier: a fundamental role in health and disease. Expert Rev Gastroenterol Hepatol. 2017;11(9):821–34.
2. Waseem T, Duxbury M, Ito H, Ashley SW, Robinson MK. Exogenous ghrelin modulates release of pro-inflammatory and anti-inflammatory cytokines in LPS-stimulated macrophages through distinct signaling pathways. Surgery. 2008;143(3):334–42.
3. Guo K, He X, Lu D, Zhang Y, Li X, Yan Z, Qin B. Cycloartane-type triterpenoids from Astragalus hoantchy French. Nat Prod Res. 2017;31(3):314–9.
4. Wang XQ, Wang L, Tu YC, Zhang YC. Traditional Chinese medicine for refractory nephrotic syndrome: strategies and promising treatments. Evid Based Complement Alternat Med. 2018;2018:8746349.
5. Kim GD, Oh J, Park HJ, Bae K, Lee SK. Magnolol inhibits angiogenesis by regulating ROS-mediated apoptosis and the PI3K/AKT/mTOR signaling pathway in mES/EB-derived endothelial-like cells. Int J Oncol. 2013;43(2): 600–10.
6. Li H, Wang P, Huang F, Jin J, Wu H, Zhang B, Wang Z, Shi H, Wu X. Astragaloside IV protects blood-brain barrier integrity from LPS-induced disruption via activating Nrf2 antioxidant signaling pathway in mice. Toxicol Appl Pharmacol. 2018;340:58–66.
7. Cui K, Zhang S, Jiang X, Xie W. Novel synergic antidiabetic effects of Astragalus polysaccharides combined with Crataegus flavonoids via improvement of islet function and liver metabolism. Mol Med Rep. 2016; 13(6):4737–44.
8. Wang Y, Chen Y, Du H, Yang J, Ming K, Song M, Liu J. Comparison of the anti-duck hepatitis a virus activities of phosphorylated and sulfated Astragalus polysaccharides. Exp Biol Med. 2017;242(3):344–53.
9. Cao Y, Shen T, Huang X, Lin Y, Chen B, Pang J, Li G, Wang Q, Zohrabian S, Duan C, et al. Astragalus polysaccharide restores autophagic flux and improves cardiomyocyte function in doxorubicin-induced cardiotoxicity. Oncotarget. 2017;8(3):4837–48.

10. Zhu X, Liu S, Zhou J, Wang H, Fu R, Wu X, Wang J, Lu F. Effect of Astragalus polysaccharides on chronic atrophic gastritis induced by N-methyl-N'-nitro-N-nitrosoguanidine in rats. Drug Res. 2013;63(11):597–602.

11. Cho CH, Mei QB, Shang P, Lee SS, So HL, Guo X, Li Y. Study of the gastrointestinal protective effects of polysaccharides from Angelica sinensis in rats. Planta Med. 2000;66(4):348–51.

12. Dai D, Gao Y, Chen J, Huang Y, Zhang Z, Xu F. Time-resolved metabolomics analysis of individual differences during the early stage of lipopolysaccharide-treated rats. Sci Rep. 2016;6:34136.

13. Nabuurs MJ, Hoogendoorn A, van der Molen EJ, van Osta AL. Villus height and crypt depth in weaned and unweaned pigs, reared under various circumstances in the Netherlands. Res Vet Sci. 1993;55(1):78–84.

14. Xiao K, Cao ST, Ie F J, Lin FH, Wang L, Hu CH. Anemonin improves intestinal barrier restoration and influences TGF-beta1 and EGFR signaling pathways in LPS-challenged piglets. Innate Immun. 2016;22(5):344–52.

15. Blikslager AT, Moeser AJ, Gookin JL, Jones SL, Odle J. Restoration of barrier function in injured intestinal mucosa. Physiol Rev. 2007;87(2):545–64.

16. Liu Y, Huang J, Hou Y, Zhu H, Zhao S, Ding B, Yin Y, Yi G, Shi J, Fan W. Dietary arginine supplementation alleviates intestinal mucosal disruption induced by Escherichia coli lipopolysaccharide in weaned pigs. Br J Nutr. 2008;100(3):552–60.

17. Oswald IP, Dozois CM, Barlagne R, Fournout S, Johansen MV, Bogh HO. Cytokine mRNA expression in pigs infected with Schistosoma japonicum. Parasitology. 2001;122(Pt 3):299–307.

18. Reddy KP, Markowitz JE, Ruchelli ED, Baldassano RN, Brown KA. Lamina propria and circulating interleukin-8 in newly and previously diagnosed pediatric inflammatory bowel disease patients. Dig Dis Sci. 2007;52(2):365–72.

19. Chen J, Gong C, Mao H, Li Z, Fang Z, Chen Q, Lin M, Jiang X, Hu Y, Wang W et al: E2F1/SP3/STAT6 axis is required for IL-4-induced epithelial-mesenchymal transition of colorectal cancer cells. Int J Oncol 2018;53(2):567–78.

20. Liu HM, Liao JF, Lee TY. Farnesoid X receptor agonist GW4064 ameliorates lipopolysaccharide-induced ileocolitis through TLR4/MyD88 pathway related mitochondrial dysfunction in mice. Biochem Biophys Res Commun. 2017;490(3):841–8.

21. Allocca M, Bonifacio C, Fiorino G, Spinelli A, Furfaro F, Balzarini L, Bonovas S, Danese S. Efficacy of tumour necrosis factor antagonists in stricturing Crohn's disease: a tertiary center real-life experience. Dig Liver Dis. 2017;49(8):872–7.

22. Collins JT, Bhimji SS: Anatomy, Abdomen, Small Intestine. In: StatPearls. edn. Treasure Island (FL); 2017.

23. Greig CJ, Cowles RA. Muscarinic acetylcholine receptors participate in small intestinal mucosal homeostasis. J Pediatr Surg. 2017;52(6):1031–4.

24. Hou Y, Wang L, Yi D, Ding B, Yang Z, Li J, Chen X, Qiu Y, Wu G. N-acetylcysteine reduces inflammation in the small intestine by regulating redox, EGF and TLR4 signaling. Amino Acids. 2013;45(3):513–22.

25. Lin HQ, Gong AG, Wang HY, Duan R, Dong TT, Zhao KJ, Tsim KW. Danggui Buxue tang (Astragali Radix and Angelicae Sinensis Radix) for menopausal symptoms: a review. J Ethnopharmacol. 2017;199:205–10.

26. Huang WM, Liang YQ, Tang LJ, Ding Y, Wang XH. Antioxidant and anti-inflammatory effects of Astragalus polysaccharide on EA.hy926 cells. Exp Ther Med. 2013;6(1):199–203.

27. Du X, Zhao B, Li J, Cao X, Diao M, Feng H, Chen X, Chen Z, Zeng X. Astragalus polysaccharides enhance immune responses of HBV DNA vaccination via promoting the dendritic cell maturation and suppressing Treg frequency in mice. Int Immunopharmacol. 2012;14(4):463–70.

28. Dang SS, Jia XL, Song P, Cheng YA, Zhang X, Sun MZ, Liu EQ. Inhibitory effect of emodin and Astragalus polysaccharide on the replication of HBV. World J Gastroenterol. 2009;15(45):5669–73.

29. Yang M, Lin HB, Gong S, Chen PY, Geng LL, Zeng YM, Li DY. Effect of Astragalus polysaccharides on expression of TNF-alpha, IL-1beta and NFATc4 in a rat model of experimental colitis. Cytokine. 2014;70(2):81–6.

30. Zhang K, Pugliese M, Pugliese A, Passantino A. Biological active ingredients of traditional Chinese herb Astragalus membranaceus on treatment of diabetes: a systematic review. Mini Rev Med Chem. 2015;15(4):315–29.

31. Sun S, Yang S, Dai M, Jia X, Wang Q, Zhang Z, Mao Y. The effect of Astragalus polysaccharides on attenuation of diabetic cardiomyopathy through inhibiting the extrinsic and intrinsic apoptotic pathways in high glucose -stimulated H9C2 cells. BMC Complement Altern Med. 2017;17(1):310.

32. Zhao HM, Wang Y, Huang XY, Huang MF, Xu R, Yue HY, Zhou BG, Huang HY, Sun QM, Liu DY. Astragalus polysaccharide attenuates rat experimental colitis by inducing regulatory T cells in intestinal Peyer's patches. World J Gastroenterol. 2016;22(11):3175–85.

Antimicrobial activities of flavonoid glycosides from *Graptophyllum grandulosum* and their mechanism of antibacterial action

Cyrille Ngoufack Tagousop[1], Jean-de-Dieu Tamokou[2]* ⓘ, Steve Endeguele Ekom[2], David Ngnokam[1]*
and Laurence Voutquenne-Nazabadioko[3]

Abstract

Background: The search for new antimicrobials should take into account drug resistance phenomenon. Medicinal plants are known as sources of potent antimicrobial compounds including flavonoids. The objective of this investigation was to evaluate the antimicrobial activities of flavonoid glycosides from *Graptophyllum grandulosum*, as well as to determine their mechanism of antibacterial action using lysis, leakage and osmotic stress assays.

Methods: The plant extracts were prepared by maceration in organic solvents. Column chromatography of the *n*-butanol extract followed by purification of different fractions led to the isolation of five flavonoid glycosides. The antimicrobial activities of extracts/compounds were evaluated using the broth microdilution method. The bacteriolytic activity was evaluated using the time-kill kinetic method. The effect of extracts on the red blood cells and bacterial cell membrane was determined by spectrophotometric methods.

Results: Chrysoeriol-7-*O*-β-D-xyloside (**1**), luteolin-7-*O*-β-D-apiofuranosyl-(1 → 2)-β-D-xylopyranoside (**2**), chrysoeriol-7-*O*-β-D-apiofuranosyl-(1 → 2)-β-D-xylopyranoside (**3**), chrysoeriol-7-*O*-α-L-rhamnopyranosyl-(1 → 6)-β-D-(4"-hydrogeno sulfate) glucopyranoside (**4**) and isorhamnetin-3-*O*-α-L-rhamnopyranosyl-(1 → 6)-β-D-glucopyranoside (**5**) were isolated from *G. grandulosum* and showed different degrees of antimicrobial activities. Their antibacterial activities against multi-drug-resistant *Vibrio cholerae* strains were in some cases equal to, or higher than those of ciprofloxacin used as reference antibiotic. The antibacterial activities of flavonoid glycosides and chloramphenicol increased under osmotic stress (5% NaCl) whereas that of vancomycin decreased under this condition. *V. cholerae* suspension treated with flavonoid glycosides, showed a significant increase in the optical density at 260 nm, suggesting that nucleic acids were lost through a damaged cytoplasmic membrane. A decrease in the optical density of *V. cholerae* NB2 suspension treated with the isolated compounds was observed, indicating the lysis of bacterial cells. The tested samples were non-toxic to normal cells highlighting their good selectivity index.

Conclusions: The results of the present study indicate that the purified flavonoids from *G. glandulosum* possess antimicrobial activities. Their mode of antibacterial activity is due to cell lysis and disruption of the cytoplasmic membrane upon membrane permeability.

Keywords: *Graptophyllum glandulosum*, Acanthaceae, Flavonoid glycosides, Antibacterial, Antifungal, Mode of action

* Correspondence: jtamokou@yahoo.fr; jean.tamokou@univ-dschang.org;
dngnokam@yahoo.fr; ngnokam@univ-dschang.org
[2]Research Unit of Microbiology and Antimicrobial Substances, Department of
Biochemistry, Faculty of Science, University of Dschang, P.O. Box 67,
Dschang, Cameroon
[1]Research Unit of Environmental and Applied Chemistry, Department of Chemistry,
Faculty of Science, University of Dschang, P.O. Box 67, Dschang, Cameroon
Full list of author information is available at the end of the article

Background

The development of resistance by microorganisms to existing antimicrobial agents has been known for a long time. In several findings, the emergence of multidrug resistant strains of *Vibrio cholerae* O1 and *Shigella flexneri* has been reported due to different genetic factors including transfer of plasmids, integrons and allelic variation in the specific genes [1]. In developing countries, fluoroquinolones, widely used for the treatment of many bacterial diseases, including cholera and shigellosis, could contribute to the emergence of multidrug resistance among potential enteric pathogens. Although significant progress has been made in microbiological research and in the control of many diseases caused by infectious microorganisms, recurrent epidemics due to drug-resistant microorganisms as well as the appearance of new microbial pathogenic strains demand the discovery of new antibiotics. The need for ecologically safe compounds as therapeutic agents against drug-resistant microorganisms has driven many studies toward medicinal plants. Literature shows thousands of plant species that have been tested in vitro against many fungal and bacterial strains, and a good number of medicinal plant extracts and pure compounds have now been proven to be active against fungi, Gram-positive and Gram-negative bacteria [2–5]. Medicinal plants contain therapeutic amount of secondary metabolites including flavonoids. These are polyphenolic and C_6-C_3-C_6 compounds in which the two C_6 groups are substituted benzene rings, and the C_3 is an aliphatic chain which contains a pyran ring [6]. They occur as *O*- or *C*-glycosides or in the free state as aglycones with hydroxyl or methoxyl groups [7]. The sugar moiety is an important factor determining their bioavailability. Flavonoids may be divided into seven types: flavones, flavonols, flavonones, flavanes, isoflavones, biflavones and chalcones [8]. Flavonoids are well documented for their pharmacological effects, including antimicrobial, anticancer, antiviral, antimutagenic and anti-inflammatory activities [9–11]. Biological properties of flavonoids are linked to their ability to act as strong antioxidants and free radical scavengers, to chelate metals, and to interact with enzymes, adenosine receptors and biomembranes [7].

Graptophyllum glandulosum Turrill (Acanthaceae) is a shrub with 4-angled, nearly glabrous branches, normal green leaves, and red-purple flowers 1 in. or more long. It is one of several shrubs and trees of *Graptophyllum* that mainly grow in West and Central Africa but also in the pacific regions [12]. This plant contains some important secondary metabolites such as polyphenols, flavonoids and glycosides [13]. Leaves, roots and other parts of *G. glandulosum*, are used in folk medicine in Cameroon to treat wounds, abscesses, skin diseases, respiratory tract infections and diarrhea. Medical importance of this plant attracted us to explore its antimicrobial properties.

Although several ethnobotanical reports have emphasized the pharmacological importance of this species for conditions that appear to be associated with microbial infections, there is very limited literature concerned with the identification of the antimicrobial compounds from this plant. However, a few reports on the in vitro antimicrobial activity of plants have been published [14, 15]. The objective of this investigation was to evaluate the antimicrobial activities of flavonoid glycosides from *G. grandulosum*, as well as to determine their mechanism of action using lysis, leakage, and osmotic stress assays.

Methods

General experimental procedures

Melting point

A Schorpp Gerätetechnik (Germany) apparatus was used to take the melting points of different compounds.

NMR analysis

The 1D (^{1}H and ^{13}C-NMR) and 2D (COSY, NOESY, HSQC and HMBC) spectra were performed in deuterated solvents (CD_3OD) on Bruker Avance III 600 spectrometer at 600 MHz/150 MHz. All chemical shifts (δ) are given in ppm units with reference to tetramethylsilane (TMS) as internal standard and the coupling constants (J) are in Hz.

Spectrometric analysis

The mass spectra (HR-TOFESIMS) were carried out on Micromass Q-TOF micro instrument (Manchester, UK). Samples were introduced by direct infusion in a solution of MeOH at a rate of 5 μL/min.

Chromatographic methods

Silica gel 60 Merck, 70–230 mesh and sephadex LH-20 were used to perform column chromatography while precoated silica gel 60 F_{254} (Merck) plates, were used to perform thin layer chromatography. The spots were visualized by an UV lamp multiband UV-254/365 nm (ModelUVGL-58 Upland CA 91786, U.S.A) followed by spraying with 50% H_2SO_4 and heating at 100 °C for 5 min.

Plant material

The aerial parts of *G. grandulosum* were harvested in a small village called Foto situated in the Menoua Division, Western region of Cameroon) in November 2015. The Plant was identified and authenticated by a Cameroonian Botanist (Mr. Fulbert Tadjouteu) at the National Herbarium where a voucher specimen was archived (N° 65631/HNC).

Extraction and isolation

The extraction and isolation of compounds were done as previously described [13]. Briefly, the aerial part of *G. grandulosum* was air-dried and powdered. The powder was macerated at room temperature with MeOH to afford the MeOH extract. Part of this extract (235 g) was suspended in water (300 mL) and successively partitioned with EtOAc and n-BuOH to yield 37 and 13 g of extracts, respectively. Column chromatography of the n-BuOH extract followed by purification of different fractions led to the isolation of five compounds.

Structural identification of the isolated compounds
The structures of isolated compounds were determined after interpretation of their physical, spectrometric and spectroscopic data summarized in this subsection.

Chrysoeriol-7-O-β-D-xyloside (1): yellow amorphous powder; molecular formula $C_{21}H_{20}O_{10}$; ^{13}C NMR (CD$_3$OD, 150 MHz) δ_C: 165.3 (C-2), 104.3 (C-3), 184.1 (C-4), 161.7 (C-5), 99.6 (C-6), 163.1 (C-7), 95.8 (C-8), 158.5 (C-9), 107.0 (C-10), 123.1 (C-1'), 110.5 (C-2'), 148.2 (C-3'), 151.0 (C-4'), 116.7 (C-5'), 121.9 (C-6'), 55.2 (C-7') for aglycone; 100.9 (C-1''), 74.4 (C-2''), 77.3 (C-3''), 70.7 (C-4''), 66.9 (C-5'') for sugar moiety. ^1H NMR data (CD$_3$OD, 600 MHz) δ_H: 6.62 (1H, s, H-3), 6.38 (1H, d, $J = 2.1$ Hz, H-6), 6.71 (1H, d, $J = 2.1$ Hz, H-8), 7.44 (1H, d, $J = 2.1$ Hz, H-2'), 6.84 (1H, d, $J = 8.4$ Hz, H-5'), 7.47 (1H, dd, $J = 8.4$ and 2.1 Hz, H-6'), 3.87 (3H, s, H-7') for aglycone; 4.95 (1H, d, $J = 7.1$ Hz, H-1''), 3.37 (1H, m, H-2''), 3.36 (1H, m, H-3''), 3.49 (1H, m, H-4''), 3.38 (1H, m, H-5''a), 3.87 (1H, m, H-5''b) for sugar moiety.

Luteolin-7-O-β-D-apiofuranosyl-(1 → 2)-β-D-xylopyranoside (2): yellow powder; molecular formula $C_{25}H_{26}O_{14}$. m.p. = 203 °C. ^{13}C NMR data (CD$_3$OD, 150 MHz) δ_C: 165.3 (C-2), 103.5 (C-3), 182.5 (C-4), 162.9 (C-5), 99.7 (C-6), 163.1 (C-7), 94.9 (C-8), 157.4 (C-9), 105.5 (C-10), 121.7 (C-1'), 114.2 (C-2'), 146.4 (C-3'), 150.5 (C-4'), 116.6 (C-5'), 119.7 (C-6') for aglycone; 99.0 (C-1''), 76.0 (C-2''), 77.0 (C-3''), 70.0 (C-4''), 66.1 (C-5''), 109.3 (C-1'''), 76.5 (C-2'''), 79.7 (C-3'''), 64.5 (C-4'''), 74.4 (C-5''') for sugar moiety. ^1H NMR data (CD$_3$OD, 600 MHz) δ_H: 6.75 (1H, s, H-3), 6.40 (1H, d, $J = 2.1$ Hz, H-6), 6.75 (1H, d, $J = 2.1$ Hz, H-8), 7.44 (1H, d, $J = 2.1$ Hz, H-2'), 6.90 (1H, d, $J = 8.4$ Hz, H-5'), 7.47 (1H, dd, $J = 8.4$ and 2.1 Hz, H-6') for aglycone; 5.18 (1H, d, $J = 7.1$ Hz, H-1''), 3.52 (1H, dd, $J = 9.0$ and 7.1 Hz, H-2''), 3.43 (1H, m, H-3''), 3.41 (1H, m, H-4''), 3.78 (1H, dd, $J = 9.7$ and 3.4 Hz, H-5''a), 3.42 (1H, dd, $J = 9.7$ and 3.4 Hz, H-5''b), 5.34 (1H, d, $J = 1.3$ Hz, H-1'''), 3.75 (1H, m, H-2'''), 3.30 (2H, d, $J = 3.4$ Hz, H-4'''), 3.88 (1H, d, $J = 9.3$ Hz, H-5'''a), 3.65 (1H, d, $J = 9.3$ Hz, H-5'''b) for sugar moiety.

Chrysoeriol-7-O-β-D-apiofuranosyl-(1 → 2)-β-D-xylopyranoside (3): yellow powder; molecular formula $C_{26}H_{28}O_4$; melting point = 181.8 °C. ^{13}C NMR (CD$_3$OD, 150 MHz) δ_C: 166.6 (C-2), 104.5 (C-3), 184.0 (C-4), 162.9 (C-5), 100.9 (C-6), 164.4 (C-7), 95.9 (C-8), 158.9 (C-9), 107.0 (C-10), 123.4 (C-1'), 110.4 (C-2'), 149.5

(C-3'), 152.3 (C-4'), 116.7 (C-5'), 121.9 (C-6'), 56.6 (C-7') for aglycone; 100.6 (C-1''), 78.6 (C-2''), 77.9 (C-3''), 70.9 (C-4''), 66.9 (C-5''), 110.0 (C-1'''), 78.1 (C-2'''), 80.7 (C-3'''), 65.8 (C-4'''), 75.4 (C-5''') for sugar moiety. ^1H NMR data (CD$_3$OD, 600 MHz) δ_H: 6.70 (1H, s, H-3), 6.45 (1H, d, $J = 2.1$ Hz, H-6), 6.77 (1H, d, $J = 2.1$ Hz, H-8), 7.52 (1H, d, $J = 2.1$ Hz, H-2'), 6.95 (1H, d, $J = 8.4$ Hz, H-5'), 7.56 (1H, dd, $J = 8.4$ and 2.1 Hz, H-6'), 3.98 (3H, s, H-7') for aglycone; 5.16 (1H, d, $J = 7.1$ Hz, H-1''), 3.68 (1H, dd, $J = 9.0$ and 7.1, H-2''), 3.63 (1H, m, H-3''), 3.62 (1H, m, H-4''), 3.98 (1H, m, H-5''a), 3.48 (1H, t, $J = 9.6$, H-5''b), 5.46 (1H, d, $J = 1.7$ Hz, H-1'''), 3.98 (1H, m, H-2'''), 3.56 (2H, brs, H-4'''), 4.05 (1H, d, $J = 9.4$, H-5'''a), 3.84 (1H, d, $J = 9.4$, H-5''' b) for sugar moiety.

Chrysoeriol-7-O-α-L-rhamnopyranosyl-(1 → 6)-β-D-(4''-hydrogenosulfate) glucopyranoside (4): yellow amorphous powder; molecular formula $C_{28}H_{31}NaO_{18}S$. ^{13}C NMR data (CD$_3$OD, 150 MHz) δ_C: 166.8 (C-2), 104.5 (C-3), 184.1 (C-4), 163.1 (C-5), 101.1 (C-6), 164.0 (C-7), 96.2 (C-8), 159.0 (C-9), 107.2 (C-10), 123.6 (C-1'), 110.8 (C-2'), 149.6 (C-3'), 152.3 (C-4'), 116.9 (C-5'), 122.0 (C-6'), 56.7 (C-7') for aglycone; 100.9 (C-1''), 74.5 (C-2''), 76.8 (C-3''), 77.5 (C-4''), 75.3 (C-5''), 67.1 (C-6''), 102.4 (C-1'''), 71.9 (C-2'''), 72.3 (C-3'''), 74.2 (C-4'''), 69.8 (C-5'''), 17.9 (C-6''') for sugar moiety. ^1H NMR data (CD$_3$OD, 600 MHz) δ_H: 6.73 (1H, s, H-3), 6.56 (1H, d, $J = 2.1$ Hz, H-6), 6.84 (1H, d, $J = 2.1$ Hz, H-8), 7.55 (1H, d, $J = 2.1$ Hz, H-2'), 6.98 (1H, d, $J = 8.4$ Hz, H-5'), 7.59 (1H, dd, $J = 8.4$ and 2.1 Hz, H-6'), 3.99 (3H, s, H-7') for aglycone; 5.15 (1H, d, $J = 7.8$ Hz, H-1''), 3.61 (1H, dd, $J = 9.1$ and 7.8 Hz, H-2''), 3.84 (1H, t, $J = 9.1$ Hz, H-3''), 4.32 (1H, dd, $J = 9.9$ and 9.1 Hz, H-4''), 3.89 (1H, m, H-5''), 4.10 (1H, m, H-6''a), 3.68 (1H, m, H-6''b), 4.75 (1H, d, $J = 1.3$ Hz, H-1'''), 3.95 (1H, dd, $J = 3.4$ and 1.3, H-2'''), 3.72 (1H, dd, $J = 9.5$ and 3.4 Hz, H-3'''), 3.32 (1H, t, $J = 9.5$ Hz, H-4'''), 3.62 (1H, m, H-5'''), 1.21 (3H, d, $J = 6.2$ Hz, H-6''') for sugar moiety.

Isorhamnetin-3-O-α-L-rhamnopyranosyl-(1 → 6)-β-D-glucopyranoside (5): yellow amorphous powder; molecular formula $C_{28}H_{32}O_{15}$. ^{13}C NMR data (CD$_3$OD, 150 MHz) δ_C: 159.8 (C-2), 135.7 (C-3), 179.8 (C-4), 162.4 (C-5), 104.3 (C-6), 160.1 (C-7), 100.2 (C-8), 157.5 (C-9), 108.6 (C-10), 123.0 (C-1'), 114.5 (C-2'), 148.4 (C-3'), 151.1 (C-4'), 116.2 (C-5'), 124.4 (C-6'), 56.7 (C-7') for aglycone; 104.0 (C-1''), 75.9 (C-2''), 78.1 (C-3''), 71.8 (C-4''), 77.4 (C-5''), 68.7 (C-6''), 102.6 (C-1'''), 72.1 (C-2'''), 72.3 (C-3'''), 73.8 (C-4'''), 69.8 (C-5'''), 18.0 (C-6''') for sugar moiety. ^1H NMR data (CD$_3$OD, 600 MHz) δ_H: 6.71 (1H, d, $J = 2.2$ Hz, H-6), 7.09 (1H, d, $J = 2.2$ Hz, H-8), 7.91 (1H, d, $J = 2.2$ Hz, H-2'), 6.95 (1H, d, $J = 8.5$ Hz, H-5'), 7.72 (1H, dd, $J = 8.5$ and 2.2 Hz, H-6'), 3.98 (3H, s, H-7') for aglycone; 5.30 (1H, d, $J = 7.6$ Hz, H-1''), 3.49 (1H, dd, $J = 9.1$ and

7.6 Hz, H-2''), 3.45 (1H, t, J = 9.1 Hz, H-3''), 3.23 (1H, t, J = 9.1 Hz, H-4''), 4.40 (1H, m, H-5''), 3.84 (1H, dd, J = 12.1 and 1.9 Hz, H-6''a), 3.42 (1H, m, H-6''b), 4.53 (1H, d, J = 1.3 Hz, H-1'''), 3.58 (1H, dd, J = 3.4 and 1.3, H-2'''), 3.47 (1H, dd, J = 9.5 and 3.4 Hz, H-3'''), 3.25 (1H, t, J = 9.5 Hz, H-4'''), 3.41 (1H, m, H-5'''), 1.10 (3H, d, J = 6.2 Hz, H-6''') for sugar moiety.

Antimicrobial assay
Microorganisms
The microorganisms used in this study were consisted of five bacterial strains namely *Staphylococcus aureus* ATCC 25923, *Vibrio cholerae* NB2, PC2, SG24 (1) and CO6 [16]. Also included were two fungi *Candida albicans* ATCC 9002 and *Cryptococcus neoformans* IP95026. These bacteria and yeasts were obtained from our local stocks.

Determination of minimum inhibitory concentration and minimum microbicidal concentration
The minimum inhibitory concentration (MIC) values were determined using the broth micro-dilution method as described earlier [17]. The MIC values were defined as the lowest sample concentration that prevented the change in color indicating a complete inhibition of microbial growth. The lowest concentrations that yielded no growth after the subculturing were taken as the minimum microbicidal concentration (MMC) values [18]. Ciprofloxacin (Sigma-Aldrich, Steinheim, Germany) and amphotericin B (Merck, Darmstadt, Germany) were used as positive controls for bacteria and yeast respectively.

Study on mode of action
MIC and MBC changes under osmotic stress condition
Osmotic stress was induced by adding 5% NaCl (w/v) to MHB. The MHB supplemented with 5% NaCl was then sterilized and used for the determination of a new MIC and MBC values of the samples as previously described [17]. The incubation time was increased from 24 to 48 h at 37 °C.

Effect of isolated compounds on cell membrane
The alteration of cell membrane of *V. cholerae* NB2 was evaluated by measuring the optical densities at 260 nm of the bacterial suspensions in the presence and absence of compounds **1–5** using the method described by Carson et al. [19]. For this purpose, the compounds were tested at their MIC using 1 mL of the bacterial suspension (approximately 10^8 CFU/mL). The mixture was then incubated at 37 °C at different time intervals (0: immediately after addition of the compound; 15; 30; 60 min), 50 μL of the mixture was taken and mixed with 1.95 mL of Phosphate Buffered Saline (PBS Buffer). The absorbance was measured on the spectrophotometer at 260 nm against the blank (PBS). For the negative control, 1 mL of bacterial suspension was incubated at 37 °C and 50 μL of the

suspension was removed at the end of the various incubation times and mixed with 1.95 mL of Buffer. The optical densities were read in the same way.

Bacteriolytic assay
The bacteriolytic activities of the isolated compounds were determined using the time-kill kinetic method as previously described [20] with slight modifications. Full growth of *V. cholerae* NB2 in MHB was diluted 100 times and incubated at 37 °C to produce an OD_{600} of 0.8 as starting inoculum. Sample solutions were added to the starting bacterial suspension to give a final concentration of 2 × MIC and incubated at 37 °C with shaking, then 100 μL was removed from each tube at 0, 15, 30, 60, and 120 min and the optical density measured at 600 nm. Vancomycin and tetracycline were used as positive controls and the tubes without isolated compounds served as negative controls.

Hemolytic assay
Whole blood (10 mL) from albino rats was collected by cardiac puncture in EDTA tubes. The study was conducted according to the ethical guidelines of the Committee for Control and Supervision of Experiments on Animals (Registration no. 173/CPCSEA, dated 28 January, 2000), Government of India, on the use of animals for scientific research. Erythrocytes were harvested by centrifugation at room temperature for 10 min at 1000 x g and were washed three times in PBS buffer [21]. The cytotoxicity was evaluated as previously described [21].

Statistical analysis
Data were analyzed by one-way analysis of variance followed by Waller-Duncan post hoc test. The experimental results were expressed as the mean ± Standard Deviation (SD). Differences between groups were considered significant when $p < 0.05$. All analyses were performed using the Statistical Package for Social Sciences (SPSS, version 12.0) software.

Results
Chemical analysis
The structures of five known flavonoid glycosides isolated from the *n*-BuOH fraction of leaves of *G. grandulosum* (Fig. 1) were determined using spectroscopic analysis and NMR spectra in conjunction with 2D experiments (COSY, NOESY, HSQC and HMBC). Direct comparison with published information led to the identification of chrysoeriol-7-*O*-β-D-xyloside **1** [22], luteolin-7-*O*-β-D-apiofuranosyl-(1 → 2)-β-D-xylopyranoside **2** [23], chrysoeriol-7-*O*-β-D-apiofuranosyl-(1 → 2)-β-D-xylopyranoside **3** [13], chrysoeriol-7-*O*-α-L-rhamnopyranosyl-(1 → 6)-β-D-(4''-hydrogeno sulfate) glucopyranoside **4** [13] and isorhamnetin-3-*O*-α-L-rhamnopyranosyl-(1 → 6)-β-D-glucopyranoside **5** [24].

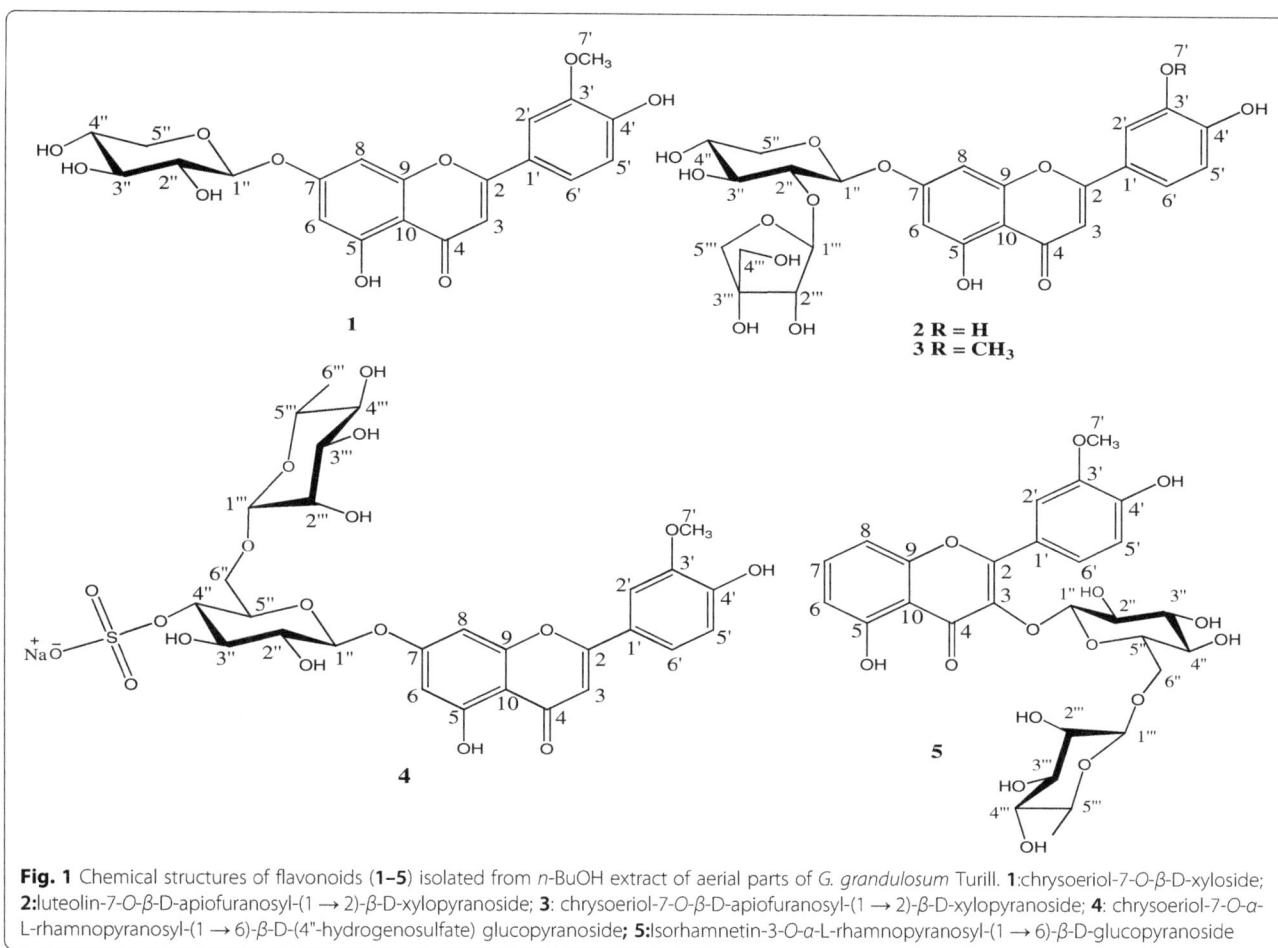

Fig. 1 Chemical structures of flavonoids (1–5) isolated from *n*-BuOH extract of aerial parts of *G. grandulosum* Turill. **1**:chrysoeriol-7-*O*-β-D-xyloside; **2**:luteolin-7-*O*-β-D-apiofuranosyl-(1 → 2)-β-D-xylopyranoside; **3**: chrysoeriol-7-*O*-β-D-apiofuranosyl-(1 → 2)-β-D-xylopyranoside; **4**: chrysoeriol-7-*O*-α-L-rhamnopyranosyl-(1 → 6)-β-D-(4"-hydrogenosulfate) glucopyranoside; **5**:Isorhamnetin-3-*O*-α-L-rhamnopyranosyl-(1 → 6)-β-D-glucopyranoside

Antimicrobial activity

The in vitro activities of MeOH, *n*-BuOH and EtOAc extracts as well as their isolated compounds against pathogenic bacteria and fungi are presented in Table 1. The test samples demonstrated varying degrees of inhibitory activities against the bacterial and fungal strains. Fungal strains were generally more susceptible to the effects of the compounds, but less susceptible to extracts. The EtOAc and *n*-BuOH extracts were active against *C. albicans* and *C. neoformans* which were not susceptible to the MeOH extract. The MIC values obtained with the EtOAc and *n*-BuOH extracts were smaller than those obtained with the MeOH extract. These observations suggest that the fractionation of the MeOH extract enhanced its antimicrobial activity. The lowest MIC values were recorded on *S. aureus*; suggesting that this microorganism was the most susceptible to all the test samples. The EtOAc extract showed the highest antimicrobial activity when compared with the MeOH and *n*-BuOH extracts.

The antimicrobial activities of the isolated compounds from *G. glandulosum* were as follows: compound 4 > compound 1 > compound 2 > compound 5 > compound 3. The

lowest MIC value of 4 µg/mL was recorded on *C. neoformans* with compound 4 and on *S. aureus* with compounds 1, 2 and 4 whereas the lowest MMC value was obtained on *S. aureus* with compound 4. However, the highest MIC value for compounds (64 µg/mL) was recorded with compound 3 against *V. cholerae* CO6, and with compounds 2 and 5 against *C. albicans*, while the highest MBC value of 128 µg/mL was obtained on *V. cholerae* CO6 with compound 3 and on *C. albicans* with compound 5.

Antibacterial activity of flavonoid glycosides under osmotic stress condition

The MIC values of flavonoid glycosides against Gram-negative and Gram-positive bacteria are reported in Table 2. The results clearly showed that the MIC values of flavonoid glycosides obtained under osmotic stress (in the presence of 5% NaCl) are smaller than those obtained under normal conditions (0% NaCl). This result suggests an increase in the activity of purified flavonoid glycosides under osmotic stress. As demonstrated under normal condition, compound 4 was still the most effective under osmotic stress, followed in decreasing order by compounds

Table 1 Antimicrobial activities of extracts, isolated compounds and reference antimicrobial drugs

Extracts/Compounds	Inhibition parameters	V. cholerae SG24 (1)	V. cholerae CO6	V. cholerae NB2	V. cholerae PC2	S. aureus ATCC 25923	C. albicans ATCC 9002	C. neoformans IP95026
MeOH extract	MIC	512	512	256	512	256	> 2048	> 2048
	MMC	512	512	512	1024	512	/	/
	MMC/MIC	1	1	2	2	2	/	/
n-BuOH extract	MIC	256	256	128	128	128	2048	2048
	MMC	256	256	128	256	128	> 2048	> 2048
	MMC/MIC	1	1	1	2	1	/	/
EtOAc extract	MIC	64	128	64	64	64	1024	512
	MMC	128	128	64	64	64	1024	1024
	MMC/MIC	2	1	1	1	1	1	2
1	MIC	16	8	8	8	4	32	8
	MMC	16	8	16	8	8	64	8
	MMC/MIC	1	1	2	1	2	2	1
2	MIC	16	16	8	8	4	64	16
	MMC	32	16	16	8	8	64	32
	MMC/MIC	2	1	2	1	2	1	2
3	MIC	32	64	32	32	8	32	16
	MMC	64	128	32	64	16	32	16
	MMC/MIC	2	2	1	2	2	1	1
4	MIC	8	8	8	8	4	8	4
	MMC	16	8	8	8	4	8	8
	MMC/MIC	2	1	1	1	1	1	2
5	MIC	32	16	16	16	8	64	32
	MMC	32	16	16	16	8	128	64
	MMC/MIC	1	1	1	1	1	2	2
Ref[a]	MIC	32	4	16	16	0.5	0.5	0.25
	MBC	32	4	16	16	0.5	0.5	0.25
	MBC/MIC	1	1	1	1	1	1	1

/: not determined; *MIC* Minimum Inhibitory Concentration, *MMC* Minimum Microbicidal Concentration; the MIC and MMC were measured in µg/mL; [a]: amphotericin B for yeasts and ciprofloxacin for bacteria

1 and 2. The MIC values of chloramphenicol determined under osmotic stress condition were smaller than those determined under normal conditions. However, all the MIC values of vancomycin determined under osmotic stress were higher than those determined under normal conditions. Table 1 further shows that under osmotic stress, the antibacterial activities of compounds **1**, **2** and **4** against *V. chorae* SG24 (1), *V. chorae* CO6, *V. chorae* NB2 and *V. chorae* PC2 were higher than that of vancomycin.

Effect of flavonoid glycosides on cell membrane
The effect of flavonoid glycosides of *G. glandulosum* was evaluated in terms of leakage of UV 260 absorbing material through the bacterial cell membrane (Fig. 2). After treatment with flavonoid glycosides at MIC values of compounds **1**, **2** and **4**, the OD_{260} values of filtrates of all test strains increased and most of the leakage

occurred during the initial period ($\leq$ 15 min), followed by a slight increase with prolonged incubation period. At the same time, the OD_{260} of the control without compound was not changed. These results suggest that flavonoid glycosides from *G. glandulosum* damage the cytoplasmic membrane and cause loss of intracellular components. The highest values of OD_{260} were recorded with compound **4** for all the *V. cholerae* strains, whereas the least OD_{260} values were noticed with compound **2**, indicating that compound **4** released the highest amounts of nucleic acids followed in decreasing order by compound **1**, then **2**.

Bacteriolytic effect of compounds 1, 2 and 4
The result on the leakage of 260 nm absorbing material was consistent with that of bacteriolysis (Fig. 3). This result showed a decrease in the optical density of

Table 2 Antibacterial activities in terms of MIC (µg/mL) of compounds 1, 3 and 4 under osmotic stress condition against bacterial strains

Bacteria	Compound 1		Compound 2		Compound 4		Chloramphenicol		Vancomycin	
	0% NaCl	5% NaCl	0% NaCl	5% NaCl	0% NaCl	5% NaCl	0% NaCl	5% NaCl	0% NaCl	5% NaCl
V. chorae SG24 (1)	16	8	16	16	8	4	4	1	16	64
V. cholerae CO6	8	4	16	4	8	2	16	2	16	32
V. cholerae NB2	8	4	8	2	8	2	64	1	32	64
V. cholerae PC2	8	4	8	2	8	2	16	1	32	64
S. aureus	4	2	4	2	4	1	32	0.5	0,5	1

suspension treated with compounds **1**, **2** and **4**. After 120 min, compounds **1**, **2** and **4** induced a decline in cell turbidity of 93.20, 94.36 and 95.16%, respectively in bacteria suspension compared to time 0, indicating the lysis of bacterial cells.

Haemolytic activity

The haemolytic activities of extracts and compounds **1–5** against red blood cells (RBCs) were investigated using Triton X-100 as a positive control. The positive control showed about 100% lysis, whereas the phosphate buffer saline (PBS) showed no lysis of RBCs. Interestingly, none of the tested samples showed haemolytic activities against RBCs at concentrations up to 256 and 2048 µg/mL for isolated compounds and extracts respectively (results not shown). This finding highlights the fact that the observed biological efficacy was not due to haemolysis.

Discussion

The antimicrobial activity of a plant extract is considered to be highly active if the MIC < 100 µg/mL; significantly active when 100 ≤ MIC ≤512 µg/mL; moderately active when 512 < MIC ≤2048 µg/mL; weakly active if MIC > 2048 µg/mL and not active when MIC > 10,000 µg/mL [25]. Hence, the EtOAc extract of *G. glandulosum* was highly active (MIC < 100 µg/mL) against *V. cholerae* SG24 (1), *V. cholerae* NB2, *V. cholerae* PC2 and *S. aureus*; significantly active (100 ≤ MIC ≤512 µg/mL) against *V. cholerae* CO6 and *C. neoformans*; moderately active (512 < MIC ≤2048 µg/mL) on *C. albicans*. The MeOH and *n*-BuOH extracts were significantly active against the test bacterial species; weakly and moderately active against the yeast cells respectively.

In this study, we also investigated if the mode of action of flavonoid compounds is bactericidal or bacteriostatic. The results of the MMC values were fourfold lesser than their corresponding MIC values. This observation suggests that the actions of extracts from *G. glandulosum* and their isolated flavonoid glycosides were bactericidal [11].

The antibacterial activities of flavonoid glycosides were in some cases equal to, or higher than those of ciprofloxacin used as reference antibiotic, suggesting that they might be effective antibiotics against these pathogenic bacteria. Taking into account the medical importance of

the test microbial species, the result can be considered as promising for the development of new antimicrobial drugs. The antimicrobial activities of purified flavonoids corroborated with those of early reports against bacteria and fungi [5, 11, 26–28]. The antibacterial activity of the samples against *V. cholerae* and *S. flexneri* are particularly noteworthy since these strains were MDR clinical isolates which were resistant to commonly used drugs such as ampicillin, streptomycin, nalidixic acid, furazolidone and co-trimoxazole [16, 29, 30].

Antimicrobial cutoff points have been defined in the literature to enable the understanding of the effectiveness of pure compounds as follows: highly active: MIC below 1 µg/mL (or 2.5 µM), significantly active: $1 \leq$ MIC ≤ 10 µg/mL (or $2.5 \leq$ MIC < 25 µM), moderately active: 10 < MIC ≤100 µg/mL (or 25 < MIC ≤250 µM), weakly active: 100 < MIC ≤1000 µg/mL (or 250 < MIC ≤2500 µM and not active: MIC > 1000 µg/mL (or > 2500 µM) [25]. Based on this, the antimicrobial activities of all the tested flavonoid glycosides could be considered as significant or moderate against the specific microorganisms.

The antimicrobial activities of the isolated compounds from *G. glandulosum* were in this order: compound **4** > compound **1** > compound **2** > compound **5** > compound **3**. Very little is known about the structure–function relationships of natural antimicrobials, but it seems that different substituent groups within the compounds had a great influence on their biophysical and biological properties [31]. Structural features such as the presence of an aromatic ring, the sugar moiety or the numbers of hydroxyl and methoxyl groups can significantly change membrane permeability and subsequent affinity to external and internal binding sites in the bacteria, thus influencing the compound's antimicrobial properties [32].

The antibacterial activities of flavonoid glycosides and chloramphenicol increased under osmotic stress (5% NaCl) whereas that of vancomycin decreased under this condition. The results were supported by the observation that certain bacterial strains (*E. coli*, *S. aureus*, *P. aeruginosa*) can survive under osmotic stress conditions [33]. At low water activity, lipid composition of bacterial cell membrane was changed [34]. This incident might lead to occurrence of more antibacterial binding site on cell membrane of bacteria and cause less resistance to

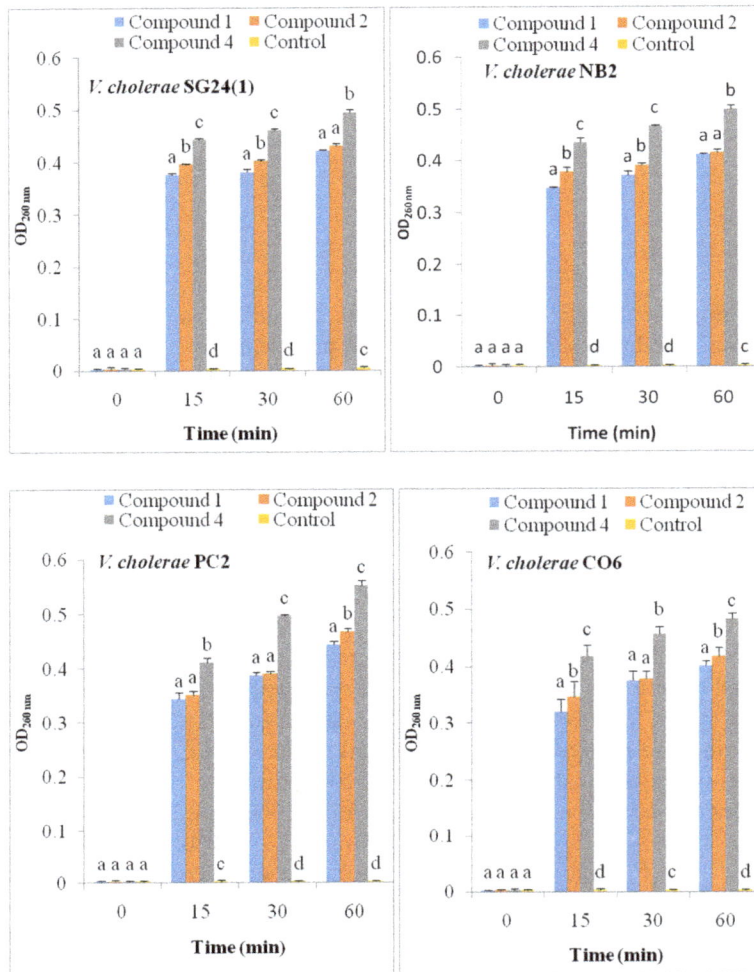

Fig. 2 Appearance of 260-nm-absorbing material in the filtrates of *V. cholerae* SG24 (1), PC2, NB2 and CO6 after treatment with compounds **1, 2** and **4**. Bars represent the mean ± standard deviation of the triplicate OD at each incubation time. At the same incubation time, letters a-d indicate significant differences between samples according to one way ANOVA and Waller Duncan test; $p < 0.05$

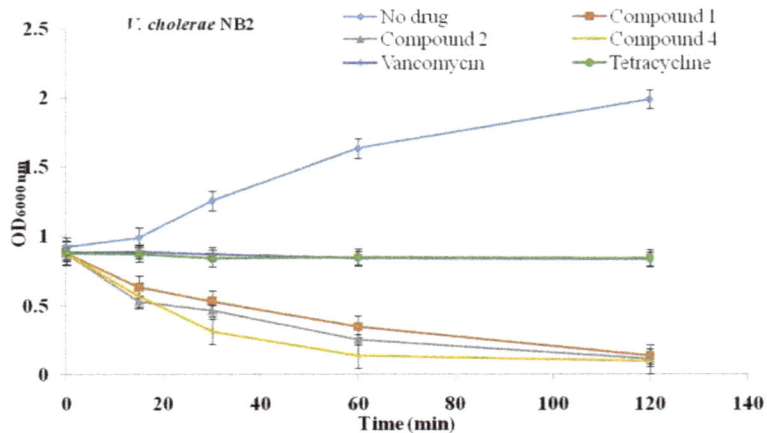

Fig. 3 Bacteriolytic effect of compounds **1**, **2** and **4** against *V. cholerae* NB2. Results represent the mean ± standard deviation of the triplicate OD at each incubation time

antibacterial substance. Therefore, the presence of the salt triggered changes in the membrane lipid composition. This is possible to increase the antibacterial activity of flavonoid glycosides and chloramphenicol. However, the mechanisms that make bacteria more sensitive to certain antibiotics under osmotic stress conditions are still unknown. The results of vancomycin activity are in agreement with those of McMahon and coworkers [35] who demonstrated a decrease in the activity of amikacin, ceftriaxone and trimethoprim against *E. coli* and *S. aureus* under osmotic stress conditions.

Marked leakage of cytoplasmic material is considered indicative of gross and irreversible damaged to the cytoplasmic membrane. Many antibacterial compounds that act on the bacterial cytoplasmic membrane induce the loss of 260 nm-absorbing materials (nucleic acids) including chlorohexidine, hexachlorophene, phenetyl alcohol, tetracycline, polymixin, α-pinene, and lemon grass oil [19]. The *V. cholerae* suspension treated with flavonoid glycosides, showed a significant increase in the optical density at 260 nm, suggesting that nucleic acids were lost through a damaged cytoplasmic membrane.

Our observations confirm that the antimicrobial activity of flavonoid glycosides results from their ability to disrupt the permeability barrier of microbial membrane structures. This mode of action is similar to that of other broad-spectrum, membrane-active disinfectants and preservatives, such as phenol derivatives, chlorohexidine and para benzoic acid derivatives [36]. Furthermore, Devi and Kapila [37], reported the antibacterial mechanism as disruption of plasma membrane by the phytochemicals in the extracts of Indian liverworts.

The fact that flavonoids-induced damage to cell membrane structure accompanied by the decline in the absorbance of bacterial cell suspension treated with compounds has confirmed it as the most likely cause of cell death. Our result is supported by the observation that other flavonoid compounds such as epigallocatechin gallate and galangin induced 3-log reduction or more in viable counts of *S. aureus* [38, 39].

Conclusions

The results of the present study indicate that the purified flavonoid glycosides from *G. glandulosum* possess antimicrobial activities. Their mode of antibacterial activity is due to cell lysis and disruption of the cytoplasmic membrane by action upon the membrane permeability leading to leakage of cellular components and eventually cell death. This will lead to improve antimicrobial formulations and to ensure the prevention of the emergence of microbial resistance. However, the possibility remains that sites of action other than the cytoplasmic membrane exist. Further work is required to expatiate fully the mechanisms involved.

Abbreviations
^{13}C-NMR: Carbon Thirteen Nuclear Magnetic Resonance; ^{1}H NMR: Proton Nuclear Magnetic Resonance; ^{2}D NMR: Two-dimension Nuclear Magnetic Resonance; ATCC: American Type Culture Collection; CC: Column Chromatography; COSY: Correlation Spectroscopy; DMSO: Dimethylsulfoxide; EtOAc: Ethyl acetate; HMBC: Heteronuclear Multiple Bond Connectivities; HNC: *Herbier National du Cameroun*; HR-EI-MS: High Resolution Electron Impact Mass Spectrometry; HR-TOFESIMS: High-Resolution Time of Flight Electrospray Ionization Mass Spectrometry; HSQC: The Heteronuclear Single Quantum Coherence; IR: Infra-red; MBC: Minimum bactericidal concentration; MDR: Multi-Drug-Resistant; MeOH: Methanol; MHA: Mueller Hinton agar; MHB: Mueller Hinton broth; MIC: Minimum inhibitory concentration; MMC: Minimum Microbicidal Concentration; NA: Nutrient agar; n-BuOH: n-Butanol; NMR: Nuclear Magnetic Resonance; Rf: Retention factor; TLC: Thin Layer Chromatography; TMS: Tetramethylsilane; TOF-ESIMS: Time of Flight Electrospray Ionization Mass Spectrometry; UV: Ultra-violet

Availability of data and materials
The datasets used and/or analyzed during the current study are available from the corresponding author on reasonable request.

Authors' contributions
CNT and SEE contributed to the data collection and analysis. JDT designated the study, did the biological assays and helped in manuscript writing and editing. JDT, DN and LVN supervised and revised the manuscript critically for important intellectual content. All authors read and agreed on the final version of the manuscript.

Competing interests
The authors declare that they have no competing interests.

Author details
^{1}Research Unit of Environmental and Applied Chemistry, Department of Chemistry, Faculty of Science, University of Dschang, P.O. Box 67, Dschang, Cameroon. ^{2}Research Unit of Microbiology and Antimicrobial Substances, Department of Biochemistry, Faculty of Science, University of Dschang, P.O. Box 67, Dschang, Cameroon. ^{3}Groupe Isolement et Structure, Institut de Chimie Moléculaire de Reims (ICMR), CNRS UMR 7312, Bat. 18 BP.1039, 51687 Reims cedex 2, France.

References
1. Nair GB, Ramamurthy T, Bhattacharya MK, Krishnan T, Ganguly S, Saha DR, et al. Emerging trends in the etiology of enteric pathogens as evidenced from an active surveillance of hospitalized diarrhoeal patients in Kolkata India. Gut Pathog. 2010;2:4.
2. Mahady GB, Huang Y, Doyle BJ, Locklear T. Natural products as antibacterial agents. Nat Prod Chem. 2008;35:423–44.
3. Tatsimo NSJ, Tamokou JD, Lamshöft M, Mouafo TF, Lannang MA, Sarkar P, et al. LC-MS guided isolation of antibacterial and cytotoxic constituents from *Clausena anisata*. Med Chem Res. 2015;24:1468–79.
4. Pagning NAL, Tamokou JD, Lateef M, Tapondjou AL, Kuiate JR, Ngnokam D, et al. New triterpene and new flavone glucoside from *Rhynchospora corymbosa* (Cyperaceae) with their antimicrobial tyrosinase and butyrylcholinesterase inhibitory activities. Phytochem Lett. 2016;16:121–8.
5. Tebou PLF, Tamokou JD, Ngnokam D, Voutquenne-Nazabadioko L, Kuiate JR, Bag PK. Flavonoids from *Maytenus buchananii* as potential cholera chemotherapeutic agents. S Afr J Bot. 2017;109:58–65.
6. Robinson T. The organic constituents of higher plants – their chemistry and interrelationships. 6th ed. North Amherst: Cordus Press; 1991.

7. Mills S, Bone K. Principles and practice of phytotherapy –modern herbal medicine. New York: Churchill Livingstone. 2000:31–4.

8. Evans WC. Trease and Evans Pharmacognosy. 15th ed. New York: W B Saunders; 2002. p. 246–8.

9. Benavente-Garcia O, Castillo J, Marin FR, Ortuno A, Del Rio JA. Uses and properties of citrus flavonoids. J Agric Food Chem. 1997;45:4505–15.

10. Vuorela S, Kreander K, Karonen M, Nieminen R, Hämäläinen M, Galkin A, et al. Preclinical evaluation of rapeseed raspberry and pine bark phenolics for health related effects. J Agric Food Chem. 2005;53:5922–31.

11. Djouossi MG, Tamokou JD, Ngnokam D, Kuiate JR, Tapondjou AL, Harakat D, et al. Antimicrobial and antioxidant flavonoids from the leaves of Oncoba spinosa Forssk (Salicaceae). BMC Complement Altern Med. 2015;15:134.

12. Barker RM. Graptophyllum nees. J Adel Bot Gard. 1986;9:156–66.

13. Ngoufack TC, Ngnokam D, Harakat D, Voutquenne-Nazabadioko L. Three new flavonoid glycosides from the aerial parts of Graptophyllum grandulosum Turril (Acanthaceae). Phytochem Lett. 2017;19:172–5.

14. Wahyuningtyas E. The Graptophylum pictum effect on acrylic resin complete denture plaque growth. Dent J (Maj Kedokt Gigi). 2005;38:201–14.

15. Jiangseubchatveera N, Liawruangrath B, Liawruangrath S, Teerawutgulrag A, Santiarwarn D, Korth J, et al. The chemical constituents and the cytotoxicity antioxidant and antibacterial activities of the essential oil of Graptophyllum pictum (L) Griff. J Essent Oil Bear Pl. 2015;18:11–7.

16. Bag PK, Bhowmik P, Hajra TK, Ramamurthy T, Sarkar P, Majumder M, et al. Putative virulence traits and pathogenicity of Vibrio cholerae non-O1 non-O139 isolated from surface waters in Kolkata India. Appl Environ Microbiol. 2008;74:5635–44.

17. Fondjo ES, Dimo KSD, Tamokou JD, Tsemeugne J, Kouamo S, Ngouanet D, et al. Synthesis characterization antimicrobial and antioxidant activities of the homocyclotrimer of 4-Oxo-4h-thieno[34-C]chromene-3diazonium sulfate. Open Med Chem J. 2016;10:21–32.

18. Joubouhi C, Tamokou JD, Ngnokam D, Voutquenne-Nazabadioko L, Kuiate JR. Iridoids from Canthium subcordatum iso-butanol fraction with potent biological activities. BMC Complement Altern Med. 2017;17:17.

19. Carson CF, Mee BJ, Riley TV. Mechanism of action of Melaleuca alternifolia (tea tree) oil on Staphylococcus aureus determined by time kill, lysis, leakage and salt tolerance assays and electron microscopy. Antimicrob Agents Chemother. 2002;46:1914–20.

20. Ooi N, Miller K, Hobbs J, Rhys-Williams W, Love W, Chopra I. XF-73 a novel antistaphylococcal membrane active agent with rapid bactericidal activity. J Antimicrob Chemother. 2009;64:735–40.

21. Situ H, Bobek LA. In vitro assessment of antifungal therapeutic potential of salivary histatin-5 two variants of histatin-5 and salivary mucin (MUC7) domain 1. Antimicrob Agents Chemother. 2000;44:1485–93.

22. Markham KR, Ternai B, Stanley R, Geiger H, Mabry TJ. Carbon-13 NMR studies of flavonoids III naturally occurring flavonoid glycosides and their acylated derivatives. Tetrahedron. 1978;34:1389–97.

23. Koffi EN, Le Guernevéc C, Lozanoa PR, MeudeccAdjéd FA, Bekrob YA, Lozanoa YF. Polyphenol extraction and characterization of Justicia secunda Vahl leaves for traditional medicinal uses. Ind Crop Prod. 2013;49:682–9.

24. Mona-Antonia B, Hanns H. Flavonol glycosides from Eschscholtzia californica. Phytochemistry. 1999;50:329–32.

25. Tamokou JD, Mbaveng TA, Kuete V. Antimicrobial activities of African medicinal spices and vegetables. In: Medicinal spices and vegetables from Africa: therapeutic potential against metabolic inflammatory infectious and systemic diseases 1st edition Elsevier chapter 8 pp 207–237 2017.

26. Tatsimo NSJ, Tamokou JD, Havyarimana L, Dezső C, Forgo P, Hohmann J, et al. Antimicrobial and antioxidant activity of kaempferol rhamnoside derivatives from Bryophyllum pinnatum. BMC Res Notes. 2012;5:158.

27. Mabou FD, Tamokou JD, Ngnokam D, Voutquenne-Nazabadioko L, Kuiate JR, Bag PK. Complex secondary metabolites from Ludwigia leptocarpa with potent antibacterial and antioxidant activities. Drug Discover Therap. 2016; 10:141–9.

28. Tatsimo NSJ, Tamokou JD, Tsague TV, Lamshoft M, Sarkar P, Bag PK, et al. Antibacterial-guided isolation of constituents from Senna alata leaves with a particular reference against multi-drug-resistant Vibrio cholerae and Shigella flexneri. Int J Biol Chem Sci. 2017;11:46–53.

29. Thakurta P, Bhowmik P, Mukherjee S, Hajra TK, Patra A, Bag PK. Antibacterial antisecretory and antihemorrhagic activity of Azadirachta indica used to treat cholera and diarrhea in India. J Ethnopharmacol. 2007;111:607–12.

30. Acharyya S, Sarkar P, Saha DR, Patra A, Ramamurthy T, Bag PK. Intracellular and membrane damaging activities of methyl gallate isolated from Terminalia chebula against multi-drug resistant Shigella species. J Med Microbiol. 2015;64:901–9.

31. Mandalari G, Bennett RN, Bisignano G, Trombetta D, Saija A, Faulds CB, et al. Antimicrobial activity of flavonoids extracted from bergamot (Citrus bergamia Risso) peel a byproduct of the essential oil industry. J Appl Microbiol. 2007;103:2056–64.

32. Fitzgerald DJ, Stratford M, Gasson MJ, Ueckert J, Bos A, Narbad A. Mode of antimicrobial action of vanillin against Escherichia coli, Lactobacillus plantarum and Listeria innocua. J Appl Microbiol. 2004;97:104–13.

33. Besten HMW, Mols M, Moezelaar R, Zwietering MH, Abee T. Phenotypic and transcriptomic analyses of mildly and severely salt-stressed Bacillus cereus ATCC 14579 cells. Appl Environ Microbiol. 2009;75:111–9.

34. Beales N. Adaptation of microorganisms to cold temperatures weak acid reservatives low pH and osmotic stress: a review. Compr Rev Food Sci Food Saf. 2004;3:1–20.

35. McMahon MAS, Xu J, Moore JE, Blair IS, McDowell DA. Environmental stress and antibiotic resistance in food-related pathogens. Appl Environ Microbiol. 2007;73:211–7.

36. Cox SD, Mann CM, Markham JL, Bell HC, Gustafson JE, Warmington JR, et al. The mode of antibacterial action of the essential oil of Melaleuca alternifolia (tea tree oil). J Appl Microbiol. 2000;88:170–5.

37. Devi K, Kapila S. Antibacterial effect of some Indian liverworts. Int J Pharm Sci Rev Res. 2013;20:219–21.

38. Cushnie TTP, Lamb AJ. Antimicrobial activity of flavonoids. Int J Antimicrob Agents. 2005;26:343–56.

39. Cushnie TTP, Lamb AJ. Recent advances in understanding the antibacterial properties of flavonoids. Int J Antimicrob Agents. 2011;38:99–107.

10-hydroxy-2-decenoic acid of royal jelly exhibits bactericide and anti-inflammatory activity in human colon cancer cells

Yuan-Chang Yang[1], Wing-Ming Chou[1], Debora Arny Widowati[1], I-Ping Lin[1,2] and Chi-Chung Peng[1]* ⓘ

Abstract

Background: Royal jelly (RJ), the exclusive food for the larva of queen honeybee, is regarded as the novel supplement to promote human health. The function of RJ may be attributed to its major and unique fatty acid, 10-hydroxy-2-decenoic acid (10-HDA). The current study investigated the anti-inflammory function of 10-HDA on human colon cancer cells, WiDr, as well as its effect on the growth of pathogenic bacterium.

Methods: The pro-inflammatory cytokines, receptor antagonist cytokine (IL-1ra) and nuclear factor-kappa B (NF-κB) in WiDr cells was analyzed by Enzyme-linked immunosorbent assay (ELISA) or western blot. The growth inhibition of 10-HDA on bacterium was evaluated by determination of minimal inhibitory concentrations (MIC) and minimal bactericide concentrations (MBC).

Results: The production of pro-inflammatory cytokines, Interleukin (IL)-8, IL-1β and tumor necrosis factor-alpha (TNF-α) in WiDr cells was modulated by 10-HDA. IL-8 were dramatically declined by 10-HDA at 3 mM, while IL-1β and TNF-α were significantly decreased. 10-HDA increased IL-1ra in a dose manner. NF-κB pathway is primarily in response to prototypical pro-inflammatory cytokines, and NF-κB was reduced after 10-HDA treatment. 10-HDA acted as potent bactericide against animal- or human-specific pathogens, including *Staphylococcus aureus, Streptococcus alactolyticus, Staphylococcus intermedius B, Staphylococcus xylosus, Salmonella cholearasuis, Vibro parahaemolyticus* and *Escherichia coli (hemolytic)*.

Conclusions: The current study showed that in vitro 10-HDA from RJ exhibited anti-inflammatory activity in WiDr cells, as well as anti-bacterial activity against animal pathogens. 10-HDA showed its potential as anti-imflammtory agent and bactericide to benefit human gastrointestinal tract.

Keywords: 10-hydroxy-2-decenoic acid, Anti-inflammation, Antimicrobial, Colon cancer cell, Cytokines

Background

In response to pathogens, the pro-inflammatory cytokines, TNF-α is induced by activated macrophages; subsequently, the spread of pathogens into the circulation is limited [1, 2]. TNF-α initiates a cascade of pro-inflammatory cytokines [3]. Among them, IL-1 a primary pro-inflammatory cytokine stimulates the expression of genes that are associated with inflammation [4]. IL-8 is rapidly induced by IL-1 or TNF-α, and used as a marker of activated inflammatory/immuno response [5]. However, the production of IL-1 is inhibited by an excess of IL-1ra [6]. The canonical NF-κB pathway has been defined primarily in response to TNF-α and IL-1 signaling, prototypical proinflammatory cytokines. The persistent, long-lasting inflammation may lead to inflammatory disease and cancer etiology [7]. The over-production of pro-inflammatory cytokines and NF-κB take important roles in the chronical inflammatory diseases such as rheumatoid arthrtitis (RA) and inflammatory bowel disease (IBD) [8]. Inflammation is generally treated with immune-suppressing drugs that reduce inflammation and painful symptoms. It was reported that non-steroidal anti-inflammatory drugs might cause the gastrointestinal complications [9]. It is thus needed to explore the natural substances that inhibit inflammation and prevent chronic inflammatory diseases with minimal toxicity [10].

* Correspondence: bocky@nfu.edu.tw
[1]Department of Biotechnology, National Formosa University, Huwei District, Yunlin, Taiwan
Full list of author information is available at the end of the article

Royal jelly (RJ), secreted by the hypopharyngeal and mandibular glands of worker honeybees (*Apis mellifera*), is supplied as the exclusive food for the larva and adult of queen honeybee. RJ well known for its novel functions to promote human health mainly comprises water, sugar, proteins, and lipids. The lipid is present in around 3 to 19% of dry RJ [11]. And approximately 90% of RJ lipids are free fatty acids, containing 8–12 carbons that are usually either hydroxyl or dicarboxylic forms. The major and unique fatty acid in RJ lipid is 10-hydroxy-2-decenoic acid (10-HDA), which was not found in other bee products [12].

The pharmacological activities of RJ were reported, including growth rate increasing [13], antitumor [14, 15], anti-inflammatory and antimicrobial activity [16–19], as well as antioxidant activity [20]. RJ has inhibitory effects toward approximately 30 bacterial species, including aerobes, anaerobes, Gram-positive and Gram-negative bacteria [21]. 10-HDA is one of the compositions responsible for the pharmacological activities of RJ. It was reported to have anti-tumor [22], collagen promoting [23], immunomodulatory [24], antimicrobial activity [16–18] and antimelanogensis [25].

In this study, we investigated the effect of 10-HDA purified from RJ on human colon adenocarcinoma cell (WiDr cells), as well as antimicrobial activity against serveral animal pathogenic bacteria. The supression of TNF-α, IL-1β, IL-8 and NF-κB pathway by 10-HDA was evaluated, as well as the induction of IL-1ra.

Methods
Preparation of 10-HDA from royal jelly
Royal jelly was provided by the Fu-Chang Beekeeping in Hualien, Taiwan. The 10-HDA was purified and quantitative analysis using the method from our previous work [25]. The highest purity of the 10-HDA sample was obtained about 92%. This sample was used on WiDr cells for the next assays.

Cell viabilities assay
The WiDR human adenocarcinoma cell (BCRC 60157) was cultured in minimum essential medium (Eagle) with 2 mM L-glutamine and Earle's BSS adjusted to contain 1.5 g/L sodium bicarbonate, 1.0 mM sodium pyruvate, 90%; fetal bovine serum, 10%, at 37 °C in a humidified atmosphere containing 5% (*v*/*v*) CO_2. To study the effect of 10-HDA on WiDr cell proliferation, the cells were seeded in 96-well plates at a density of 1×10^4 cells/well. After one night, the cells were then treated with different doses of 10-HDA, ranging from 0.1 to 5 mM, for 24 h. After the 24-h treatment, the supernatant were collected. Cell viability was evaluated by the MTT (methyl

thiazol tetrazolium bromide) assay as described previously [25]. The optical density was determined at 570 nm (OD_{570}).

Cytokines analysis
The cytokines production of TNF-α, IL-1β, IL-8 and IL-1ra in the cell culture supernatants collected after 24 h of cultivation were determined by ELISA kit (DUO Set, R&D systems, Abingdon, UK) according to the manufacturer's instructions. Capture antibody (1:180 dilution) was added into each well of a 96-well microplate, incubated overnight at room temperature. In the following day, after washing, block buffer was added and incubated for 1 h. The wells were washed again, then the standards and the culture supernatant of the 10-HDA-treated cells was added and incubated at room temperature for 2 h. After washing, the detection antibody (1:180 dilution) was added to each well. After incubated for 2 h, Streptavidin horseradish-peroxidase (HRP: reagent diluent = 1: 200) was added, then kept away from light for 20 min. Finally, substrate solution was added to each well, kept for 20 min before adding 50 μL stop solution to each well. The optical density was determined at 450 nm (OD_{450}).

NF-κB western assays
The NF-κB production in the cell were determined by western blot as described previously [8]. The cells were lysed in RIPA buffer (pH 7.4, 50 mM tris, 0.1% SDS, 50 mM NaCl, 1% NP-40, 1 mM PMSF, 10 μg/mL aprotinin and 10 μg/mL leupeptin) and collected its nuclear fraction. Protein quantified by Bradford assay using BSA as the standard and the proteins were separated by 10% SDS-PAGE, transferred onto hybond-C Extra nitrocellulose membrane (Amersham Biotscience, U.K.). The membranes were blocked overnight in block solution (TBS-T buffer containing 5% non-fat skim milk). The membrane was then incubated with rabbit polyclonal anti-NF-κB and antiβ-actin antibodies as an internal control. The membranes were further incubated with HRP conjugated anti-rabbit goat polyclonal secondary antibody. Proteins were detected by chemilluminescent with Super Signal® West Pico Chemiluminescent Substrate (ECL) (Thermo Scientific). The signal density of each band was measure and analyzed using a densitometer system Gel Doc TM / Chemi Doc TM Universal hood II (Bio-Rad).

Antimicrobial activity assay
Antimicrobial activity were evaluated by against four Gram-positive bacteria, *Staphylococcus aureus*, *S. intermedius B*, *S. xylosus*, and *Streptococcus alactolyticus*, and four Gram-negative bacteria, *hemolytic Escherichia coli*, *Pseudomonas aeruginosa*, *Salmonella*

cholearasuis, and *Vibrio parahaemolyticus* [19]. The MIC and MBC of 10-HDA was measured using the method according our previous work [26]. 10-HDA was dissolved in dimethyl sulphoxide (DMSO) at a final concentration of 100 μM. The assay solution contain 100 μl of 10-HDA dilution, 100 μl of culture medium (Tryptone Soya Broth (TSB)) and 100μl of a 10× suspension of each microorganism in 96-well microtiter plate (Iwaki Inc., Japan). Each assay and growth control well was inoculate with final concentration of a bacterial is $1–5 \times 10^5$ CFU/well. Bacterial growth was detected by optical density (OD) (ELISA reader, μQuant microplate spectroplate, Bio-TEK, VT, USA).

Statistical analysis

Data are presented as mean ± SD. Statistical analysis was performed using SigmaPlot software (Systat Software Inc., San Jose, CA, USA). Significant differences were evaluated using one way ANOVA followed by the Dunnett's multiple comparison test. Values of $p \leq 0.05$ or less were considered as statistically significance.

Results

10-HDA inhibited growth of WiDr cells

The MTT assay was performed to assess the rate of proliferation of WiDr human colon cancer cells after treatment with various concentrations of 10-HDA (0.1–5 mM). Fig. 1 shows that the inhibitory effect of 10-HDA on WiDr cell proliferation is dose-dependent. The inhibitory effects of 10-HDA were more pronounced at the higher dose (5 mM), which has cytotoxic effect and could kill the WiDr cells directly. 10-HDA at a concentration of 3 mM

inhibited significantly about 82.82% of the cell proliferation compared to the control group as the 100%, but it was not cytotoxic to the WiDr cells. Lower doses of 10-HDA did not inhibited the cells

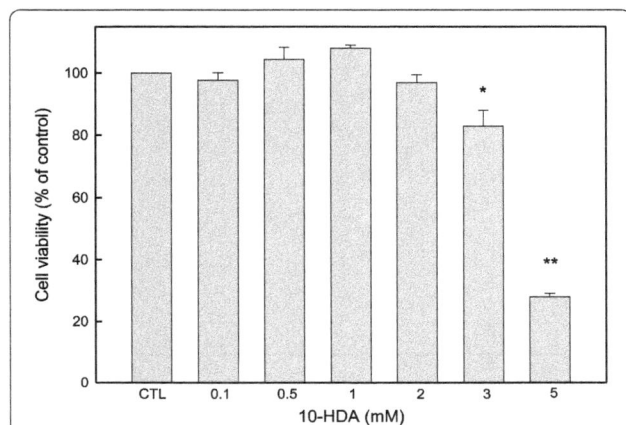

Fig. 2 Effect of 10-HDA on human TNF-α, IL-1β and IL-8 production in WiDr cells. Supernatants of WiDr cultures, treated with or without 10-HDA (0.1, 0.5, 1, 2 and 3 mM), were collected after 24 h and tested by ELISA for detecting TNF-α (**a**), IL-1β (**b**) and IL-8 (**c**). CTL represents the control group (without 10-HDA). Each point is a mean ± SD of the triplicates from one representative experiment. * = $p \leq 0.05$; ** = $p \leq 0.01$ compared to control

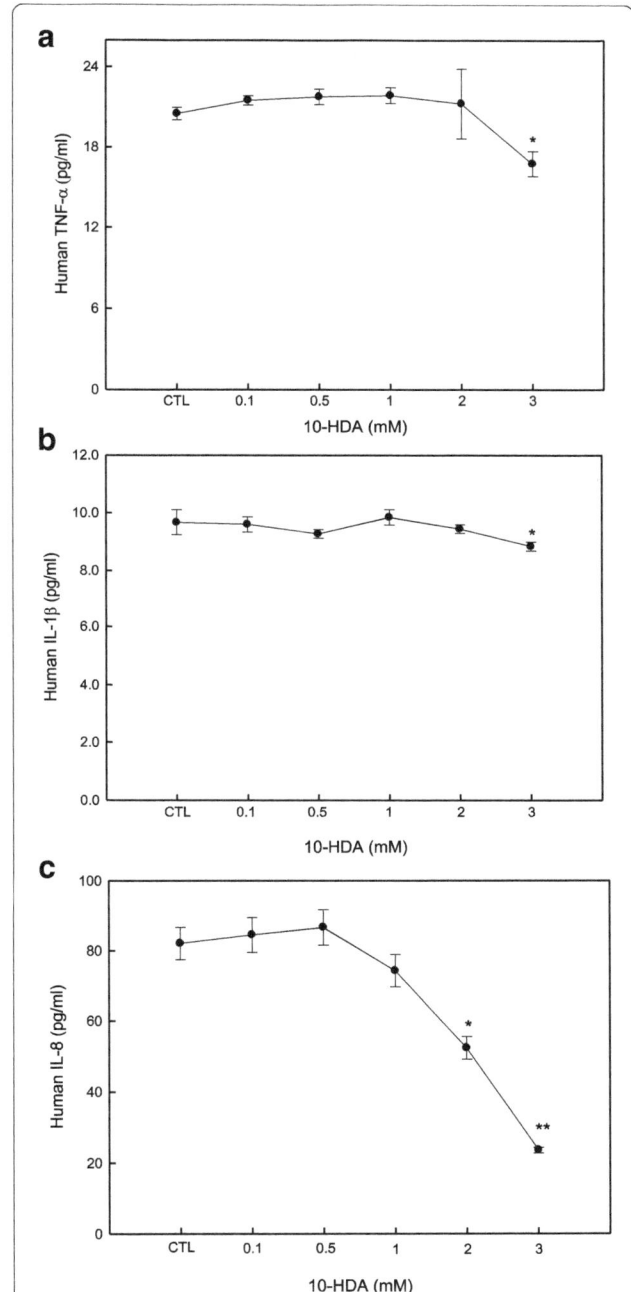

Fig. 1 Percent cell viability of WiDr colon cancer cells after 10-HDA treatment (0.1, 0.5, 1, 2, 3, and 5 mM) for 24 h. CTL represents the control group (without 10-HDA). Each bar is a mean ± SD of the triplicates from one representative experiment. * = $p \leq 0.05$; ** = $p \leq 0.01$ compared to control

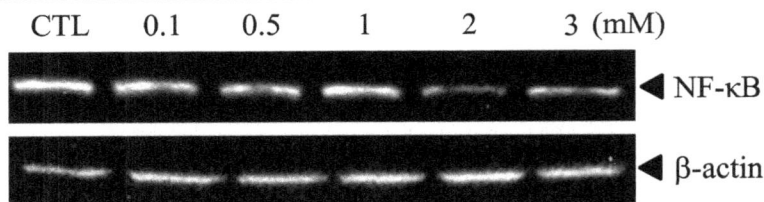

Fig. 3 Effect of 10-HDA on human NF-κB production in WiDr cells. Supernatants of WiDr cultures, treated with or without 10-HDA (0.1, 0.5, 1, 2 and 3 mM), were collected after 24 h and tested by Western Blotting to detect the presence of NF-κB. CTL represents the control group (without 10-HDA). Results are expressed as relative percentages of NF-κB activation compared to the control group (100%)

significantly. The maximum growth inhibitory effect of 10-HDA was observed at the 5 mM concentration after 24 h of treatment.

10-HDA inhibited TNF-α, IL-1β and IL-8 production in WiDr cells

We investigated the effects of 10-HDA on TNF-α, IL-1β, IL-8 and IL-1ra production in WiDr cells by ELISA. After examining the effec of 10-HDA on human TNF-α production, it was observed that 10-HDA inhibited TNF-α at a concentration of 3 mM 10-HDA, about 81.79% compared to the control. The level of TNF-α secreted by the control group was about 20.50 pg/mL, whereas in the group treated with a concentraion of 10-HDA at 3 mM, the TNF-α secretion level was reduced to 16.76 pg/mL (Fig. 2a). Further results indicated that 10-HDA inhibited human IL-1β secretion at 24 h in WiDr cells. The WiDr cells in the control group produced 9.66 pg/mL IL-1β, but the IL-1β secretion decreased to 8.83 pg/mL when the cells were treated with a concentration of 10-HDA at 3 mM (Fig. 2b). Fig. 2c shows that 10-HDA markedly inhibited IL-8 secretion at non-cytotoxic concentrations (2 and 3 mM) at 24 h treatment. In the control group, the WiDr cells produced 82.08 pg/mL IL-8, and the treatement in 2 mM and 3 mM 10-HDA reduced the human IL-8 production by 72.31 and 43.57%, respectively.

10-HDA inhibited NF-κB expression in WiDr cells

To investigate the effect of 10-HDA on NF-κB expression, we examined this effect using WiDr cells. The result (Fig. 3) was observed that 10-HDA inhibited the NF-κB expression, the inhibition rate were approximately ranging from 6.56 to 68.9% compared to the control. This result suggested that 10-HDA would modulate the inflammatory response in a dose-dependent manner.

10-HDA induced IL-1ra production in WiDr cells

IL-1ra is one of the major anti-inflammatory cytokine [27]. The results on Fig. 4 indicated that 10-HDA stimulated the human IL-1ra production in WiDr cells. 10-HDA concentration at 1, 2 and 3 mM showed the significant stimulation activity on the IL-1ra secretion (57.97, 62.95, and 57.97 pg/mL, respectively) compared to the control, in which the WiDr cells only produced 34.26 pg/mL of IL-1ra.

Antibacterial activity of 10-HDA

10-HDA was assayed for bactericidal and bacteriostatic activities against eight strains of Gram-positive and Gram-negative bacteria (Table 1). Result showed that the MIC of 10-HDA against Gram-positive bcateria was 23–44 μM, and MBC was 33–66 μM. The MIC and MBC of 10-HDA against Gram-negative bcateria were in the ranges of 40–43 μM and 74–78 μM, respectively. However, the growth of the Gram-negative bcateria, *Pseudomonas aeruginosa*, was not affected by 10-HDA at all. 10-HDA has higher

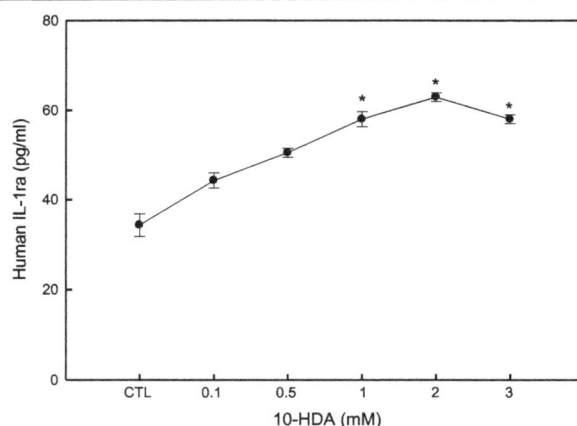

Fig. 4 Effect of 10-HDA on human IL-1ra production in WiDr cells. Supernatants of WiDr cultures, treated with or without 10-HDA (0.1, 0.5, 1, 2, 3, and 5 mM), were collected after 24 h and tested by ELISA for detecting IL-1ra. CTL represents the control group (without 10-HDA). Each point is a mean ± SD of the triplicates from one representative experiment. * = $p \leq 0.05$ compared to control

Table 1 Bacteriostatic and Bactericidal Activities of 10-HDA against Eight Different Animal- and Human-Specific Pathogens

Bacteria	MIC (μM)	MBC (μM)
Staphylococcus aureus (+)	23	53
Streptococcus alactolyticus(+)	44	66
Staphylococcus intermediusB(+)	23	33
Staphylococcus xylosus(+)	24	36
Pseudomonas aeruginosa(−)	NI	ND
Salmonella cholearasuis(−)	42	74
Vibro parahaemolyticus(−)	40	76
Escherichia coli (hemolytic)	43	78

*NI: No inhibition activity
*ND: Not Detected

antibacterial activity against most of the Gram-positive bacteria as well as several Gram-negative bacteria.

Discussion

In this study, 10-HDA was showed to inhibit the production of pro-inflammatory cytokines, TNF-α, IL-1β and IL-8 in WiDr cells. In contrast, 10-HDA effectively induced the production of IL-1ra at a dose, from 0.1 to 3 mM. Consequently, abundant of IL-1ra restrained the production of IL-1β. The production of IL-8 was siginficantly reduced in a dose-dependent manner at a dose, from 0.5 to 3.0 mM of 10-HDA. 10-HDA inhibited the production of NF-κB in WiDr cells as well. In summary, 10-HDA exhibited anti-inflammation function in WiDr cells. To our knowledge, it is the first time to show that 10-HDA also has in vitro anti-inflammory activity in the human colon cancer cells.

10-HDA was reported to have pharmacological functions potentially due to its anti-tumor [28–30], angiogenesis–inhibition [22], and immunomodulatory activities [31]. The pro-inflammatory cytokines such as TNF-a, IL-1β, IL-8 and TGF-β may trigger inflammatory diseases.10-HDA could act as Histone deacetylase inhibitor (HDACI) to inhibit the proliferation of FLS cells from RA, a systemic chronic inflammatory disease [31]. HDACIs have emerged as potent anti-inflammatory drugs to treat inflammatory diseases [32].

The chronic inflammation is considered as a major cause in cancer etiology [7]. Either IL-8 or IL-1 could stimulate the proliferation of melanoma, pancreatic carcinoma and colon carcinoma cell lines [33]; while IL-1ra could inhibit tumor growth [20]. It was reported that serum IL-1ra were reduced in colorectal cancer patients [34]. Inhibition of NF-κB expression is one of strategies to prevent carcinogenesis. 10-HDA inhibited the production of TNF-α, IL-1β, IL-8, and NF-κB in WiDr cells; whereas it

increased the amount of IL-1ra. Hence, 10-HDA perhaps can be supplied as a chemopreventive agent for chronic inflammation and carcinogenesis. Nevertheless, more study should be done to address whether 10-HDA has in vivo anti-inflammatory and anti-tumor activities in human gastrointestinal tract.

RJ possesses antimicrobial activity attributing to its antimicrobial peptide and fatty acids [35]. The potency of anti-bacterial properties of RJ could be from its unique fatty acid, 10-HDA [17, 35]. The results revealed that 10-HDA has high anti-bacterial activity toward animal- and human-specific pathogens, including S. aureus, S. alactolyticus, S. intermedius B, S. xylosus, S.cholearasuis, V. parahaemolyticus and E. coli (hemolytic). 10-HDA, one of the active compounds in RJ, is responsible for the novel functions of RJ. And more studies should be conducted to verify that 10-HDA may benefit our gastrointestinal tract from chronic inflammation and pathogen infection.

Conclusion

The production of pro-inflammatory cytokines, TNF-α, IL-1β and IL-8 in WiDr cells was inhibited by 10-HDA. In contrast, 10-HDA effectively induced the production of IL-1ra at a dose, from 0.1 to 3 mM. The production of IL-8 was significantly reduced in a dose-dependent manner at a dose, from 0.5 to 3.0 mM of 10-HDA. Abundant of IL-1ra subsequently suppressed the production of IL-1β, which was reduced after 10-HDA treatment at 3 mM. 10-HDA inhibited NF-κB in WiDr cells as well. 10-HDA also possessed high anti-bacterial activity against animal pathogens. These results suggested that 10-HDA in RJ could benefit human gastrointestinal tract via its anti-inflammatory and anti-bacterial activities.

Abbreviations
10-HDA: 10-hydroxy-2-decenoic acid; ELISA: Enzyme-linked immunosorbent assay; IBD: inflammatory bowel disease; IL-1ra: receptor antagonist cytokine; MBC: minimal bactericide concentrations; MIC: minimal inhibitory concentrations; MTT: methyl thiazol tetrazolium bromide; NF-κB: nuclear facctor-kappa B; RJ: royal jelly; TNF-α: tumor necrosis factor-alpha; TSB: Tryptone Soya Broth

Acknowledgements
We thank Mr. Jen-Chieh Li of the Honey Bee Town Co., Ltd. for preparing royal jelly.

Funding
This research was supported by the Ministry of Science and Technology, Taiwan, ROC (MOST 103–2313-B-150 -001 -MY2 to C. C. Peng) and National Formosa University (EN105D-D3001 to C. C. Peng). The funder had no role in study design, data collection and analysis, decision to publish, or preparation of the manuscript.

Availability of data and materials
All data generated or analyzed during this study are included in this published article and its supplementary information files.

Authors' contributions

CCP, YCY, and WMC conceived and designed the experiments. YCY and DAW performed the experiments. CCP, YCY and WMC contributed reagents/materials/analysis tools. CCP, WMC and IPL contributed to the analyses of data, manuscript preparation and made critical revisions. CCP, WMC and IPL wrote and revised the paper. All authors read and approved the final version of the manuscript.

Authors' information

YCY, Doctor in Life science, assistant professor at Department of Biotechnology, National Formosa University. WMC, Doctor in Biotechnology, associate professor at Department of Biotechnology, National Formosa University. DAW, Master in Biotechnology, graduate from Department of Biotechnology, National Formosa University. IPL, Doctor in Biotechnology, Manager at Department of Research and Development, Challenge Bioproducts Co., Ltd. CCP, Doctor in Biotechnology, associate professor at Department of Biotechnology, National Formosa University.

Competing interests

The authors declare that they have no competing interests.

Author details

¹Department of Biotechnology, National Formosa University, Huwei District, Yunlin, Taiwan. ²Department of Research and Development, Challenge Bioproducts Co., Ltd., Yunlin, Taiwan.

References

1. Wang WY, Tan MS, Yu JT, Tan L. Role of pro-inflammatory cytokines released from microglia in Alzheimer's disease. Ann Transl Med. 2015; 3:136. https://doi.org/10.3978/j.issn.2305-5839.2015.03.49.
2. Torraca V, Masud S, Spaink HP, Meijer AH. Macrophage-pathogen interactions in infectious diseases: new therapeutic insights from the zebrafish host model. Dis Model Mech. 2014;7:785–97.
3. Parameswaran N, Patial S. Tumor necrosis factor-α signaling in macrophages. Crit Rev Eukaryot Gene Expr. 2010;20:87–103.
4. Garlanda C, Dinarello CA, Mantovani A. The Interleukin-1 family: back to the future. Immunity. 2013;39:1003–18.
5. Turner MD, Nedjai B, Hurst T, Pennington DJ. Cytokines and chemokines: at the crossroads of cell signalling and inflammatory disease. BBA- Molecular Cell Research. 2014;1843:2563–82.
6. Schiff MH. Role of interleukin 1 and interleukin 1 receptor antagonist in the mediation of rheumatoid arthritis. Ann Rheum Dis. 2000;59:103–8.
7. Coussens LM, Werb Z. Inflammation and cancer. Nature. 2002;420:860–7.
8. Williams RO, Paleolog E, Feldmann M. Cytokine inhibitors in rheumatoid arthritis and other autoimmune diseases. Curr Opin Pharmacol. 2007;7:412–7.
9. Henry D, McGettigan P. Epidemiology overview of gastrointestinal and renal toxicity of NSAIDs. Int J Clin Pract. 2003;135:43–9.
10. Kim EJ, Lee YJ, Shin HK, Park JH. Induction of apoptosis by the aqueous extract of Rubus coreanum in HT-29 human colon cancer cells. Nutrition. 2005;21:1141–8.
11. Melliou E, Chinou I. Chemistry and bioactivity of Royal Jelly from Greece. J Agric Food Chem. 2006;53:8987–92.
12. Honda Y, Araki Y, Hata T, Ichihara K, Ito M, Tanaka M, Honda S. 10-Hydroxy-2-decenoic acid, the major lipid component of royal jelly, extends the lifespan of Caenorhabditis elegans through dietary restriction and target of rapamycin signaling. J Aging Res. 2015;2015: 425261. https://doi.org/10.1155/2015/425261.
13. Honda Y, Fujita Y, Maruyama H, Araki Y, Ichihara K, Sato A, Kojima T, Tanaka M, Nozawa Y, Ito M, Honda S. Lifespan-extending effects of royal jelly and its related substances on the nematode Caenorhabditis elegans. PLoS One. 2011;6(6):e23527. https://doi.org/10.1371/journal. pone.0023527.
14. Hiroshi I, Masamitsu S, Kazuhiro T, Yoko A, Satoshi M, Hideaki H. Bee products prevent VEGF-induced angiogenesis in human umbilical vein endothelial cells. BMC Complement Altern Med. 2009;9:1–10.
15. Pasupuleti VR, Sammugam L, Ramesh N, Gan SH. Honey, propolis, and royal jelly: a comprehensive review of their biological actions and health benefits. Oxidative Med Cell Longev. 2017;2017:1259510. https://doi.org/10.1155/ 2017/1259510.
16. Fujii A, Kobayashi S, Kuboyama N, Kuboyama N, Furukawa Y, Kaneko Y, Ishihama S, Yamamoto H, Tamura T. Augmentation of wound healing by royal jelly (RJ) in streptozotocin-diabetic rats. Jpn J Pharmacol. 1990;53:331–7.
17. Genc M, Aslan A. Determination of trans-10-hydroxy-2-decenoic acid content in pure royal jelly and royal jelly products by column liquid chromatography. J Chromatogr. 1999;839:265–8.
18. Kitahara T, Sato N, Ohya Y, Shinta H, Hori K. The inhibitory effect of ω-hydroxy acids in royal jelly extract on sebaceous gland lipogenesis. J Dermatol Sci. 1995;10:75–9.
19. Tseng JM, Huang JR, Huang HC, Tzen JTC, Chou WM, Peng CC. Facilitative production of an antimicrobial peptide royalisin and its antibody via an artificial oil-body system. Biotechnol Prog. 2010;27: 153–61.
20. Liu JR, Yang YC, Shi LS, Peng CC. Antioxidant properties of royal jelly associated with larval age and time of harvest. J Agric Food Chem. 2008;56: 11447–52.
21. Eshraghi S, Seifollahi F. Antibacterial effect of royal jelly on different strains of bacteria. Iran J Public Health. 2003;32:25–30.
22. Izuta H, Chikaraishi Y, Shimazawa M, Mishima S, Hara H. 10-Hydroxy-2-decenoic Acid, a major fatty acid from Royal Jelly, inhibits VEGF induced angiogenesis in human umbilical vein endothelial cells. Evid Based Complement Alternat Med. 2009;6:489–94.
23. Satomi KM, Okamoto I, Ushio S, Iwaki K, Ikeda M, Kurimoto M. Identification of a collagen production-promoting factor from an extract of royal jelly and its possible mechanism. Biosci Biotechnol Biochem. 2004;68:767–73.
24. Dzopalic T, Vucevic D, Tomic S, Djokic J, Chinou I, Colic M. 3,10-Dihydroxy-decanoic acid, isolated from royal jelly, stimulates Th1 polarising capability of human monocyte-derived dendritic cells. Food Chem. 2011;126:1211–7.
25. Peng CC, Sun HT, Lin IP, Kuo PC, Li JC. The functional property of royal jelly 10-hydroxy-2-decenoic acid as a melanogenesis inhibitor. BMC Complement Altern Med. 2017;17:392.
26. Bílikova K, Huang SC, Lin IP, Simuth J, Peng CC. Structure and antimicrobial activity relationship of royalisin, anantimicrobial peptide from royal jelly of Apis mellifera. Peptides. 2015;68:190–6.
27. Townsend GF, Morgan JF, Hazlett B. Activity of 10-hydroxydecenoic acid from royal jelly against experimental leukaemia and ascitic tumours. Nature. 1959;183:1270–1.
28. Townsend GF, Morgan JF, Tolnai S, Hazlett B, Morton HJ, Shuel RW. Studies on the in vitro antitumor activity of fatty acids. I. 10-Hydroxy-2-decenoic acid from royal jelly. Cancer Res. 1960;20:503–10.
29. Townsend GF, Brown WH, Felauer EE, Hazlett B. Studies on the in vitro antitumor activity of fatty acids. IV. The esters of acids closely related to 10-hydroxy-2-decenoic acids from royal jelly against transplantable mouse leukemia. Can J Biochem Physiol. 1961;39:1765–70.
30. Yang XY, Yang DS, Wei Z, Wang JM, Li CY, Hui Y, Lei KF, Chen XF, Shen NH, Jin LQ, Wang JG. 10-Hydroxy-2-decenoic acid from royal jelly: a potential medicine for RA. J Ethnopharmacol. 2010;128:314–21.
31. Sugiyama T, Takahashi K, Mori H. Royal jelly acid, 10-hydroxy-trans 2-decenoic acid, as modulator of the innate immune response. Endocrine, Metabolic & Immune Disorders - drug. Targets. 2012;12: 368–76.
32. Mukaida N, Ketlinsky SA, Matsushima K. Interleukin-8 and other CXC chemokines. In: Thomson AW, Lotze MT, editors. The cytokine handbook. 4th ed. London: Elsevier Science Ltd; 2003. p. 1049–81.
33. Ito H, Miki C. Profile of circulating levels of interleukin-1 receptor antagonist and interleukin-6 in colorectal cancer patients. Scand J Gastroenterol. 1999; 34:1139–43.
34. Cooper MA, Caligiuri MA. Cytokines and cancer. In: Thomson AW, Lotze MT, editors. The cytokine handbook. 4th ed. London: Elsevier Science Ltd; 2003. p. 1213–32.
35. Alreshoodi FM, Sultanbawa Y. Antimicrobial activity of royal jelly. Anti-Infective Agents. 2015;13:50–9.

11

Five traditional Nigerian Polyherbal remedies protect against high fructose fed, Streptozotocin-induced type 2 diabetes in male Wistar rats

O. E. Kale[1]* ⓘ, O. B. Akinpelu[2], A. A. Bakare[2], F. O. Yusuf[2], R. Gomba[2], D. C. Araka[2], T. O. Ogundare[1], A. C. Okolie[2], O. Adebawo[2] and O. Odutola[2]

Abstract

Background: This present study sought to assess the modulatory effects of five Nigerian traditional polyherbal in high fructose-fed, streptozotocin-induced (HF-STZ) Type 2 diabetes (T2D) in rats. T2D was achieved via fructose feeding ($20\%^{W/V}$) ad libitum for 2 weeks and streptozotocin (STZ, 40 mg/kg) (15th Day) intraperitoneally.

Methods: Seventy-two hours after STZ injection, fourty-eight diabetic rats were divided into eight of 6 rats/group: Diabetic normal untreated, glibenclamide (GBLI, 0.07 mL/kg) or yoyo (YB, 0.43), ruzu (RB, 0.08), fajik (FJB, 0.20), oroki (OB, 0.16), and fidson (FB, 0.43)/ mL/kg bitters respectively. Controls normal and diabetic untreated groups received intragastric carboxylmethylcellulose (CMC, 1 mL/kg) for eleven days.

Results: T2D was characterized in rats by an increased ($p < 0.001–0.05$) blood glucose levels (BGL), total cholesterol, triglycerides, low-density lipoprotein and alanine aminotransferase compared with control CMC group. Similarly, hepatic and pancreatic malondialdehyde (MDA) were increased by 180 and 97% respectively. Polyherbal treatments demonstrated efficacies on BGL as follow: YB (55.6%, 160.7 mg/dL); RB (59.7%, 145.2 mg/dL); FJB (59.8%, 243.4 mg/dL); OB (60.8%, 194.5 mg/dL) and FB (61.3%, 203.3 mg/dL) respectively by day 11 (versus GBLI, 65.1%) compared with control untreated diabetic rats. Also, elevated TC, LDL cholesterol, ALT were lowered ($p < 0.05$) by YB, FJB, and FB respectively in rats. YB, FJB, and OB lowered MDA levels in treated rats. Further, YB, RB, FJB and FB restored changes in liver, and pancreas histopathology. Predominant non-polar bioactive include oleic, hexadecanoic, octadecanoic among others following gas chromatography-mass spectrophotometry analyses.

Conclusion: Overall, these present results demonstrate anti-hyperglycemic potentials, although with cautions, of some polyherbal in T2D rats, which may, in part, be antioxidants mediated.

Keywords: Type 2 diabetes mellitus, Polyherbal, Fructose, Streptozotocin, Oxidative stress

Background

In most developing countries and even some developed, over the counter use of polyherbal is on the high side and the manufacturers claimed a complete cure for diabetes mellitus (type 2 diabetes, T2D). A polyherbal mixture is composed of different plants constituents and unpurified extracts with medicinal properties in maintaining good health and for treatment of different aliments [1]. As a result of cost effectiveness and the notions for fewer side effects, these concoctions have been reportedly used in the treatment of metabolic syndrome risk factors particularly T2D, although, not many have undergone careful scientific evaluation [2]. T2D is an endocrine pathological disorder characterized by two significant conditions resulting from defects in insulin secretion or reduced sensitivity of the tissue to insulin (insulin resistance) and pancreas β-cells dysfunction [3]. Other metabolic syndrome comorbidities have also been found in the vicinity

* Correspondence: kaleo@babcock.edu.ng; kalefemi@gmail.com
[1]Department of Pharmacology, Benjamin S. Carson (Snr.) School of Medicine, Babcock University, Ilishan-Remo, Ogun State, PMB, Ikeja 21244, Nigeria
Full list of author information is available at the end of the article

of T2D and may be responsible for increased metabolic syndrome risks factors [1, 2]. Several medicinal plants have birthed active drugs which are considered as useful resources capable of preventing and improving metabolic syndrome diseases [3]. Up to now, there have been increases in the search for new anti-diabetic agents which are cheaper with greater effectiveness and lesser side effects due to the fact that many of the available synthetic oral hypoglycemic agents are costly and produce predictable adverse drug reactions [4]. Also, some noxious actions of hypoglycemic agents have led many to turn to the use of herbs in the treatment of diabetes [5]. Yearly, several herbs are scientifically reported to have anti-diabetic effects as well as significant antioxidant activity and this has led to the formulation of polyherbal based on these hypotheses. In respect, a combination of herbs is believed to work synergistically and may have a more beneficial effect than in single preparation [6]. The five most commonly paraded bitters in Nigeria for T2D are Yoyo bitters (YB), Oroki herbal mixture (OB), Ruzu Bitters (RB), Fijk flusher (FB), and Fidson Bitter (FB) respectively. Although, each of this preparation has claimed for several indications, however, this study sought to verify this aspect predicated solely on T2D. Interestingly, for any medicinal plant to be present and used in a formulation, many of the individual constituents of these agents have been investigated extensively and reported in the literature. The following compounds have been reported given these combinations with very wide applications: YB (*Acinos arvensis, Chenopodium murale, Citrus aurantifolia, Aloe vera* and *Cinnamomum aromaticum* [7], OB (*Sorghum bicolor, Khaya grandifoliola, Cassia sieberiana, Staudtia stipitata, Alstonia cognensis, Ocimum basillicum, Mangifera indica, Cythula prostrate, Securidaca longepedunculata, Saccharum officinarum* and water [8]. RB (*Uvarie chamae, Curculigo pilosa* and *Colocythis citrullis*) [9], FJB (*Cassia alata, Citrus medica var. acida* (Roxb.), *Aloe barbaris, Aloe vera, Cassia angustifolia*) and FB (*Ginseng, Phyllanthus niruri, Aloe vera, Tephrosia purpurea, Eclipta alba, Swertia chirata* (Buch-Ham.), *Casssia angustifolia, Cinnamomum zeylanicum*). In respect, some of their characteristic phytomedicines or bioactive components have also been confirmed by different studies. For instance, *Acinos arvensis* (Lamiaceae) commonly referred to as basil thyme has been reported to contain a number of compounds such as germacrene, hexadecanoic acid, β-bourbonene, pulegone, izomenthone, phytol, linarin [10]. *Aloe vera* (Liliaceae) is one of the oldest medicinal plants with diversifying medicinal effects which have been explored and reviewed [11]. Many of its compounds possess anti-tumor, anti-arthritic, anti-rheumatoid, anti-cancer, anti-diabetic, antioxidant, anti-microbial, anti-viral, anti-hyperlipidermic, anti-ulcer, hepatoprotective and immunomodulatory properties [12]. Glucomannan, a water-soluble fiber from this plant, possesses anti-hyperglycemic and

insulin sensitizing activity [13]. Thus, evidence abounds that *Aloe vera* improved the survival of islet cells of rat pancreas, increased insulin levels and decreased the production of reactive oxygen species [12, 14]. *Citrus aurantifolia* (Rutaceae) is referred to as key lime or "osan wewe" in South Western Nigeria [15]. Lime juice has numerous numbers of nutrients and phytochemical substances such as citric acid, ascorbic acid, minerals, and flavonoids. Further derivative includes hesperedin, apigenin, naringenin, quercetin, rutin etc. [16]. It has been reported to possess antibacterial, anti-cancer, anti-diabetic, anti-fungal, anti-hypertensive, anti-inflammatory, anti-lipidemic and antioxidant properties [16]. *Chenopodium murale* (Chenopodiaceae) grows on waste a land which is commonly referred to as nettle- leaf goose foot. *Chenopodium murale* has yielded analgesics, anti-inflammatory, anti-fungal, anti-bacterial, anti-oxidant, hypotensive and hepatoprotective molecules [17]. *Cinnamomum aromaticum*, commonly called *Cinnamon cassia* or Chinese cinnamon belongs to the Lauraceae family and it serves as a spice, flavoring agent, preservative, oral health agent as well as an anti-termitic, nematicidal, insecticidal [18]. Phytochemical studies have revealed the presence of volatile oils such as cinnamaldehyde, weitechin, cinnamylacetate, cinnamyl alcohol, cinnamic acid, lignans. Cinnamaldehyde is effective against metabolic disorder and diabetes-induced renal damage. *Cinnamomum aromaticum* shows biological effects such as anti-microbial, antioxidant, anti-inflammatory, anti-ulcerogenic, anticancer, analgesic, lipid-lowering, cardiovascular disease lowering, coagulating and anti-diabetic effects [18]. It has also been reported to have activity against neurological disorders such as Parkinson's and Alzheimer's disease. *Curculigo pilosa* of the genus curculigo belongs to the family Hypoxidacea and also known as ground squirrel groundnut or "Epakun" in Yoruba land, Nigeria [19]. *Curculigo pilosa* is used in the treatment of gastrointestinal diseases and cardiovascular heart related diseases due to its good anti-oxidant properties [19]. *Colocynthis citrullus* belongs to the family Cucurbitaceae which is referred to locally as bitter apple cucumber and Egusi baara by the Yorubas. It has been reported to enhance the activity of glucokinase/ hexokinase pathway in the liver [20]. *Phyllanthus niruri* aids memory enhancement, help to reduce fatigue and possess anti-ageing and anti-stress properties [21]. Also, *Aloe vera, Tephrosia purpurea* and *Eclipta alba* have hepatoprotection, blood cleansing synergy and also help in managing gastrointestinal integrity and heart burn [22]. *Eclipta alba, Aloe vera, Tephrosia purpurea* and *Phyllanthus niruri* together offer hepatoprotection weight loss therapy. *Swertia chirata, Phyllanthus niruri, Casssia angustifolia, Cinnamomum zeylanicum, Aloe vera* and *Tephrosia purpurea* are said to aid digestion, regulate bowel movement and for correction of urinary disorders [23]. *Cinnamomum zeylanicum, Swerta chirata, Aloe vera* and ginseng combination will help regulate blood glucose levels [23]. Despite the great relevance placed on polyherbal, several of these popular plants used traditionally for the treatment of diabetes have received criticism elsewhere [24, 25]. Thus, standardization of polyherbal is essential for several reasons. These include verify the manufacturers' claims, assess the quality of products as well as document the detail toxicological profiles based on the concentration of their active principles [26]. Therefore, this study assessed five Nigerian popular yoyo, ruzu, fajik, oroki, and fidson herbal remedies in high fructose-fed, streptozotocin-induced T2D in male Wistar rats.

Methods

Drugs and chemicals

Yoyo bitters® was purchased at Romitel Pharmacy limited at Mowe, Ogun State, Nigeria. Ruzu Bitters® was purchase from Ruzu Natural Health Products and services (Egan-Igando, Lagos Nigeria). Oroki herbal mixture® was purchased from Nured industrial and commercial company limited located in Lagos Nigeria. Fijk Flusher® was purchased from De-Fayus Organization Igando Market Igando Rd., Alimosho, Lagos (Nigeria). Fidson Bitters® was purchased from Fidson Pharmaceutical Limited, Nigeria. Streptozotocin was purchased from Sigma Aldrich respectively and Fructose from Burgoyne Reagents (India), Reduced glutathione (GSH), metaphosphoric acid and trichloroacetic acid (TCA) were purchased from J.I. Baker (Center Valley, PA, U.S.A.). Thiobarbituric acid (TBA) was purchased from Sigma Chemical Company (USA). Alanine aminotransferase (ALT), aspartate aminotransferase (AST), alkaline phosphatase (ALP), total cholesterol (TC), and triglyceride (TG) assay kits were obtained from Randox Laboratory (Crumlin, UK), 5^l, 5^l-dithiobis-2-nitrobenzoate (Ellman's reagent) from Sigma (USA) and sodium hydroxide from Merck (Germany). Other chemicals and reagents used were of analytical grade.

Experimental animals

The study was carried out in compliance with established guidelines for biomedical research as approved by the Babcock University, Ogun State, Nigeria in conjunction with the organization for Animal Care and Use in Research, Education and Testing (ACURET.ORG). An ethical clearance was obtained from the Babcock University Human Research Ethics Committee (BUHREC 308/17). The study was carried out in the Department of Biochemistry, Benjamin Carson (Snr.) School of Medicine, Babcock University, Nigeria. Healthy adult male Wistar rats (160 ± 40 g) were obtained from a commercial private colony in Ibadan, Oyo-State, Nigeria and housed in the Babcock University Laboratory animal (Ilishan, Ogun State, Nigeria) facility. They were housed in a unisexual group of 4 in metallic cages (60 × 45 × 25 cm)

under a reversed light-dark cycle (12 h/ 12 dark scheduled) and controlled temperature (22 ± 3 °C). The animals were acclimatized for 2 weeks. They were fed with commercially available pelleted diet (Vita Feeds, Jos, Plateau State, Nigeria) and water ad libitum during the period of acclimatization and throughout the period of the experiment. The investigation conforms to the Guide for the Care and Use of Laboratory Animals published by the U. S. National Institutes of Health (NIH Publication No. 85–23, revised 1996) for studies involving experimental animals and the procedures as documented by Kilkenny et al. [27] for reporting animal research.

Extraction and bioactive compound identification

The fractionation process was carried out according to the method described by Onyeaghala et al. [28] with slight modifications. Briefly, 2 × 200 mL of the bitters was exhaustively extracted using n-hexane. The extraction was carried out in a ratio of 1:1 (polyherbal: hexane). The vortexed mixture of bitters and hexane was put into a separating funnel, vortexes and allowed to stand for about 45 min to ensure complete extraction of the non-polar components. The non-polar portion was separated by funnels, concentrated at 40 °C under reduced pressure using a rotary evaporator [29] and stored at − 4 °C until needed. Gas Chromatography-Mass Spectrometry (GC-MS) analysis of polyherbal from non-polar components was carried out using an Agilent HP- 7890A gas chromatograph (Agilent Technologies, Palo Alto, CA, USA) with HP-5MS 5% phenylmethylsiloxane capillary column (30 m × 0.25 mm, 0. 25 lm film thickness; Restek, Bellefonte, PA) equipped with an MSD detector and characterized as previously described (Adams, 2001) and Proestos et al. (2006) with some modifications as reported elsewhere Okolie et al. [30].

Induction of diabetes

T2D was achieved via the method of Wilson & Islam [31] as modified by Okolie et al. [30] by fructose feeding ($20\%^{W/V}$) ad libitum for 2 weeks and streptozotocin (40 mg/kg $i.p.$) to rats. Seventy-two house following STZ injection, fourty-eight (48) diabetic rats were divided into eight of 6 rats/group: Diabetic normal untreated, glibenclamide (0.07 mg/kg), and yoyo (YB, 0.43), ruzu (RB, 0.08), fajik (FB, 0.20), oroki (OB, 0.16), and fidson (FB, 0.43), mL/kg bitters respectively. All bitters were administered via the oral route. Controls normal and diabetic untreated groups received intragastric carboxylmethylcellulose (1 mL/kg) for two weeks.

Necropsy

Animals were sacrificed by cervical dislocation 24 h after the last treatment, and blood was collected by cardiac puncture into plain bottles. Serum was separated by centrifugation at 4200 rpm at room temperature for 5 min.

The pancreas and liver were carefully excised, cleared of adhering tissues, and weighed. Weight was recorded in grams and expressed as g/g body weight. A small portion of the excised pancreas and liver were fixed in 10% formaldehyde and subsequently prepared for histology. The remaining portion of the excised pancreas and liver were weighed and homogenized in four volumes of 100 mM of phosphate buffer (pH 7.4). The plasma and liver homogenates obtained from each animal were then analyzed to assess pancreas and liver function and other biochemical parameters.

Biochemical assessment of hepatic function, lipid parameters, and antioxidants enzymes

Serum aspartate and alanine aminotransferases (AST and ALT) and alkaline phosphatase (ALP) activities were assessed for liver function. AST and ALT activities were determined according to the principle described by Reitman and Frankel [32] while the ALP activity was carried out according to the method described by Roy [33]. Total Cholesterol (TC) and Triglyceride (TG) concentrations were estimated following the principle described by Trinder [34] using commercial kits obtained from Randox Laboratories Ltd. (Crumlin, UK). Uric acid was also determined using Randox kit following the principle described by Fossati et al. [35]. The method described by Warnick and Albers [36] was used to determine High-Density Lipoprotein (HDL) while Freidewald formula [37] was used to extrapolate serum low-density lipoprotein (LDL). GSH level was estimated at 412 nm following the method of Beutler et al. [38]. Lipid peroxidation was estimated spectrophotometrically by the thiobarbituric acid reactive substance (TBARS) method as described by Varshney and Kale [39] and expressed in terms of malondialdehyde (MDA) formed per mg protein.

Statistic

All data were expressed as mean ± S.E.M. Significant differences among the group were determined by T-test and one-way analysis of variance (ANOVA) using statistical package for social science student (version 20). Data were converted to figures using Graph Pad Prism (6.0). Results were considered to be significant at $p \leq 0.05$.

Results

The effects of polyherbal on fasting blood glucose (FBGL) levels

Figure 1 shows effects of polyherbal on fasting blood glucose (FBGL) levels in normal and diabetic rats. The control normal CMC group, baseline, shows no significant change in FBGLs in all rats. However, at 72 h following STZ intoxication to high fructose fed rats, there were increased FBGL ($p < 0.001–0.05$) when compared with control CMC group. However, following treatments, glibenclamide (GBLI), an anti-diabetic drug, lowered FBGL ($p < 0.05$) by 56.5% (day 4), 50% (day 7) and 65.1% (day 11) respectively when compared with control untreated diabetic rats. Similarly, polyherbal demonstrated efficacies as follow: YB 39.4% (day 4), 14.5% (day 7), 55.6% (day 11); RB 49.2% (day 4), 2.8% (day 7), 59.7% (day 11); FJB 13.2% (day 4), 15.1% (day 7), 69.8% (day 11); OB 59.8% (day 4), 43.2% (day 7), 60.8% (day 11) and FB 47.5% (day 4), 14.9% (day 7), 61.3% (day 11) respectively compared with control untreated diabetic rats. FBGL remains unchanged in untreated diabetic rats when compared with baseline.

The effects of polyherbal on body weight

Figure 2 shows effects of polyherbal on body weight in normal and diabetic rats. The baseline shows no significant change in body weight of rats. Assessment of body weight on day 4, 7 and 10th of treatments did not show any significant change in body weight when compared

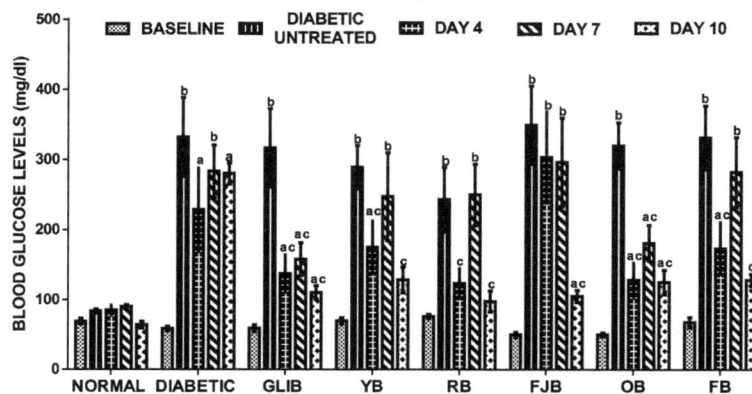

Fig. 1 effects of polyherbals on fasting blood glucose (FBGL) levels in normal and diabetic rats. Results represented as Mean ± S.E.M. $n = 6$. $^{a}p < 0.05$ or $^{b} < 0.001$ different from control normal CMC group. $^{c}p < 0.05$ or $^{d} < 0.001$ different from control Untreated Diabetic group. CMC: Carboxylmethyl cellulose; YB: Yoyo bitters; RB: Ruzu bitters; FB: fajik bitters; OB: Oroki bitters; FB: Fidson bitters

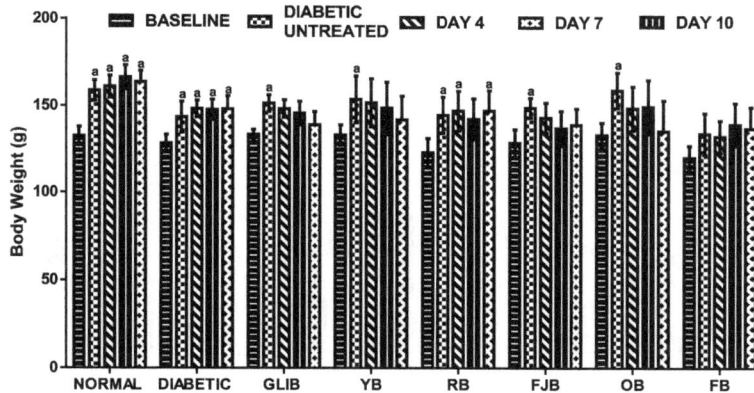

Fig. 2 effects of polyherbals on body weight in normal and diabetic rats. Results represented as Mean ± S.E.M. n = 6. $^{a}p < 0.05$ different from control normal CMC group. CMC: Carboxylmethyl cellulose; YB: Yoyo bitters; RB: Ruzu bitters; FB: fajik bitters; OB: Oroki bitters; FB: Fidson bitters

with controls. However, slight but insignificantly increased ($p > 0.05$) body weight in rats treated with OB (day 4, 19.4%), RB (day 7, 18.1%) and YB (day 10, 18.1%) when compared with control normal CMC group.

The effects of polyherbal on lipid parameters

Figure 3 results show effects of polyherbal on lipid parameters in normal and diabetic rats. Diabetic rats showed increased ($p < 0.05$) in serum total cholesterol (102.7%), triglycerides (85.4%), and low density lipoprotein (38.5%) when compared with control normal rats. Also, RB, FJB, OB elevated TC by 82.6, 47.8 and 41.6% respectively. In addition, RB increased ($p > 0.05$) LDL in treated rats. However, TG was reduced in treated rats: Glib (40.2%, $p < 0.05$), YB (30.2%, p < 0.05), RB (25.6%, p > 0.05), FJB (30.9%, p < 0.05), OB (17.2%, p > 0.05) and FB (23.1%, p > 0.05) respectively. YB, RB and OB increased HDL by 22.5% ($p > 0.05$), 49.3% ($p < 0.05$) and 12.8% ($p > 0.05$)

respectively when compared with control normal rats. In addition, TC and LDL cholesterol levels were reduced ($p < 0.05$) by GLIB (28.1, 38.9%), YB (41.5, 48.9%), FJB (27.1, 49.1%), OB (34.99, 36.3%), and FB (41.5, 43.3%) by respectively when compared with control untreated diabetic group. YB, RB and OB increased (p < 0.05) HDL by 92.6, 134.7 and 77.4% respectively in the treated rats when compared with control untreated diabetic group.

The effects of different polyherbal on liver function enzymes

Figure 4 results show effects of different polyherbal on liver function enzymes in normal and diabetic rats. Untreated diabetic rats showed increased ($p < 0.001$) ALT by 760.9% when compared with control normal group. GLIB lowered ALT level ($p < 0.05$, 54.96%) and AST ($p > 0.05$, 30.2%) respectively when compared with control untreated diabetic group. Similarly, polyherbal YB, RB,

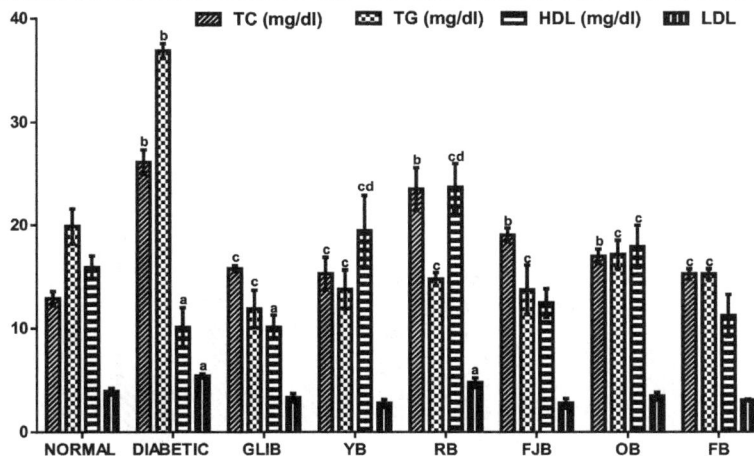

Fig. 3 effects of polyherbals on lipid parameters in normal and diabetic rats. Results represented as Mean ± S.E.M. n = 6. $^{a}p < 0.05$ or $^{b} < 0.001$ different from control normal CMC group. $^{c}p < 0.05$ or $^{d} < 0.001$ different from control Untreated Diabetic group. CMC: Carboxylmethyl cellulose; YB: Yoyo bitters; RB: Ruzu bitters; FB: fajik bitters; OB: Oroki bitters; FB: Fidson bitters

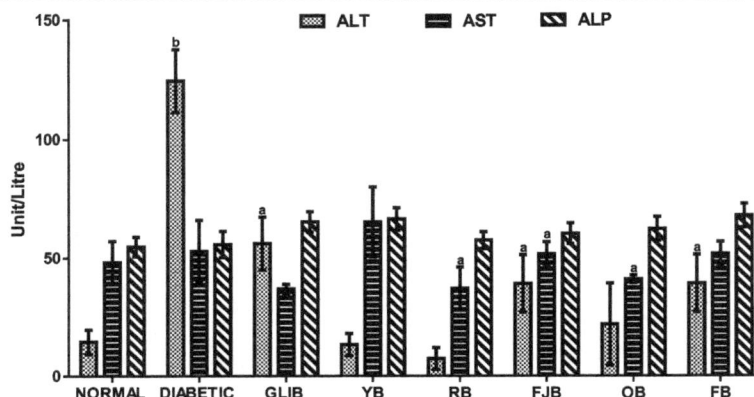

Fig. 4 effects of polyherbals on plasma ALT, AST and ALP levels in normal and diabetic rats. Results represented as Mean ± S.E.M. n = 6. [a]$p < 0.05$ or [b] < 0.001 different from control normal CMC group. [c]$p < 0.05$ or [d] < 0.001 different from control Untreated Diabetic group. CMC: Carboxylmethyl cellulose; YB: Yoyo bitters; RB: Ruzu bitters; FB: fajik bitters; OB: Oroki bitters; FB: Fidson bitters. ALT and AST: Alanine and aspartate aminotransferases; ALP: Alkaline phosphatase

FJB, OB and FB lowered ($p < 0.05$) ALT levels by 89.4, 94.1, 68.7, 82.5, and 68.7% respectively. Also, YB elevated ($p > 0.05$, 23.3%) AST levels in treated rats.

The effects of polyherbal on hepatic and pancreatic lipid peroxidation levels

Figure 5 results show effects of polyherbal on hepatic and pancreatic lipid peroxidation levels in normal and diabetic rats. In the untreated diabetic group, hepatic and pancreatic malondialdehyde (MDA) increased ($p < 0.05$) by 180 and 97% respectively. Administration of GLIB, YB, FJB, and OB lowered ($p < 0.05$) hepatic MDA when compared with control untreated diabetic rats. GLIB, YB, OB reduced ($p < 0.05$) pancreatic MDA by 42, 42, and 36.2% respectively when compared with control untreated diabetic group.

The effects of polyherbal on hepatic and pancreatic reduced glutathione (GSH) levels

Figure 6 results show effects of polyherbal on hepatic and pancreatic reduced glutathione (GSH) levels in normal and diabetic rats. In the untreated diabetic group, hepatic reduced glutathione (GSH) level was lowered by 9.97% when compared with control normal group. In contrast, increased ($p < 0.05$) hepatic and pancreatic GSH levels were obtained in rats that received FJB (60.5, 49.8%), OB (60.5, 84.9%), and FB (57.1, 65.5%) respectively when compared with control untreated diabetic group. Similarly, GLIB and YB increased although insignificantly by 21.7 and 27.2% respectively.

Histological sections of the liver and pancreas

Representative photomicrographs of liver and pancreas histology of rats in all treatment groups are presented in

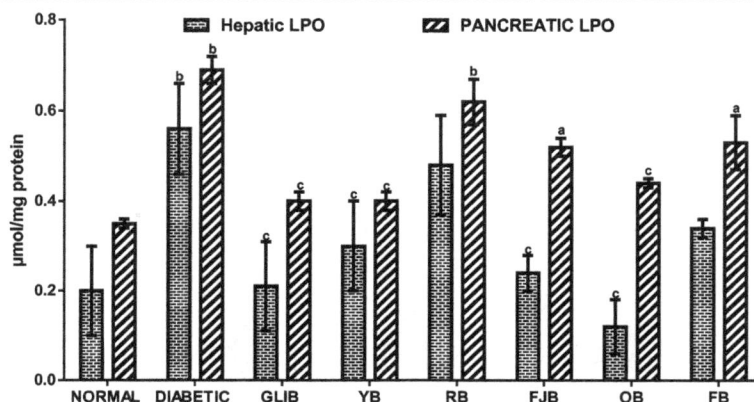

Fig. 5 effects of polyherbals on hepatic and pancreatic lipid peroxidation (MDA) levels in normal and diabetic rats. Results represented as Mean ± S.E.M. n = 6. [a]$p < 0.05$ or [b] < 0.001 different from control normal CMC group. [c]$p < 0.05$ or [d] < 0.001 different from control Untreated Diabetic group. CMC: Carboxylmethyl cellulose; YB: Yoyo bitters; RB: Ruzu bitters; FB: fajik bitters; OB: Oroki bitters; FB: Fidson bitters. MDA: Malondialdehyde

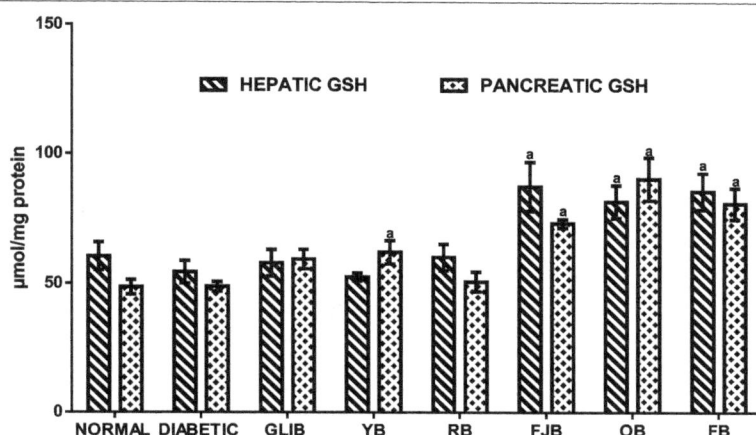

Fig. 6 effects of polyherbals on hepatic and pancreatic reduced glutathione (GSH) levels in normal and diabetic rats. Results represented as Mean ± S.E.M. n = 6. $^ap < 0.05$ or $^b < 0.001$ different from control normal CMC group. $^cp < 0.05$ or $^d < 0.001$ different from control Untreated Diabetic group. CMC: Carboxylmethyl cellulose; YB: Yoyo bitters; RB: Ruzu bitters; FB: fajik bitters; OB: Oroki bitters; FB: Fidson bitters

Figs. 7 and 8 respectively. T2D rats liver and pancreas treated with HF-STZ showed sinusoidal congestion of radial plates of hepatocytes and shrunk cellular islets surrounded by normal appearing exocrine acini with near-to-normal necrosis. However, different polyherbals administered in treated rats showed some modulatory roles.

12iscussion

Scientists all over the world have worried over the population that roams the health centers over T2D which has become pandemic over decades [40]. Although prevalence studies present divergent reports, however suggestions are that concerted efforts are required to increase the life span of the people [41]. According to the World Health Organization, the prevalence of DM is projected to rise to 300 million within 2025 [41]. In view of the increasing prevalence, there is a growing need to develop integrated approaches toward the management and prevention of DM by exploring the potentials offered by the traditional, complementary and alternative medicines. A very large percentage of the drugs in circulation are plant derivatives [11]. The insulin injection and hypoglycemic agents continue to thrive for T2D management. However, there have been concerns over several adverse effects associated with their application. In respect, the search for effective compounds with lower side effects in treating this ailment has been on the increase [30]. Herbal medicines have in recent time contributes immensely as an alternative or complementary sources. Several studies have investigated anti-diabetic activities of various plants used in Nigeria, and have confirmed potentials for therapeutic efficacies [25, 42]. Since the manufacturers of polyherbal most especially YB, RB, FJB, OB and FB engaged in a high-quality public advertisement that has enabled high demand in

pharmacies which boost their sales especially among patients with chronic diseases including diabetes and cardiovascular disorders. One major reason why this study is very important to the population is that some still indulge in drug-herb combination which may place them at a high risk since this may result in interactions which may possibly alter the bioavailability or clinical effectiveness of a conventional drug when given concurrently. Interestingly, several of the constituents of these polyherbal have scientific evidence for their uses. For instance, over thirty compounds have been synthesized from *Mangifera indica* following bioactivity guided fractionations in order to identify the active anti-diabetic constituents. Several of compounds obtained including penta-O-galloyl-β-d-glucose, 3-β taraxerol etc. have shown potentials for managing the hyperglycemic state in rodents [43, 44]. The flavonoid, epiafzelechin, was also isolated and fully characterized from the root bark of *Cassia sieberiana* and *Khaya grandifoliola* for its antioxidant activity demonstrated diabetic animals [45] and so on. Although, not all ingredients possess anti-diabetic effects, however, evidence abounds for anti-hyperglycemic effects of *Citrus aurantifolia, Aloe vera* and *Cinnamomum aromaticum* found in YB [46], *Sorghum bicolor* stem, *Khaya grandifoliola* bark, *Cassia sieberiana* root, *Alstonia cognensis* bark, *Ocimum basillicum* leaves, *Mangifera indica* leaves, *Cythula prostrate* Leaves, *Securidaca longepedunculata* root, *Saccharum officinarum* stem and water in OB [47, 48]. *Uvarie chamae, Curculigo pilosa* and *citrullis Colocythis* in RB [9, 42, 49], *Cassia alata, Citrus medica var. acida* (Roxb.), *Aloe vera, Cassia angustifolia* in FJB [46] and *ginseng, Phyllanthus niruri, Aloe vera, Tephrosia purpurea, Eclipta alba, Swertia chirata* (Buch-Ham.), *Casssia angustifolia, Cinnamomum zeylanicum* found in FB [50]. This present study investigated on the potentials of five traditional of

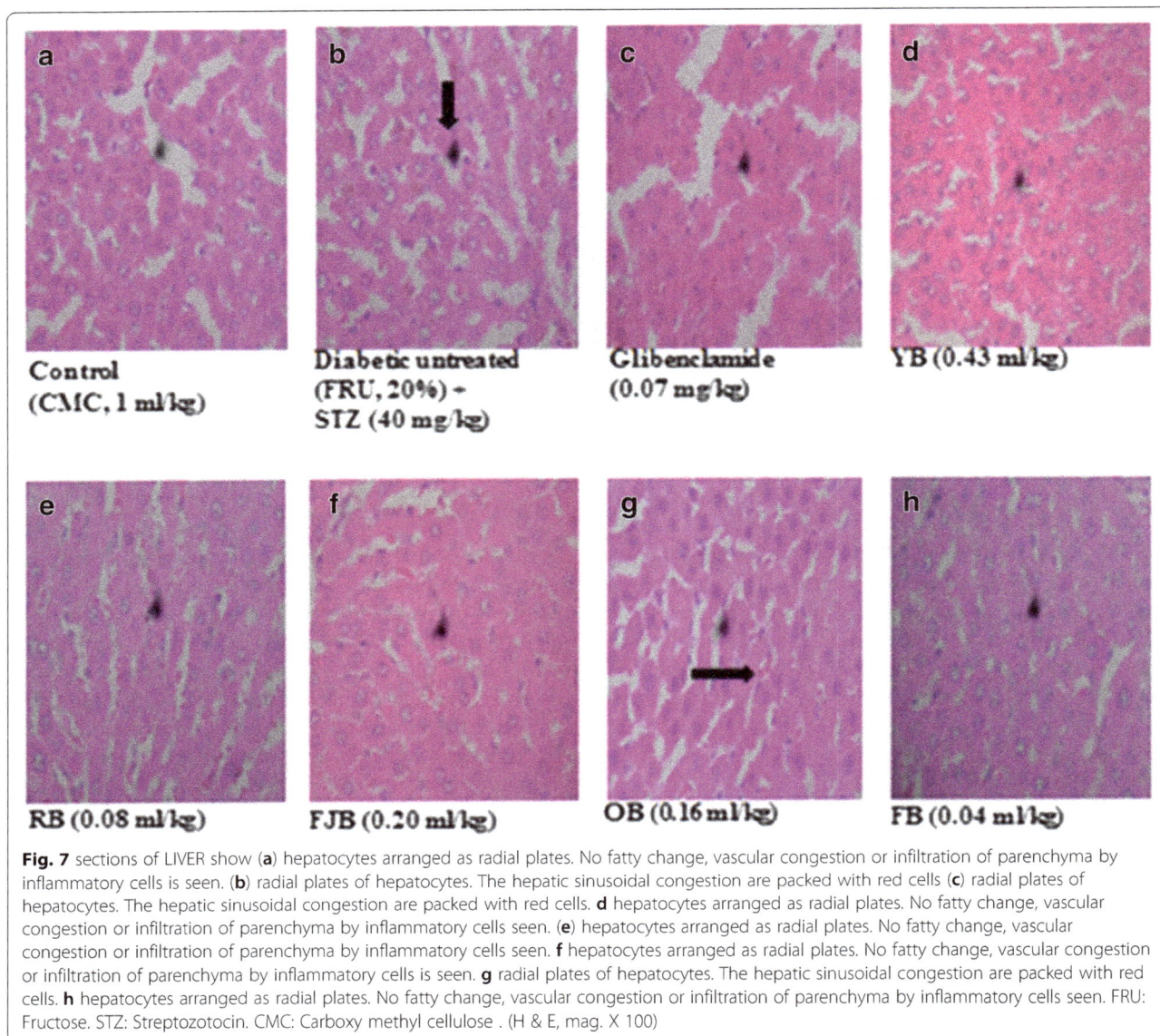

Fig. 7 sections of LIVER show (**a**) hepatocytes arranged as radial plates. No fatty change, vascular congestion or infiltration of parenchyma by inflammatory cells is seen. (**b**) radial plates of hepatocytes. The hepatic sinusoidal congestion are packed with red cells (**c**) radial plates of hepatocytes. The hepatic sinusoidal congestion are packed with red cells. **d** hepatocytes arranged as radial plates. No fatty change, vascular congestion or infiltration of parenchyma by inflammatory cells seen. (**e**) hepatocytes arranged as radial plates. No fatty change, vascular congestion or infiltration of parenchyma by inflammatory cells seen. **f** hepatocytes arranged as radial plates. No fatty change, vascular congestion or infiltration of parenchyma by inflammatory cells is seen. **g** radial plates of hepatocytes. The hepatic sinusoidal congestion are packed with red cells. **h** hepatocytes arranged as radial plates. No fatty change, vascular congestion or infiltration of parenchyma by inflammatory cells seen. FRU: Fructose. STZ: Streptozotocin. CMC: Carboxy methyl cellulose . (H & E, mag. X 100)

Nigerian polyherbal remedies against high fructose-fed, streptozotocin-induced type 2 diabetes in male Wistar rats in order to ascertain their herbo-therapeutic effects. Obtaining experimental T2D in rodents has taken different routes. However, the use of high-fat diet and streptozotocin model has been on the forefront. This is because fructose-induced insulin resistance and hyperinsulinaemia in normal rats are complemented by pancreatic β-cells dysfunction that impedes insulin production. Thus, an ideal model for T2D which would closely reflect natural history and metabolic characteristics of human T2D is mimicked. Diabetic untreated rats in this study demonstrated elevated blood glucose levels (Fig. 1) accompanied by an increased lipid peroxidation in pancreas and liver respectively. In addition, the histopathology of the liver (Fig. 7) and pancreas (Fig. 8) following HF-STZ in rats

resulted in sinusoidal congestion of radial plates of hepatocytes and shrunk cellular islets surrounded by normal appearing exocrine acini with near-to-normal necrosis. Similarly, there were increased serum total cholesterol, triglycerides, and low-density lipoprotein respectively in diabetic rats. These evidence of its suitability were the major reasons why HF-STZ was employed for use. Assessment of body weight at day fourth, seventh and eleventh of treatments did not show any significant change when compared with controls, although, a slight increase was observed in rats treated with OB, RB, and YB respectively. There are convergent studies that show the link between lipid and glucose profile as well as diabetic complications [51]. Polyherbal administration improved lipid parameters in diabetic rats. However, hypercholesterolemia persists in diabetic rats treated with RB and FJB respectively. In

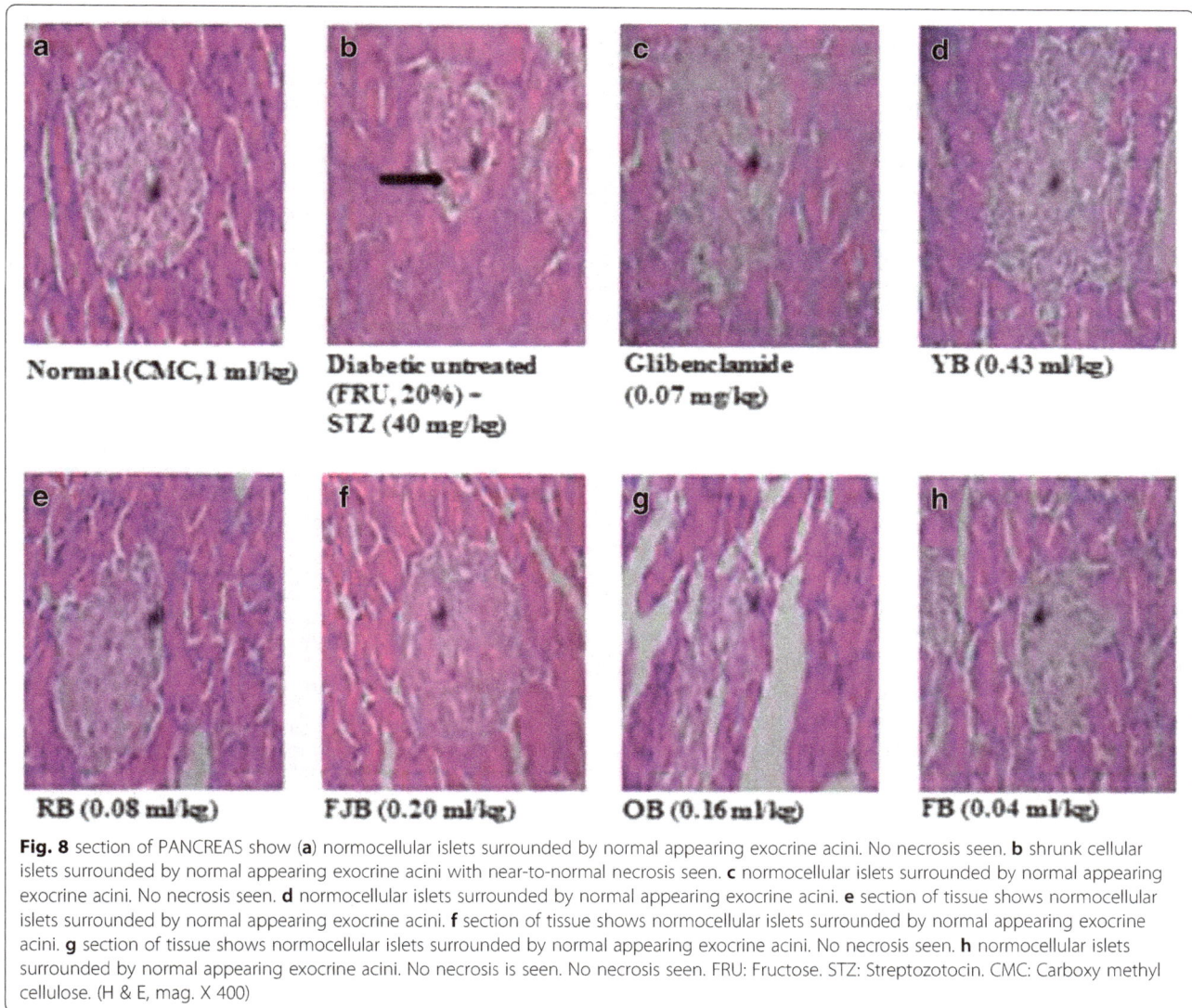

Fig. 8 section of PANCREAS show (**a**) normocellular islets surrounded by normal appearing exocrine acini. No necrosis seen. **b** shrunk cellular islets surrounded by normal appearing exocrine acini with near-to-normal necrosis seen. **c** normocellular islets surrounded by normal appearing exocrine acini. No necrosis seen. **d** normocellular islets surrounded by normal appearing exocrine acini. **e** section of tissue shows normocellular islets surrounded by normal appearing exocrine acini. **f** section of tissue shows normocellular islets surrounded by normal appearing exocrine acini. **g** section of tissue shows normocellular islets surrounded by normal appearing exocrine acini. No necrosis seen. **h** normocellular islets surrounded by normal appearing exocrine acini. No necrosis is seen. No necrosis seen. FRU: Fructose. STZ: Streptozotocin. CMC: Carboxy methyl cellulose. (H & E, mag. X 400)

addition, RB increased LDL in treated rats. Thus, caution to avoid rebound dyslipidemia by dosage regulation and optimum compliance may enable effectiveness in RB users. In contrast, hypertriglyceremia were reduced in rats treated YB, RB, FJB, OB and FB respectively compared with controls. Treatments with YB, RB, and OB increased antioxidant lipids HDL in rats. More so, both serum TC and LDL cholesterol levels were reduced YB, FJB, OB, and FB respectively compared with control. Effects of different polyherbal on liver function enzymes in normal and diabetic rats were demonstrated. An increased alanine aminotransferase level was evident in untreated diabetic rats. Polyherbal YB, RB, FJB, OB and FB lowered ALT levels in rats. However, treatment with YB elevated AST levels in rats. Lipid peroxidation metabolite is usually measured to score damage biochemically since insulin secretion is also closely associated with lipoxygenase derived peroxides [51]. Oxidative stress has been implicated in diabetes both

type 1 and 2 by increasing level of lipid peroxidation [52]. This results in generation of free radicals in pancreas and vital organs including the liver. An increase in lipid peroxidation level may initiate cellular infiltration and islet cell damage in diabetes [52]. Thus, elevation of MDA or hydroxydobenenal levels in the tissues of diabetic animals may be associated with oxidative stress. In this study, hepatic and pancreatic lipid peroxidation (LPO) levels were assessed in normal and diabetic rats and following polyherbal treatments. There were elevated hepatic and pancreatic malondialdehyde (MDA), a metabolite of LPO, in diabetic rats. Similar to anti-diabetic drug, GLIB, administration of, YB, FJB, and OB lowered reversed hepatic MDA while YB, OB reduced pancreatic MDA respectively in treated diabetic group. More so, reduced glutathione constitutes one of the antioxidant capacities that help to combat oxidative stress in diabetes by its reducing power in the cytoplasm [53]. GSH protects against toxic effects of lipid peroxidation metabolites. From the results obtained in this present study, hepatic reduced glutathione (GSH) remained low in untreated diabetic rats. In contrast, increased hepatic and pancreatic GSH levels were elevated in rats that received FJB, OB and FB respectively, although, YB shows increased but insignificantly compared with control. Further, administrations of different polyherbals however demonstrated some levels of efficacy in the treated rats, although, complete histoarchitectural status was not attained. In spite of the potential postreatment actions of these polyherbals in T2D diabetes, such subacute administration may not necessarily translate into a complete amelioration as observed in this study.

Conclusion

The results from this present study demonstrate antihyperglycemic potentials of most commonly used polyherbal in Nigeria in experimental T2D rats. Although specific mechanisms of actions were not determined, however, it appears to be, in part, antioxidants mediated. Also, there is also an urgent need for caution and or monitoring because RB, FJB, and OB could elevate serum TC while RB shows a tendency to increase LDL cholesterol in rats. In addition, a holistic toxicological evaluation of these polyherbals is essential.

Acknowledgements
The technical assistance of Mr. Gisarin O.O. of the Department of Biochemistry, Babcock University, Nigeria, is gratefully acknowledged.

Authors' contributions
OO, AO and KOE designed and coordinated all laboratory experiments. KOE, AOB, BAA, YFO, GR, ADC, OTO, OAC conducted all experiments, statistical analysis, drafted the manuscript and both authors interpreted the results. All authors funded, read and approved the manuscript.

Competing of interest
The authors declare that there is no conflict of interests.

Author details
[1]Department of Pharmacology, Benjamin S. Carson (Snr.) School of Medicine, Babcock University, Ilishan-Remo, Ogun State, PMB, Ikeja 21244, Nigeria. [2]Department of Biochemistry, Benjamin S. Carson (Snr.) School of Medicine, Babcock University, Ilishan-Remo, Ogun State, PMB, Ikeja 21244, Nigeria.

References
1. Jordan SA, Cunningham DG, Marles RJ. Assessment of herbal medicinal products: challenges, and opportunities to increase the knowledge base for safety assessment. Toxicol Appl Pharmacol. 2010;243(2):198–216.
2. Keter LK, Mutiso PC. Ethnobotanical studies of medicinal plants used by traditional health practitioners in the management of diabetes in lower Eastern Province, Kenya. J Ethnopharmacology. 2012;139(1):74–80.
3. Boden G, Shulman GI. Free fatty acids in obesity and type 2 diabetes: defining their role in the development of insulin resistance and β-cell dysfunction. Eur J Clin Investig. 2002;32(s3):14–23.
4. Rodriguez-Fragoso L, Reyes-Esparza J, Burchiel SW, Herrera-Ruiz D, Torres E. Risks and benefits of commonly used herbal medicines in Mexico. Toxicol Appl Pharmacol. 2008;227(1):125–35.
5. Murad MH, Coto-Yglesias F, Wang AT, Sheidaee N, Mullan RJ, Elamin MB, Montori VM. Drug-induced hypoglycemia: a systematic review. J Clin Endocrin Metabolism. 2009;94(3):741–5.
6. Li S, Zhang B, Zhang N. Network target for screening synergistic drug combinations with application to traditional Chinese medicine. BMC Syst Biol. 2011;5(1):S10.
7. Adeyemi OS, Fambegbe M, Daniyan OR, Nwajei I. Yoyo bitters, a polyherbal formulation influenced some biochemical parameters in Wistar rats. J Basic Clin Physiol Pharmacol. 2012;23(4):135–8.
8. Oreagba IA, Oshikoya KA, Amachree M. Herbal medicine use among urban residents in Lagos, Nigeria. BMC Complement Altern Med. 2011;11(1):117.
9. Emordi JE, Agbaje EO, Oreagba IA, Iribhogbe OI. Antidiabetic and hypolipidemic activities of hydroethanolic root extract of Uvaria chamae in streptozotocin induced diabetic albino rats. BMC Complement Altern Med. 2016;16(1):468.
10. Stojanović G, Golubović T, Palić R. Acinos species: chemical composition, antimicrobial and antioxidative activity. J Med Plants Res. 2009;3(13):1240–7.
11. Sharma P, Kharkwal AC, Kharkwal H, Abdin MZ, Varma A. A review on pharmacological properties of Aloe vera. Int J Pharm Sci Rev Res. 2014;29(2):31–7.
12. Radha MH, Laxmipriya NP. Evaluation of biological properties and clinical effectiveness of Aloe vera: a systematic review. J traditional complementary med. 2015;5(1):21–6.
13. Cefalu WT, Ribnicky D. Modulation of insulin action by botanical therapeutics. Obesity Weight Management. 2009;5(6):277–81.
14. Mohamed AE, Abdel-Aziz AF, El-Sherbiny EM, Mors R. Anti-diabetic effect of Aloe vera juice and evaluation of thyroid function in female diabetic rats. Biosci Res. 2009;6:28–34.
15. Odugbemi TO, Akinsulire OR, Aibinu IE, Fabeku PO. Medicinal plants useful for malaria therapy in Okeigbo, Ondo state, Southwest Nigeria. Afr J Tradit Complement Altern Med. 2007;4(2):191–8.
16. Benavente-Garcia O, Castillo J. Update on uses and properties of citrus flavonoids: new findings in anticancer, cardiovascular, and anti-inflammatory activity. J Agric Food Chem. 2008;56(15):6185–205.
17. Calzada F, Yépez-Mulia L, Aguilar A. In vitro susceptibility of Entamoeba histolytica and Giardia lamblia to plants used in Mexican traditional medicine for the treatment of gastrointestinal disorders. J Ethnopharmacol. 2006;108(3):367–70.
18. Nabavi SF, Di Lorenzo A, Izadi M, Sobarzo-Sánchez E, Daglia M, Nabavi SM. Antibacterial effects of cinnamon: from farm to food, cosmetic and pharmaceutical industries. Nutrients. 2015;7(9):7729–48.
19. Sofidiya MO, Oduwole B, Bamgbade E, Odukoya O, Adenekan S. Nutritional composition and antioxidant activities of Curculigo pilosa (Hypoxidaceae) rhizome. Afr J Biotechnol. 2011;10(75):17275–81.
20. Murali R, Saravanan R. Antidiabetic effect of d-limonene, a monoterpene in streptozotocin-induced diabetic rats. Biomedicine & Preventive Nutrition. 2012;2(4):269–75.
21. Syamasundar KV, Singh B, Thakur RS, Husain A, Yoshinobu K, Hiroshi H. Antihepatotoxic principles of Phyllanthus niruri herbs. J Ethnopharmacol. 1985;14(1):41–4.
22. Bansal J, Kumar N, Malviya R, Sharma PK. Hepatoprotective models and various natural product used in Hepatoprotective agents: a review. Pharmacognosy Communications. 2014;4(3):2.
23. Balachandran P, Govindarajan R. Ayurvedic drug discovery. Expert Opin Drug Discovery. 2007;2(12):1631–52.
24. Ekor M. The growing use of herbal medicines: issues relating to adverse reactions and challenges in monitoring safety. Front Pharmacol. 2014;4:177.
25. Ezuruike UF, Prieto JM. The use of plants in the traditional management of diabetes in Nigeria: pharmacological and toxicological considerations. J Ethnopharmacol. 2014;155(2):857–924.
26. Kale OE, Awodele O. Safety evaluation of bon-santé cleanser® polyherbal in male Wistar rats. BMC Complement Altern Med. 2016;16(1):188.
27. Kilkenny C, Browne WJ, Cuthill IC, Emerson M, Altman DG. Improving bioscience research reporting: the ARRIVE guidelines for reporting animal research. PLoS Biol. 2010;8(6):e1000412.
28. Onyeaghala AA, Omotosho IO, Shivashankara AR. Cytotoxicity of various fractions of compounds extracted from Yoyo bitters on human cervical Cancer cells. European J Med Plants. 2015;7(2):46–58.

29. Proestos C, Sereli D, Komaitis M. Determination of phenolic compounds in aromatic plants by RP-HPLC and GC-MS. Food Chem. 2006;95(1):44–52.

30. Okolie AC, Kale OE, Osilesi O. Chemoprotective effects of butanol fraction of Buchholzia Coriacea (Capparidaceae) against type 2 diabetes and oxidative stress in male Wistar rats. Biosci Rep. BSR20170665. 2017; https://doi.org/10.1042/BSR20170665.

31. Wilson R, Islam M. (2012). Fructose-fed Streptozotocin injected rat; an alternative model for type 2 diabetes. *Pharm.*

32. Reitman S, Frankel SA. Colorimetric method for the determination of serum glutamate oxaloacetate and pyruvate transaminases. Am J Clin Pathol. 1957; 28:56–63.

33. Roy AV. Rapid method for determining alkaline phosphatase activity in serum with thymolphthalein monophosphate. Clin Chem. 1970;16(5):431–6.

34. Trinder P. Quantitative determination of triglyceride using GPO-PAP method. Annals Clin Biochem. 1969;6:24–7.

35. Fossati P, Prencipe L, Berti G. Enzymic creatinine assay: a new colorimetric method based on hydrogen peroxide measurement. Clin Chem. 1983;29(8): 1494–6.

36. Warnick GR, Albers JJ. A comprehensive evaluation of the heparinmanganese precipitation procedure for estimating high density lipoprotein cholesterol. J Lipid Res. 1978;19:65–76.

37. Friedewald WT, Levy RI, Fredrickson DS. Estimation of the concentration of low-density lipoprotein cholesterol in plasma, without use of the preparative ultracentrifuge. Clin Chem. 1972;18:499–502.

38. Beutler E, Duron O, Kelly BM. Improved method for the determination of blood glutathione. J Lab Clin Med. 1963;61:882–8.

39. Varshney R, Kale RK. Effect of calmodulin antagonist on radiation induced lipid peroxidation in microsomes. Inter J Radiation Biol. 1990;58(5):733–43.

40. Shaw JE, Sicree RA, Zimmet PZ. Global estimates of the prevalence of diabetes for 2010 and 2030. Diabetes Res Clin Pract. 2010;87(1):4–14.

41. Whiting DR, Guariguata L, Weil C, Shaw J. IDF diabetes atlas: global estimates of the prevalence of diabetes for 2011 and 2030. Diabetes Res Clin Pract. 2011;94(3):311–21.

42. Gbolade AA. Inventory of antidiabetic plants in selected districts of Lagos state Nigeria. *J Ethnopharmacology.* 2009;121(1):135–9.

43. Mohan CG, Viswanatha GL, Savinay G, Rajendra CE, Halemani PD. 1, 2, 3, 4, 6 Penta-O-galloyl-β-d-glucose, a bioactivity guided isolated compound from Mangifera indica inhibits 11β-HSD-1 and ameliorates high fat diet-induced diabetes in C57BL/6 mice. Phytomedicine. 2013;20(5):417–26.

44. Sangeetha KN, Sujatha S, Muthusamy VS, Anand S, Nithya N, Velmurugan D, Lakshmi BS. 3β-taraxerol of Mangifera indica, a PI3K dependent dual activator of glucose transport and glycogen synthesis in 3T3-L1 adipocytes. Biochimica et Biophysica Acta (BBA)-General Subjects. 2010;1800(3):359–66.

45. Zhu F. Chemical composition and health effects of Tartary buckwheat. Food Chem. 2016;203:231–45.

46. Sreekeesoon DP, Mahomoodally MF. Ethnopharmacological analysis of medicinal plants and animals used in the treatment and management of pain in Mauritius. J Ethnopharmacol. 2014;157:181–200.

47. Farrar JL, Hartle DK, Hargrove JL, Greenspan P. A novel nutraceutical property of select sorghum (Sorghum bicolor) brans: inhibition of protein glycation. Phytother Res. 2008;22(8):1052–6.

48. Patel DK, Kumar R, Laloo D, Hemalatha S. Natural medicines from plant source used for therapy of diabetes mellitus: an overview of its pharmacological aspects. Asian Pacific J Tropical Disease. 2012;2(3):239–50.

49. Soladoye MO, Chukwuma EC, Owa FP. An 'Avalanche'of plant species for the traditional cure of diabetes mellitus in south-western Nigeria. J Nat Prod Plant Resour. 2012;2(1):60–72.

50. Boaduo NKK, Katerere D, Eloff JN, Naidoo V. Evaluation of six plant species used traditionally in the treatment and control of diabetes mellitus in South Africa using in vitro methods. Pharm Biol. 2014;52(6):756–61.

51. Tuhin RH, Begum MM, Rahman MS, Karim R, Begum T, Ahmed SU, Begum R, Mostofa R, Hossain A, Abdel-Daim M, Begum R. Wound healing effect of Euphorbia hirta Linn.(Euphorbiaceae) in alloxan induced diabetic rats. *BMC complementary and alternative medicine.* 2017;17(1):423.

52. Brownlee M. Biochemistry and molecular cell biology of diabetic complications. Nature. 2001;414(6865):813–20.

53. Rahimi R, Nikfar S, Larijani B, Abdollahi M. A review on the role of antioxidants in the management of diabetes and its complications. Biomed Pharmacother. 2005;59(7):365–73.

12

Paediatric massage for treatment of acute diarrhoea in children

Li Gao, Chunhua Jia*⊙ and Huiwen Huang

Abstract

Background: Massage therapy has been used by many traditional Chinese medicine physicians to treat acute diarrhoea in children. Since no relevant systematic reviews assessed the clinical effectiveness or the risk of massage therapy, in this study, a meta-analysis was conducted to evaluate the efficacy of paediatric massage for the treatment of acute diarrhoea in children.

Methods: In this meta-analysis, paediatric patients who were diagnosed with acute diarrhoea were included. Interventions using massage therapy alone or combined with other non-pharmacological approaches were included, while in the control groups, patients received pharmacotherapy. The primary outcome was clinical effective rate. Seven databases were used in our research, and the following search terms were used: (massage OR tui na OR manipulation OR acupressure) AND (infant OR child OR baby OR paediatrics) AND (diarrhoea OR diarrhoea) AND (randomized controlled trial). The search date was up to April 30, 2018.

Results: A total of 26 studies encompassing 2644 patients were included in this meta-analysis. It was shown that paediatric massage was significantly better than pharmacotherapy in treating acute diarrhoea in children in terms of clinical effective rate ($n = 2213$, RR = 1.20, 95% CI: 1.14 to 1.27), clinical cure rate ($n = 345$, RR = 1.37, 95% CI: 1.19 to 1.57), and cure time ($n = 513$, MD = − 0.77, 95% CI: -0.89 to − 0.64). However, the quality of evidence for this finding was low due to high risk of bias of the included studies.

Conclusions: The present work supported paediatric massage in treating acute diarrhoea in children. More well-designed randomized controlled trials are still needed to further evaluate the efficacy of paediatric massage.

Keywords: Massage therapy, Children, Acute diarrhoea, Meta-analysis

Background

Acute diarrhoea is a common disease in children in developing countries, especially for those younger than five years old [1]. There are many causes for acute diarrhoea in children [2], such as viruses or bacterial infection, malabsorption, and inflammatory bowel disease. Delayed treatment may cause dehydration, electrolyte imbalance, or even death. Currently, the main treatment for acute diarrhoea is pharmacotherapy, such as oral rehydration salts, Zinc supplement [3], probiotics, or loperamide [4].

In addition to pharmacotherapy, in China, massage therapy is also used by many traditional Chinese medicine (TCM) physicians to treat acute diarrhoea in children. Massage therapy is defined as the manipulation

of the soft tissue of the body, and it is part of the complementary and alternative medicine. Most commonly, massage therapy is conducted on meridians and acupuncture points. The theory behind this therapy was outlined in Huangdi Neijing, which is an ancient Chinese medical book. Over the centuries, massage therapy has been used for emotional and physical healing [5, 6]. There are many benefits of massage therapy [7–10], such as enhancing immune function, unblocking meridians and collateral, activating Qi and blood, and improving the flow of Qi through the meridians. As a result, self-healing in the body is promoted. Paediatric massage is the massage therapy for children that aims to promote health [8, 11].

Many studies have assessed the effects of massage therapy. Vickers et al. [12] conducted a meta-analysis to assess the effects of massage therapy for improving

* Correspondence: chjia11@163.com
Beijing University of Chinese Medicine, No. 11 North 3rd Ring East Road, Chaoyang District, Beijing 100029, China

health and development in preterm birth and low birth weight infants. The results showed that infants who received massage therapy demonstrated improved weight gain (5 g/d) and shorter hospital stays (4–5 days) compared to control groups who did not receive daily massage. Beider et al. [13] conducted a review to examine the effectiveness of massage therapy, and it was shown that massage therapy has real value to the paediatric population, such as a considerable impact on the state of anxiety. Moyer et al. [5] conducted a meta-analysis of randomized studies to test the effectiveness of massage therapy, and the results showed that massage therapy was superior in reducing anxiety and depression. Furthermore, several studies [14–16] have suggested that massage therapy is beneficial to children because it improves blood flow, normalizes function of the central nervous system, and reduces tissue stiffness.

For the treatment of acute diarrhoea in children, many clinical studies have reported beneficial effects of massage therapy. The theorized mechanism of massage therapy on acute diarrhoea is that it promotes gastrointestinal motility, regulates gastric acid secretion, and improves spontaneous bowel movements by stimulating acupuncture points [17–19], although the actual mechanism is still unclear. Considering no relevant systematic reviews have assessed the clinical effectiveness or the risk of paediatric massage therapy, in this study, a meta-analysis was conducted to assess the efficacy of paediatric massage for the treatment of acute diarrhoea in children.

Methods
The protocol of this study was registered in PROSPERO with a registration number CRD42017056523.

Database and search strategies
Relevant studies were searched in the following electronic databases: Cochrane Library, Web of Science, PubMed, Chinese Biomedical Literature Database, Chinese National Knowledge Infrastructure, Chinese Scientific Journal Database, and Wan-fang Database up to April 30, 2018. The following search terms were used: (massage OR tui na OR manipulation OR acupressure) AND (infant OR child OR baby OR paediatrics) AND (diarrhea OR diarrhoea) AND (randomized controlled trial). There were no language limitations.

Inclusion criteria
Included studies must all be randomized controlled trials (RCTs).

Participants
Paediatric patients who were diagnosed with acute diarrhoea. Acute diarrhoea is a disease defined as more stools than normal, and there are some changes in the stool traits, such as loose stool, or watery stool. Usually, course of the disease lasts less than 14 days.

Interventions
Interventions using massage therapy alone or combined with other non-pharmacological approaches were included. Interventions using massage therapy combined with pharmacological therapies, such as montmorillonite, were excluded.

Comparators
In the control groups, patients received pharmacotherapy.

Outcomes
Clinical effective rate was the primary outcome. Some other outcomes included clinical cure rate, and cure time.

Exclusion criteria
Patients with chronic diarrhoea were excluded. Studies lacking data for course of disease were excluded, because it is impossible to judge patients were in acute diarrhoea. Non-RCTs, unpublished or repeated literature, case studies, qualitative studies, and experience summaries were excluded.

Data extraction and quality assessment
Three reviewers (Gao, Jia, and Huang) independently extracted the data and conducted quality assessments. Statistical analysis was conducted using the RevMan 5.3 software, and risk of bias was assessed using the Cochrane tool. Any disagreement was resolved by discussions among the reviewers.

Results
Description of included studies
In this meta-analysis, 813 potentially eligible studies were identified, of which 787 were excluded, including 431 repeated publications, 145 irrelevant studies, 63 studies that combined pharmacological therapy in the intervention group, 110 studies that included patients with chronic diarrhoea, 17 studies that lacked data for the course of disease, 12 studies that did not meet inclusion criteria in the control group, and 9 studies that were not RCTs. Thus, a total of 26 studies [20–45] encompassing 2644 participants (1462 in the intervention group and 1182 in the control group) were included in the meta-analysis, and all were published in Chinese Journal Literature

Databases. The screening process is summarized in a flow diagram (Fig. 1).

Details of the 26 studies are summarized in Table 1. All the children were under 5 years old, and disease course of the participants was less than 14 days. In the intervention group, massage therapy was used alone or combining with other non-pharmacological approaches to treat acute diarrhoea. There are many different treatment methods in the intervention group, and details of the interventions of the included studies are shown in additional file 1. In general, these interventions can be classified into several categories. According to the book Massage [46] in China, there were some basic manipulations suggested for the treatment of acute diarrhoea, including pushing Pijing, Dachang upward, rubbing the abdomen, kneading navel, pushing Qijiegu upward, and Pinching spine. Almost all the studies used the basic massage treatment. Furthermore, in the aim of increasing efficacy, many physicians utilized acupressure (Pressing some acupuncture points), while some physicians performed an individual massage treatment, some other physicians used the acupuncture therapy. In the control group, all the studies used pharmacotherapy; fourteen studies [21, 23, 25, 26, 28–30, 34, 36–38, 42–44] used montmorillonite alone, while other studies used combined therapy.

Ten studies [21, 24, 26, 30, 34–36, 38, 40, 42] reported using standard of Diagnosis and treatment proposal for diarrhoea in China [47] for the definition of acute diarrhoea. This standard provides a diagnostic basis for acute diarrhoea, that is more stools than usual, some changes in the stool traits, and lasting less than 2 weeks. Seven studies [25, 28, 29, 33, 37, 43, 44] adopt a standard in traditional Chinese medicine [48], while other studies did not report any standards cited in the inclusion criteria. However, their definitions of acute diarrhoea in the inclusion criteria were similar to the standard of Diagnosis and treatment proposal for diarrhoea in China.

Risk of bias

The risk of bias was high in the included studies (Fig. 2). All the studies used randomization, but only seven [22, 30, 35, 38, 40, 44, 45] of these studies reported using an appropriate method of random sequence generation, while three [25, 31, 36] of these studies reported using inappropriate methods. None of the studies described the method for allocation concealment and blinding of the outcome assessment. Most of the included studies had a high risk of performance bias,

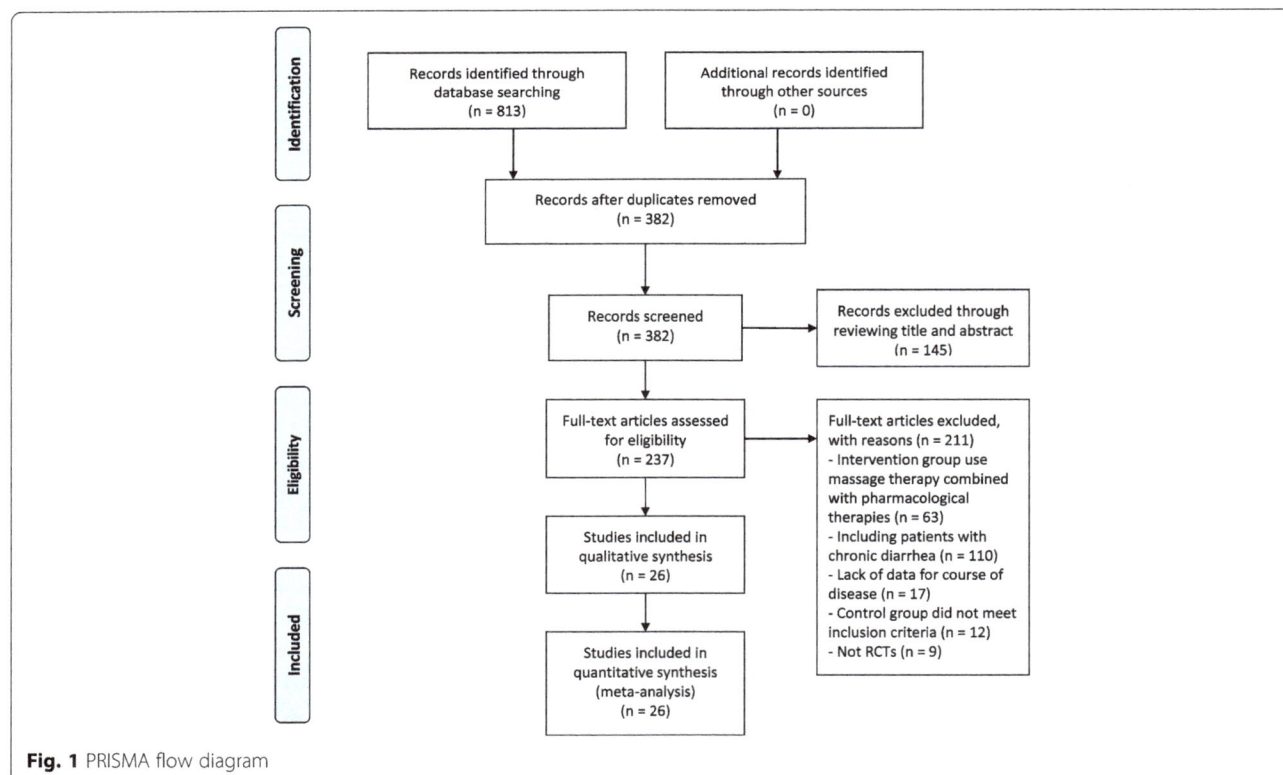

Fig. 1 PRISMA flow diagram

Table 1 Details of the 26 included studies

Study	Sample size	Age	Course of disease	Intervention group	General classification of the massage therapy	Control group
Cheng (2014)	72 (36/36)	1.9 ± 0.5 y	3.6 ± 1.1 d	massage 3 d	BMT + PSAP	(1) montmorillonite (2) combined bacillus subtilis and enterococcus faecium 3 d
Du (2009)	100 (52/48)	19 ± 5 m	1.2 ± 0.5 d	massage 3 d	BMT + PSAP	montmorillonite 3 d
Gao (2005)	60 (30/30)	18 ± 6 m / 17 ± 6.5 m	1.3 ± 0.5 d / 1.2 ± 0.6 d	massage 3 d	BMT + PSAP	(1) montmorillonite (2) combined bacillus subtilis and enterococcus faecium 3 d
Leng (2011)	26 (20/6)	3 m to 5 y	≤1w	massage 3 d	BMT + PSAP	montmorillonite 3 d
Li K (2013)	61 (30/31)	< 3 y	< 2 w	massage 3 d	BMT + PSAP	(1) Cangling antidiarrhea oral solution (2) montmorillonite (3) bifidobacterium 3 d
Li X (2015)	176 (87/89)	2 m to 3 y / 1.5 m to 2 y and 11 m	< 2 w	massage 5 d	IMT	montmorillonite 5 d
Ma (2016)	80 (40/40)	3 m to 4 y	< 1 w	massage 3 d	BMT + PSAP	montmorillonite 3 d
Ni (2018)	70 (35/35)	1.67 ± 1.41 y / 1.64 ± 1.39 y	3.16 ± 0.82 d / 3.19 ± 0.87 d	massage 7 d	BMT + PSAP	norfloxacin 7d
Peng (2011)	240 (180/60)	3 m to 5 y	2.81 ± 1.61 d / 2.78 ± 1.39 d	massage 3 d	BMT + PSAP	montmorillonite 3 d
Shao (2006)	120 (68/52)	18 ± 6 m / 17 ± 6 m	1.3 ± 0.5 d / 1.2 ± 0.6 d	massage 3 d	BMT + PSAP	montmorillonite 3 d
Tang (2014)	135 (67/68)	1.84 ± 0.33 y / 1.87 ± 0.37 y	6.84 ± 2.21 d / 6.58 ± 2.13 d	massage	BMT + PSAP	montmorillonite
Tao (2015)	60 (30/30)	2.03 ± 1.21 y / 2.30 ± 1.16 y	2.81 ± 1.31 d / 2.70 ± 1.20 d	massage 3 d	BMT + PSAP	(1) montmorillonite (2) clostridium butyricum 3 d
Wang (2004)	88 (48/40)	6 m to 3 y	all were acute diarrhea	massage 3 d	BMT + PSAP	(1) intravenous drip ribavirin (2) montmorillonite (3) lactobacillus 3 d
Wang (2014)	86 (43/43)	1.75 ± 0.37 y / 1.25 ± 0.14 y	3.47 ± 0.34 d / 3.41 ± 0.24 d	massage 3 d	BMT + PSAP	(1) norfloxacin (2) ciprofloxacin 5 d
Yang (2016)	80 (40/40)	1.60 ± 0.72 y / 1.81 ± 0.68 y	< 1 w	massage 3 d	BMT + PSAP	montmorillonite 3 d
Yang (2013)	69 (36/33)	6 m to 3 y / 6 m to 3.5 y	1–5 d / 1–6 d	massage 6 d	BMT + PSAP	(1) montmorillonite (2) combined bacillus subtilis and enterococcus faecium (3) bifidobacterium 6 d
Yin (2000)	50 (30/20)	< 3 y	< 3 d	massage 3 d	BMT + PSAP	montmorillonite 3 d
Yin (2009)	315 (190/125)	2 m to 5 y	< 48 h	massage 3 d	IMT	montmorillonite 3 d
You (2013)	55 (32/23)	11.55 ± 4.68 m / 10.58 ± 5.05 m	3.25 ± 1.06 d / 3.39 ± 1.15 d	massage 3 d	BMT + PSAP	montmorillonite 3 d
Zhang (2016)	180 (90/90)	2.41 ± 1.6 y / 2.5 ± 1.2 y	2.8 ± 1.4 d / 2.9 ± 1.2 d	massage 6 d	BMT + PSAP	(1) montmorillonite (2) bifidobacterium 6 d
Zhang	64 (32/32)	< 3 y	1 to 3 d	massage 3 d	BMT + PSAP	(1) probiotics (2) mucosal protection 3 d

Table 1 Details of the 26 included studies (Continued)

Study	Sample size	Age	Course of disease	Intervention group	General classification of the massage therapy	Control group
(2011)						
Zhao (2016)	80 (40/40)	3.1 ± 0.6 y 3.3 ± 0.7 y	14.2 ± 2.1 h 13.2 ± 1.7 h	massage 3 d	BMT + PSAP	(1) enterococcus faecium (2) bifidobacterium (3) montmorillonite 3 d
Zhu (2004)	90 (60/30)	< 3 y	≤3 d	massage 3 d	BMT + PSAP	montmorillonite 3 d
Li G (2013)	120 (60/60)	1.5 ± 0.3 y	< 3 d	massage + acupuncture 3 d	IMT + Acupuncture	montmorillonite 3 d
Wang (2003)	99 (52/47)	1.7 ± 1.1 y 1.8 ± 1.2 y	< 3 d	massage + acupuncture 3 d	BMT + IMT + Acupuncture	montmorillonite 3 d
Wei (2016)	68 (34/34)	12.6 ± 5.7 m 11.9 ± 5.3 m	3.1 ± 0.3 d 3.2 ± 0.4 d	massage + acupuncture 7 d	BMT + IMT + Acupuncture	combined bacillus subtilis and enterococcus faecium 7 d

y: years; m: months; w: weeks; d days; h hours; BMT Basic massage treatment; PSAP Pressing some acupuncture points; IMT Individual massage treatment

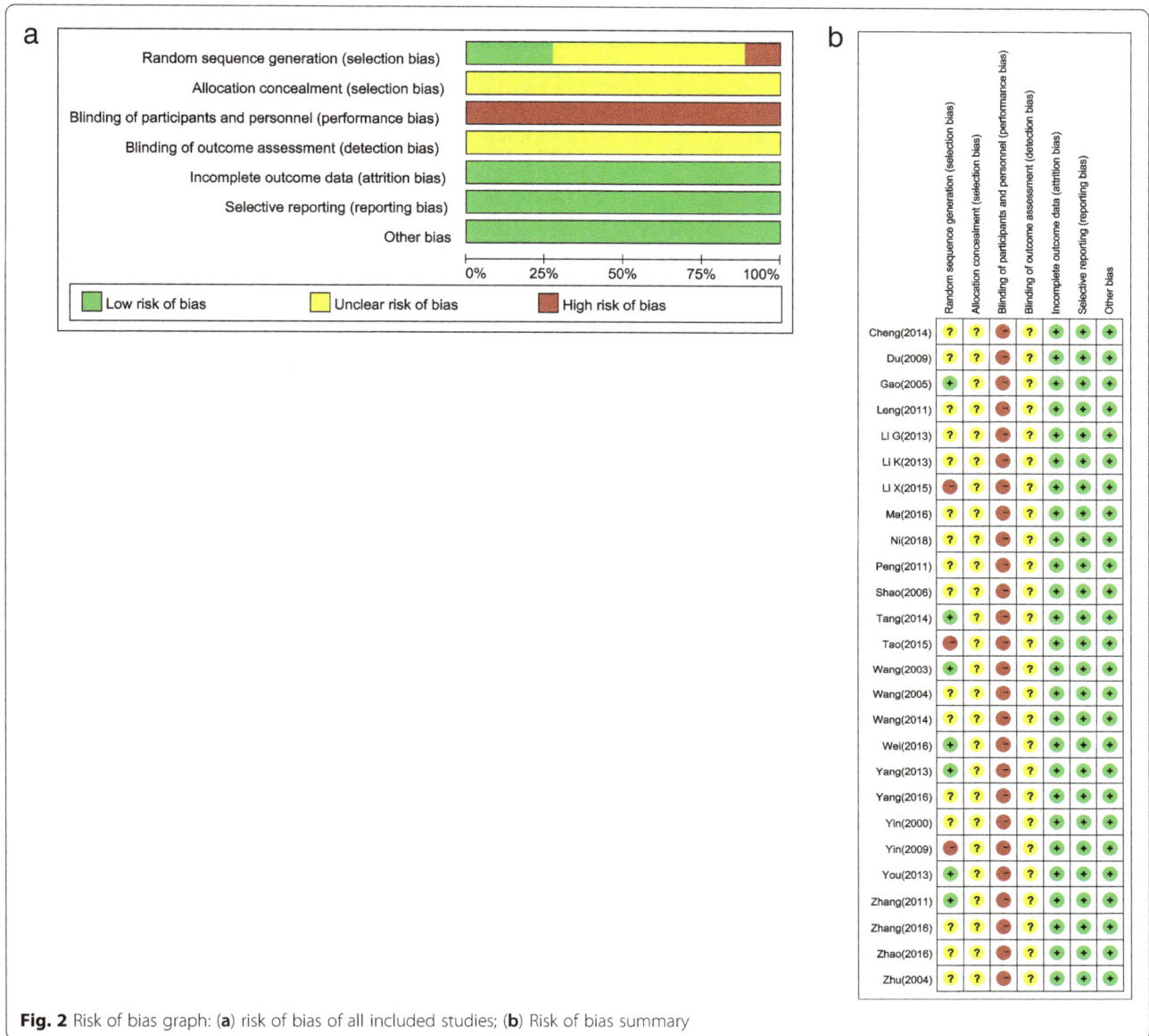

Fig. 2 Risk of bias graph: (**a**) risk of bias of all included studies; (**b**) Risk of bias summary

because both the physicians and the patients clearly knew which treatment was given.

Outcome measurements

Clinical effective rate

According to the standard of Diagnosis and treatment proposal for diarrhoea in China [47], effective was defined as that there is significant improvement in stool traits after 72 h of treatment, and the frequency of stools reduced by 50%. Only four of all studies did not use this standard to define effective. They adopt a similar method, the difference is that two studies [35, 39] did the evaluation after 6 days

of treatment, while two studies [27, 45] did the evaluation after 7 days of treatment.

Twenty-two studies showed that massage therapy had a higher clinical effective rate compared with pharmacotherapy. Since high heterogeneity was observed in the meta-analysis ($I^2 = 64\%$, which is higher than 50%), a random-effects model was used to calculate the pooled estimation with analysis of dichotomous data using relative risk (RR), including 95% confidence intervals (CIs). The meta-analysis showed favourable effects of massage therapy in clinical effective rate ($n = 2213$, RR = 1.20, 95% CI: 1.14 to 1.27, $P < 0.01$) compared with the control group (Fig. 3). A subgroup analysis was conducted for massage therapy alone and massage combined with

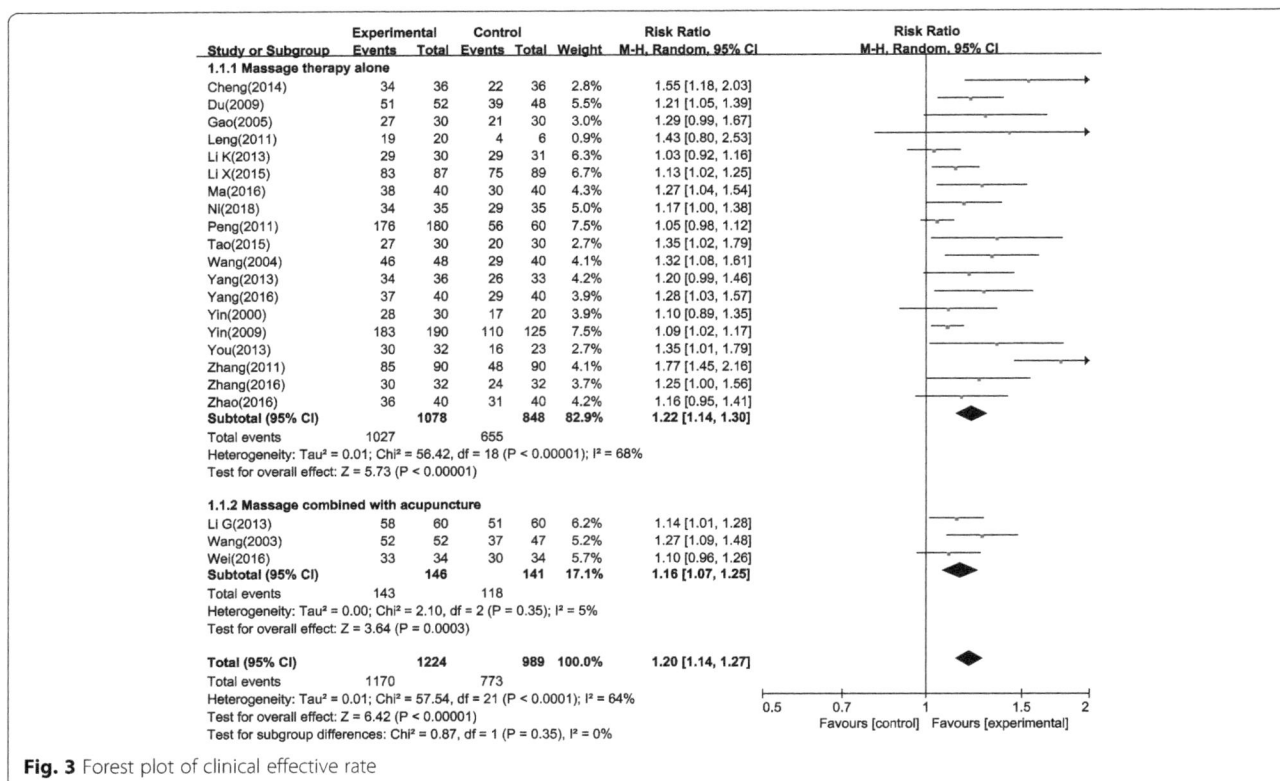

Fig. 3 Forest plot of clinical effective rate

acupuncture. The results showed high heterogeneity in the subgroup massage therapy alone, with $I^2 = 68\%$. While there was low heterogeneity for subgroup differences, with $I^2 = 0\%$.

The reason for the high heterogeneity in the subgroup massage therapy alone may be due to different pharmacotherapies in the control group. Since several studies used montmorillonite alone in the control group, a subgroup analysis was also performed for montmorillonite alone and combined therapy, as shown in Fig. 4. The subgroup of montmorillonite had 1122 patients, with RR = 1.13, 95% CI: 1.07 to 1.20, $P < 0.01$. The subgroup with combined therapy had 804 patients, with RR = 1.28, 95% CI: 1.13 to 1.45, P < 0.01. Heterogeneity in the subgroup montmorillonite was low ($I^2 = 32\%$), while heterogeneity in the subgroup of combined therapy was high ($I^2 = 74\%$), which resulted in a significant difference between these two subgroups, with $I^2 = 68.5\%$. Thus, it can be concluded that the differences in the pharmacotherapies in the control group was a main reason for the high heterogeneity.

Clinical cure rate

Cure was defined as that the stool traits and frequency returned to normal within 72 h of treatment. Three

studies [29, 30, 42] showed that massage therapy had a higher clinical cure rate compared with pharmacotherapy ($n = 345$, RR = 1.37, 95% CI: 1.19 to 1.57, $I^2 = 0\%$), as shown in Fig. 5.

Cure time

Cure time was defined as the length of treatment time spent before the patient is completely cured. Six studies [21, 30, 33, 35, 38, 45] reported data on cure time. The meta-analysis of cure time shows a mean difference (MD) of − 0.77 (95% CI: -0.89 to − 0.64) with a low heterogeneity ($I^2 = 37\%$), as shown in Fig. 6, which means that the participants receiving massage therapy had shorter cure time than those with pharmacotherapy.

Discussion

In TCM, paediatric massage therapy takes into consideration each child's individual physical development and has been found to have many benefits through manipulation on acupoints, such as improving digestive system [49], promoting mental and physical health [11], and increasing body weight in premature infants [50]. However, massage therapy should be carried out by medical staff with enough training, for inaccurate

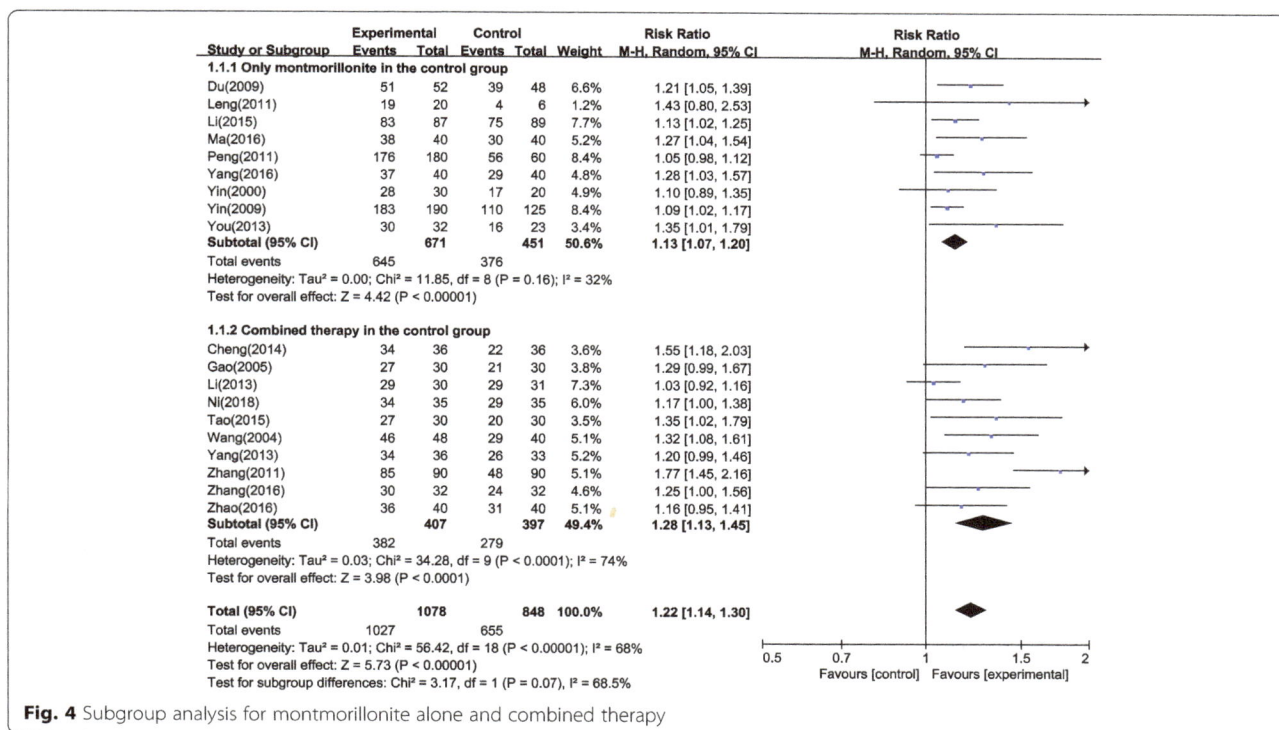

Fig. 4 Subgroup analysis for montmorillonite alone and combined therapy

treatment may reduce the clinical effects. As a complementary and alternative medicine, massage therapy benefits the body in a way that is quick, easy, and inexpensive. It was reported that paediatric massage therapy has been used for treating diseases in children for thousands of years [51]. In recent years, many physicians have reported that paediatric massage therapy can effectively improve the function of the spleen and stomach by stimulating some specific acupoints [19, 49]. However, clinical effectiveness and risk have not been systematically assessed. This study reported a meta-analysis of massage therapy for the treatment of acute diarrhoea in children.

In the treatment of acute diarrhoea in children, massage therapy acts on the on meridians and acupuncture points, activating the flow of Qi and nourishing spleen and stomach. As a result, the function of the digestive system is improved. In addition,

several studies have reported that massage therapy has a positive effect on emotional state of children [52, 53], and as we know, a good emotional state has benefits for improving immune function. It is reasonable to think that part of the rationale for massage therapy to address acute diarrhoea is improving emotional state in paediatric patients.

High heterogeneity was found in clinical effective rate, with $I^2 = 64\%$. Reasons may include different pharmacotherapies used in different control groups. For example, Du [21] used montmorillonite in the control group for the treatment of diarrhoea, while Zhang [40] used probiotics and mucosal protection. These different therapies make the efficacy of massage therapy hard to assess. We conducted a subgroup analysis for montmorillonite alone and combined therapy. It was shown that heterogeneity in the subgroup montmorillonite was low ($I^2 = 32\%$),

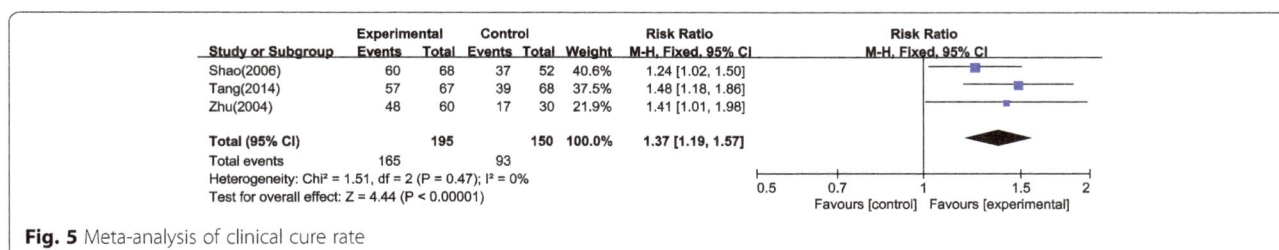

Fig. 5 Meta-analysis of clinical cure rate

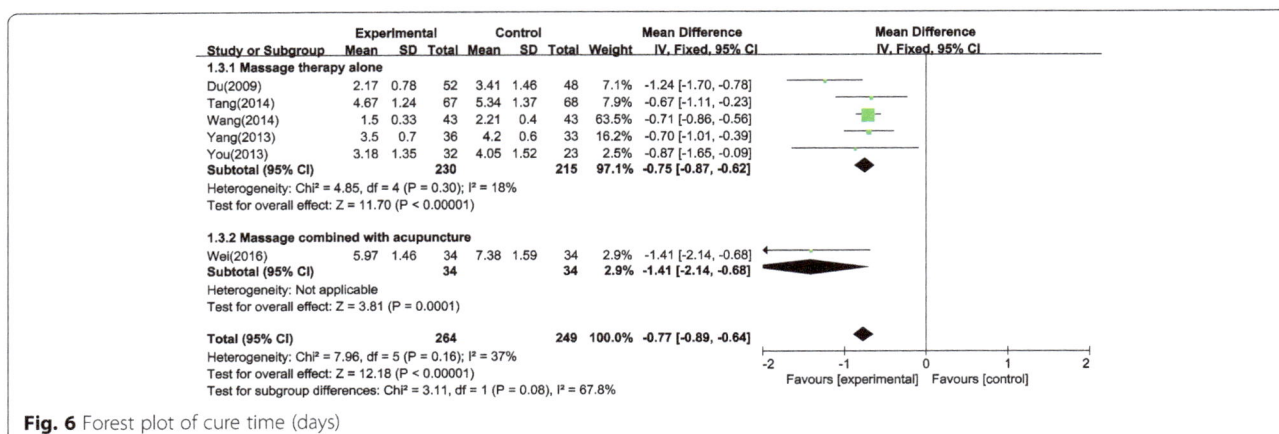

Fig. 6 Forest plot of cure time (days)

while heterogeneity in the subgroup combined therapy was high ($I^2 = 74\%$), resulting in a significant difference between these two subgroups. It can be concluded that the differences in pharmacotherapies in the control group was a main reason for the high heterogeneity. Second,

In addition, another reason for high heterogeneity was that different massage techniques were used by different TCM physicians (as shown in additional file 1). In these studies, some basic manipulations were utilized by all the physicians. However, more manipulations were conducted in different ways, massaged parts of body, manipulation order, and manipulation frequency are usually different. Furthermore, diarrhoea is classified into different types by different TCM physicians, such as cold damp type, spleen deficiency type, and damp hot type; thus, different massage therapy techniques were applied to different types of diarrhoea.

The methodological quality for this finding was low because of high risk of bias. There are several limitations in this systematic review. First, for most of the included studies, the methods for randomization, allocation concealment, and blinding were not reported clearly. Due to the characteristics of TCM, both the physicians and the patients clearly knew which treatment was been given, making blinding methods difficult. Second, in the 26 included studies, only 8 studies had sample sizes greater than 100 trials; small sample sizes in most studies made it hard to draw a meaningful conclusion. Third, clinical effective rate was the main outcome measurement for most studies, and thus, bias from the physicians might decrease reliability and validity of the studies. Fourth, limited information about adverse effects was reported by the included studies; therefore, conclusions on the safety of massage therapy on treatment of acute diarrhoea should be seriously considered. Fifth, all the studies

were conducted in China, which may limit generalization of the findings. Considering the limitations in this meta-analysis, it is strongly recommended that more rigorous RCTs with large sample sizes should be used to further evaluate the clinical efficacy and adverse effects of paediatric massage in treating acute diarrhoea in children.

Conclusions

A total of 26 studies encompassing 2644 patients were included in this meta-analysis that compared paediatric massage and pharmacotherapy for treating acute diarrhoea in children. The results of the meta-analysis suggest that massage therapy was superior to pharmacotherapy. However, the studies analysed to date are of relatively low quality. More rigorous RCTs with large sample sizes are recommended to further evaluate the clinical efficacy and adverse effects of paediatric massage in treating acute diarrhoea in children.

Funding

This study was funded by the National Natural Science Foundation of China (Grant No. 81373770).

Authors' contributions

LG contributed to conception, acquisition, analysis, and interpretation; CJ contributed to conception, design, and analysis; HH contributed to conception, and analysis. All authors drafted manuscript, revised manuscript, gave final approval, agreed to be accountable for all aspects of work ensuring integrity and accuracy.

Competing interests

The authors declare that they have no competing interests.

References

1. Vos T, Barber RM, Bell B, Bertozzi-Villa A, Biryukov S, et al. Global, regional, and national incidence, prevalence, and years lived with disability for 301 acute and chronic diseases and injuries in 188 countries, 1990–2013: a systematic analysis for the global burden of disease study 2013. Lancet. 2015;386(9995):743–800.
2. Caramia G, Silvi S, Verdenelli MC, Coman MM. Treatment of acute diarrhoea: past and now. Int J Enteric Pathog. 2015;3(4):e28612.

3. Lamberti LM, Walker CLF, Chan KY, Jian WY, Black RE. Oral zinc supplementation for the treatment of acute diarrhea in children: a systematic review and meta-analysis. Nutrients. 2013;5(11):4715–40.

4. Li ST, Grossman DC, Cummings P. Loperamide therapy for acute diarrhea in children: systematic review and meta-analysis. PLoS Med. 2007;4(3):e98.

5. Moyer CA, Rounds J, Hannum JW. A meta-analysis of massage therapy research. Psychol Bull. 2004;130(1):3–18.

6. Furlan AD, Giraldo M, Baskwill A, Irvin E, Imamura M. Massage for low-back pain. Cochrane Database Syst Rev. 2015;9:CD001929.

7. Lee MS, Kim JI, Ernst E. Massage therapy for children with autism spectrum disorders: a systematic review. J Clin Psychiat. 2011;72(3):406–11.

8. Beider S, Mahrer NE, Gold JI. Pediatric massage therapy: an overview for clinicians. Pediatr Clin N Am. 2007;54(6):1025–41.

9. Lämås K, Häger C, Lindgren L, Wester P, Brulin C. Does touch massage facilitate recovery after stroke? A study protocol of a randomized controlled trial. BMC Complem Altern M. 2015;16:50.

10. Kania-Richmond A, Reece BF, Suter E, Verhoef MJ. The professional role of massage therapists in patient care in Canadian urban hospitals – a mixed methods study. BMC Complem Altern M. 2015;15:20.

11. Bennett C, Underdown A, Barlow J. Massage for promoting mental and physical health in typically developing infants under the age of six months. Cochrane Database Syst Rev. 2013;4:CD005038.

12. Vickers A, Ohlsson A, Lacy JB, Horsley A. Massage for promoting growth and development of preterm and/or low birth-weight infants. Cochrane Database Syst Rev. 2000;41(2):CD000390.

13. Beider S, Moyer CA. Randomized controlled trials of pediatric massage: a review. Evid Based Complement Alternat Med. 2007;4(1):23–34.

14. Diego MA, Field T, Hernandezreif M. Vagal activity, gastric motility, and weight gain in massaged preterm neonates. J Pediatr. 2005;147(1):50–5.

15. Mcgrath JM. Touch and massage in the newborn period: effects on biomarkers and brain development. J Perinat Neonat Nur. 2009;23(4):304–6.

16. Procianoy RS, Mendes EW, Silveira RC. Massage therapy improves neurodevelopment outcome at two years corrected age for very low birth weight infants. Early Hum Dev. 2010;86(1):7–11.

17. Hui Z, Ying L, Wei Z, Fang Z, Zhou SY, et al. Electroacupuncture for patients with diarrhea-predominant irritable bowel syndrome or functional diarrhea: a randomized controlled trial. Medicine. 2016;95(24):e3884.

18. Qin Z, Li B, Wu J, Tian J, Xie S, et al. Acupuncture for chronic diarrhea in adults:protocol for a systematic review. Medicine. 2017;96(4):e5952.

19. Wei R, Chen Z, Yan J. "Four-step massage" in treating childhood spleen-deficiency diarrhea. Journal of Acupuncture and Tuina Science. 2006;4(5):271–3.

20. Cheng G. Clinical study of massage in the treatment of 36 cases of pediatric noninfectious diarrhea. J North Phar. 2014;11(7):83.

21. Du L. Traditional massage therapy for treating 52 cases of infantile autumn diarrhea. Chinese Journal of Ethnomedicine and Ethnopharmacy. 2009;24:111–3.

22. Gao G. Clinical observation of massage therapy for treating children rotaviral enteritis. Clinical Journal of Traditional Chinese Medicine. 2005;17(3):267–8.

23. Leng L, Zhang J, Wang D, Chen Z, Xing F, et al. Clinical effect observation of massage therapy for treating 20 cases of children cold diarrhea. Nei Mongo Journal of Traditional Chinese Medicine. 2011;8:13.

24. Li K, Xie Y, Ying X. Tuina therapy for treating infant damp-heat diarrhea. Journal of Beijing University of Traditional Chinese Medicine (Clinical Medicine). 2013;20(5):26–30.

25. Li X, Yan Y, Dian Y. Clinical effective observation on treating diarrhea in the acute phase in infants by massage. Clinical Journal of Chinese Medicine. 2015;7(35):22–3.

26. Ma B. Clinical analysis of anterograde and retrograde massage therapy for treatment of children rotaviral enteritis. Modern Health. 2016;18:86.

27. Ni Y. Clinical efficacy observation of massage therapy on acute diarrhea in children. Diet Health. 2018;5(6):84–5.

28. Peng Y, Leng L, Chen Z, Zhang J, Wang D, et al. Acute infantile diarrhea treated with infantile Tuina: a multicentre randomized controlled trial. Chinese Acupuncture & Moxibustion. 2011;31(12):1116–20.

29. Shao X, Wei G, Liu Y. Clinical observation of Liu massage therapy for treatment of 68 cases of children rotaviral enteritis. New Journal of Traditional Chinese Medicine. 2006;38(3):67–8.

30. Tang Y, Shang Q, Yan X. Clinical studies in children with diarrhea by tonifying spleen qi manipulation. China Journal of Chinese Medicine. 2014;29(3):444–5.

31. Tao H, Li Z, Ling X. Clinical efficacy of massage in treatment of infantile indigestion diarrhea caused by improper diet: a report of 30 cases. Journal of Anhui University of Chinese Medicine. 2015;34(6):33–5.

32. Wang T, Jiang W. Massage therapy for treatment of 48 cases of children rotaviral enteritis. Shaanxi Journal of Traditional Chinese Medicine. 2004;5:445.

33. Wang Y. Clinical observation of massage therapy for treating 43 cases of children diarrhea. Chinese Journal of Ethnomedicine and Ethnopharmacy. 2014;21:33.

34. Yang J, Yang T. Clinical study of anterograde and retrograde massage therapy for treatment of children rotaviral enteritis. Practical Clinical Journal of Integrated Traditional Chinese and Western Medicine. 2016;16(2):36–7.

35. Yang Y, Zhang Y. Clinical study of massage in the treatment of pediatric noninfectious diarrhea. China Journal of Chinese Medicine. 2013;28(11):1763–5.

36. Yin C, Xiao Z. Observation and care of massage therapy for treatment of children diarrhea. Today Nurse. 2009;9:61–3.

37. Yin M, Chen X, Han X, Wu Y. Massage therapy for treating 30 cases of children rotaviral enteritis. Journal of Nanjing University of Traditional Chinese Medicine (Natural Science). 2000;16(1):40–1.

38. You X. Massage therapy for treating 32 cases of infantile diarrhea. Chinese Pediatrics of Integrated Traditional and Western Medicine. 2013;5(5):423–5.

39. Zhang J. Clinical effect study of massage therapy in combination with diet instruction for treating children diarrhea. Guangming Journal of Chinese Medicine. 2016;31(14):2078–80.

40. Zhang Z, Shen H, Wang X. Clinical efficacy of transporting massage and stopping diarrhea in the treatment of children rotavirus enteritis. Liaoning Journal of Traditional Chinese Medicine. 2011;38(5):967–8.

41. Zhao W, Song J, Junfeng S. Syndrome differentiation of traditional Chinese medicine massage therapy in clinical application in the treatment of infantile diarrhea. Contemporary Medical Symposium. 2016;14(8):24–5.

42. Zhu Q, Hou D, Zheng Y. Clinical observation of massage therapy in combination with finger pressing for treating children diarrhea. Hubei Journal of Traditional Chinese Medicine. 2004;26(5):49–50.

43. Li G. Treatment of 60 cases of autumn diarrhea in children with acupuncture and massage. Henan Traditional Chinese Medicine. 2013; 33(10):1690–1.

44. Wang X, Bian D, Ma Q. Clinical observation on treating autumn diarrhea in children with acupuncture and massage. Liaoning Journal of Traditional Chinese Medicine. 2003;30(6):492–3.

45. Wei H. Observation on the therapeutic effect of treating children with diarrhea with acupuncture and massage. Journal of Clinical Acupuncture and Moxibustion. 2016;32(7):33–4.

46. Yu D. Massage Science. Shanghai: Shanghai Science and Technology Press; 1995.

47. Fang H, Wei C, Duan S, Dong X, Dong Y, et al. Diagnosis and treatment proposal for diarrhea in China. Chinese Journal of Practical Pediatrics. 1998; 13(6):381–4.

48. State Administration of Traditional Chinese Medicine: Criteria of diagnosis and therapeutic effect of paediatric diseases and syndromes in traditional Chinese medicine. 1994.

49. Xia Q, Feng Z, Ping C. Evaluating the efficacy of Tui Na in treatment of childhood anorexia: a meta-analysis. Altern Ther Health Med. 2014;20(5):45–52.

50. Chen L, Su Y, Su C, Lin H, Kuo H. Acupressure and meridian massage: combined effects on increasing body weight in premature infants. J Clin Nurs. 2008;17(9):1174–81.

51. Badr LK, Abdallah B, Kahale L. A meta-analysis of preterm infant massage: an ancient practice with contemporary applications. Mcn the American Journal of Maternal Child Nursing. 2015;40(6):341–7.

52. Suresh S, Wang S, Porfyris S, Kamasinski-SOL R, Steinhorn D. Massage therapy in outpatient pediatric chronic pain patients: do they facilitate significant reductions in levels of distress, pain, tension, discomfort, and mood alterations? Pediatr Anesth. 2008;18(9):884–7.

53. Kemper K, Shannon S. Complementary and alternative medicine therapies to promote healthy moods. Pediatr Clin N Am. 2007;54(6):901–26.

13

Anti-cancer activity of *Angelica gigas* by increasing immune response and stimulating natural killer and natural killer T cells

Seo Hyun Kim[1†], Sung Won Lee[2†], Hyun Jung Park[2†], Sang Hee Lee[1], Won Kyun Im[1], Young Dong Kim[1], Kyung Hee Kim[3], Sang Jae Park[3], Seokmann Hong[2*] and Sung Ho Jeon[1*]

Abstract

Background: The polysaccharide component of *Angelica gigas* induces immuno-stimulatory effects on innate immune cells. However, it is unclear whether *A. gigas'* adjuvant activity on the immune system can elicit anti-cancer responses.

Methods: A water-soluble immuno-stimulatory component of *A. gigas* was prepared. How this ISAg modulated the activation of innate immune cells such as dendritic cells (DCs) was examined. ISAg-induced cytotoxic activity via natural killer (NK) and NKT cells was also tested using a tumor-bearing mouse model.

Results: ISAg treatment induced nitric oxide (NO) production and cytokine gene expression involved in innate immune responses. ISAg activated macrophages and DCs to secrete cytokine IL-12, through the TLR4 signaling pathway. IL-12 plays a crucial role in ISAg-mediated NK and NKT cell activation. Thus, the anti-cancer activity of NK and NKT cells induced ISAg-mediated cytotoxicity of B16 melanoma cells in mice.

Conclusions: These results indicated that the natural ingredient, ISAg, has adjuvant activity to induce strong anti-cancer activity of NK and NKT cells in vivo.

Keywords: *Angelica gigas*, Immuno-stimulatory polysaccharide fraction, Activation of innate immunity, NK cells, NKT cells, Anti-cancer activity

Background

Angelica gigas Nakai (i.e., Korean angelica or Dang Gui) is used as a traditional medicinal herb in East Asian countries. Decursin and decursinol angelate are major coumarinic components of the *A. gigas* root, which has anti-cancer [1–3], neuroprotective [4], anti-platelet [5], prevention of obesity [6] and bone-loss [7], and anti-inflammatory [8, 9] properties. Angelan (*A. gigas* peptic polysaccharide) is

obtained from water-soluble fraction of *A. gigas* extracts [10]. It has immuno-stimulatory effects through the activation of the innate and adaptive immune systems [11, 12].

Angelan induces splenic lymphocyte proliferation and increases interferon (IFN)-γ production and the immuno-stimulatory cytokine interleukin (IL)-6 during the early stages of treatment [12]. Therefore, macrophages and natural killer (NK) cells in splenocytes might be the main cellular targets directly affected by angelan. Angelan also activates dendritic cell (DC) maturation via the toll-like receptor 4 (TLR4) signaling pathways [11]. Its mechanism of action in lipopolysaccharide (LPS)-induced macrophage activation through the mitogen-activated protein kinase (MAPK) and NF-κB/Rel is well-understood [13]. Angelan also prevents tumor

---

* Correspondence: shong@sejong.ac.kr; sjeon@hallym.ac.kr
†Seo Hyun Kim, Sung Won Lee and Hyun Jung Park contributed equally to this work.
2Department of Integrative Bioscience and Biotechnology, Institute of Anticancer Medicine Development, Sejong University, Seoul 05006, South Korea
1Department of Life Science, Multidisciplinary Genome Institute, Hallym University, Chuncheon, Gangwon 24252, South Korea
Full list of author information is available at the end of the article

growth and metastasis [14], but the mechanisms via which cells are directly involved in anti-cancer activity are poorly understood. Angelan increases the migration of DCs to lymph nodes; these DCs enhance the anti-tumor activity of the lymphocytes [15]. Release of IL-12 cytokine is one of the effector cell functions of active DCs and macrophages. IL-12 is required for the activation of NK and natural killer T (NKT) cells [16, 17]. NK and NKT cells have major roles in the anti-cancer activity of innate immunity. Infiltration of NK and NKT cells into tumors is closely associated with augmented cytotoxicity against tumor cells, and a much higher survival rate in mice [18, 19].

During the development of natural ingredients for functional food, we separated the water-soluble polysaccharide fraction of *A. gigas* that has immuno-stimulating effects (immuno-stimulatory fraction of *A. gigas*; ISAg). The polysaccharide composition of ISAg is similar to that of angelan [10]. However, ISAg contains a higher fraction of glucose (44.7% of total polysaccharides), which is involved in the TLR4 signaling pathways of macrophages. The objective of this study was to investigate the possible roles of ISAg in induction of the innate immune response and stimulation of the anti-cancer activity of NK and NKT cells.

Methods

Preparation of *A. gigas* extract

Angelica gigas Nakai root was obtained from Gangwon province, Korea. The voucher specimen (*Y.D. Kim* et al. *TG-20090258*) was deposited at the Herbarium of Hallym University (Chuncheon, Korea). The ISAg was prepared by adding five times greater v/v % water to *A. gigas* root and extracting twice at 80 °C for 6 h, and then filtered (pore size, 0.45 μm). The resulting extract was concentrated in vacuo and dissolved in 5 to 8 times 70% ethanol at 55 °C for 2 h with stirring. The ethanol-insoluble precipitates were obtained after centrifugation. The phenol-sulfuric acid method was used to measure the total carbohydrate content of the ISAg [20]. Briefly, 200 μl ISAg was mixed with 1 ml 5% phenol; 5 ml H_2SO_4 was then added and mixed well on a vortex mixer. After a 20-min incubation, the color intensity was measured at 490 nm using a Microplate reader (Thermo Fisher Scientific, Waltham, MA, USA). To investigate the constituent sugars, the ISAg was hydrolyzed with H_2SO_4 and subjected to anion-exchange high performance liquid chromatography (ICS-5000, Dionex Co., USA) for quantitative analysis.

Mice and chemical reagents

Wild-type (WT) C57BL/6 (B6), C3H/HeN (TLR4-WT), and C3H/HeJ (TLR4-mutant) mice were obtained from Jung Ang Lab Animal Inc. (Seoul, Korea). IL-12p40

reporter (Yet40) and IL-12p35 knockout (KO) B6 were provided by Dr. R. Locksley (University of California at San Francisco, CA, USA). All mice used in this study were maintained at Hallym University or Sejong University. The animal experiments were approved by the Institutional Animal Care and Use Committee (IACUC) at Hallym University (Hallym 2016–34) and Sejong University (SJ-20160705). All experiments were performed blindly and randomly using age- and sex-matched mice. For sacrifice, mice were euthanized by CO_2 asphyxiation. The CpG oligodeoxynucleotides (CpG ODN type B 1826) were manufactured by Bioneer (Daejeon, Korea). LPS was obtained from Sigma-Aldrich (St. Louis, MO, USA). Alpha-galactosylceramide (α-GalCer) was obtained from Enzo Life Sciences (Farmingdale, NY, USA).

Cell culture and cell viability determination

Murine macrophage, RAW264.7 cells were grown in Dulbecco's modified Eagle's medium (DMEM; Gibco, Carlsbad, CA, USA) containing 10% fetal bovine serum (FBS, Gibco) supplemented with 2 mM glutamine and 100 units/mL penicillin-streptomycin. Cell viability was measured by using CellTiter 96® AQueous assay kit (Promega, Fitchburg, WI, USA). The cultured cells (5×10^4 cells/well) on 96-well plates were treated with serial dilutions of ISAg for 24 h. MTS tetrazolium was added to the plates and incubated at 37 °C for 1 h. Absorbance was measured at 490 nm using a microplate reader.

Nitrite assay and enzyme-linked immunosorbent assay (ELISA)

RAW264.7 cells were incubated with LPS (1 μg/mL) or various amounts of ISAg (0.125–2 μg/mL) at 37 °C for 24 h. The amount of nitrite (NO_2^-) in the culture supernatant was measured by Griess Reagent System (Promega). The amounts of IL-6, tumor necrosis factor (TNF)-α, and IL-1β secreted to the culture medium were quantified using an ELISA kits (KOMA Biotech, Seoul, Korea).

Quantitative reverse transcriptase-polymerase chain reaction (qRT-PCR)

Total RNA from RAW264.7 cells was isolated with TRIzol reagent (Invitrogen, Waltham, MA, USA). The relative amount of specific mRNA was assessed by RT-PCR using amfiRivert cDNA Synthesis Platinum Master Mix (GenDEPOT, Baker, TX, USA). Quantification of mRNA was performed using qRT-PCR. The AccuPower® 2X GreenStar™ qPCR Master Mix (Bioneer) and the Exicycler™ 96 PCR system (Bioneer) were used according to the manufacturer's instructions. The sequences of the sense- and antisense-strand primers used for PCR amplification were inducible nitric oxide synthase (iNOS), 5'-GCTACCACA

TTGAAGAAGCTGGTG-3′, 5′-CCATAGGAAAAGACT GCACCGAAG-3′; cyclooxygenase-2 (COX-2), 5′-GTCT CTCAATGAGTACCGCAAACG-3′, 5′-CTACCATGGTC TCCCCAAAGATAG-3′; IL-6, 5′-GCCAGAGTCCTTCA GAGAGATACA-3′, 5′-ATTGGATGGTCTTGGTCCTTA GCC-3′; IL-1β, 5′-CCTGTGTAATGAAAGACGGCACA C-3′, 5′-CTTGTGAGGTGCTG ATGTACCAGT-3′; TNF-α, 5′-TCTCATCAGTTCTATGGCCCAGAC-3′, 5′-GGCACCA CTAGTTGGTTGTCTTTG-3′. As a control, glyceraldehyde-3-phosphate dehydrogenase (GAPDH) gene was also amplified using 5′-GACATCAAGAAGGTGGTGAAGCA G-3′, 5′-CCCTGTTGCTGTAGCCGTATTCAT-3′.

Immunoblot analysis of MAPK

Total cell lysates were extracted using CytoBuster™ Protein Extraction Reagent (Novagen). Equal amounts of protein were separated on 10 to 15% sodium dodecyl sulfate-polyacrylamide gel electrophoresis (SDS-PAGE) gels at 300 mA for 20 min. They were then transferred to Immobilon-P polyvinylidene difluoride (PVDF) membranes (Millipore Sigma, Billerica, MA, USA) using a trans-blot SD Semi-Dry Transfer Cell (Bio-Rad, Hercules, CA, USA). After transfer, the membranes were incubated in Tris buffered saline (TBS), 5% dry milk, and 0.2% Tween 20 for 1 h. They were then further incubated in TBS and 0.2% Tween 20 with specific antibodies at 4 °C overnight. After washing, a horseradish peroxidase (HRP)-labeled secondary antibody was applied and the membranes were incubated for 2 h. Immunoblot detection was performed using Immobilon Western HRP Substrate (Millipore Sigma). The following antibodies from Cell Signaling Technology were used: anti-protein kinase B (PBK/Akt), anti-phospho-Akt (Ser473), anti-c-jun N-terminal kinase (JNK), anti-phospho-JNK, anti-p38, anti-phospho-p38, anti-p44/42 extracellular signal-related kinase (ERK), anti-phospho-p44/42 ERK, and anti-GAPDH.

Generation of bone marrow-derived DCs (BMDCs)

BMDCs were generated from the bone marrow (BM) cells of Yet40 B6 mice, as previously described [21]. Briefly, BM cells were harvested from femurs and tibiae of mice by flushing with Roswell Park Memorial Institute (RPMI) 1640 medium (Gibco). Red blood cells were removed by adding ACK lysis buffer (0.15 M NH_4Cl, 10 mM $KHCO_3$, and 2 mM EDTA in distilled water), and remaining cells were washed with phosphate buffered saline (PBS) and cultured at a concentration of 1×10^6 cells/well in complete RPMI 1640 medium containing recombinant mouse fms-related tyrosine kinase 3 ligand (Flt3L) (100 ng/ml; R&D Systems, Minneapolis, MN, USA). Fresh cytokine-included culture medium was added on day 5 to generate BMDCs. Five days later, the BMDCs were harvested and stimulated for 16 h with

vehicle or ISAg (125 to 2000 ng/ml). The purity of cluster of differentiation (CD)11c$^+$ cells of these cultures was > 92%.

Flow cytometry and intracellular cytokine staining

The following monoclonal antibodies (mAbs) were obtained from BD Biosciences (San Jose, CA, USA): PE-Cy7-, or allophycocyanin (APC)-conjugated anti-CD11c (clone HL3); phycoerythrin (PE)-, or APC-conjugated anti-NK1.1 (clone PK-136); biotin-conjugated anti-TRAIL; PE-Cy7- or APC-conjugated anti-CD3ε (clone 145-2C11); PE-Cy7-conjugated anti-CD11b (clone M1/70); biotin-conjugated anti-CD45 (clone PC61); PE-conjugated anti-IL-12p40 (clone C15.6); biotin-conjugated CD86 (clone GL1); PE-conjugated anti-TNF-α (clone XP6-XT22); PE-conjugated anti-IgG1 (κ isotype control). The following mAbs from Thermo Fisher Scientific were used: PE-conjugated anti-FasL (clone MFL3); APC-conjugated anti-F4/80 (clone BM8); PE-conjugated anti-perforin (clone eBioOMAK-D); PE-conjugated anti-IFN-γ (clone XMG1.2). Flow cytometric data were acquired using a FACSCalibur (Becton Dickinson Inc., San Jose, CA, USA) and were analyzed with FlowJo analysis tool (Tree Star Inc., Ashland, OR, USA). For surface antibody staining, the cells were collected and washed twice with fluorescence-activated cell sorting (FACS) buffer (PBS containing 0.5% bovine serum albumin). The cells were pre-incubated with purified anti-CD16/CD32 mAbs (BD Bioscience, Bedford, MA, USA) on ice for 10 min for blocking non-specific binding to Fc receptors, and were then stained with fluorescence-labeled mAbs. For intracellular staining, splenocytes were incubated with brefeldin A in RPMI 1640 medium (10 μg/ml) at 37 °C for 2 h. Cells were stained for specific surface markers and fixed with 1% paraformaldehyde. After permeabilization with 0.5% saponin (Sigma-Aldrich), cells were stained with the indicated mAbs (PE-conjugated anti-IL-12p40, anti-TNF-α, anti-IFN-γ, and ant-Perforin; PE-conjugated isotype control rat IgG mAbs) for 30 min. More than 5000 events per sample were acquired using the FACSCalibur.

Cell enrichment using magnetic activated cell sorting (MACS) and cell culture

NK1.1$^+$ cells were enriched from total splenocytes isolated from B6 mice using positive selection with anti-APC MACS (Miltenyi Biotec, Bergisch Gladbach, Germany), after staining with APC-conjugated anti-NK1.1 mAb. The cell populations included > 92% NK1.1$^+$ cells among all the MACS-purified populations. Splenocytes were prepared as single cell suspensions and cultured in complete RPMI 1640 medium containing 10% FBS supplemented with 5 mM 2-mercaptoethanol,

2 mM L-glutamine, 10 mM HEPES, and 100 units/mL penicillin-streptomycin.

Cytotoxicity assay

The flow cytometric 7-amino actinomycin D (7-AAD)/ carboxyfluorescein succinimidyl ester (CFSE) cytotoxicity assay was used as previously described [22]. NK1.1$^+$ cells were isolated as described above and were suspended in complete RPMI 1640 medium. B16 melanoma cells (3×10^6) were stained with CFSE (50 μM) in a 2 ml Hanks' Balanced Salt Solution at 37 °C for 10 min. NK1.1$^+$ cells were incubated with the CFSE-labeled target cells (20,000 cells) at different effector/target (E:T) ratios (27:1, 9:1, 3:1, and 1:1). After a 10-h incubation, the cells were stained with 0.25 μg/ml 7-AAD and were incubated at 37 °C for 10 min. After two washes with PBS containing 1% FBS, cells were resuspended in FACS buffer and their cytotoxicity was evaluated using flow cytometry.

In vivo ISAg injection procedure

To evaluate the dose-dependent effects of ISAg on innate immune responses, Yet40 B6 mice were given ISAg via oral gavage at doses of 0.5, 1, 2, or 4 mg/mouse, three times per week for 4 weeks. In addition, to measure the time-dependent effects of ISAg on innate immune responses, Yet40 B6 mice were received oral ISAg (4 mg/injection) three times per week for the indicated times (1 to 4 weeks). For experiments to test the involvement of TLR4 signaling in ISAg-mediated innate immune responses, C3H/HeN and C3H/HeJ mice were orally administered ISAg (4 mg/injection) three times per week for 4 weeks. Besides, to investigate whether ISAg-mediated innate immune responses are IL-12 dependent, WT or IL-12p35 KO mice were orally administered ISAg (4 mg/injection) three times per week for 4 weeks. In all the aforementioned experiments, LPS (2 μg/mouse) was used as a positive control to inject mice intraperitoneally (i.p.) once a week for a total of 4 weeks.

Tumor injection and isolation of tumor-infiltrating leukocytes

To examine in vivo anti-tumor effects of ISAg, Yet40 mice ($n = 5$/group) received subcutaneous (s.c.) injections of 5×10^5 B16 melanoma cells. One week later, these mice were treated orally using oral gavage with either ISAg (4 mg/injection) or PBS three times per week for the following 2 weeks. As a positive control for anti-tumor immune responses, α-GalCer (2 μg) was injected via the intraperitoneal route two times per week starting 7 days after tumor injection, for a total of 2 weeks. On day 21 after tumor injection, groups of mice were euthanized and tumor tissues were excised for immunological analysis.

Tumor-infiltrating leukocytes were isolated using the following procedure: small pieces tumor tissues were digested (15 min, 37 °C) using 2.5 mg/ml collagenase type IV (Sigma-Aldrich) and 1 mg/ml DNase I (Promega). After incubation, the digested tissues were dissociated into single-cell suspensions using a gentleMACS Dissociator and C Tubes (Miltenyi). The cell-containing suspension was passed through a 70-μm pore nylon cell strainer (BD Bioscience, Bedford, MA, USA), and put on ice. The tumor-infiltrating leukocytes were harvested from the interface of a 40/70% Percoll (GE Healthcare, Little Chalfont, UK) gradient after centrifugation at 1000 g for 20 min.

Statistical analysis

Statistical significance was analyzed using the Excel statistical analysis tool (Microsoft, Redmond, WA, USA). The comparison of two groups was performed by the Student's t-test. Values of *$P < 0.05$ and **$P < 0.01$ were considered to indicate a statistically significant result in the Student's t-test. VassarStats statistical software (http://vassarstats.net/anova2u.html) was used for two-way analysis of variance (ANOVA). Values of #$P < 0.05$ and ##$P < 0.01$ indicates a statistically significant result in the two-way ANOVA.

Results

ISAg stimulated innate immune activity of macrophages

A water-soluble polysaccharide fraction of *A. gigas*, ISAg, was obtained as described in the Methods section. The final product consisted of 63.7% total carbohydrate, 17.4% protein, 0.38% lipid, and inorganic compounds. The maximum content of crude polysaccharide was > 20% of the total extracts. The content of uronic acid, which is a major component of pectin, was 15.1%. The result for the composition of monomeric carbohydrate present in the polysaccharides is presented in Table 1. Glucose was the main polysaccharide component (69.5% of total carbohydrate). The other major sugar constituents were galactose (17.4%) and arabinose (9.0%), Rhamnose, mannose and xylose were also detected as minor components.

To investigate the immuno-stimulatory activity of ISAg, we examined the ISAg-treated mouse macrophage cell line, RAW264.7. ISAg increased NO production of macrophages in a dose-dependent manner, compared with LPS used as a positive control (Fig. 1a). The inducible isoform of nitric oxide synthase (iNOS), which produces NO as an innate immune response defense mechanism, also increased after exposure to ISAg (Fig. 1b). NO stimulates gene expression of COX-2, which converts arachidonic acid to prostaglandin. The transcript level of COX-2 was also increased by the ISAg treatment (Fig. 1c). The high ISAg concentrations

Table 1 Chemical composition of ISAg and its major monosaccharide components

Chemical composition	Molar ratio (w/w %)
Total saccharides	63.7 ± 1.7
Uronic acid	15.1 ± 0.7
Total protein	17.4 ± 0.6
Total lipid	0.4 ± 0.0
Moisture	1.8 ± 0.0
Ash[a]	16.6 ± 0.2
Component Saccharide	Contents (Mole%)[b]
Glucose	69.5 ± 0.6
Galactose	17.4 ± 0.2
Arabinose	9.0 ± 0.2
Rhamnose	2.6 ± 0.2
Mannose	1.2 ± 0.2
Xylose	0.3 ± 0.0

[a]Ash is the non-gaseous, non-liquid residue after complete combustion
[b]Mole% was calculated from the detected total carbohydrate

(up to 2000 ng/ml) used in all experiments did not induce cytotoxic effects (Fig. 1d).

ISAg also induced macrophages to express the pro-inflammatory cytokine genes IL-6, IL-1β, and TNF-α (Fig. 2). Both the RNA transcripts (Fig. 2a–c) and proteins secreted in the culture medium (Fig. 2d–f) were increased by ISAg treatment. These cytokines activate innate immune responses of pathogen-infected host cells. The immuno-stimulatory effects of ISAg on the production of NO and cytokines might be due to the induction of phosphoinositide 3 kinase (PI3K)/Akt signal transduction pathways and MAPK activity. ISAg significantly induced phosphorylation of Akt and JNK in a dose dependent manner (Fig. 3). Other MAPKs, such as ERK-1/2 and p38, were also phosphorylated after exposure to ISAg. This result was consistent with previously reported results [15].

ISAg induced IL-12 production in antigen-presenting cells via TLR4 signaling

Angelan stimulation of DC maturation and migration has anti-cancer effects [11, 15]. Little is known about the details of the cytotoxic process or how it affects the tumor cells. To investigate whether ISAg possessed adjuvant-like ability to stimulate DCs, BMDCs derived

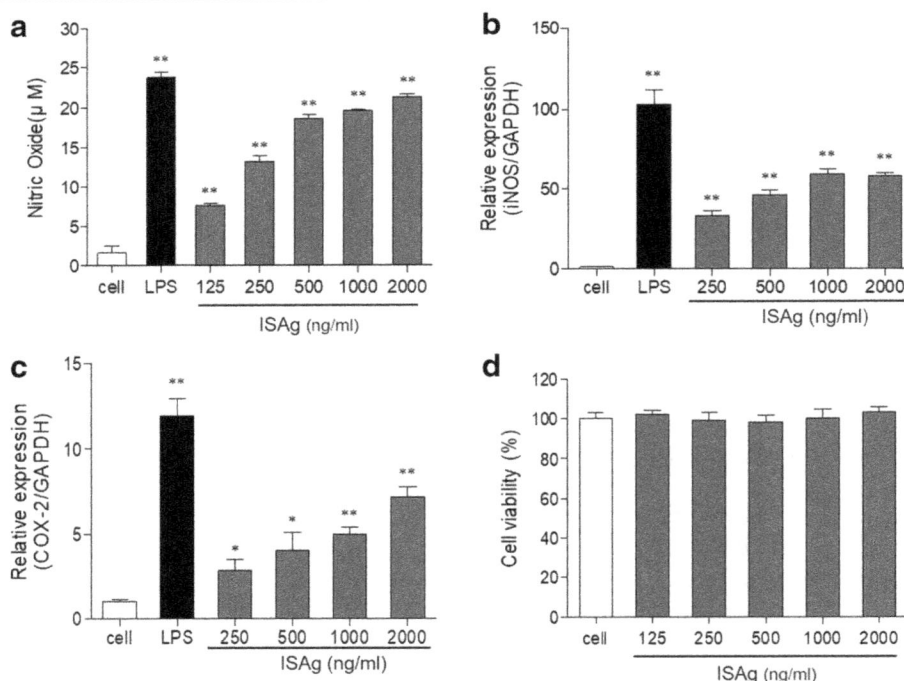

Fig. 1 ISAg induced NO production and COX-2 gene expression in murine peritoneal macrophages. **a** RAW264.7 cells were treated with LPS (1 μg/mL) or indicated concentrations of ISAg for 24 h. The amount of NO production was then measured using Griess reagents and an ELISA kit. Gene expression levels of (**b**) iNOS and (**c**) COX-2 relative to GAPDH were analyzed using qRT-PCR. **d** In all experiments, no significant toxic effects of ISAg were detected in the cells. The mean ± standard deviation values are presented (n = 3 per group; Student's t-test; *P < 0.05, **P < 0.01)

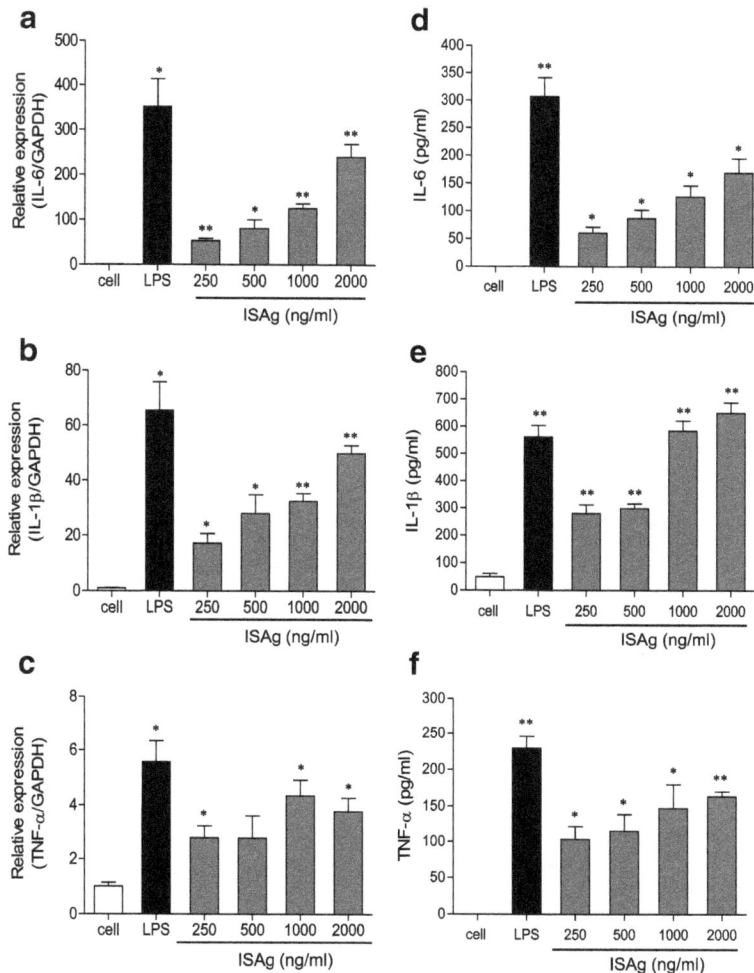

Fig. 2 ISAg treatment induced secretion of immuno-stimulatory cytokines from macrophages. **a–c** RAW264.7 cells were treated with LPS or indicated concentrations of ISAg. Gene expression levels of (**a**) IL-6, (**b**) IL-1β, and (**c**) TNF-α relative to GAPDH were compared using qRT-PCR. **d–f** The levels of each protein secreted in the culture medium were quantified using an ELISA kit. The mean ± standard deviation values are presented (n = 3 per group; Student's t-test; *$P < 0.05$, **$P < 0.01$)

from Yet40 B6 mice were prepared and subsequently stimulated with ISAg in vitro. Sixteen hours later, both CD86 expression and cytokine production (IL-12p40 and TNF-α) in BMDCs were examined using flow cytometric analysis. ISAg-treated BMDCs significantly increased the expression of the co-stimulatory molecule CD86 and cytokine production (IL-12p40 and TNF-α) (Fig. 4a–d). Taken together, these results indicated that ISAg had a priming effect during activation of the DCs.

Based on these results, we investigated whether in vivo treatment with ISAg might modulate innate immune cells, including DCs and macrophages. To test this hypothesis, we delivered ISAg into Yet40 mice and then examined the expression of IL-12p40 [yellow fluorescent protein (YFP)] using splenic DCs and macrophages isolated from ISAg-treated mice. We found that in vivo treatment with ISAg caused a statistically significant

dose-dependent increase in IL-12 secretion (Fig. 5a, b). Next, to examine the kinetics of ISAg-induced IL-12 production in antigen-presenting cells (APCs), we measured IL-12 production in splenic DCs and macrophages from Yet40 B6 mice fed ISAg (4 mg/injection) three times per week for 1 to 4 weeks. We found that a significant increase in IL-12 secretion by DCs and macrophages was saturated after 2 weeks post-ISAg treatment (Fig. 5c). To further understand how ISAg affects IL-12 production in mouse APCs, we used TLR4-mutant C3H/HeJ and TLR4-sufficient C3H/HeN mice to examine whether TLR4 was responsible for ISAg-mediated IL-12 expression. We found that the enhancing effect of ISAg on IL-12 production was not present in APCs from TLR4-mutant C3H/HeJ mice (Fig. 5d). This result suggested that ISAg-induced IL-12 production in APCs was dependent on the TLR4 signaling pathway.

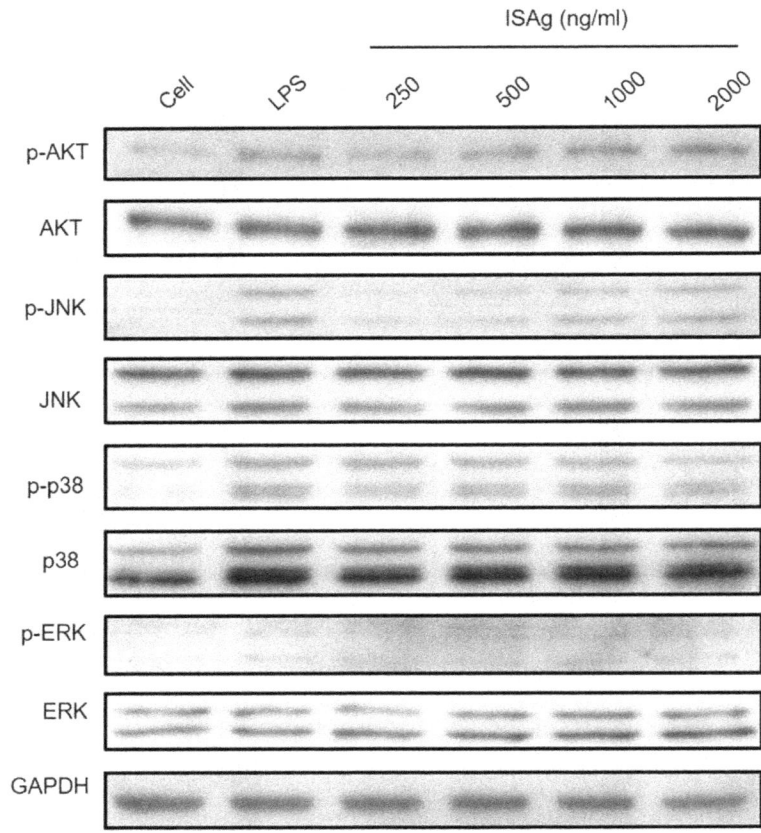

Fig. 3 The PBK/Akt and MAPK signaling pathways of macrophages were activated by ISAg treatment. Total cell lysates from RAW264.7 cells treated with LPS or ISAg were separated using SDS-PAGE gel and transferred to PVDF membranes. Phosphorylated-Akt, -JNK, -p38, and -ERK were detected using immunoblot and specific antibodies. GAPDH and the non-phosphorylated form of each protein were used as controls

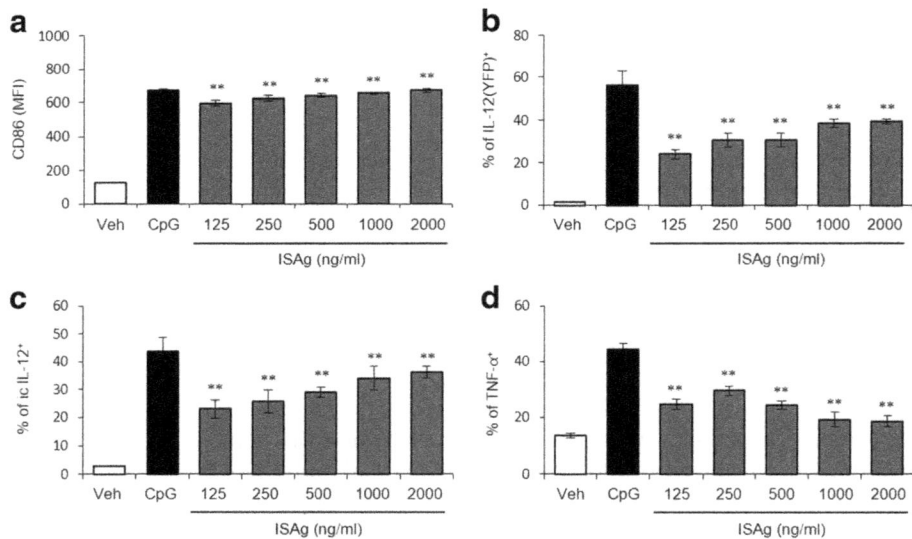

Fig. 4 ISAg enhanced production of Th1-type cytokines in BMDCs. Flt3L-cultured BMDCs from Yet40 B6 mice were stimulated for 16 h using a vehicle or the indicated concentration of ISAg. As a positive control, BMDCs were treated with CpG (5 μg/mL). Subsequently, (**a**) the surface expression of CD86 and the production of (**b**) IL-12p40 (YFP), (**c**) intracellular IL-12p40, and (**d**) TNF-α were assessed in CD11c[+] BMDCs using flow cytometry. The mean ± standard deviation values are presented ($n = 3$ per group; Student's t-test; **$P < 0.01$)

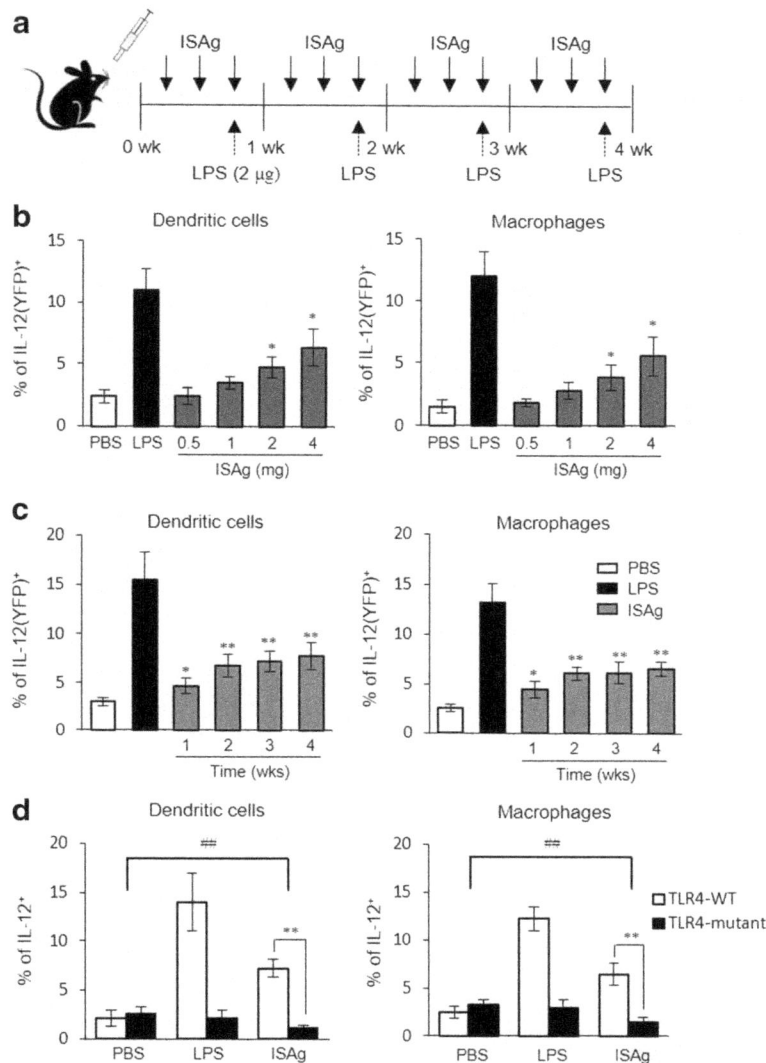

Fig. 5 Oral administration of ISAg induced IL-12 production in antigen-presenting cells via TLR4 signaling. **a** Yet40 B6 mice were exposed via the oral route using gavage with ISAg (0.5, 1, 2, or 4 mg/injection) or PBS three times per week for 4 weeks. As a positive control, mice were injected (i.p.) with LPS (2 μg) once per week for 4 weeks. **b** Four weeks later, IL-12p40 (YFP) productions in splenic DCs (CD11c$^+$) and macrophages (CD11c$^-$CD11b$^+$F4/80$^+$) were assessed using flow cytometry. **c** Yet40 B6 mice were received oral ISAg (4 mg/injection) three times per week for 1 to 4 weeks. At the indicated times, IL-12p40 (YFP) productions in splenic DCs and macrophages were assessed using flow cytometry. **d** C3H/HeN and C3H/HeJ mice were exposed via the oral route to ISAg (4 mg/injection) or PBS three times per week for 4 weeks. Four weeks later, intracellular IL-12p40 production was analyzed in splenic DCs and macrophages using flow cytometry. The mean ± standard deviation values are presented ($n = 4$ per group; Student's t-test; *$P < 0.05$, **$P < 0.01$). Two-way ANOVA (genotype × treatment) revealed the presence of an interaction between these two factors ($^{##}P < 0.01$)

ISAg activated NK receptor-expressing innate immune cells via IL-12

Our results indicated that ISAg had stimulatory effects on APC activation. However, the effects of ISAg on cytotoxic immune cell (e.g., NK1.1$^+$ cells including NK and NKT cells) function have not been studied. To examine these effects, we measured the levels of inflammatory cytokine (IFN-γ and TNF-α) production using splenic NK and NKT cells from Yet40 mice given orally administered ISAg (from 0.5 to 4 mg/mouse). In vivo

ISAg treatment showed a statistically significant ($p <$ 0.05) increase of NK1.1$^+$ cells expressing IFN-γ and TNF-α in Yet40 mice (Fig. 6a, b). We hypothesized that ISAg-associated NK and NKT cell activation is mediated by IL-12. To confirm this, WT or IL-12p35 KO mice were orally administered ISAg and the activation of NK and NKT cells was examined by flow cytometry. The production of inflammatory cytokines in NK and NKT cells of IL-12p35 KO mice was significantly reduced compared to that of WT mice (Fig. 6c, d). These results indicated that IL-12 is required for ISAg-mediated NK and NKT cell activation in vivo. We also examined whether oral administration of ISAg could enhance cytotoxicity and cytokine secretion in NK and NKT cells. NK1.1$^+$ cells isolated from PBS- or ISAg-injected WT B6 mice were used as effector cells for the cytotoxicity assay against B16 melanoma cells. We found that in vivo ISAg treatment increased cytotoxicity of NK1.1$^+$ cells against the tumor cells (Fig. 6e, f). Based on these results, we propose that NK1.1$^+$ cells activated by ISAg treatment can eliminate tumors more efficiently through enhanced effector functions such as cytotoxicity.

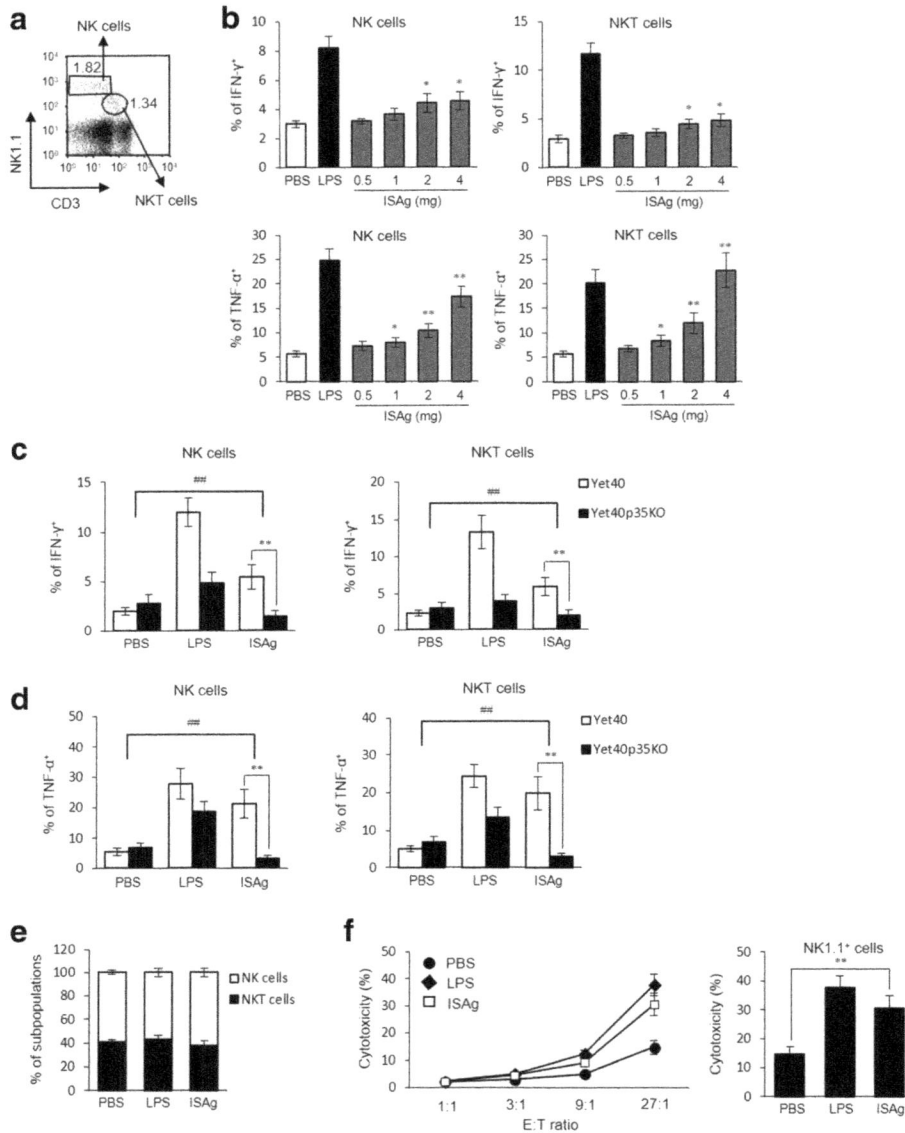

Fig. 6 ISAg activated NK receptor-expressing innate immune cells via DC-derived IL-12. **a** The percentages of NK (NK1.1$^+$CD3$^-$) and NKT cells (NK1.1$^+$CD3$^+$) among the total splenocytes from Yet40 B6 mice were plotted. **b** Yet40 B6 mice were treated via the oral route with ISAg (0.5, 1, 2, or 4 mg/injection) or PBS three times per week for 4 weeks. As a positive control, mice were injected (i.p.) with LPS (2 μg) once per week for 4 weeks. Intracellular productions of IFN-γ and TNF-α were analyzed in NK and NKT cells. **c, d** Yet40 and Yet40p35KO mice were treated via the oral route with ISAg (4 mg/injection) or PBS three times per week for 4 weeks; intracellular production of (**c**) IFN-γ and (**d**) TNF-α were then analyzed in NK and NKT cells. (**e**) NK1.1$^+$ cells were isolated from total splenocytes of WT B6 mice treated with ISAg (4 mg/injection), PBS, or LPS [2 μg/injection (i.p.)]. The percentages of NK and NKT cells among the purified NK1.1$^+$ cells were measured using flow cytometry. **f** Purified NK1.1$^+$ cells were co-cultured with CFSE-labeled B16 tumor cells (2 × 10^4) at the indicated E:T ratios. After 10 h of co-culture, cytotoxicity was evaluated by calculating the percentage of 7-AAD$^+$ (dead) cells, compared with the CFSE$^+$ target cells. The mean ± standard deviation values are presented (n = 3 per group; Student's t-test; *$P < 0.05$, **$P < 0.01$). Two-way ANOVA (genotype × treatment) revealed there was an interaction between these two factors ($^{##}P < 0.01$)

Anti-tumor effects by ISAg were associated with increased cytotoxicity of NK receptor-expressing innate immune cells

Based on the results of the in vitro experiments that examined activation of NK receptor-expressing innate immune cells via IL-12, we hypothesized that in vivo ISAg treatment can inhibit tumor growth in mice. To examine in vivo anti-tumor activity of ISAg, Yet40 mice were inoculated (s.c.) with B16 melanoma. One week later ISAg was orally injected to these mice. ISAg-injected mice had a significant decrease in tumor growth, compared with PBS-injected mice (Fig. 7a, b). To examine whether the increased accumulation of NK and NKT cells was correlated with a decrease in tumor mass, we compared the numbers of NK and NKT cells infiltrated into the tumors between PBS- and ISAg-injected mice. There was a marked increase in accumulation of NK and NKT cells in B16 tumors after ISAg treatment, compared with the PBS-treated mice (Fig. 7c, d). Next, we examined whether there was any change in the expression of cytotoxic molecules such as perforin, TRAIL, or FasL, following ISAg administration. All these molecules were significantly increased in NK and NKT cells after ISAg treatment in vivo (Fig. 8a–c). These results indicated that the cytotoxicity of ISAg treatment against B16 tumor cells in mice was mainly due to the anti-cancer activity of NK and NKT cells.

Discussion

Natural compounds obtained from the same plant using different kinds of solvents (usually water-soluble versus water-insoluble) often have opposite effects on human and experimental animal physiology [8, 11]. However, contradictory (immuno-stimulatory or inhibitory) regulation of immune responses induced by these extracts can achieve the same goal of anti-cancer activity. Decursin induces direct cytotoxic effects on tumor cells through cell cycle arrest [23] or activation of the protein kinase C and reactive oxygen species signaling pathways [24]. Our study found that the polysaccharide component of A. gigas induced the death of target tumor cells through activation of the immune system.

Depending on the microenvironment, macrophages can be polarized into either an M1 phenotype with anti-tumor properties or an alternative M2 phenotype with pro-tumor properties [25]. Components of A. gigas extract can induce distinct immune responses that are pro-inflammatory or anti-inflammatory [11, 26]; our

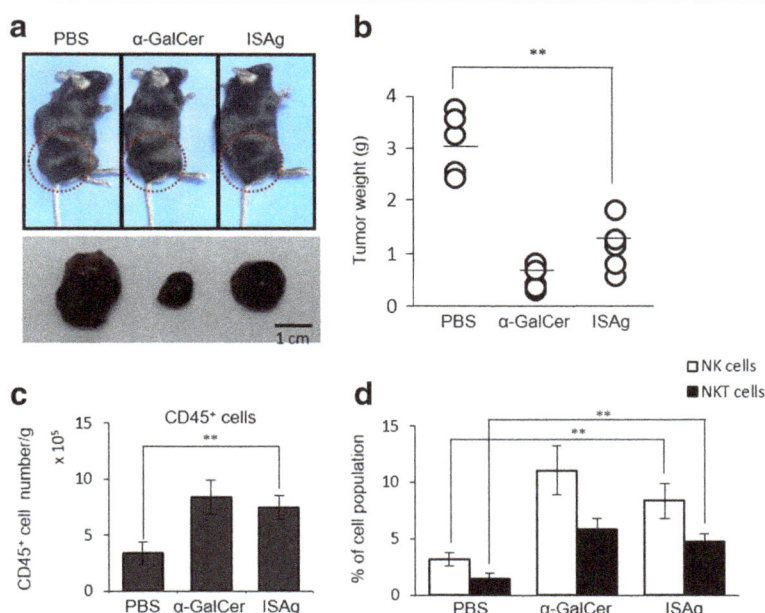

Fig. 7 Anti-tumor effects by ISAg were associated with boosted cytotoxicity of NK receptor-expressing innate immune cells. Yet40 B6 mice were treated via the oral route with ISAg (4 mg/injection) or PBS three times per week beginning 1 week after tumor injection and ending at 3 weeks. As a positive control, mice were injected (i.p.) two times per week beginning at 1 week after tumor injection until 3 weeks with α-GalCer (2 μg) dissolved in PBS. The mice were euthanized at day 21 after B16 tumor cell injection. The spleen and tumor tissues were excised from each mouse. **a** Representative photographs of a mouse from each treatment, 21 days after tumor injection (top row). Photographs of the tumors from each of the mice in the top row (bottom row). **b** The weights of the tumors from individual mice are presented mean ± standard deviation values ($n = 5$ per group; Student's t-test; **$P < 0.01$). **c, d** On day 21 after injection, mononuclear cells were isolated from the tumors of mice in the indicated treatment groups using a Percoll gradient. **c** The absolute numbers of CD45$^+$ cells per gram of tumor tissue were assessed using flow cytometry. **d** The frequencies of the NK and NKT cells among the CD45$^+$ cells from the tumors were evaluated using flow cytometric analysis

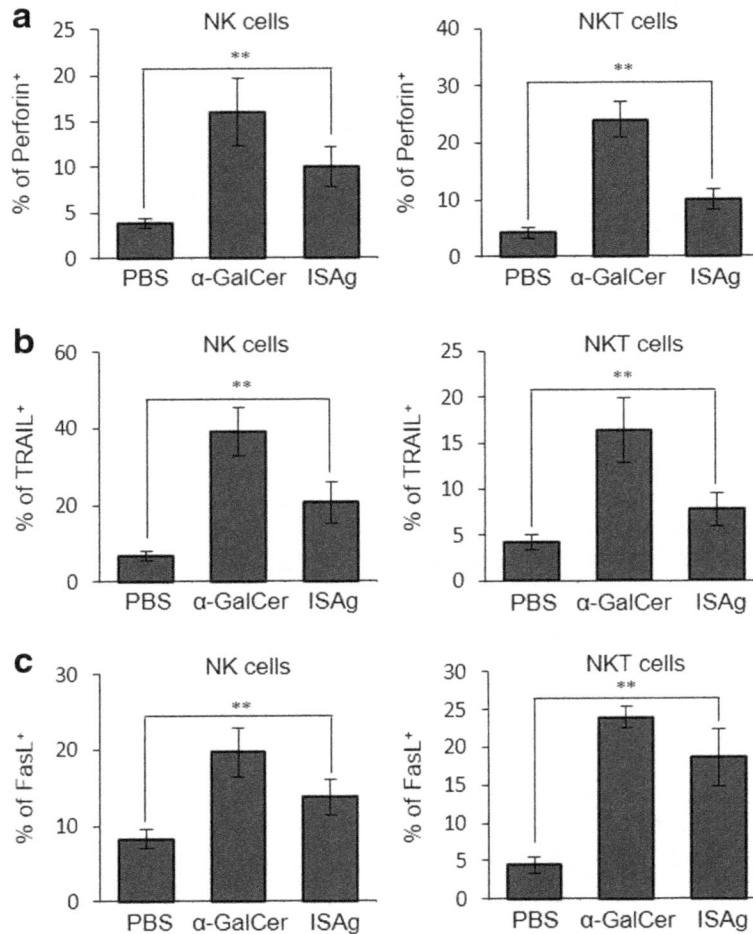

Fig. 8 ISAg induced expression of cytotoxic molecules in NK and NKT cells. The preparation of splenic NK1.1$^+$ cells is described in the Fig. 7 legend. Expressions of (**a**) perforin, (**b**) TRAIL, and (**c**) FasL by splenic NK and NKT cells were evaluated using flow cytometry. The mean ± standard deviation values are presented (n = 5 per group; Student's t-test; **$P < 0.01$)

study revealed that ISAg treatment preferentially differentiated macrophages toward the M1 phenotype (producer of TNF-α and IL-12), but not the M2 phenotype (producer of IL-10). These results indicated that the M1 polarization of macrophages by ISAg treatment is a mechanism that elicits an optimal anti-tumor response. Angelan increases the maturation of DCs via TLR4 [11], but the signaling pathway of ISAg is unclear because the major components of ISAg polysaccharide are quite different. In conclusion, we found that macrophages and DCs were activated by ISAg through TLR4 signaling pathway and subsequently secreted IL-12 cytokine.

NK and NKT cells are activated via ISAg-induced IL-12, which results in increased levels of cytolytic molecules including perforin, TRAIL, and FasL. Thus, TLR4- and IL-12-dependent NK and NKT cell activation by ISAg ultimately results in enhanced cytotoxicity against tumor cells. Previous studies found that angelan induces

proliferation of splenic B lymphocytes [12], but T-cells can be indirectly activated [15]. Regulatory T (Treg) cells are required for suppression of the innate anti-tumor immunity of NK and NKT cells [27, 28]. Inversely, activated NK and NKT cells can inhibit the development of Treg cells via IFN-γ production [29, 30]. Consistent with the results of previous studies, our results indicated that ISAg increased IFN-γ production by NK and NKT cells, resulting in a significant decrease in the Treg population within the tumor tissue (data not shown). This result suggested that enhanced anti-tumor function by ISAg treatment might be related to the suppression of Treg cells resulting from activation of NK and NKT cells. Moreover, our previous results indicated that anti-tumor effects of human T helper type 1 (Th1)-type cytokine (IL-32γ) are attributed to induction of DC maturation followed by consequent enhancement of NK and NKT cell cytotoxicity [31] via DC-derived IL-12 manner [16].

Therefore, it will be of interest to apply ISAg as an immune adjuvant or functional food ingredient to boost anti-cancer immune responses.

Conclusions

This study suggests the following scenario in which ISAg can induce more effective anti-tumor immunity. First, oral administration of ISAg initiates phenotypic changes in innate immune cells such as macrophages and DCs. These results lead to polarization of macrophages to the M1 phenotype as well as DCs to the immunostimulatory phenotype. Second, such ISAg-induced IL-12 subsequently activates NK and NKT cells in order to produce cytotoxic cytokines, especially IFN-γ and TNF-α. Consequently, in vivo ISAg treatment could effectively elicit anti-tumor immune responses. Taken together, our findings strongly suggest that ISAg is an excellent natural product that helps boost the anti-cancer immune responses.

Abbreviations
7-ADD: 7-amino actinomycin D; ACK: Ammonium-chloride-potassium; APC: Allophycocyanin; APCs: Antigen-presenting cells; B6: C57BL/6; BMDCs: Bone marrow-derived dendritic cells; CD: Cluster of differentiation; CFSE: Carboxyfluorescein succinimidyl ester; COX-2: Cyclooxygenase-2; DCs: Dendritic cells; DMEM: Dulbecco's modified Eagle's medium; ELISA: Enzyme linked immunoabsorbance assay; ERK: Extracellular signal-related kinase; FACS: Fluorescence-activated cell sorting; FBS: Fetal bovine serum; Flt3L: Fms-related tyrosine kinase 3 ligand; GAPDH: Glyceraldehyde-3-phosphate dehydrogenase; HRP: Horseradish peroxidase; i.p.: Intraperitoneally; IFN: Interferon; IL: Interleukin; iNOS: Inducible nitric oxide synthase; ISAg: Immuno-Stimulatory fraction of A. gigas; JNK: c-jun N-terminal kinase; LPS: Lipopolysaccharide; mAbs: Monoclonal antibodies; MACS: Magnetic activated cell sorting; MAPK: Mitogen-activated protein kinase; NK: Natural killer; NKT: Natural killer T; NO: Nitric oxide; PBK/Akt: Protein kinase B; PBS: Phosphate buffered saline; PE: Phycoerythrin; PI3K: Phosphoinositide 3 kinase; PVDF: Polyvinylidene difluoride; RPMI: Roswell Park Memorial Institute; s.c.: Subcutaneous; SDS-PAGE: Sodium dodecyl sulfate-polyacrylamide gel electrophoresis; TBS: Tris buffered saline; Th1: T helper type 1; TLR4: Toll-like receptor 4; TNF: Tumor necrosis factor; Treg: Regulatory T; YFP: Yellow fluorescent protein; α-GalCer: Alpha-galactosylceramide

Funding
Financial support for this study was received from the Ministry of Trade, Industry and Energy (MOTIE) and the Korea Institute for Advancement of Technology (KIAT) through a Research and Development for Regional Industry grant (# R0003864) to SHJ and SJP.

Authors' contributions
SHK, SWL, and HJP contributed equally to all of the experiments, data analysis of this study, and the drafting of the manuscript. YDK identified the original specimen. KHK and SJP prepared the extraction of plant materials. SHL and WKI carried out data analysis and interpretation. SH and SHJ contributed to not only the experimental design and data interpretation of this study but also the drafting and editing of the manuscript. All authors read and approved the final manuscript.

Competing interests
The authors declare that they have no competing interests

Author details
[1]Department of Life Science, Multidisciplinary Genome Institute, Hallym University, Chuncheon, Gangwon 24252, South Korea. [2]Department of Integrative Bioscience and Biotechnology, Institute of Anticancer Medicine Development, Sejong University, Seoul 05006, South Korea. [3]Medience Co., Ltd., 301, Chuncheon Bioindustry Foundation, Chuncheon, Gangwon 24232, South Korea.

References
1. Ahn KS, Sim WS, Kim IH. Decursin: a cytotoxic agent and protein kinase C activator from the root of Angelica gigas. Planta Med. 1996;62(1):7–9.
2. Ahn KS, Sim WS, Lee IK, Seu YB, Kim IH. Decursinol angelate: a cytotoxic and protein kinase C activating agent from the root of Angelica gigas. Planta Med. 1997;63(4):360–1.
3. Lee HJ, Lee HJ, Lee EO, Lee JH, Lee KS, Kim KH, Kim SH, Lu J. In vivo anti-cancer activity of Korean Angelica gigas and its major pyranocoumarin decursin. Am J Chin Med. 2009;37(1):127–42.
4. Kang SY, Lee KY, Sung SH, Kim YC. Four new neuroprotective dihydropyranocoumarins from Angelica gigas. J Nat Prod. 2005;68(1):56–9.
5. Lee YY, Lee S, Jin JL, Yun-Choi HS. Platelet anti-aggregatory effects of coumarins from the roots of Angelica genuflexa and A. Gigas. Arch Pharm Res. 2003;26(9):723–6.
6. Hwang JT, Kim SH, Hur HJ, Kim HJ, Park JH, Sung MJ, Yang HJ, Ryu SY, Kim YS, Cha MR, et al. Decursin, an active compound isolated from Angelica gigas, inhibits fat accumulation, reduces adipocytokine secretion and improves glucose tolerance in mice fed a high-fat diet. Phytother Res. 2012; 26(5):633–8.
7. Wang X, Zheng T, Kang JH, Li H, Cho H, Jeon R, Ryu JH, Yim M. Decursin from Angelica gigas suppresses RANKL-induced osteoclast formation and bone loss. Eur J Pharmacol. 2016;774:34–42.
8. Kim JH, Jeong JH, Jeon ST, Kim H, Ock J, Suk K, Kim SI, Song KS, Lee WH. Decursin inhibits induction of inflammatory mediators by blocking nuclear factor-kappaB activation in macrophages. Mol Pharmacol. 2006;69(6):1783–90.
9. Ohshiro T, Namatame I, Lee EW, Kawagishi H, Tomoda H. Molecular target of decursins in the inhibition of lipid droplet accumulation in macrophages. Biol Pharm Bull. 2006;29(5):981–4.
10. Ahn KS, Sim WS, Kim HM, Han SB, Kim IH. Immunostimulating components from the root of Angelica gigas Nakai. Kor J Pharmacogn. 1996;27(3):254–61.
11. Kim JY, Yoon YD, Ahn JM, Kang JS, Park SK, Lee K, Song KB, Kim HM, Han SB. Angelan isolated from Angelica gigas Nakai induces dendritic cell maturation through toll-like receptor 4. Int Immunopharmacol. 2007;7(1):78–87.
12. Han SB, Kim YH, Lee CW, Park SM, Lee HY, Ahn KS, Kim IH, Kim HM. Characteristic immunostimulation by angelan isolated from Angelica gigas Nakai. Immunopharmacology. 1998;40(1):39–48.
13. Jeon YJ, Kim HM. Experimental evidences and signal transduction pathways involved in the activation of NF-kappa B/Rel by angelan in murine macrophages. Int Immunopharmacol. 2001;1(7):1331–9.
14. Han SB, Lee CW, Kang MR, Yoon YD, Kang JS, Lee KH, Yoon WK, Lee K, Park SK, Kim HM. Pectic polysaccharide isolated from Angelica gigas Nakai inhibits melanoma cell metastasis and growth by directly preventing cell adhesion and activating host immune functions. Cancer Lett. 2006;243(2): 264–73.
15. Kim JY, Kim YJ, Kim JS, Ryu HS, Lee HK, Kang JS, Kim HM, Hong JT, Kim Y, Han SB. Adjuvant effect of a natural TLR4 ligand on dendritic cell-based cancer immunotherapy. Cancer Lett. 2011;313(2):226–34.
16. Lee SW, Park HJ, Lee KS, Park SH, Kim S, Jeon SH, Hong S. IL32gamma activates natural killer receptor-expressing innate immune cells to produce IFNgamma via dendritic cell-derived IL12. Biochem Biophys Res Commun. 2015;461(1):86–94.
17. Zhang C, Zhang J, Niu J, Zhou Z, Tian Z. Interleukin-12 improves cytotoxicity of natural killer cells via upregulated expression of NKG2D. Hum Immunol. 2008;69(8):490–500.

18. Wendel M, Galani IE, Suri-Payer E, Cerwenka A. Natural killer cell accumulation in tumors is dependent on IFN-gamma and CXCR3 ligands. Cancer Res. 2008;68(20):8437–45.

19. Song L, Asgharzadeh S, Salo J, Engell K, Wu HW, Sposto R, Ara T, Silverman AM, DeClerck YA, Seeger RC, et al. Valpha24-invariant NKT cells mediate antitumor activity via killing of tumor-associated macrophages. J Clin Invest. 2009;119(6):1524–36.

20. Nielsen SS. Phenol-Sulfuric acid method for total carbohydrates. In: Nielsen SS, editors. Food analysis laboratory manual. Food Science Texts Series. Boston: Springer; 2010. p. 47–53. https://doi.org/10.1007/978-1-4419-1463-7_6.

21. Gilliet M, Boonstra A, Paturel C, Antonenko S, Xu XL, Trinchieri G, O'Garra A, Liu YJ. The development of murine plasmacytoid dendritic cell precursors is differentially regulated by FLT3-ligand and granulocyte/macrophage colony-stimulating factor. J Exp Med. 2002;195(7):953–8.

22. Lecoeur H, Fevrier M, Garcia S, Riviere Y, Gougeon ML. A novel flow cytometric assay for quantitation and multiparametric characterization of cell-mediated cytotoxicity. J Immunol Methods. 2001;253(1–2):177–87.

23. Yim D, Singh RP, Agarwal C, Lee S, Chi H, Agarwal R. A novel anticancer agent, decursin, induces G1 arrest and apoptosis in human prostate carcinoma cells. Cancer Res. 2005;65(3):1035–44.

24. Kim HH, Sik Bang S, Seok Choi J, Han H, Kim IH. Involvement of PKC and ROS in the cytotoxic mechanism of anti-leukemic decursin and its derivatives and their structure-activity relationship in human K562 erythroleukemia and U937 myeloleukemia cells. Cancer Lett. 2005;223(2): 191–201.

25. Biswas SK, Mantovani A. Macrophage plasticity and interaction with lymphocyte subsets: cancer as a paradigm. Nat Immunol. 2010;11(10):889–96.

26. Cho JH, Kwon JE, Cho Y, Kim I, Kang SC. Anti-inflammatory effect of Angelica gigas via Heme oxygenase (HO)-1 expression. Nutrients. 2015;7(6): 4862–74.

27. Ghiringhelli F, Menard C, Terme M, Flament C, Taieb J, Chaput N, Puig PE, Novault S, Escudier B, Vivier E, et al. CD4+CD25+ regulatory T cells inhibit natural killer cell functions in a transforming growth factor-beta-dependent manner. J Exp Med. 2005;202(8):1075–85.

28. Hong H, Gu Y, Zhang H, Simon AK, Chen X, Wu C, Xu XN, Jiang S. Depletion of CD4+CD25+ regulatory T cells enhances natural killer T cell-mediated anti-tumour immunity in a murine mammary breast cancer model. Clin Exp Immunol. 2010;159(1):93–9.

29. Brillard E, Pallandre JR, Chalmers D, Ryffel B, Radlovic A, Seilles E, Rohrlich PS, Pivot X, Tiberghien P, Saas P, et al. Natural killer cells prevent CD28-mediated Foxp3 transcription in CD4+CD25- T lymphocytes. Exp Hematol. 2007;35(3):416–25.

30. Oh KH, Lee C, Lee SW, Jeon SH, Park SH, Seong RH, Hong S. Activation of natural killer T cells inhibits the development of induced regulatory T cells via IFNgamma. Biochem Biophys Res Commun. 2011;411(3):599–606.

31. Park MH, Song MJ, Cho MC, Moon DC, Yoon DY, Han SB, Hong JT. Interleukin-32 enhances cytotoxic effect of natural killer cells to cancer cells via activation of death receptor 3. Immunology. 2012;135(1):63–72.

14

Homoharringtonine regulates the alternative splicing of Bcl-x and caspase 9 through a protein phosphatase 1-dependent mechanism

Qi Sun[1], Shiyue Li[1], Junjun Li[1], Qiuxia Fu[1], Zhongyuan Wang[1], Bo Li[2], Shan-Shan Liu[1], Zijie Su[1], Jiaxing Song[1] and Desheng Lu[1]* (iD)

Abstract

Background: Homoharringtonine (HHT) is a natural alkaloid with potent antitumor activity, but its precise mechanism of action is still poorly understood.

Methods: We examined the effect of HHT on alternative splicing of Bcl-x and Caspase 9 in various cells using semi-quantitative reverse transcriptase-polymerase chain reaction (RT-PCR). The mechanism of HHT-affected alternative splicing in these cells was investigated by treatment with protein phosphatase inhibitors and overexpression of a protein phosphatase.

Results: Treatment with HHT downregulated the levels of anti-apoptotic Bcl-xL and Caspase 9b mRNA with a concomitant increase in the mRNA levels of pro-apoptotic Bcl-xS and Caspase 9a in a dose- and time-dependent manner. Calyculin A, an inhibitor of protein phosphatase 1 (PP1) and protein phosphatase 2A (PP2A), significantly inhibited the effects of HHT on the alternative splicing of Bcl-x and Caspase 9, in contrast to okadaic acid, a specific inhibitor of PP2A. Overexpression of PP1 resulted in a decrease in the ratio of Bcl-xL/xS and an increase in the ratio of Caspase 9a/9b. Moreover, the effects of HHT on Bcl-x and Caspase 9 splicing were enhanced in response to PP1 overexpression. These results suggest that HHT-induced alternative splicing of Bcl-x and Caspase 9 is dependent on PP1 activation. In addition, overexpression of PP1 could induce apoptosis and sensitize MCF7 cells to apoptosis induced by HHT.

Conclusion: Homoharringtonine regulates the alternative splicing of Bcl-x and Caspase 9 through a PP1-dependent mechanism. Our study reveals a novel mechanism underlying the antitumor activities of HHT.

Keywords: Homoharringtonine, Alternative splicing, Bcl-x, Caspase 9, Protein phosphatase 1, Apoptosis

Background

Alternative splicing of mRNA is a key molecular event that allows the generation of multiple mRNAs from a single gene, coding for protein isoforms with different structural and functional properties. Approximately 90% of human genes produce more than one transcript through alternative splicing [1]. This process is highly regulated by a complex interplay between *trans*-splicing factors and *cis*-responsive elements within exons and surrounding introns in normal growth and development [2–4]. Dysregulation of alternative splicing has been found to be associated with various human diseases, including cancer [5–8].

Programmed cell death or apoptosis is a common mechanism to eliminate unnecessary or damaged cells in the development and homeostasis of multicellular organisms. The balance between cell proliferation and apoptosis plays an important role in the control of tissue homeostasis. A failure in apoptosis can lead to the

---
* Correspondence: delu@szu.edu.cn
[1]Guangdong Key Laboratory for Genome Stability & Disease Prevention, Carson International Cancer Center, Department of Pharmacology, Shenzhen University Health Science Center, Shenzhen 518060, Guangdong, China
Full list of author information is available at the end of the article

development of neoplasia. Abnormal expressions of apoptosis-related factors are frequently associated with resistance to apoptosis. It is widely observed that many apoptotic genes encode for splice variants with opposing effects on apoptotic regulation. Bcl-x is an anti-apoptotic member of the Bcl-2 gene family and plays a critical role in regulating apoptosis in mammalian cells. Alternative splicing of the Bcl-x gene generates two protein isoforms with opposing functions, anti-apoptotic Bcl-xL and pro-apoptotic Bcl-xS. Relative expressions of these two isoforms control the susceptibility of cells to apoptotic stimuli [9–11]. Caspase 9 is one of the most important initiators of the intrinsic apoptotic pathway and is activated upon the formation of the Apaf-1/cytochrome c complex, termed the apoptosome [12]. The pro-apoptotic Caspase 9a and anti-apoptotic Caspase 9b are derived from the alternative splicing of the Caspase 9 gene. The Caspase 9b isoform lacks catalytic activity and acts as an endogenous inhibitor of Caspase 9a by interfering with the formation of a functional apoptosome complex between Apaf-1 and Caspase 9 [13, 14]. The alternative splicing of Bcl-x and Caspase 9 can be regulated by several small molecules. Chalfant et al. demonstrated the ability of ceramide to induce pro-apoptotic Bcl-xS and Caspase 9a through activation of alternative splicing [15]. Emetine, an inhibitor of protein synthesis, was shown to be able to regulate the alternative splicing of Bcl-x and Caspase 9 in tumor cells [16, 17]. Chang et al. showed that the antihypertensive drug amiloride could modulate the alternative splicing of various cancer genes, including Bcl-x, HIPK3, and BCR/ABL, in leukemia cells [18, 19]. The manipulation of the alternative splicing of Bcl-x and Caspase 9 may have therapeutic potential in cancer treatment.

Homoharringtonine (HHT) is a natural alkaloid derived from various Cephalotaxus species and has been used in the treatment of hematological malignancies for the past 30 years in China [20]. In 2012, the US FDA approved the use of HHT for treating patients with chronic or accelerated phase chronic myeloid leukemia (CML) [21]. In multiple myeloma (MM) cells, HHT showed anti-myeloma effect with concomitant targeting of the myeloma-promoting molecules, Mcl-1, XIAP, and beta-catenin [22]. Recently, Chen et al. reported that HHT could inhibit the proliferation of acute myeloid leukemia (AML) cells by targeting Smad3/TGF-β pathway [23]. Although HHT has been shown to exert its anticancer activity partly through inhibition of protein synthesis and promotion of apoptosis, its detailed molecular mechanism remains unknown. In this study, we demonstrated for the first time that HHT could regulate the alternative splicing of Bcl-x and Caspase 9 pre-mRNA in several human cancer cells. We further demonstrated that the effect of HHT on alternative splicing is mediated by PP1.

Methods

Compounds

Homoharringtonine (Fig. 1a) was purchased from Sigma (St. Louis, MO, USA). Phosphatase inhibitors calyculin A and okadaic acid were purchased from Cell Signaling Technology (Boston, MA, USA).

Cell culture

Human cancer cell lines MCF7, A549, UACC903 were purchased from the Chinese Academy of Sciences Cell Bank (Shanghai, China). Human breast cancer MCF7, MCF-7/Bobi and MCF-7/PP1 cells were maintained in Dulbecco's modified Eagle's media (DMEM), supplemented with 10% fetal bovine serum (FBS), L-Glutamine and penicillin-streptomycin. Adenocarcinoma lung cancer cells A549 were grown in DMEM/nutrient mixture F-12 (Ham) supplemented with 10% FBS, L-Glutamine and penicillin-streptomycin. Human melanoma UACC903 cells were cultured in Roswell Park Memorial Institute (RPMI1640) with 10% FBS, L-glutamine and penicillin-streptomycin. All cultures were maintained in a humidified 5% CO_2 incubator at 37 °C and routinely passed when 80–90% confluent.

HHT treatment

Homoharringtonine was dissolved in DMSO, with the stock solution concentration at 5 mM. The stock solution was diluted with the cell-specific media and the final DMSO concentration is < 0.1%. HHT was used at concentrations less than 50% inhibitory concentration (IC_{50}) in the studies. At 24 h prior to HHT treatment, the cells were plated in 2 ml of medium in 6-well plates at a density of 200,000 cells/well. The cells were treated with different concentrations of HHT for 24 h for the dose-dependent study. For the time course experiment, the cells were treated with 0.5 μM of HHT for various durations in MCF7 cells.

Treatment with protein phosphatase inhibitors

MCF7, A549 and UACC903 cells were pretreated with calyculin A (2 nM) or okadaic acid (5 nM) for 1 h, after which the media was removed. Fresh media with HHT was then added to the cells for 24 h. Semi-quantitative RT-PCR was performed to evaluate Bcl-x and Caspase 9 splicing.

Semi-quantitative RT-PCR

Total RNA was extracted from cultured MCF7, A549 and UACC903 cells using Trizol reagent (Takara, Shiga, Japan) according to the manufacturer's instruction. Reverse transcription was carried out with 0.5 μg total RNA using the PrimerScript™ RT reagent kit (Takara, Shiga, Japan). After incubation for 1 h at 42 °C, the reactions were terminated by heating at 70 °C for 15 min. To

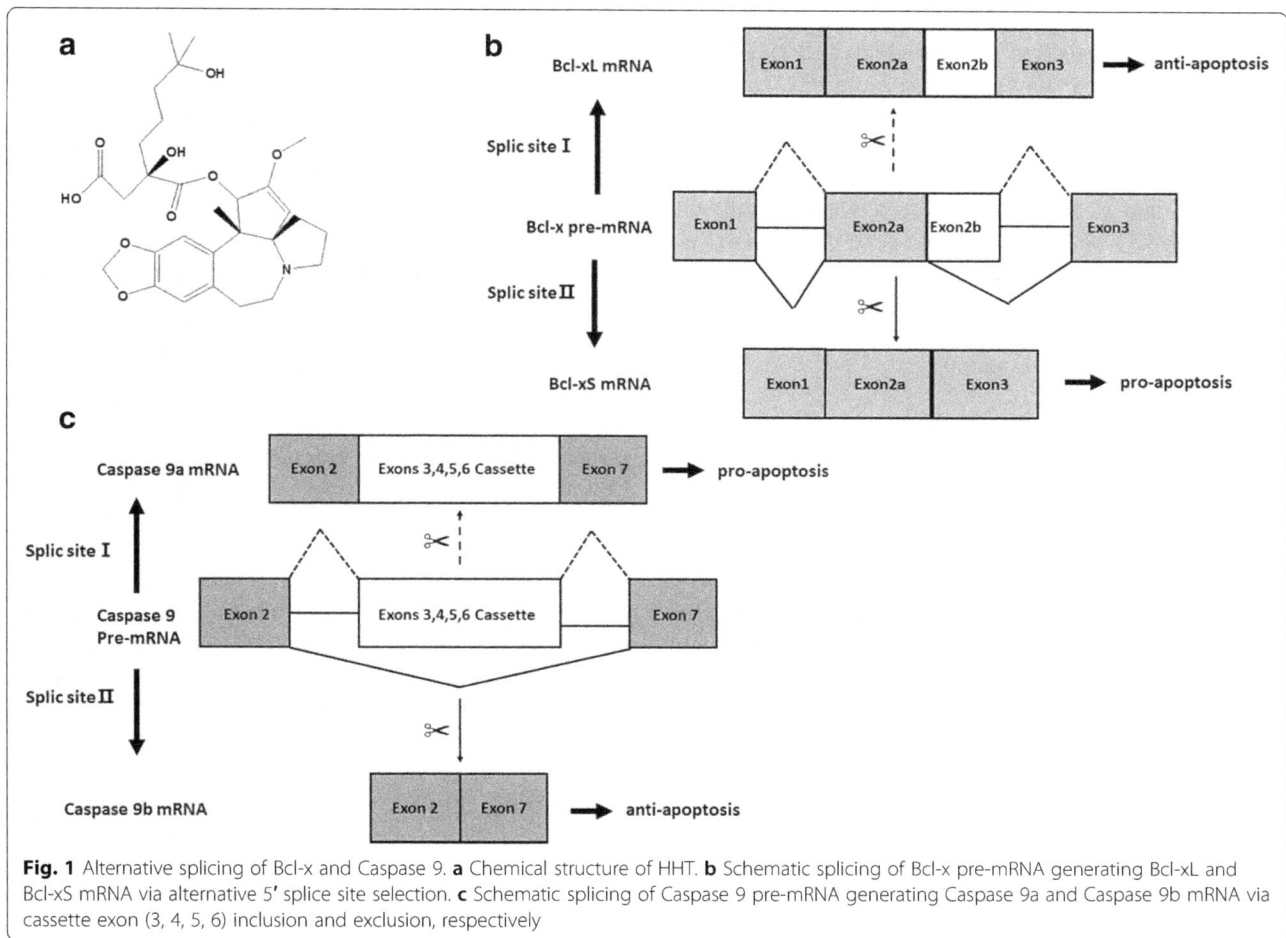

Fig. 1 Alternative splicing of Bcl-x and Caspase 9. **a** Chemical structure of HHT. **b** Schematic splicing of Bcl-x pre-mRNA generating Bcl-xL and Bcl-xS mRNA via alternative 5' splice site selection. **c** Schematic splicing of Caspase 9 pre-mRNA generating Caspase 9a and Caspase 9b mRNA via cassette exon (3, 4, 5, 6) inclusion and exclusion, respectively

analyze alternative splicing of exon 2 in the Bcl-x gene, 5' primer to Bcl-x (5'-GAGGCAGGCGACGAGTTTG AA-3') and 3' primer (5'-TGGGAGGGTAGAGTGGATG GT-3') were used for PCR amplification (30 cycles, 94 °C, 30s; 56 °C, 30s; 72 °C, 1 min) with 2xEasy Taq superMix (Transgen Biotech, China). The length of splicing variants of Bcl-xL and Bcl-xS are 460 bp and 271 bp respectively. To analyze alternative splicing of exon 3, 4, 5, 6 in the Caspase 9 gene, 5' primer to Caspase 9 (5'- GCTCTTCCT TTGTTCATCTCC -3') and 3' primer (5'- CATCTGGCT CGGGGTTACTGC -3') were used for PCR amplification (30 cycles, 94 °C, 30s; 54 °C, 30s; 72 °C, 1 min). The length of splicing variants of Caspase 9a and Caspase 9b are 742 bp and 292 bp, respectively. PCR products were separated and analyzed on agarose gels, with the bands of the Bcl-x and Caspase 9 splicing variants being confirmed by DNA sequencing.

Western blotting

MCF7, A549, UACC903 cells were treated with control or HHT for 24 h, then harvested and sonicated in lysis buffer buffer (20 mM Tris·HCl pH 7.4, 150 mM NaCl,

1 mM EDTA, 1 mM EGTA, 1% Triton X-100, 2.5 mM sodium pyrophosphate, 1 mM β-glycerol phosphate, 1 mM sodium orthovanadate, 2 µg/mL leupeptin, and 1 mM PMSF). Equal amount of proteins were resolved by SDS/PAGE, followed by immunoblotting with a specific Bcl-xL antibody (Cell Signaling Technology).

PP1 cloning, lentiviral vector production and infection

In order to construct the stable overexpression of PP1 in MCF7 cells, a lentiviral vector pBobi was used for gene delivery. The human PP1 gene (XM_001348279.1) was amplified by PCR from a complementary deoxyribonucleic acid (cDNA) library. Following the addition of 10 µl of the PCR products onto a 1% agarose gel with ethidium bromide (0.5 mg/ml) and electrophoresis, images were captured by ultraviolet transillumination. The plasmid was doubly digested with Kpnl and Xba1 (Thermo Fisher Scientific, San Jose, CA, USA). The PCR products and plasmid were purified and ligated, and the resultant mixture was transformed into competent *Escherichia coli* DH5α cells (Transgen Biotech, China). Clones were selected for PCR validation and the recombinant plasmid was extracted for sequencing. The lentivirus packaging system is consisted of 3 plasmids: pMDLg/pRRE, pRSV-Rev, and pVSV-G. To produce the PP1 lentivirus, the recombinant pBobi vector was cotransfected with pMDLg/pRRE, pRSV-Rev, pVSV-G into HEK293T cells. The culture supernatants containing the virus were collected 48 h and 72 h after transfection. For infection with lentivirus, MCF7 cells were cultured with the lentiviral solution for 24 h in the presence of 1 μg/mL Polybrene (Sigma, St. Louis, MO, USA). The resulting cell line was named MCF7-PP1. The control cell line MCF7-Bobi was transfected with an empty vector.

Annexin V-PE /7-Aminoactinomycin D (7-AAD) staining
MCF7-Bobi and MCF7-PP1 cells treated with 5 μM HHT for 24 h were collected and incubated with Annexin V-PE and 7-Aminoactinomycin D (7-AAD) fluorescein solutions (Multi Sciences, China) according to the manufacturer's protocol. The FACSCalibur™ (BD Biosciences, San Jose, CA, USA) fluorescent-activated cell-sorting (FACS) instrument was used for quantitative fluorescent sorting, and FlowJo v10.0.8 (TreeStar Inc., Ashland, OR, USA) was used for subsequent analysis.

Statistical analyses
Student's t-test was used to compare means between groups and all data are represented as the mean ± SEM. Differences at $P < 0.05$ were considered statistically significant.

Results
Homoharringtonine regulates the alternative splicing of Bcl-x and caspase 9 pre-mRNA in breast cancer MCF7 cells
We explored the effects of some natural products on the alternative splicing of Bcl-x using semi-quantitative RT-PCR in MCF7 cells. Alternative splicing of the Bcl-x gene generates Bcl-xL and Bcl-xS variants by using the alternative 5′ splice site within exon 2 (Fig. 1b). Our preliminary results indicate that HHT might affect the alternative splicing of Bcl-x. To further validate the effect of HHT on Bcl-x splicing, MCF7 cells were treated with various concentrations of HHT for 24 h (Fig. 2a-b) or with 0.5 μM HHT for different time durations (Fig. 2c-d). We observed a decrease in the ratio of Bcl-xL/xS from 9.9 in the DMSO control to 4.4, 3.4, 3.0, 2.6, and 2.5 with HHT at 0.05, 0.1, 0.5, 1.0, 5.0 μM, respectively (Fig. 2a-b). Moreover, HHT significantly reduced the ratio of Bcl-xL/xS in a time-dependent manner (Fig. 2c-d).

We further tested the effect of HHT on Caspase 9 splicing in MCF7 cells (Fig. 2e-h). The two splice variants of caspase-9 (Caspase 9a and Caspase 9b) can be generated by either the inclusion or exclusion of the exon 3,4,5,6 cassette in the mature caspase-9 mRNA

(Fig. 1b). As shown in Fig. 2e and f, HHT treatment increased pro-apoptotic Caspase 9a with a concomitant decrease of the anti-apoptotic smaller Caspase 9b, resulting in an increase in the ratio of the Caspase 9a/9b isoform. Importantly, the effect of HHT on the alternative splicing of Caspase 9 is concentration- (Fig. 2e-f) and time-dependent (Fig. 2g-h).

The effects of HHT on the alternative splicing of Bcl-x and caspase 9 in A549 and UACC903 cells
To explore whether HHT-induced alternative splicing has potential relevance in cancer treatment, we examined the effect of HHT on the alternative splicing of Bcl-x and Caspase 9 in human non-small cell lung cancer A549 cells and human malignant melanoma UACC903 cells (Fig. 3). A549 and UACC903 cells were significantly more sensitive to HHT. The dramatic change in the alternative splicing of Bcl-x can be achieved with doses much lower than those required to affect Bcl-x splicing in MCF7 cells. As shown in Fig. 3, 50 nM HHT induced profound effects on the alternative splicing of Bcl-x, decreasing the ratio of Bcl-xL/xS from 13.3 to 2.9 in A549 cells (Fig. 3a-b) and from 44.3 to 2.6 in UACC903 cells (Fig. 3e-f). For Caspase 9, 50 nM HHT induced a significant increase in the ratio of Caspase 9a/9b from 6.0 to 12.3 in UACC903 cells (Fig. 3g-h). However, treatment with HHT had no effect on Caspase 9 splicing in A549 cells (Fig. 3c-d), suggesting that the regulation of the alternative splicing of Caspase 9 in response to HHT may be cell line-specific.

Homoharringtonine decreases the protein expression of Bcl-xL in MCF7, A549 and UACC903 cells
To examine the effect of HHT on protein level of Bcl-xL, a Bcl-xL specific antibody was used to detect the protein expression of Bcl-xL in MCF7, A549 and UACC903 cells. Western blotting showed that HHT decreased the protein level of Bcl-xL in a dose-dependent manner (Fig. 4), which is consistent with its effect of downregulating Bcl-xL mRNA level.

Homoharringtonine exerts its effect on the alternative splicing of Bcl-x and caspase 9 via PP1
Previous studies showed that ceramide and emetine modulate the alternative splicing of Bcl-x and Caspase 9 by affecting PP1. To test whether PP1 mediates the effects of HHT on the alternative splicing of Bcl-x and Caspase 9, MCF7, A549 and UACC903 cells were pretreated for 1 h with 2 nM calyculin A, an inhibitor of both PP1 and PP2A, or 5 nM okadaic acid, a selective PP2A inhibitor, prior to HHT treatment. Calyculin A partially inhibited the effects of HHT on Bcl-x splicing, while pretreatment with okadaic acid had no effect on

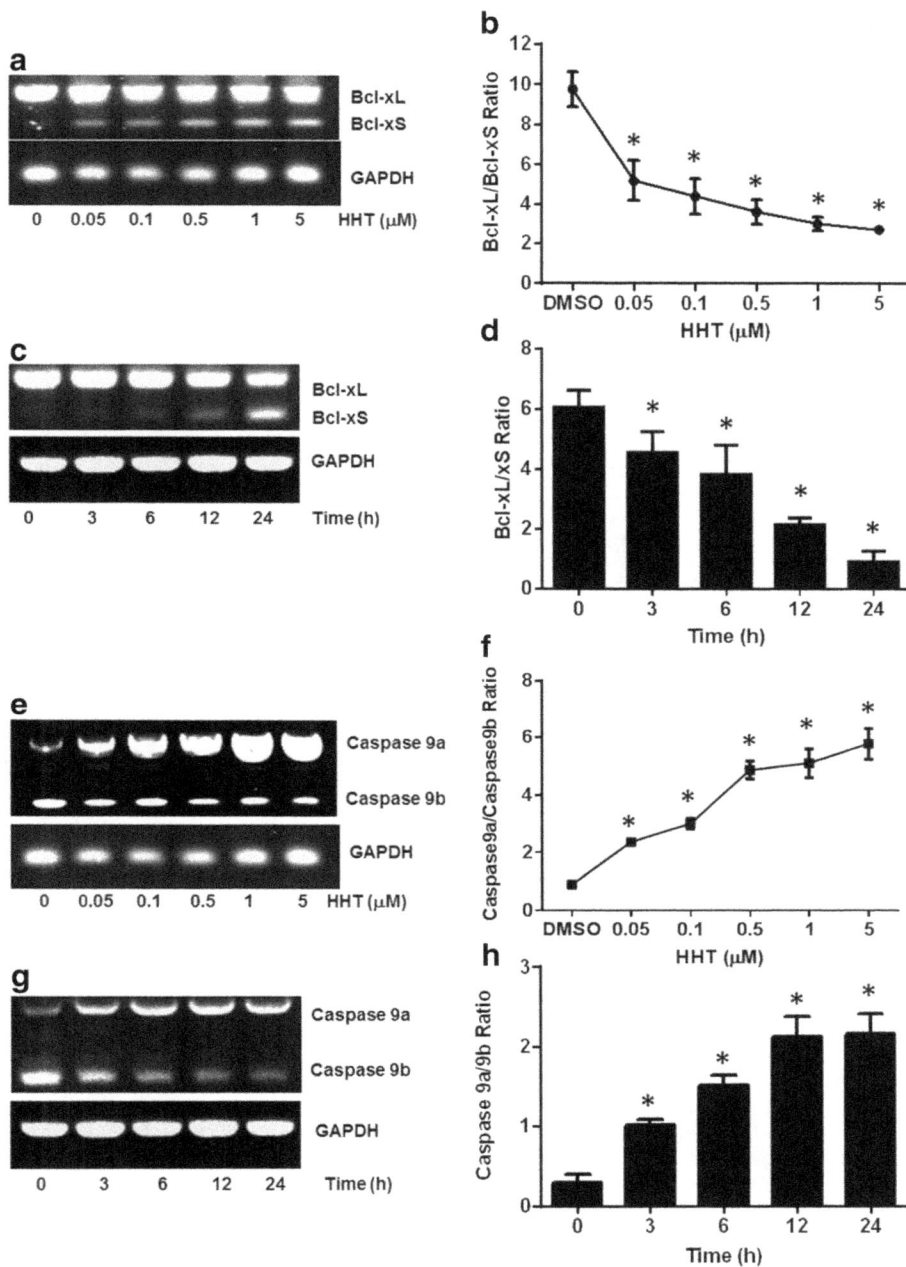

Fig. 2 HHT regulates Bcl-x and Caspase 9 splicing in MCF7 cells. MCF7 cells were treated with HHT. Total RNA was extracted and analyzed by semi-quantitative RT-PCR for the alternative splicing of Bcl-x and Caspase 9. **a** Decrease of Bcl-xL and increase of Bcl-xS is correlated with HHT concentration. **b** Densitometric analysis of the ratio of Bcl-xL/xS ($*P < 0.05$ compared to cells treated with control). **c** and **d** Cells were treated with 0.5 μM HHT for different durations. Semi-quantitative RT-PCR was performed to quantify Bcl-x splicing ($*P < 0.05$ compared to cells at 0 h). **e** Decrease of Caspase 9b and increase of Caspase 9a is correlated with HHT concentration. **f** Densitometric analysis of the ratio of Caspase 9a/9b ($*P < 0.05$ compared to cells treated with control). **g** and **h** Cells were treated with 0.5 μM HHT for different durations. Semi-quantitative RT-PCR was then performed to quantify the alternative spliced products of Caspase 9 ($*P < 0.05$ compared to cells at 0 h)

Bcl-x splicing in all three cell lines (Fig. 5a-d). These results suggest that PP1 mediates the effects of HHT on the alternative splicing of Bcl-x.

In the case of Caspase 9, calyculin A blocked the effect of HHT on Caspase 9 splicing in MCF7 (Fig. 5e-f) and UACC903 cells (Fig. 5g-h). However, okadaic acid pretreatment slightly relieved the effects of HHT on Caspase 9 splicing in MCF7 and UACC903 cells, suggesting that PP2A may also be involved in the HHT-mediated splicing of Caspase 9.

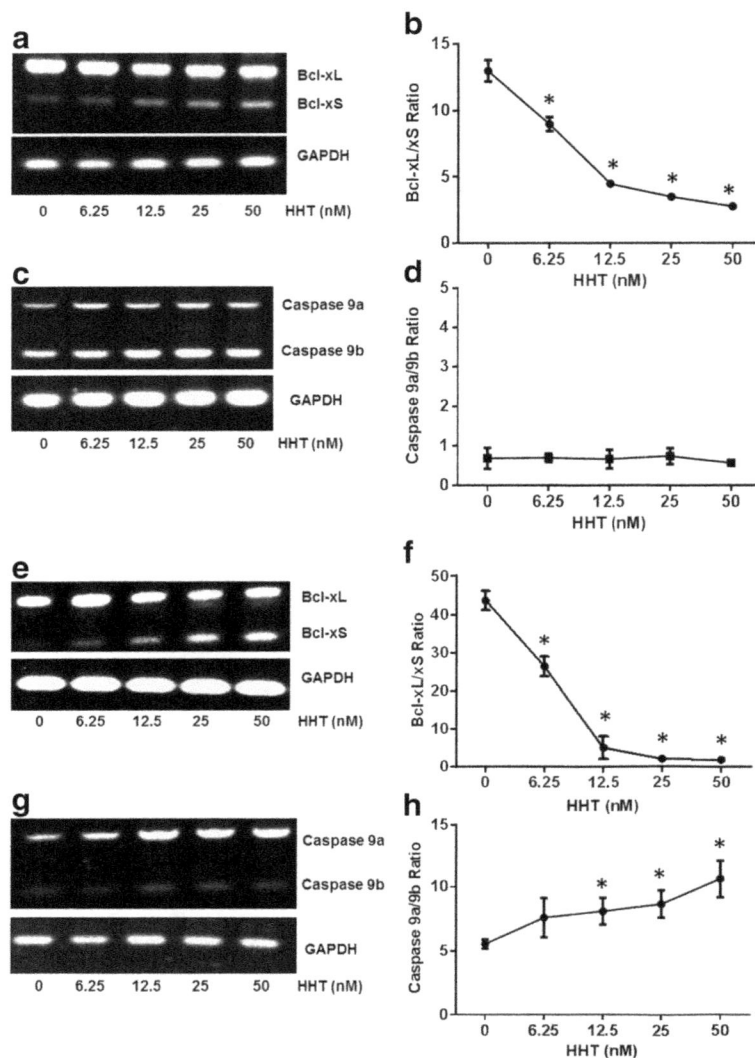

Fig. 3 HHT regulates Bcl-x and Caspase 9 splicing in A549 and UACC903 cells. Total RNA was extracted from A549 cells and UACC903 cells treated with HHT. The alternative splicing of Bcl-x and Caspase 9 was then analyzed by semi-quantitative RT-PCR. **a** Semi-quantitative RT-PCR analysis of Bcl-x splicing from A549 cells treated with different concentrations of HHT. **b** Densitometric analysis of the ratio of Bcl-xL/xS in A549 cells treated by HHT (*$P < 0.05$ compared to cells treated with control). **c** Semi-quantitative RT-PCR analysis of Caspase 9 splicing from A549 cells treated with different concentrations of HHT. **d** Densitometric analysis of the ratio of Caspase 9a/9b in A549 cells treated by HHT. **e** Semi-quantitative RT-PCR analysis of Bcl-x splicing from UACC903 cells treated with different concentrations of HHT. (f) Densitometric analysis of the ratio of Bcl-xL/xS in UACC903 cells treated by HHT (*$P < 0.05$ compared to cells treated with control). **g** Semi-quantitative RT-PCR analysis of Caspase 9 splicing from UACC903 cells treated with different concentrations of HHT. **h** Densitometric analysis of the ratio of Caspase 9a/9b in UACC903 cells treated by HHT (*$P < 0.05$ compared to cells treated with control)

Overexpression of PP1 enhances the effects of HHT on Bcl-x and caspase 9 splicing and sensitizes MCF7 cells to apoptosis induced by HHT

To verify the role of PP1 in HHT-mediated alternative splicing, we constructed a stable MCF7 cell line overexpressing PP1 using a lentiviral system (Fig. 6a). Significant changes in the alternative splicing of Caspase 9 and Bcl-x were observed in the MCF7 cells overexpressing PP1, with a decrease in the ratio of Bcl-xL/xS and an increase in the ratio of Caspase 9a/9b compared with the

MCF7 control cells (Fig. 6b-d). Moreover, the effects of HHT on Bcl-x and Caspase 9 splicing were further enhanced in response to PP1 overexpression.

We next examined the effect of HHT on apoptosis in the PP1 overexpressing MCF7 cell line and parental MCF7 cell line. Cellular apoptosis was evaluated by measurement of the exposure of phosphatidylserine on the cell membrane by using Annexin V-PE and 7-AAD staining. Figure 6e showed that HHT induced apoptosis in MCF7 cells. About 22.54% cells were apoptotic when

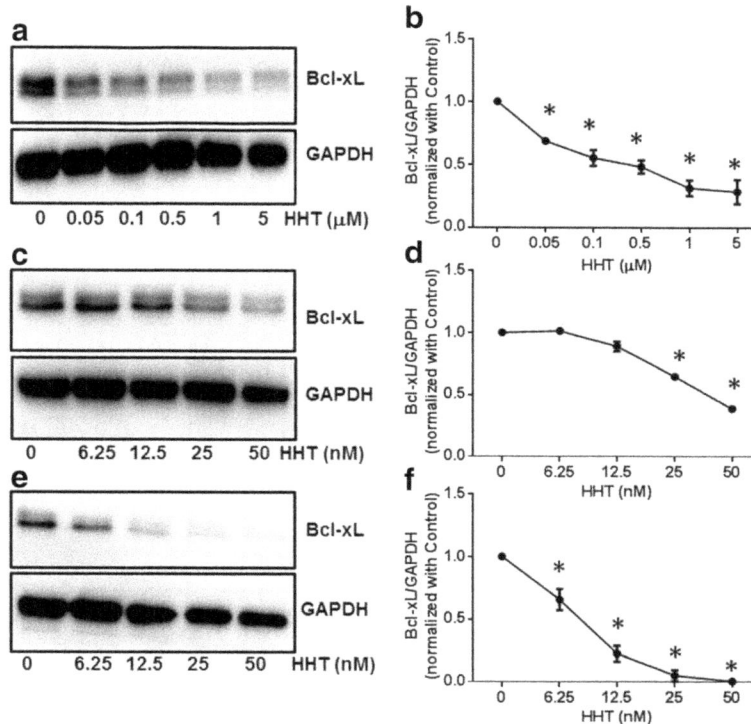

Fig. 4 HHT effects on the protein expression of Bcl-xL in MCF7, A549 and UACC903 cells. MCF7 (**a**), A549 (**c**) and UACC903 (**e**) cells were treated with control or HHT for 24 h. Total cell lystates were isolated and assayed for expression by western blotting using a specific Bcl-xL antibody. Densitometric analysis of the Bcl-xL protein expression in MCF7 (**b**), A549 (**d**), UACC903 (**f**) (*$P < 0.05$ compared to cells treated with control)

treated with HHT, while the apoptotic rate was 6.44% in the untreated cells (Fig. 6e). Overexpression of PP1 also induced apoptosis and sensitized MCF7 cells to apoptosis induced by HHT. Treatment with HHT induced an apoptotic rate of 31.41% in the PP1 overexpressing MCF7 cells (Fig. 6e).

Discussion

Homoharringtonine has been widely used to treat hematopoietic malignant disorders, such as AML and CML [24, 25]. A number of clinical studies have confirmed its clinical therapeutic effect. However, the mechanism underlying the antitumor activities of HHT is still poorly understood. HHT is a potent apoptosis inducer in a variety of leukemia cells. The apoptosis-inducing ability of HHT might account for its main therapeutic potential in the treatment of patients with leukemia. Increasing evidence showed that HHT could induce cell apoptosis through various intrinsic and extrinsic apoptotic pathways, including down-regulation of myeloid cell leukemia-1 (Mcl-1), XIAP and survivin [22, 26], and the activation of caspase-3, caspase-8, caspase-9 and PARP [27, 28]. Several studies have demonstrated that HHT could induce apoptosis via inhibition of protein synthesis and down-regulation of Mcl-1 in chronic lymphocytic

leukemia and myeloid leukemia cells [26, 29, 30]. Meng et al., reported that HHT inhibited AKT phosphorylation and downregulated the expression of several AKT target genes, including NF-κB, XIAP, cIAP and Cyclin D1 in MM cells [31]. Recently, HHT has been shown to induce apoptosis and suppress STAT3 via IL-6/JAK1/STAT3 signal pathway in Gefitinib-resistant lung cancer cells [32]. Moreover, Yin et al. noted that HHT treatment significantly decreased the levels of Bcl-xL and identified Bcl-xL as a dominant anti-apoptotic protein that inhibits HHT-induced apoptosis in leukemia cells [33]. In the present study, we showed that HHT could regulate the alternative splicing of Bcl-x and Caspase 9, resulting in a decrease in the levels of anti-apoptotic Bcl-xL and Caspase 9b mRNA with a concomitant increase in the mRNA levels of pro-apoptotic Bcl-xS and Caspase 9a in several cancer cells. Our study thus identifies a novel mechanism of antitumor action for HHT (Fig. 7).

Phosphatase inhibitors calyculin A and okadaic acid were used to investigate the role of PP1 in HHT-induced alternative splicing. Calyculin A is an inhibitor of both PP1 and PP2A, while okadaic acid selectively inhibits PP2A. Our results showed that calyculin A, but not okadaic acid, significantly inhibits the effects of HHT on the alternative splicing of Bcl-x in MCF7, A549 and UACC903 cells. In MCF7

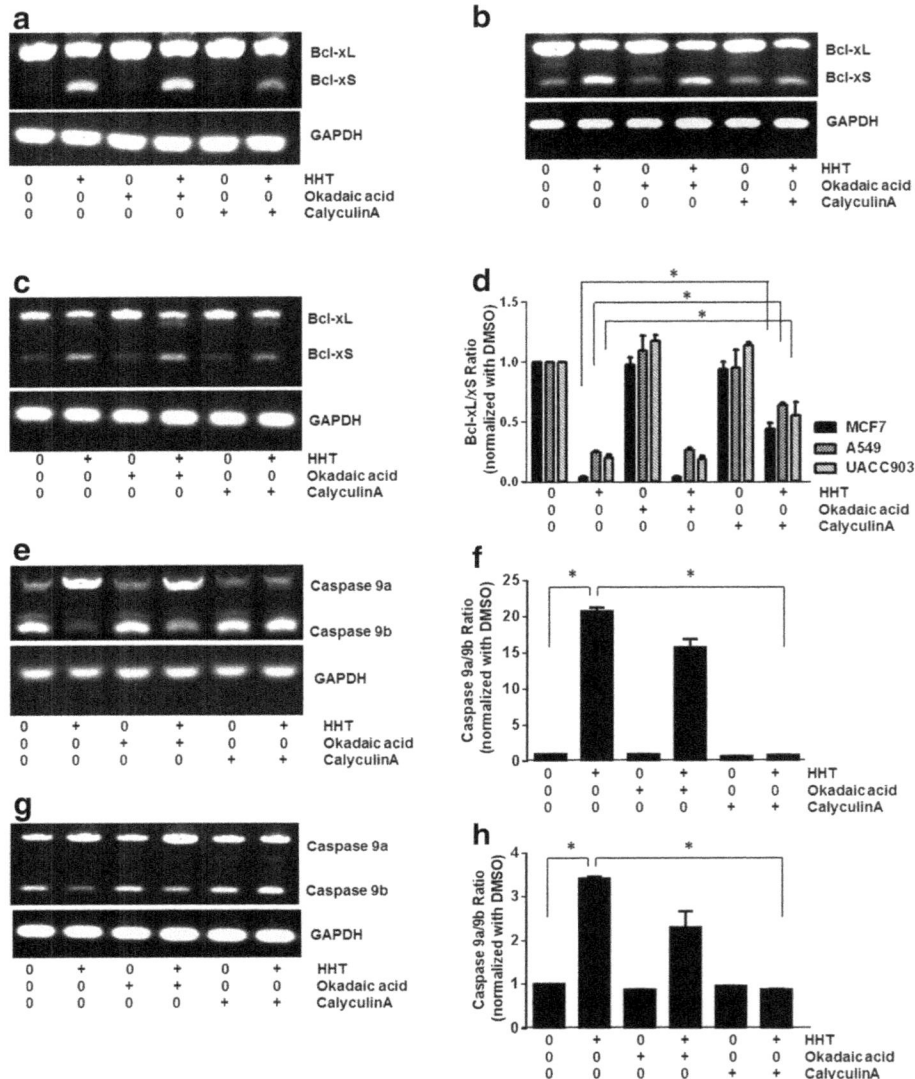

Fig. 5 CalyculinA blocks effects of HHT on Bcl-x and Caspase 9 splicing. Cells were pretreated with either 2 nM calyculin A or with 5 nM okadaic acid, and then exposed to the indicated concentration of HHT for 24 h. Semi-quantitative RT-PCR was performed. **a** Effects of calyculin A on HHT-induced Bcl-x splicing in MCF7 cells. **b** Effects of calyculin A on HHT-induced Bcl-x splicing in A549 cells. **c** Effects of calyculin A on HHT-induced Bcl-x splicing in UACC903 cells. **d** Densitometric analysis of the ratio of Bcl-xL/xS in MCF7, A549 and UACC903 cells (*$P < 0.05$). **e** Effects of calyculin A on HHT-induced Caspase 9 splicing in MCF7 cells. **f** Densitometric analysis of the ratio of Caspase 9a/9b in MCF7 (*$P < 0.05$). **g** Effects of calyculin A on HHT-induced Caspase 9 splicing in UACC903 cells. **h** Densitometric analysis of the ratio of Caspase 9a/9b in UACC903. +, with HHT, okadaic acid or calyculin A; −, without HHT, okadaic acid or calyculin A (*$P < 0.05$)

cells, HHT regulated the alternative splicing of Caspase 9 through a similar mechanism. To investigate the role of PP1 in HHT-mediated alternative splicing, we generated a stable MCF7 cell line overexpressing PP1. Overexpression of PP1 resulted in a decrease in the ratio of Bcl-xL/xS and an increase in the ratio of Caspase 9a/9b. Importantly, the effects of HHT on Bcl-x and Caspase 9 splicing were further enhanced in response to PP1 overexpression. These results indicated that HHT-induced alternative splicing of Bcl-x and Caspase 9 depends on the activation of PP1. Several studies have demonstrated other small molecules,

such as ceramide and emetine, could regulate the alternative splicing of Bcl-x and Caspase 9 through a PP1-mediated splicing mechanism [15–17]. The effects of amiloride on the alternative splicing of both Bcl-x and HIPK3 might partially be mediated by PP1 through the dephosphorylation of SR proteins [18, 19]. Lamond and co-workers showed that dephosphorylation of SR proteins with PP1 induced alternative 5′ splice site selection in vitro [34]. SR proteins belong to a family of arginine–serine-rich domain containing proteins that are required for alternative splicing. The dephosphorylation of SR proteins with PP1 is critical to

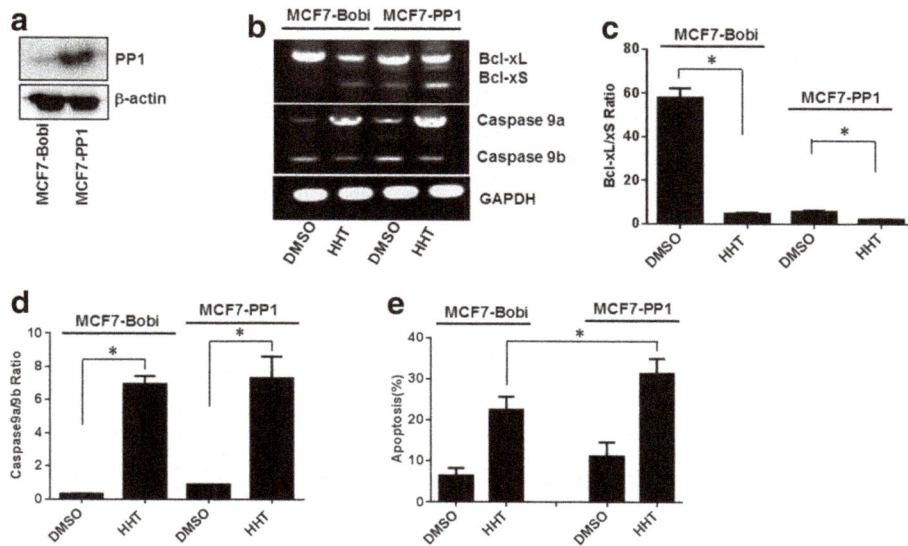

Fig. 6 Overexpression of PP1 increases alternative splicing and promotes tumor cell apoptosis induced by HHT. A stable MCF7 cell line overexpressing PP1 was constructed with a lentiviral expression system. MCF7-Bobi and MCF7-PP1 cells were treated with 0.5 μM HHT. Total RNA was extracted and analyzed by semi-quantitative RT-PCR for the splicing of Bcl-x and Caspase 9. **a** Overexpression of PP1 in MCF7 cells. **b** Semi-quantitative RT-PCR analysis of Bcl-x and Caspase 9 splicing from MCF7-Bobi and MCF7-PP1 cells treated with 0.5 μM HHT. **c** and **d** Ratio of Bcl-xL/xS and Caspase 9a/9b in MCF7-Bobi and MCF7-PP1 cells (*P < 0.05). **e** Apoptosis induced by 5 μM HHT in MCF7-Bobi and MCF7-PP1 cells (*P < 0.05)

the splicing reaction [35, 36]. Future studies are needed to investigate the role of SR proteins in HHT-induced alternative splicing.

Previous studies have demonstrated that ceramide increases the pro-apoptotic Bcl-xS and Caspase 9a isoforms by regulating alternative splicing in A549 cells [15]. Consistent with this finding, emetine regulated alternative splicing of Bcl-x, increasing the pro-apoptotic Bcl-xS isoform and decreasing the anti-apoptotic Bcl-xL isoform [16]. However, emetine had an opposite effect on the alternative splicing of Caspase 9 in different tumor cell lines. In PC3 cells, emetine increased pro-apoptotic Caspase 9a with a concomitant decrease of anti-apoptotic Caspase 9b, while emetine increased anti-apoptotic Caspase 9b with a decrease of the pro-apoptotic Caspase 9a in C33A and MCF-7 cells [17].

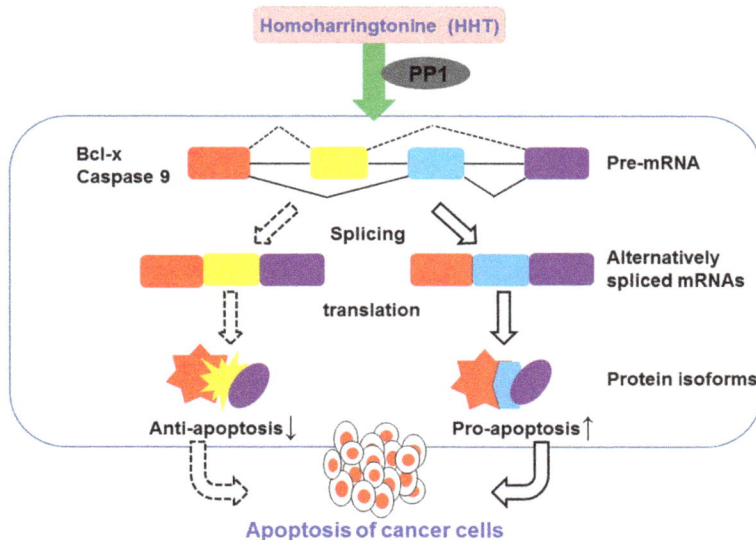

Fig. 7 A novel mechanism underlying the antitumor activities of HHT. Homoharringtonine regulates the alternative splicing of Bcl-x and Caspase 9 through a PP1-dependent mechanism, resulting in a decreased expression of anti-apoptotic Bcl-xL and Caspase 9b with a concomitant increase in the levels of pro-apoptotic Bcl-xS and Caspase 9a in various cancer cells

In this study, HHT exhibited a cell type-specific effect on Caspase 9 splicing. HHT induced a significant increase in the ratio of Caspase 9a/9b in MCF7 and UACC903 cells, but had no effect on Caspase 9 splicing in A549 cells. These results suggest that HHT may mediate the alternative splicing of Bcl-x and Caspase 9 via different mechanisms. In accordance with this hypothesis, PP2A inhibitor okadaic acid partially relieved the effects of HHT on Caspase 9 splicing, but had no effect on Bcl-x splicing in MCF7 and UACC903 cells. It will be very interesting to address whether or not PP2A is involved in the HHT-induced alternative splicing of Caspase 9 in the future.

Conclusions

Homoharringtonine regulates the alternative splicing of Bcl-x and Caspase 9, resulting in a decreased expression of anti-apoptotic Bcl-xL and Caspase 9b with a concomitant increase in the levels of pro-apoptoticBcl-xS and Caspase 9a in various cancer cells. Furthermore, the effect of HHT on alternative splicing is mediated by PP1. This study reveals a novel mechanism underlying the antitumor activities of HHT.

Abbreviations
7-AAD: 7-Aminoactinomycin D; AML: Acute myeloid leukemia; cDNA: Deoxyribonucleic acid; CML: Chronic myeloid leukemia; DMEM: Dulbecco's modified Eagle's media; FBS: Fetal bovine serum; HHT: Homoharringtonine; MM: Multiple myeloma; PP1: Protein phosphatase 1; PP2A: Protein phosphatase 2A; RPMI1640: Roswell Park Memorial Institute 1640; Semi-quantitative RT-PCR: Semi-quantitative reverse transcriptase-polymerase chain reaction

Acknowledgements
The authors would like to thank Carson International Cancer Center, Department of Pharmacology, Shenzhen University Health Science Center for providing the facilities to carry out this study.

Funding
This work was supported by Nature Science Foundation of Guangdong Province (Grant No.2017A030310329), Shenzhen Basic Research Program (Grant No. JCYJ20170302143447936 and JCYJ20170817094611664), National Nature Science Foundation of China (Grant No. 81372342, 31501143 and 81700153), Shenzhen Peacock Innovation Team Project (Grant No. KQTD2014063010658078), Shenzhen Peacock Plan (Grant No.827000186), Shenzhen University Research Project (Grant No. 2016085).

Authors' contributions
DL conceived, designed, and supervised the study; QS, SL, JL, QF, ZW, and BL performed research; QS, SSL, ZS, JS and DL did data analysis and interpretation; QS and DL wrote the paper. All authors have read and approved the final manuscript.

Competing interests
The authors declare that they have no competing interests.

Author details
[1]Guangdong Key Laboratory for Genome Stability & Disease Prevention, Carson International Cancer Center, Department of Pharmacology, Shenzhen University Health Science Center, Shenzhen 518060, Guangdong, China. [2]Key Laboratory of Systems Bioengineering (Ministry of Education), Tianjin University, Tianjin 300072, China.

References
1. Pan Q, Shai O, Lee LJ, Frey BJ, Blencowe BJ. Deep surveying of alternative splicing complexity in the human transcriptome by high-throughput sequencing. Nat Genet. 2008;40(12):1413–5.
2. Black DL. Protein diversity from alternative splicing: a challenge for bioinformatics and post-genome biology. Cell. 2000;103(3):367–70.
3. Keren H, Lev-Maor G, Ast G. Alternative splicing and evolution: diversification, exon definition and function. Nat Rev Genet. 2010;11(5):345–55.
4. Nilsen TW, Graveley BR. Expansion of the eukaryotic proteome by alternative splicing. Nature. 2010;463(7280):457–63.
5. David CJ, Manley JL. Alternative pre-mRNA splicing regulation in cancer: pathways and programs unhinged. Genes Dev. 2010;24(21):2343–64.
6. Chen J, Weiss WA. Alternative splicing in cancer: implications for biology and therapy. Oncogene. 2015;34(1):1–14.
7. Wang BD, Ceniccola K, Hwang S, Andrawis R, Horvath A, Freedman JA, Olender J, Knapp S, Ching T, Garmire L, et al. Alternative splicing promotes tumour aggressiveness and drug resistance in African American prostate cancer. Nat Commun. 2017;8:15921.
8. Pio R, Montuenga LM. Alternative splicing in lung cancer. J Thorac Oncol. 2009;4(6):674–8.
9. Akgul C, Moulding DA, Edwards SW. Alternative splicing of Bcl-2-related genes: functional consequences and potential therapeutic applications. Cell Mol Life Sci. 2004;61(17):2189–99.
10. Wu L, Mao C, Ming X. Modulation of Bcl-x alternative splicing induces apoptosis of human hepatic stellate cells. Biomed Res Int. 2016;2016:7478650.
11. Mercatante DR, Bortner CD, Cidlowski JA, Kole R. Modification of alternative splicing of Bcl-x pre-mRNA in prostate and breast cancer cells. Analysis of apoptosis and cell death. J Biol Chem. 2001;276(19):16411–7.
12. Li P, Nijhawan D, Budihardjo I, Srinivasula SM, Ahmad M, Alnemri ES, Wang X. Cytochrome c and dATP-dependent formation of Apaf-1/caspase-9 complex initiates an apoptotic protease cascade. Cell. 1997; 91(4):479–89.
13. Seol DW, Billiar TR. A caspase-9 variant missing the catalytic site is an endogenous inhibitor of apoptosis. J Biol Chem. 1999;274(4):2072–6.
14. Srinivasula SM, Ahmad M, Guo Y, Zhan Y, Lazebnik Y, Fernandes-Alnemri T, Alnemri ES. Identification of an endogenous dominant-negative short isoform of caspase-9 that can regulate apoptosis. Cancer Res. 1999;59(5):999–1002.
15. Chalfant CE, Rathman K, Pinkerman RL, Wood RE, Obeid LM, Ogretmen B, Hannun YA. De novo ceramide regulates the alternative splicing of caspase 9 and Bcl-x in A549 lung adenocarcinoma cells. Dependence on protein phosphatase-1. J Biol Chem. 2002;277(15):12587–95.
16. Boon-Unge K, Yu Q, Zou T, Zhou A, Govitrapong P, Zhou J. Emetine regulates the alternative splicing of Bcl-x through a protein phosphatase 1-dependent mechanism. Chem Biol. 2007;14(12):1386–92.
17. Pan D, Boon-Unge K, Govitrapong P, Zhou J. Emetine regulates the alternative splicing of caspase 9 in tumor cells. Oncol Lett. 2011;2(6):1309–12.
18. Chang WH, Liu TC, Yang WK, Lee CC, Lin YH, Chen TY, Chang JG. Amiloride modulates alternative splicing in leukemic cells and resensitizes Bcr-AblT315I mutant cells to imatinib. Cancer Res. 2011;71(2):383–92.
19. Chang JG, Yang DM, Chang WH, Chow LP, Chan WL, Lin HH, Huang HD, Chang YS, Hung CH, Yang WK. Small molecule amiloride modulates oncogenic RNA alternative splicing to devitalize human cancer cells. PLoS One. 2011;6(6):e18643.
20. Kantarjian HM, Talpaz M, Santini V, Murgo A, Cheson B, O'Brien SM. Homoharringtonine: history, current research, and future direction. Cancer. 2001;92(6):1591–605.
21. Kantarjian HM, O'Brien S, Cortes J. Homoharringtonine/omacetaxine mepesuccinate: the long and winding road to food and drug administration approval. Clin Lymphoma Myeloma Leuk. 2013;13(5):530–3.
22. Kuroda J, Kamitsuji Y, Kimura S, Ashihara E, Kawata E, Nakagawa Y, Takeuichi M, Murotani Y, Yokota A, Tanaka R, et al. Anti-myeloma effect of homoharringtonine with concomitant targeting of the myeloma-

promoting molecules, Mcl-1, XIAP, and beta-catenin. Int J Hematol. 2008;87(5):507–15.

23. Chen J, Mu Q, Li X, Yin X, Yu M, Jin J, Li C, Zhou Y, Zhou J, Suo S, et al. Homoharringtonine targets Smad3 and TGF-beta pathway to inhibit the proliferation of acute myeloid leukemia cells. Oncotarget. 2017;8(25):40318–26.

24. Lu S, Wang J. Homoharringtonine and omacetaxine for myeloid hematological malignancies. J Hematol Oncol. 2014;7:2.

25. Yu W, Mao L, Qian J, Qian W, Meng H, Mai W, Tong H, Tong Y, Jin J. Homoharringtonine in combination with cytarabine and aclarubicin in the treatment of refractory/relapsed acute myeloid leukemia: a single-center experience. Ann Hematol. 2013;92(8):1091–100.

26. Chen R, Guo L, Chen Y, Jiang Y, Wierda WG, Plunkett W. Homoharringtonine reduced Mcl-1 expression and induced apoptosis in chronic lymphocytic leukemia. Blood. 2011;117(1):156–64.

27. Yinjun L, Jie J, Weilai X, Xiangming T. Homoharringtonine mediates myeloid cell apoptosis via upregulation of pro-apoptotic bax and inducing caspase-3-mediated cleavage of poly(ADP-ribose) polymerase (PARP). Am J Hematol. 2004;76(3):199–204.

28. Lou YJ, Qian WB, Jin J. Homoharringtonine induces apoptosis and growth arrest in human myeloma cells. Leuk Lymphoma. 2007;48(7):1400–6.

29. Novotny L, Al-Tannak NF, Hunakova L. Protein synthesis inhibitors of natural origin for CML therapy: semisynthetic homoharringtonine (Omacetaxine mepesuccinate). Neoplasma. 2016;63(4):495–503.

30. Tang R, Faussat AM, Majdak P, Marzac C, Dubrulle S, Marjanovic Z, Legrand O, Marie JP. Semisynthetic homoharringtonine induces apoptosis via inhibition of protein synthesis and triggers rapid myeloid cell leukemia-1 down-regulation in myeloid leukemia cells. Mol Cancer Ther. 2006;5(3):723–31.

31. Meng H, Yang C, Jin J, Zhou Y, Qian W. Homoharringtonine inhibits the AKT pathway and induces in vitro and in vivo cytotoxicity in human multiple myeloma cells. Leuk Lymphoma. 2008;49(10):1954–62.

32. Cao W, Liu Y, Zhang R, Zhang B, Wang T, Zhu X, Mei L, Chen H, Zhang H, Ming P, et al. Homoharringtonine induces apoptosis and inhibits STAT3 via IL-6/JAK1/STAT3 signal pathway in Gefitinib-resistant lung cancer cells. Sci Rep. 2015;5:8477.

33. Yin S, Wang R, Zhou F, Zhang H, Jing Y. Bcl-xL is a dominant antiapoptotic protein that inhibits homoharringtonine-induced apoptosis in leukemia cells. Mol Pharmacol. 2011;79(6):1072–83.

34. Mermoud JE, Cohen PT, Lamond AI. Regulation of mammalian spliceosome assembly by a protein phosphorylation mechanism. EMBO J. 1994;13(23): 5679–88.

35. Ma CT, Ghosh G, Fu XD, Adams JA. Mechanism of dephosphorylation of the SR protein ASF/SF2 by protein phosphatase 1. J Mol Biol. 2010;403(3):386–404.

36. Chalfant CE, Ogretmen B, Galadari S, Kroesen BJ, Pettus BJ, Hannun YA. FAS activation induces dephosphorylation of SR proteins; dependence on the de novo generation of ceramide and activation of protein phosphatase 1. J Biol Chem. 2001;276(48):44848–55.

15

Weipixiao attenuate early angiogenesis in rats with gastric precancerous lesions

Jinhao Zeng[1], Ran Yan[1], Huafeng Pan[2*], Fengming You[1*] ⓘ, Tiantian Cai[2], Wei Liu[2], Chuan Zheng[1], Ziming Zhao[3], Daoyin Gong[1], Longhui Chen[4] and Yi Zhang[1]

Abstract

Background: Angiogenesis is a pathobiological hallmark of gastric cancer. However, rare studies focus on angiogenesis in gastric precancerous lesions (GPL). Weipixiao (WPX), a Chinese herbal preparation, is proved clinically effective in treating GPL. Here, we evaluated WPX's anti-angiogenic potential for GPL, and also investigated the possibility of its anti-angiogenic mechanisms.

Methods: HPLC analysis was applied to screen the major chemical components of WPX. After modeling N-methyl-N '-nitro-N-nitrosoguanidine (MNNG)-induced GPL in male Sprague-Dawley rats, different doses of WPX were administrated orally for 10 weeks. Next, we performed histopathological examination using routine H&E staining and HID-AB-PAS staining. In parallel, we assessed angiogenesis revealed by microvessel density (MVD) using CD34 immunostaining, and subsequently observe microvessel ultrastructure in gastric mucosa under Transmission Electron Microscope. Finally, we detect expression of angiogenesis-associated markers VEGF and HIF-1α using immunohistochemistry. Moreover, mRNA expressions of ERK1, ERK2, Cylin D1 as well as HIF-1α in gastric mucosa were determined by quantitative real-time reverse transcription- polymerase chain reaction.

Results: We observed the appearance of active angiogenesis in GPL rats, and demonstrated that WPX could reduce microvascular abnormalities and attenuate early angiogenesis in most of GPL specimens with a concomitant regression of most intestinal metaplasia (IM) and a portion of gastric epithelial dysplasia (GED). In parallel, WPX could suppress HIF-1α mRNA expression ($P < 0.01$) as well as protein expression (although without statistical significance), and could markedly inhibit VEGF protein expression in GPL rats. Mechanistically, WPX intervention, especially at low dose, caused a significant decrease in the ERK1 and Cylin D1 mRNA levels. However, WPX might probably have no regulatory effect on ERK2 amplification.

Conclusions: WPX could attenuate early angiogenesis and temper microvascular abnormalities in GPL rats. This might be partly achieved by inhibiting on the angiogenesis-associated markers HIF-1α and VEGF, and on the ERK1/Cylin D1 aberrant activation.

Keywords: Gastric precancerous lesions, ERK signaling, VEGF, HIF-1α, Herbal medicine, Weipixiao

Background

Gastric precancerous lesions (GPL) are generally defined as intestinal metaplasia (IM) and gastric epithelial dysplasia (GED). A direct link has been sought between gastric cancer and high prevalence of GPL worldwide [1–3], especially in Asia. Thus, blocking of gastric precancerosis toward malignant transformation is crucial to reducing the gastric cancer incidence. Nowadays, endoscopic mucosal resection is clinically applied only to severe GED and definite intramucosal carcinoma, yet most cases of GPL are not amenable to the endoscopic resection [4]. Moreover, vitacoenzyme tablet, a chemopreventive agent used in China, has been reported to be beneficial in treating atrophic gastritis and metaplasia lesion [5, 6]. Its therapeutic effect against GPL, however, was not completely confirmed. Therefore, the pursuit to discover alternative therapies to treat GPL is of high concern. In China, early

* Correspondence: gzphf@gzucm.edu.cn; yfmdoc@163.com
[2]Guangzhou University of Chinese Medicine, Guangzhou 510405, China
[1]Chengdu University of Traditional Chinese Medicine, Chengdu 610075, China
Full list of author information is available at the end of the article

herbal intervention has proved to be effective in halting and even reversing the majority of GPL [7, 8].

Angiogenesis, the sprouting of new capillaries from pre-existing vessels, is a fundamental process accelerating gastric cancer progression. Considerable evidence has demonstrated that excessive angiogenesis is significantly correlated with enhanced migratory and invasive activity, and therefore with poor prognosis [9–11]. Hence, targeting angiogenesis has been a central focus in gastric cancer treatment [12]. Angiogenesis is generally resulted from hypoxia orchestrated by multiple transcriptional activators, aiming at restoring intratumoral O_2 delivery to hypoxic regions, thereby sustaining tumor growth [13]. Hypoxia inducible factor-1α (HIF-1α) has been proved to be a key regulator of cellular adaptation to hypoxia involved in angiogenesis process, and the process is frequently accompanied by a concomitant aberrant activation of vascular endothelial growth factor (VEGF) [14], which is essential for vascular development and can induce proliferation, differentiation and apoptosis of endothelial cells. Extracellular signal-regulated kinase (ERK), which may serve as specific effectors of VEGF signaling, play a vital role in sprouting endothelial cells during vascular development [15]. Aberrant activation of ERK signaling is closely linked to the carcinogenesis and development of gastric cancer [16]. ERK1 has been reported to overexpressed in 52.98% (231/436) cases of human gastric tumor, and high level of ERK1 protein expression was significantly correlated with age, tumor location, depth of invasion, Lauren's classification, lymph node metastasis and tumor node metastasis (TNM) stage [17]. ERK2 is similarly important for predicting the prognosis of gastric cancer. The positive occurrence of ERK2 mRNA expression is 64.0% (32/50) in tumor tissues from patients with gastric cancer, which is markedly higher than that in non-cancerous tissues showing 18.0% (9/50) [18]. Furthermore, ERK2 expression level is significantly increased from TNM stage II to stage IV, suggesting a closely relationship between elevated ERK2 level and tumor invasion and TNM stage [18]. Cyclin D1 is involved in G1-S point of cell cycle, and thus induces cell proliferation and migration coexisted with angiogenesis. Cyclin D1 is frequently overexpressed in a substantial proportion of gastric cancer, and its expression may be governed by the ERK signaling [19, 20]. Although studies reported in recent years have addressed the pro-angiogenic role of the molecules in gastric cancer, it is unclear what role the molecules may play in gastric precancerosis.

Weipixiao (WPX) is a Chinese herbal prescription consisting of six herbs including *Astragalus Membranaceus, Pseudostellaria Heterophylla, Atractylodis Macrocephalae, Curcuma zedoaria, Salvia Miltiorrhiza* and *Hedyotis Diffusa Willd*. WPX prescription has been widely used in clinical for more than 15 years, and it shows satisfactory effects against "non-progressive GPL". In previous clinical trials, different teams demonstrated that WPX possesses excellent abilities at relieving the clinical symptoms, reducing the precursor lesions (through gastroscopic and pathohistological examination), as well as partially eradicating *Helicobacter pylori* in GPL patients, and shows no toxic or side effects [21–23]. Experimentally, some WPX individuals exhibited potential anti-angiogenesis activities in several solid tumors. Extracts from *Astragalus membranaceus*, a "Yi Qi Hua Yu" herb (function to tonify qi and activate blood) belonging to WPX, could reduce angiogenesis-related molecules vascular endothelial growth factor and cyclooxygenase-2 in ovarian tumor-bearing mice [24]. Another active compound of *Astragalus membranaceus*, named formononetin, has been reported to repress hypoxia-induced retinal angiogenesis via the HIF-1α/VEGF signaling pathway [25]. Essential oil from another member *Curcuma zedoaria*, a widely used "Hua Yu Tong Luo" herb (function to dissipate blood stasis and free the collateral vessels), presented the anti-angiogenic activity, which therefore contributed to suppressing melanoma growth and lung metastasis [26]. A recent study suggested that Danshensu, a major water-soluble compound from *Salvia miltiorrhiza*, could improve microcirculation and remodel tumor vasculature, thereby enhancing the radioresponse for Lewis lung carcinoma xenografts in mice [27]. The aforementioned researchers revealed the anti-angiogenesis properties of several herbs from WPX. However, the anti-angiogenic potential of WPX in GPL treating, and the possibility of its anti-angiogenic mechanisms still remain unclear.

In this study, we tested whether early angiogenesis existed in N-methyl-N′-nitro-N-nitrosoguanidine (MNNG)-induced GPL rats. Also, we determined whether WPX had the ability against hyper- angiogenesis. In parallel, we screened potential anti-GPL constituents of WPX. More importantly, the hypothesis we wished to test was that the anti-angiogenesis property of WPX was associated with its regulatory effects on the angiogenesis-associated markers HIF-1α and VEGF, and on the ERK/Cylin D1 signal transduction pathway.

Methods
Animals
Male Sprague-Dawley rats weighting 150–170 g were obtained from Experimental Animal Center of Sun Yat-sen University (certificate No. 0111909). Animals were housed in a specific pathogen-free animal room, kept under optimal condition at 23 ± 1 °C and 40–60% humidity with a 12 h light-dark cycle, and fed with standard rat chow. All procedures relating to animal care and the animal research protocols conformed to the guidelines for the Care and Use of Laboratory Animal, issued by the Ministry of Science and Technology of China. This experiment was conducted in Guangdong

Provincial Institute of Traditional Chinese Medicine, and was presented to the institutional ethical review board for approval (Ethic No. GDPITCM111018).

Drugs and reagents

WPX comprises the following components: Huangqi (*Astragalus Membranaceus*)30 g, Taizishen (*Pseudostellaria Heterophylla*)15 g, Baishu (*Atractylodis Macrocephalae*)15 g, Eshu (*Curcuma zedoaria*)10 g, Danshen (*Salvia Miltiorrhiza*)10 g and Baihuasheshecao (*Hedyotis Diffusa Willd*)30 g. The herbs were provided and authenticated by the First Affiliated Hosipital of Guangzhou University of Chinese Medicine. The medical herbs were boiled with distilled water, and concentrated into a mixture containing crude drugs 1.5 g/mL. MNNG was supplied by Tokyo Kabushiki Kaisha, Japan (No. ZG4T1-FP). CD34 antibody was abtained from R&D Systems, USA (lot ZDP0112111); VEGF antibody was supplied by Abcam, UK (lot GR-116031-1); HIF-1α antibody was purchased from Santa Cruz Biotechnology, USA (lot L1212). Maxima™ SYBR Green/Fluorescein qPCR Master Mix (2X) was supplied by Fermentas, USA.

High performance liquid chromatography (HPLC) analysis

HPLC analysis was performed to screen the potential chemical constituents of WPX preparation. Condition optimization of fingerprint: JADE-PAK ODS-AQ column (250 × 4.6 mm, 5 μm) and Inertsil ODS-SP column (4.6 × 150 mm, 5 μm) were utilized, with acetonitrile 0.1% phosphoric acid solution and acetonitrile 0.4% phosphoric acid solution as the mobile phase respectively, under full wavelength detection. The following chromatographic analysis conditions were determined: the separation was determined on Inertsil ODS-SP column (4.6 × 150 mm, 5 μm) with a mobile phase of acetonitrile (solvent A) 0.4% phosphoric acid solution (solvent B). For HPLC analysis, a 10 μL sample was injected into the column and eluted at a flow rate of 1.0 ml/min under room temperature. The detective wavelength was 203 nm.

Grouping, modeling and treatment

SD rats were randomly divided into six experimental groups: control group ($n = 9$), model group ($n = 11$), model + vitacoenzyme group (VIT, $n = 9$, 0.2 g/kg/d), model + high-dose WPX group (H-WPX, $n = 9$, 15 g/kg/d), model + medium-dose WPX group (M-WPX, $n = 9$, 7.5 g/kg/d), and model + low-dose WPX group (L-WPX, $n = 9$, 3.75 g/kg/d). Based on the literatures [8, 28, 29], the GPL rat model was set up with minor modifications. Briefly, All the rats, except for control rats, were allowed to drink MNNG solution (200 μg·ml^{-1}) ad libitum, and underwent hunger-satiety shift every other day. At the end of 15th week, 2 random rats in the model group were humanely terminated with sodium pentobarbital

(140 mg/kg i.p.) and examined for IM/GED. At the beginning of 16th week, the treated rats were administered WPX or VIT by gastrogavage for 10 consecutive weeks, while the control and the model rats were given 2 mL distilled water by gastrogavage once daily.

Pathological examination

Animals were humanely euthanized with sodium pentobarbital (140 mg/kg i.p.) after 12 h fasting, and the stomachs were removed immediately, incised along the greater curvature, and fixed in 10% neutralized formalin solution. Then, each sample was embedded in paraffin wax and serially sectioned at 3 μm thick. The sections were stained with hematoxylin and eosin (H-E staining), and with high-iron diamine-alcian blue-periodic acid Schiff (HID-AB-PAS staining). Gastric tissues were examined macroscopically to identify IM and GED lesions in rats.

Evaluation of microvessel density

To evaluate microvessel density (MVD) in gastric mucosa, CD34 expression was determined using EnVision immunohistochemistry. Quantification of MVD was specified by Weidner et al. [30]. Briefly, area of highest angiogenesis (also called hot-spot) were identified under low-power magnification (40× and 100×), and stained microvessels in three random views of the 'hot-spot' area were counted under high-power magnification (200×). The mean value of the three 200× field counts was recorded as MVD for each case. Any brown staining endothelial cell or cell cluster that was clearly separated from adjacent microvessels or other connective tissue was considered a single countable microvessel.

Microvessel ultrastructure

The gastric mucosa tissue were sliced into 1 mm^3 pieces and fixed with 2.5% glutaraldehyde in phosphate buffer for 2.5 h, and then re-fixed in 1% osmium tetroxide in phosphate buffer for 2 h. The tissues were dehydrated in a graded series of ethanol solutions and then immersion in a mixture of acetone and epoxy resin twice (2:1 for 3 h in the first time, 1:2 for overnight in the second time). Finally, the tissues were embedded in epoxy resin-filled capsules and heated at 70 °C overnight, ultrathin sections (60–80 nm) were sliced with LKB microtome. The sections were viewed and photographed under a transmission electron microscope (JEOL 100C, JEOL, Tokyo, Japan).

Levels of ERK1, ERK2, Cyclin D1 and HIF-1α by RT-qPCR

The mRNA levels of ERK1, ERK2, Cyclin D1 and HIF-1α were determined by quantitative real-time reverse transcription-polymerase chain reaction (RT-qPCR) method using Maxima™ SYBR Green/Fluorescein qPCR Master Mix

(Fermentas, USA) via IQ™5 real-time PCR detection system (Bio-Rad, USA). The PCR primers used were as follows: ERK1 (GenBank accession no. NM_011952; 104 bp) forward, 5′-CGGATTGCTGACCCT-3′ and reverse 5′-GTGTAGCC CTTGGAGTT-3′; ERK2 (GenBank accession no. NM_053842; 113 bp) forward, 5′-CAACCTCCTGCTGAA C-3′ and reverse 5′-GCGTGGCTACATACTC-3′; Cyclin D1 (GenBank accession no. NM_171992; 191 bp) forward, 5′-GCAGAAGTGCGAAGAGG-3′ and reverse 5′-GGCG GATAGAGTTGTCAGT-3′; HIF-1α (GenBank accession no. NM_024359; 132 bp) forward, 5′-CAACTGCCACCAC TGATG-3′ and reverse 5′-CACTGTATGCTGATGCCTT AG-3′; 18S (GenBank accession no. M11188; 204 bp) forward, 5′-TCAGCCACCCGAGATT-3′ and reverse 5′-GCT TATGACCCGCACTTA-3′. The level of 18 s mRNA transcript was used to normalize all reported gene expression levels, and the data were analyzed using $2^{-\triangle\triangle Ct}$ method.

Expression of VEGF and HIF-1α by immunohistochemistry

Formalinfixed and paraffin-embedded gastric tissues were cut at 3 μm thick. The EnVision immunohistochemical technology was utilized, VEGF protein immunoreactivity was shown as brown color in the cytosolic and perinuclear regions of gastric epithelial cells. HIF-1α positive staining was brown or brown yellow and was detected predominantly in the cytoplasm and nucleus. To access the protein expression levels of VEGF and HIF-1α, three visual fields were randomly selected from each slice under light microscope (100×), and then images were acquired and analyzed by Image Pro Plus 6.0 software. Quantification of VEGF and HIF-1α levels was determined using mean of integrated optical density (IOD).

Statistical analysis

Data were presented as mean ± standard deviation (SD). Statistical analysis was performed using IBM SPSS 19.0 software (SPSS, Chicago, IL). One-way analysis of variance (ANOVA) was applied to analyze the comparisons among multiple groups. The comparison between two groups was performed with SNK method for the homogeneous variances, while the variances were heterogeneous, Dunnett's T3 method should be adopted. A P value of less than 0.05 was considered as significant.

Results

HPLC profile

WPX possessed an excellent ability against GPL revealed by our previous clinical trials and animal testing, so we are curious about the major constituents of WPX polyherbal mixture. Figure 1 shows the HPLC chromatograms of WPX test sample (A) and reference sample (B). The retention times of the major chemical constituents were 20.5 min (Calycosin-7- glucoside), 34.8 min (ginsenoside-Rg1), 48.3 min (ginsenoside-Rb1), 49.5 min

(astragaloside IV), 59.0 min (atractylenolide III), 71.7 min (atractylenolide II), and 81.7 min (atractylenolide I) (Fig. 1).

WPX efficiently blocked and even reversed gastric intestinal metaplasia

We evaluated the degree of IM lesion in gastric tissues by HID-AB-PAS staining. As depicted in Fig. 2, neutral mucins present in normal mucosa were stained red, gastric specimens from controls didn't exhibit IM lesion. In model rats, sialomucins expressed only in small intestinal-type metaplasia (S-IM) were stained blue, and sulfomucins present in colonic-type metaplasia (C-IM) were stained brown, indicating that both S-IM and C-IM were widespread. In treated rats, IM lesion was regressed slightly in VIT-treated rats. Comparatively, IM lesion was regressed visibly in WPX-treated rats. Our observation revealed that WPX has a potent anti-IM capacity in GPL rats (Fig. 2).

WPX partly ameliorated gastric epithelial dysplasia

To further investigate the anti-GPL effect of WPX, we also examined the GED lesion in H&E stained sections of gastric tissues. Histologically, the control gland and cell structure of gastric epithelium remained intact. By contrast, almost all model rats displayed GED pathology. In detail, gastric epithelium was characterized by architectural abnormalities showing splitting, elongated, crowded glands and back-to-back tubular structure, and also by cytological atypia with hyperchromatic nuclei, increased nuclear-cytoplasmic ratio, loss of nuclear polarity and occasional binucleation. Inflammatory infiltration was variable, and sometimes extensive. Occasionally, two model rats exhibited mild dysplasia, due to the multifocal nature of the dysplastic lesion. In most cases of WPX-treated rats, GED lesion alterations, especially tubular structure irregularities and inflammatory infiltration, were regressed in varying degrees. However, the treatment was not able to restore the GED pathology near to the normal tissues. In contrast, this GED-rescuing effect was not presented in most VIT-treated rats. These observations suggested that WPX could partly halt and even reverse dysplastic process, especially the "non-progressive GED" (Fig. 3).

WPX reduced the CD34+ MVD level in GPL tissues

In order to identify whether early angiogenesis occur in GPL, we examined the angiogenic state in gastric tissues using CD34-labelled sections. As visualized by light microscopy, an increased number of CD34+ microvessels, which were suggestive of active angiogenesis, could be found in most cases of GPL tissues, whereas those in control tissues were minimal. Moreover, we found more GEDs with a higher number of microvessels than IMs, and more severe GEDs than mild or moderate GEDs.

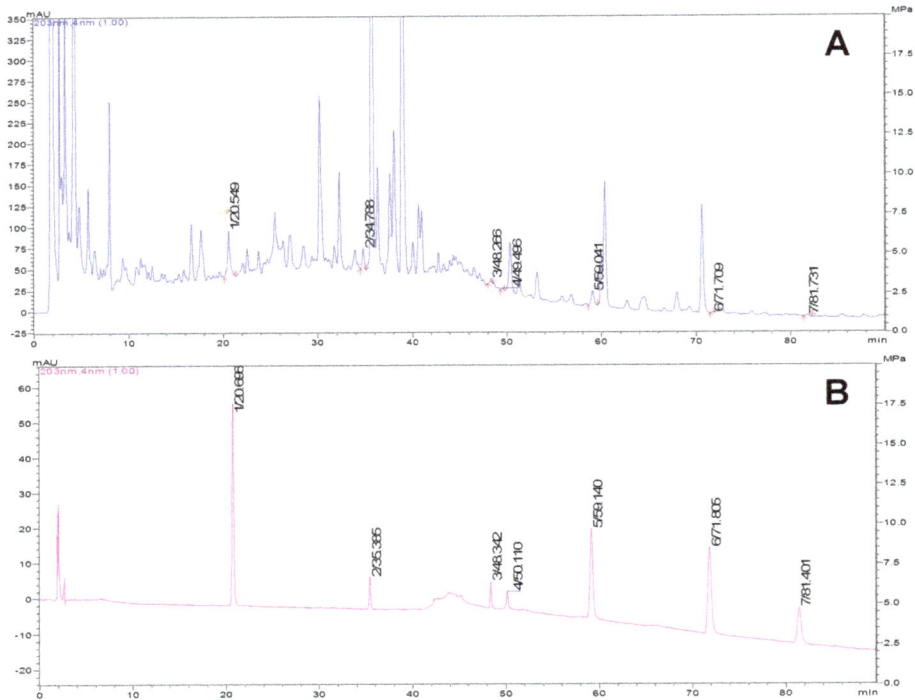

Fig. 1 HPLC chromatogram of WPX test sample (**a**) and reference sample (**b**). Notes: Peak: 1, Calycosin-7-glucoside; 2, ginsenoside-Rg1; 3, ginsenoside-Rb1; 4, astragaloside IV; 5–7, atractylenolide III, II, and I, respectively

Occasionally, CD34+ microvessels were apparently abundant and distributed diffusely in two model rats all diagnosed with severe GED. By contrast, we observed a clear decreased CD34+ microvessel count in many cases of WPX-treated rats. Our data showed a statistic significant increase of CD34+ MVD level in model rats comparing to controls. But it dropped by at least half after WPX intervention, when in comparison to the non-treatment rats. Thus, WPX could effectively inhibit active angiogenesis in GPL rats (Fig. 4).

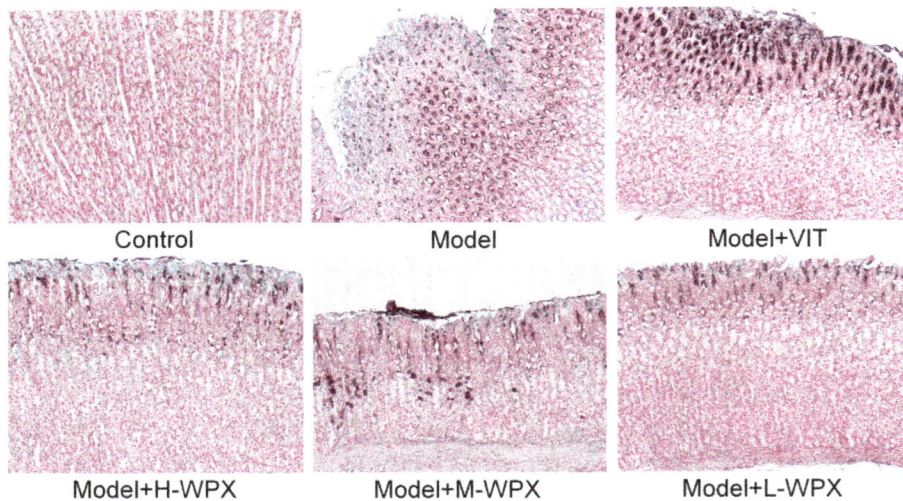

Fig. 2 Histological evaluation of gastric intestinal metaplasia. Neutral mucins present in normal mucosa were stained red. Sialomucins expressed only in small intestinal-type metaplasia (S-IM) were stained blue, and sulfomucins present in colonic-type metaplasia (C-IM) were stained brown. Images of model gastric epithelium depicted prominent S-IM and C-IM lesions, which were dramatically reduced after WPX administration. $n = 9$ in each group. (HID-AB-PAS staining, 100×)

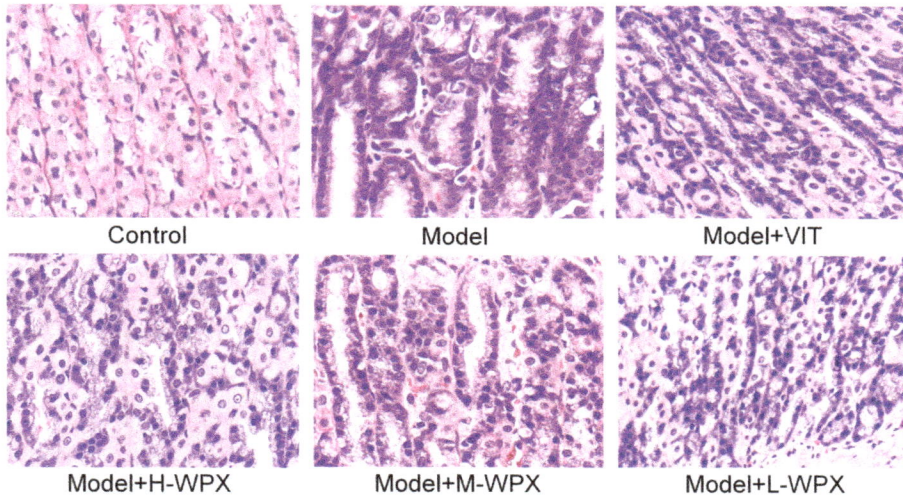

Fig. 3 Histological evaluation of gastric epithelial dysplasia. Model gastric epithelium displayed GED pathology characterized by glandular architectural abnormalities such as splitting, elongated and crowded glands, back to back formation, as well as by cytological atypia with rounded, pleomorphic nuclei that display prominent nucleoli and loss of polarity. After WPX intervention, these GED pathological alterations, especially irregularities of glandular structure, were regressed in varying degrees. $n = 9$ in each group. (H&E staining, 100×)

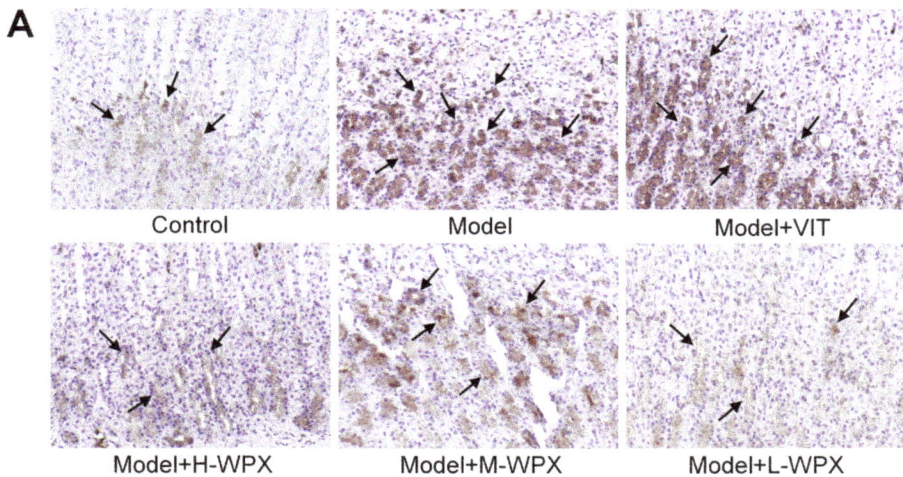

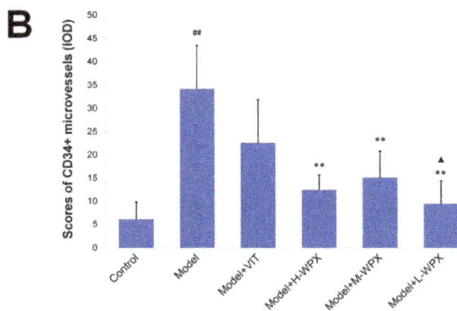

Fig. 4 Evaluation of CD34-labelled microvessel density in gastric mucosa. **a** CD34-labelled microvessels in gastric mucosa from various groups. Some representative microvessels are indicated by black arrows. **b** Scores of CD34+ MVD levels. The results are expressed as mean ± SD ($n = 9$ in each group). Note: [##]$P < 0.01$, vs Control; [**]$P < 0.01$, vs Model; [▲]$P < 0.05$, vs VIT. (IHC, 200×)

WPX tempered microvascular abnormalities in GPL tissues

We further examined the morphological changes of microvessels in gastric mucosa under transmission electron microscope. In control rats, microvessels were clearly demarcated from the surrounding connective tissues. The microvessels appeared a normal vascular inner diameter, smooth basal lamina with uniform thickness, and also showed a complete and clear structure of basal lamina with homogeneous electron-density. Endothelial cell bordering the basal lamina was morphologically flat or elongated, with smooth and clear nuclear membrane and normal chromatin distribution.

In model rats, intervascular boundaries were ill-defined or invisible. Remodeled microvessels showed dilated vascular lumen but with a markedly decreased inner diameter, accompanied with clearly thickened, rough basal lamina which was often coated by abundant high-density granules aggregation. Some vascular lumens were partly or completely occluded by erythrocytes and neutrophils. Apart from these, features such as segmental breakup of basal lumina and increased vascular permeability also existed. Furthermore, endothelial cells displayed severe swelling and were shaped like grapes,

with debased cytoplasm electron-density, nucleus chromatin condensation, as well as abundant pinocytotic vesicles. Abnormalitiesof vascular lumen, basal lamina and endothelial cell were still prominent in VIT-treated rats.

In WPX-treated rats, vascular lumen showed a mild-moderate decrease in inner diameter. Basal lamina coated by some high-density granule aggregation was still a little rough, and also with occasional breakup. Endothelial cells exhibited slight swelling and mild vacuolisation. Most of the nuclear membrane became clear and complete, and nucleus chromatin distribution also became normalized. Accordingly, WPX intervention could normalize ultrastructural alterations of vascular lumen, basal lamina and endothelial cell, thus showing the potent rescuing effect of WPX on microvascular abnormalities in GPL rats (Fig. 5).

Effect of WPX on HIF-1α mRNA levels

HIF-1α plays an important role in hypoxic responses and induces the transcription of various genes responsible for tumor angiogenesis, invasion and metastasis. Thus, we texted whether WPX possessed a regulatory ability on hypoxic responses in GPL rats through classic HIF-1α marker detection. Figure 6 clearly showed that

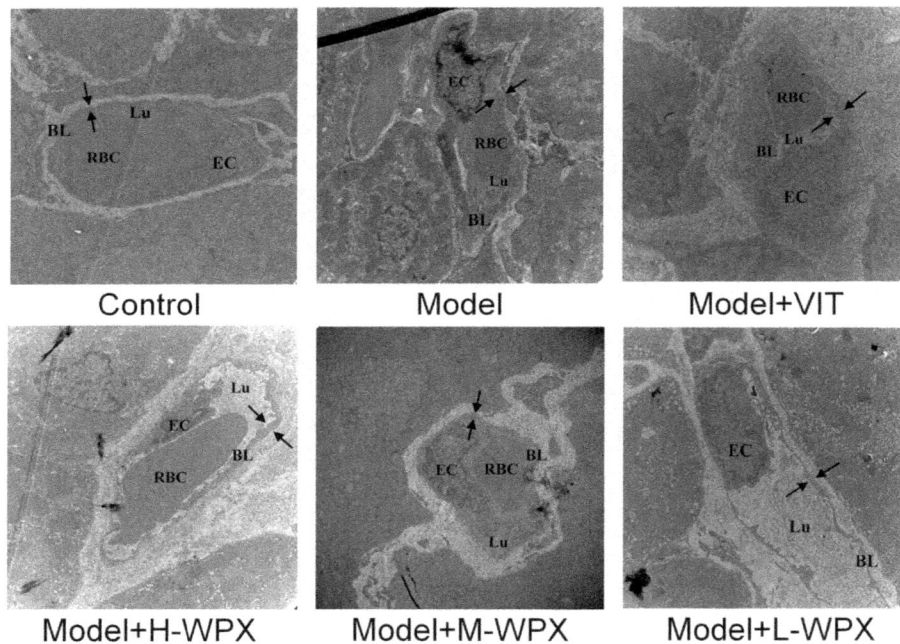

Fig. 5 Representative electron micrographs of microvessels in gastric mucosa. **Control group**: TEM observation of control microvessel ultrastructures appeared intact, in terms of vascular lumen, basal lamina and endothelial cell. **Model group**: Microvessels lost their typical structures. Vascular lumen, frequently plugged by erythrocytes, was dilated but with a markedly decreased inner diameter. Clearly thickened, rough basal lamina was coated by abundant high-density granules aggregation. Segmental breakup of basal lumina and increased vascular permeability were also existed. Endothelial cells were conglobated and shaped as grapes, characterized by debased cytoplasm electron-density, nucleus chromatin condensation, as well as numerous pinocytotic vesicles. **Treatment group**: Microvascular abnormalities were still prominent in VIT-treated tissues. However, the abnormalities reversed markedly in WPX-treated tissues, especially in terms of vascular lumen and basal lamina. Even in a few cases, the microvessels were detected to ultrastructurally resemble the normal ones. Note: Opposing arrows mark the thickness of basal lamina; EC, endothelial cell; BL, basal lamina; Lu, lumen; RBC, red blood cell. $n = 9$ in each group. (10000×)

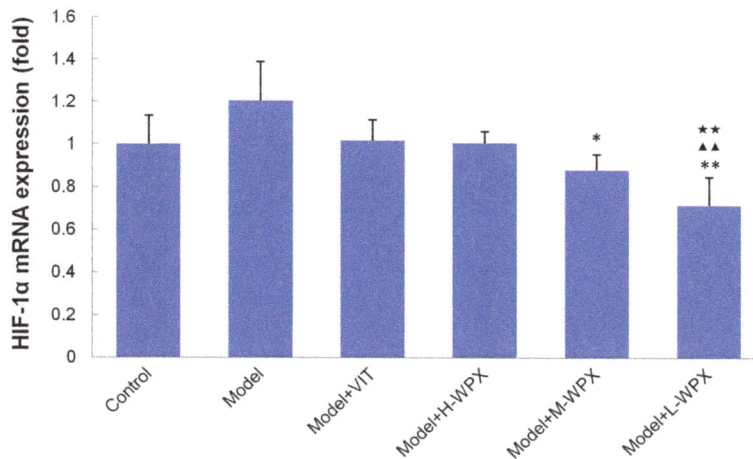

Fig. 6 Effect of WPX on HIF-1α mRNA levels in gastric epithelial cells. The results are expressed as mean ± SD ($n = 9$ in each group). Note: $^{**}P < 0.01$, $^{*}P < 0.05$, vs Model; ▲▲$P < 0.01$, vs VIT; ★★$P < 0.01$, vs H-WPX

HIF-1α mRNA level was elevated in GPL rats when compared with those of controls (although without statistical significance). Compared with model rats, HIF-1α mRNA levels in rats were significantly diminished by medium and low doses of WPX. By comparison, treatment with low dose of WPX led to a marked reduction in HIF-1α mRNA level. The data suggest that WPX, especially at low dose, could efficiently inhibit HIF-1α mRNA expression in GPL rats (Fig. 6).

Effect of WPX on HIF-1α protein expressions

We subsequently applied immunohistochemistry to visualize activation of presumptive HIF-1α marker in gastric mucosa. By immunostaining, HIF-1α was sparsely expressed in normal gastric mucosa, whereas HIF-1α positive cells were found relatively abundant in most GPL tissues. Moreover, we found that WPX could visually reduce the number of HIF-1α positive cells in majority of GPL tissues, as shown in Fig. 7a. Semiquantitatively, elevated HIF-1α protein expression was observed in GPL mucosa as compared to normal mucosa. After WPX intervention, we found a clearly downtrend, although without statistical significance, of HIF-1α levels in gastric mucosa. Our results indicated that WPX treatment may produce regulatory effects on hypoxic responses in GPL gastric mucosa (Fig. 7).

Effect of WPX on VEGF protein expressions

VEGF is generally considered as a vital driving force behind the angiogenesis process, thus we next tested whether VEGF inhibition was of relevance for WPX's anti-angiogenic capacity. As shown in Fig. 8a, normal gastric mucosa did not or barely express VEGF marker, while diffuse and intense cytoplasmic labeling, found in most cases of GPL rats, could be markedly diminished by WPX. Statistically, GPL rats displayed an increased

VEGF protein expression compared with negative controls, whereas WPX treatment reduced the over-expression. In addition, we observed a stronger inhibition effect of L-WPX on VEGF over-expression than that of VIT treatment. Intriguingly, we found HIF-1α and VEGF reduction was frequently along with the attenuation of CD34+ angiogenesis in GPL tissues, indicating that HIF-1α and VEGF inhibition may play a beneficial role in WPX-alleviated angiogenesis (Fig. 8).

Effect of WPX on ERK1, ERK2 and Cyclin D1 mRNA levels

To identify the possible mechanism underlying the anti-angiogenesis activity of WPX on GPL rats, we examined the key targets ERK1, ERK2 and Cyclin D1, which are closely related to the HIF-1α and EVGF signals. As described above, ERK is a specific effector of VEGF signaling and plays a pro-angiogenic role in sprouting [12], thereby instrumental in the progression of gastric cancer. As shown in Fig. 9, we found the gastric precancerous tissues with dramatically elevated ERK1 mRNA levels, which could be reversed by varying concentrations of WPXs. In addition, low dose WPX was found to be markedly superior to VIT in reducing mucosal ERK1 levels. We also noted an elevated ERK2 mRNA levels in GPL tissues, when in comparison to normal gastric tissues. However, in most cases of WPX-treated rats, upregulated ERK2 mRNA levels remained.

We then analyzed mRNA levels of Cyclin D1, a downstream molecule related to ERK signals. Real-time PCR results revealed that GPL rats exhibited notably elevated Cyclin D1 levels compared with the controls. Importantly, WPX treatment caused a marked drop of Cyclin D1 levels in GPL tissues. Similar to ERK1, the inhibitory activity on Cyclin D1 by WPX was more distinct at low dose. Taken together, our findings implicated that the

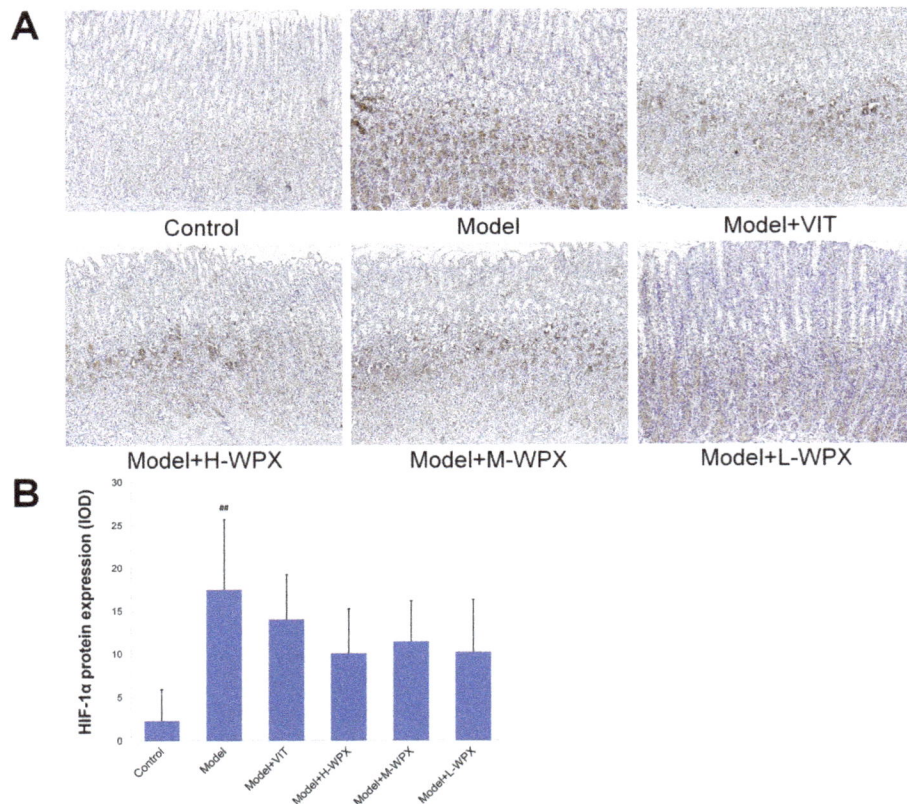

Fig. 7 Effect of WPX on HIF-1α protein expressions in gastric epithelium. **a** HIF-1α protein expressions in gastric epithelium from different groups. **b** IOD scores of HIF-1α protein levels. The results are expressed as mean ± SD ($n = 9$ in each group). Note: [##]$P < 0.01$, vs Control. (IHC, 100×)

anti-angiogenesis effect of WPX was achieved partly by suppressing ERK1 and Cyclin D1 activation, and its inhibitory effect was identified to be more potent than that of VIT. However, WPX may have little effect on ERK2 amplification (Fig. 9).

Discussion

It is well established that gastric carcinogenesis is a complex and multifactorial process, in which accumulation of multiple genetic changes may be implicated. The recognized human model [31] of gastric carcinogenesis comprises the following precancerous steps: superficial gastritis → multifocal atrophic gastritis → intestinal metaplasia → dysplasia. Based on differences in the magnitude of the malignant risk, GPL could be categorized into (1) "non-progressive GPL" (mainly contains S-IM, mild and moderate dysplasia), remaining a comparatively stable status and with a reduced risk of evolving into gastric carcinoma [32, 33], and (2) "progressive GPL" (comprises some cases of C-IM and severe dysplasia), which is more ominous due to a relatively high risk of malignant transformation and requires advisably interval endoscopic and histologic controls [34, 35]. The vast majority of GPL represents a stage within a

prolonged process and remains stable, thereby providing an opportunity to block and even reverse the precursors. WPX is a typical Chinese herbal prescription proved clinically effective in treating GPL.

In this project, almost all model rats exhibited GPL pathology, which ranged from moderate IM to severe GED lesion. After WPX administration, IM lesion (including S-IM and C-IM) were markedly regressed in most cases of GPL rats. We also found that WPX could halt and even reverse the majority of mild and moderate dysplasia. However, 4 WPX-treated rats (two M-WPX rats, one H-WPX rat, one L-WPX rat) displayed moderate or severe GED pathology, suggesting that a refractory state to WPX administration might have developed in a certain percentage of "progressive GPL". Our observations reinforce the view that a few advanced GED and early gastric cancer are partly similar, in terms of cell proliferative activity and cell atypia. Thus, some cases of "progressive GPL" might be difficult to block and reverse.

Microvasculature serves to circulate and transport oxygen and nutrients, which is imperative to various tissues including gastric mucosa. In contrast to the normal microvasculature, cancer-related angiogenesis, which is continually activated and unregulated [36], is a fundamental

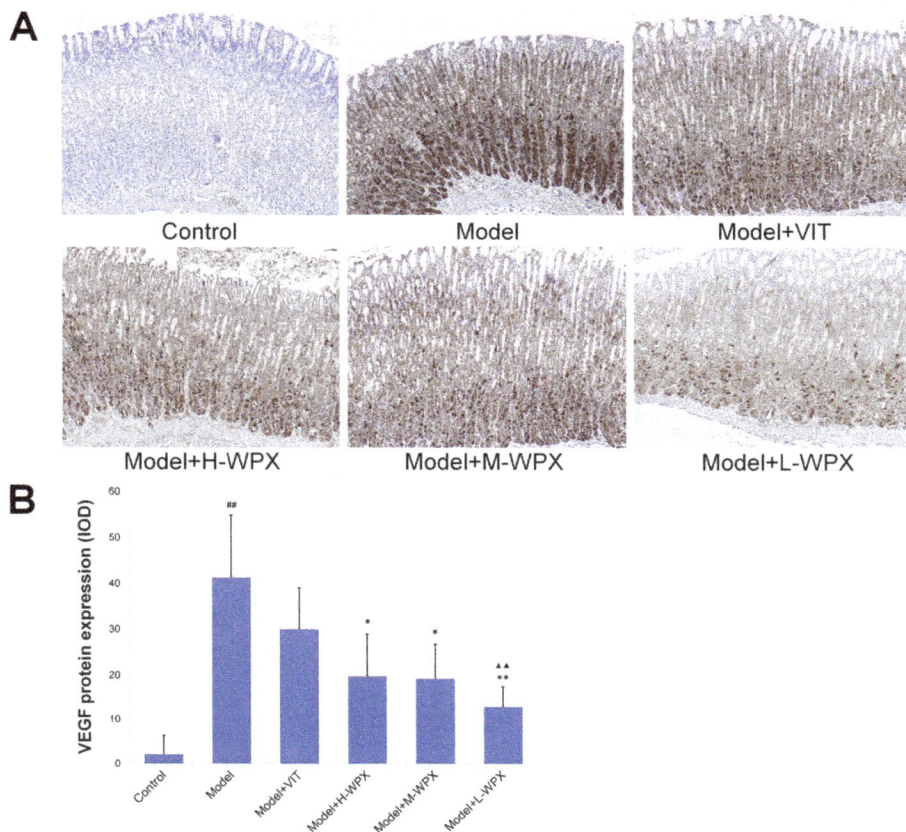

Fig. 8 Effect of WPX on VEGF protein expressions in gastric epithelium. **a** VEGF protein expressions in gastric epithelium in various groups. **b** IOD scores of HIF-1α protein levels. The results are expressed as mean ± SD ($n = 9$ in each group). Note: $^{\#\#}P < 0.01$, vs Control; $^{**}P < 0.01$, $^{*}P < 0.05$, vs Model; $^{\blacktriangle\blacktriangle}P < 0.01$, vs VIT. (IHC, 100×)

pathobiological process. It develops a new but malfunctional microvasculature [37], aiming at facilitating oxygen and nutrients supply, and thereby fuels tumor fast-growth. However, the occurrence of angiogenic activity in GPL, and microvessel morphological changes still remain unclear. In this study, we found that CD34+ microvessels were distributed sparsely in normal gastric mucosa, while their number increased significantly in GPL tissue, supporting the hypothesis that early angiogenesis is existed in GPL rats. Interestingly, in more advanced lesions, gastric mucosa frequently exhibited a higher CD34+ microvessel count. We found more GEDs with a higher number of microvessels than IMs, and more severe GEDs than mild or moderate GEDs. Notably, the most numerous CD34+ microvessels were detected in two model rats with severe GED. The above mentioned phenomena may reveal that gastric precancerosis were frequently heterogeneous in angiogenic behavior, and that a significant higher angiogenic state may imply an increased potential biological attitude towards malignancy, which is in agreement with a previous study [38]. Micromorphologically, the microvessel ultrastructural alterations found in GPL tissue were mainly characterized by dilated vascular lumen, clearly thickened and rough basal lamina, and also by conglobated, degenerated endothelial cell. These characteristics suggest that microvascular abnormalities and hypoxia vasodilation often co-existed in GPL rats. This subsequently induces hypoxia stress together with the activation of hypoxia-inducible factors [39], which stimulate secretion of VEGF and angiogenesis. Hence, angiogenesis may be an adaptive pathobiological response, often accompanying with microvascular abnormalities, triggered by microenvironmental hypoxia in gastric mucosa, aiming at restoring O_2 delivery to hypoxic regions. We speculated that chronic inflammation is a prominent inducer, which could result in microvascular injury [40] and also render gastric tissues more hypoxic [41], and therefore drive angiogenesis [42]. (inflammatory infiltration and altered expressions of inflammatory cytokines TNF-α and IL-4 were observed in GPL rats revealed by our previous study [43]). Nonetheless, these were just our preliminary findings, detailed information concerning microcirculation blood flow, inflammation-induced hypoxia and angiogenesis in GPL tissues became our next focus.

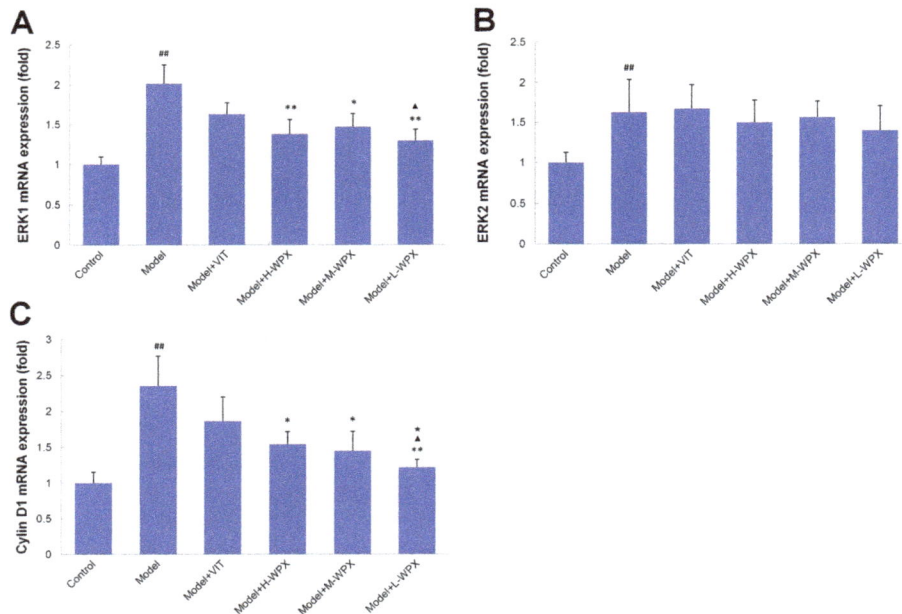

Fig. 9 Effect of WPX on the mRNA levels of ERK1, ERK2 and Cyclin D1 in gastric epithelial cells. **a** ERK1 mRNA levels of gastric epithelium in various groups. **b** ERK2 mRNA levels of gastric epithelium in various groups. **c** Cyclin D1 mRNA levels of gastric epithelium in various groups. The results are expressed as mean ± SD ($n = 9$ in each group). Note: $^{##}P < 0.01$, vs Control; $^{**}P < 0.01$, $^{*}P < 0.05$, vs Model; $^{▲}P < 0.05$, vs VIT; $^{★}P < 0.05$, vs H-WPX

Interestingly, WPX administration could rescue microvascular abnormalities and attenuate early angiogenesis in most of the specimens with a concomitant regression of IM and GED lesions. These findings suggested that WPX might possess multi-functions in blocking the GPL aggravation, not only by its anti-angiogenesis ability revealed by a marked drop of MVD level, but also, probably the most important, by ameliorating the microvascular abnormalities and the subsequent microcirculatory dysfunction. HIF-1α and VEGF have been implicated as classic factors controlling multiple proangiogenic processes hijacked by hypoxic tumors, aimed at normalizing blood flow [13]. In this study, we noted that early angiogenesis observed in GPL tissue is paralleled by HIF-1α and VEGF activation. More importantly, WPX could suppress the hypoxia-triggered accumulation of HIF-1α and the VEGF activation, this result supports the hypothesis that HIF-1α and VEGF inhibition plays a beneficial role in WPX-alleviated angiogenesis. While HIF-1α mRNA levels were elevated in GPL tissues, and the number of HIF-1α positive cells was visually reduced after WPX treatment, we archived no statistically significant differences. Given the hypoxia was a heterogeneous concept with uneven oxygen tensions in localized regions [44], spatial maldistribution of HIF-1α activation in GPL tissues may factor in these non-significant differences. Besides, sample size limitation may be another possible contributor.

Angiogenesis is a complex multistep process regulated by compounding factors. It is proposed that ERK/Cyclin D1 could act as specific effectors of VEGF signaling to elicit excessive angiogenesis behavior, and thus facilitated cell proliferation, suggesting a crucial role of the molecules in the initiation and progression of gastric cancer. However, what role the molecules may play in GPL is less clear. In this study, as expected, up-regulated mRNA expressions of ERK1, ERK2 and Cyclin D1 were observed in gastric mucosa from GPL rats as compared to normal mucosa. Our results bring a crucial contribution by evidencing that hyper-angiogenesis observed in GPL is driven, in part, through aberrant activation of ERK-related molecules, suggesting their involvement in the malignant transformation. We were also curious as to whether inhibition of ERK signals is involved in the underlying mechanisms of WPX-mediated attenuation of angiogenesis. Interestingly, after WPX intervention, a decrease in ERK1levels was frequently concurrent with the reduction of CD34+ microvessels. Hence, this ERK mitigating effect might be contributed to the anti-angiogenic activity of WPX against precursor lesions. In addition, no significant decrease in ERK2 levels was observed in WPX-treated rats, which might be due to sample size limitation, or to the speculation that ERK2 might not be the potential therapeutic target for GPL with WPX.

Previously, we have found that H-WPX and M-WPX were more superior to L-WPX in ameliorating gastric precancerosis [45], as well as suppressing cell proliferation and promoting apoptosis [46]. In this study, conversely,

L-WPX showed a relatively better anti-GPL activity by attenuating early angiogenesis, and by regulating ERK-related molecules as compared to those of H-WPX and M-WPX. We speculate that different treatment duration (10 weeks in the present study, 4 weeks in the previous studies) might be responsible for the inconsistency. It remains possible that WPX, at low dose, might be more efficient for long-term intervention of GPL when compared with that at high and medium doses. However, due to the small sample size, the speculation need to be further validated in larger scale studies. Our HPLC analysis revealed that Calycosin-7-glucoside, ginsenoside-Rg1, ginsenoside-Rvb1, astragaloside IV, as well as atractylenolide III, II and I might be the potential anti-angiogenic candidates of WPX. Ginsenoside Rg1 has been reported to suppress the vascular neointimal hyperplasia by inhibiting on ERK2 signaling [47]. Ginsenoside Rb1 displayed anti-angiogenesis through suppressing the formation of endothelial tube-like structures [48]. Besides, atractylenolide I displayed a potent inhibitory effect on angiogenesis driven by chronic inflammation in vivo and vitro [49]. Although the aforementioned reports likely support the anti-angiogenesis capacity of WPX, there are some caveats. For instance, there have been conflicting reports regarding the pro-angiogenic role [50, 51] or anti-angiogenic role [52] of astragaloside IV. Thus, much more work remains to be addressed in order to fully exploit anti-angiogenic potential of the compounds in MNNG-induced GPL rats and other GPL models in the future.

Conclusion

In summary, WPX could attenuate the angiogenic response and temper microvascular abnormalities in GPL rats. The anti-angiogenesis property might be related to inhibition on the angiogenesis-associated markers HIF-1α and VEGF, and on the ERK1/Cylin D1 aberrant activation. Additional files 1, 2, 3, 4, 5, 6 and 7.

Additional files

Additional file 1: CD34 (IHC-IOD). Raw data for Fig. 4

Additional file 2: HIF-1alpha (PCR). Raw data for Fig. 6

Additional file 3: HIF-1alpha (IHC-IOD). Raw data for Fig. 7

Additional file 4: VEGF (IHC-IOD). Raw data for Fig. 8

Additional file 5: ERK1 (PCR). Raw data for Fig. 9

Additional file 6: ERK2 (PCR). Raw data for Fig. 9

Additional file 7: Cyclin-D1(PCR). Raw data for Fig. 9

Abbreviations

ANOVA: Analysis of variance; ERK: Extracellular signal-regulated kinase; GED: Gastric epithelial dysplasia; GPL: Gastric precancerous lesions; H&E: Hematoxylin and eosin; HID-AB-PAS: High-iron diamine- alcian blue-periodic acid schiff; HIF-1α: Hypoxia inducible factor-1α; HPLC: High performance liquid chromatography; IM: Intestinal metaplasia; IOD: Integrated optical density.; MNNG: N-methyl-N′-nitro-N-nitrosoguanidine; MVD: Microvessel density; RT-qPCR: Quantitative real-time reverse transcription-polymerase chain reaction; TEM: Transmission electron microscope; TNM: Tumor node metastasis; VEGF: Vascular endothelial growth factor; VIT: Vitacoenzyme; WPX: Weipixiao

Funding

This work was supported by National Natural Science Foundation of China (Nos. 81473620, 81673946, 81774284), and by Science and Technology Developmental Foundation of Affiliated Hospital of Chengdu University of TCM (2016-D-YY-34).

Authors' contributions

JHZ and TTC carried out the experiments. HFP and FMY designed the work. ZMZ and WL prepared for WPX and preformed the HPLC analysis. DYG and RY performed histopathological examination. CZ, LHC and YZ provided helpful advice for the manuscript. All authors agree to be accountable for all aspects of the work.

Ethics approval and consent to participate

All procedures relating to animal care and the animal research protocols conformed to the guidelines for the Care and Use of Laboratory Animal, issued by the Ministry of Science and Technology of China. The animal experiments were agreed by the institutional ethical review board of Guangdong Provincial Institute of Traditional Chinese Medicine (Ethic No. GDPITCM111018).

Competing interests

The authors declare that they have no competing interests.

Author details

[1]Chengdu University of Traditional Chinese Medicine, Chengdu 610075, China. [2]Guangzhou University of Chinese Medicine, Guangzhou 510405, China. [3]Guangdong Provincial Institute of Chinese Medicine, Guangzhou 510095, China. [4]Guangzhou Institutes of Biomedicine and Health, Chinese Academy of Sciences, Guangzhou 510530, China.

References

1. Joo YE, Park HK, Myung DS, Baik GH, Shin JE, Seo GS, Kim GH, Kim HU, Kim HY, Cho SI, Kim N. Prevalence and risk factors of atrophic gastritis and intestinal metaplasia: a nationwide multicenter prospective study in Korea. Gut Liver. 2013;7(3):303–10.
2. de Vries AC, van Grieken NC, Looman CW, Casparie MK, de Vries E, Meijer GA, Kuipers EJ. Gastric cancer risk in patients with premalignant gastric lesions: a nationwide cohort study in the Netherlands. Gastroenterology. 2008;134(4):945–52.
3. Sun SB, Chen ZT, Zheng D, Huang ML, Xu D, Zhang H, Wang P, Wu J. Clinical pathology and recent follow-up study on gastric intraepithelial neoplasia and gastric mucosal lesions. Hepatogastroenterology. 2013; 60(127):1597–601.
4. Srivastava A, Lauwers GY. Gastric epithelial dysplasia: the Western perspective. Dig Liver Dis. 2008;40(8):641–9.
5. Zhang RF, Li JT, He SB, Xiao ZD. Effects of vitacoenzyme on atrophic and intestinal metaplastic lesions in chronic atrophic gastritis--pathologic and histochemical studies of 94 cases. Acad J Sun Yat-Sen Univ Med Sci. 1987;8(2):1–5.

6. Chen XT, Jiang YH, Chen LH, Li XQ, Kuang ZS, Xie YH, Fang YQ. Effects of Weiyankang plus vitacoenzyme on gastric precancerous lesions and its possible mechanism. Acad J Tradit Chin Med. 2004;22(9):1703–4.

7. Deng X, Liu ZW, Wu FS, Li LH, Liang J. A clinical study of weining granules in the treatment of gastric precancerous lesions. J Tradit Chin Med. 2012; 32(2):164–72.

8. Li HZ, Wang H, Wang GQ, Liu J, Zhao SM, Chen J, Song QW, Gao W, Qi XZ, Gao Q. Treatment of gastric precancerous lesions with Weiansan. World J Gastroenterol. 2006;12(33):5389–92.

9. Zhang X, Zheng Z, Shin YK, Kim KY, Rha SY, Noh SH, Chung HC, Jeung HC. Angiogenic factor thymidine phosphorylase associates with angiogenesis and lymphangiogenesis in the intestinal-type gastric cancer. Pathology. 2014;46(4):316–24.

10. Gao LM, Wang F, Zheng Y, Fu ZZ, Zheng L, Chen LL. Roles of fibroblast activation protein and hepatocyte growth factor expressions in angiogenesis and metastasis of gastric cancer. Pathol Oncol Res. 2017; https://doi.org/10.1007/s12253-017-0359-3.

11. Maeda K, Chung YS, Takatsuka S, Ogawa Y, Onoda N, Sawada T, Kato Y, Nitta A, Arimoto Y, Kondo Y. Tumour angiogenesis and tumour cell proliferation as prognostic indicators in gastric carcinoma. Br J Cancer. 1995; 72(2):319–23.

12. Pinto MP, Owen GI, Retamal I, Garrido M. Angiogenesis inhibitors in early development for gastric cancer. Expert Opin Investig Drugs. 2017; 26(9):1007–17.

13. Rey S, Schito L, Wouters BG, Eliasof S, Kerbel RS. Targeting hypoxia-inducible factors for antiangiogenic cancer therapy. Trends Cancer. 2017;3(7):529–41.

14. Arany Z, Foo SY, Ma Y, Ruas JL, Bommi-Reddy A, Girnun G, Cooper M, Laznik D, Chinsomboon J, Rangwala SM, Baek KH, Rosenzweig A, Spiegelman BM. HIF-independent regulation of VEGF and angiogenesis by the transcriptional coactivator PGC-1alpha. Nature. 2008;451(7181):1008–12.

15. Shin M, Beane TJ, Quillien A, Male I, Zhu LJ, Lawson ND. Vegfa signals through ERK to promote angiogenesis, but not artery differentiation. Development. 2016;143(20):3796–805.

16. Yang JJ, Cho LY, Ma SH, Ko KP, Shin A, Choi BY, Han DS, Song KS, Kim YS, Chang SH, Shin HR, Kang D, Yoo KY, Park SK. Oncogenic CagA promotes gastric cancer risk via activating ERK signaling pathways: a nested case-control study. PLoS One. 2011;6(6):e21155.

17. Luo ZY, Wang YY, Zhao ZS, Li B, Chen JF. The expression of TMPRSS4 and Erk1 correlates with metastasis and poor prognosis in Chinese patients with gastric cancer. PLoS One. 2013;8(7):e70311.

18. Yang D, Fan X, Yin P, Wen Q, Yan F, Yuan S, Liu B, Zhuang G, Liu Z. Significance of decoy receptor 3 (Dcr3) and external-signal regulated kinase 1/2 (Erk1/2) in gastric cancer. BMC Immunol. 2012;13:28.

19. Modi PK, Komaravelli N, Singh N, Sharma P. Interplay between MEK-ERK signaling, cyclin D1, and cyclin-dependent kinase 5 regulates cell cycle reentry and apoptosis of neurons. Mol Biol Cell. 2012;23(18):3722–30.

20. Weber JD, Raben DM, Phillips PJ, Baldassare JJ. Sustained activation of extracellular-signal- regulated kinase 1 (ERK1) is required for the continued expression of cyclin D1 in G1 phase. Biochem J. 1997;326(Pt 1):61–8.

21. Guo YL, Rao J, Pan HF, Fang J. Effect of the treatment of Jianpi Huayu Jiedu for patients with chronic atrophic gastritis and its influence on cyclin E protein expression. Chin J Exp Tradit Med Form. 2013;19(11):292–5.

22. He JJ, Zhang BP, Zhao XY. Clinical efficacy of Weipixiao in treating chonic atrophic gastritis. J Guangzhou Univ Tradit Chin Med. 2017;34(6):823–7.

23. Zhang SL. Clinical efficacy of Weipixiao in treating chonic atrophic gastritis (spleen-stomach weakness, syndrome type of TCM): a randomized clinical trial. J Pr Tradit Chin Intern Med. 2017;31(9):12–4.

24. Yin G, Tang D, Dai J, Liu M, Wu M, Sun YU, Yang Z, Hoffman RM, Li L, Zhang S, Guo X. Combination efficacy of Astragalus membranaceus and Curcuma wenyujin at different stages of tumor progression in an imageable orthotopic nude mouse model of metastatic human ovarian cancer expressing red fluorescent protein. Anticancer Res. 2015;35(6):3193–207.

25. Wu J, Ke X, Ma N, Wang W, Fu W, Zhang H, Zhao M, Gao X, Hao X, Zhang Z. Formononetin, an active compound of Astragalus membranaceus (Fisch) Bunge, inhibits hypoxia-induced retinal neovascularization via the HIF-1alpha/VEGF signaling pathway. Drug Des Devel Ther. 2016;10:3071–81.

26. Chen W, Lu Y, Gao M, Wu J, Wang A, Shi R. Anti-angiogenesis effect of essential oil from Curcuma zedoaria in vitro and in vivo. J Ethnopharmacol. 2011;133(1):220–6.

27. Cao HY, Ding RL, Li M, Yang MN, Yang LL, Wu JB, Yang B, Wang J, Luo CL, Wen QL. Danshensu, a major water-soluble component of Salvia miltiorrhiza, enhances the radioresponse for Lewis lung carcinoma xenografts in mice. Oncol Lett. 2017;13(2):605–12.

28. Saito T, Inokuchi K, Takayama S, Sugimura T. Sequential morphological changes in N-methyl-N'-nitro-N-nitrosoguanidine carcinogenesis in the glandular stomach of rats. J Natl Cancer Inst. 1970;44(4):769–83.

29. Tatematsu M, Aoki T, Inoue T, Mutai M, Furihata C, Ito N. Coefficient induction of pepsinogen 1-decreased pyloric glands and gastric cancers in five different strains of rats treated with N-methyl-N'-nitro-N-nitrosoguanidine. Carcinogenesis. 1988;9(3):495–8.

30. Weidner N, Semple JP, Welch WR, Folkman J. Tumor angiogenesis and metastasis-correlation in invasive breast carcinoma. N Engl J Med. 1991; 324(1):1–8.

31. Correa P. A human model of gastric carcinogenesis. Cancer Res. 1988;48(13): 3554–60.

32. Dinis-Ribeiro M, Lopes C, da Costa-Pereira A, Guilherme M, Barbosa J, Lomba-Viana H, Silva R, Moreira-Dias L. A follow up model for patients with atrophic chronic gastritis and intestinal metaplasia. J Clin Pathol. 2004;57(2):177–82.

33. Li D, Bautista MC, Jiang SF, Daryani P, Brackett M, Armstrong MA, Hung YY, Postlethwaite D, Ladabaum U. Risks and predictors of gastric adenocarcinoma in patients with gastric intestinal metaplasia and dysplasia: a population-based study. Am J Gastroenterol. 2016;111(8):1104–13.

34. Di Gregorio C, Morandi P, Fante R, De Gaetani C. Gastric dysplasia. A follow-up study. Am J Gastroenterol. 1993;88(10):1714–9.

35. Gonzalez CA, Sanz-Anquela JM, Companioni O, Bonet C, Berdasco M, López C, Mendoza J, Martín-Arranz MD, Rey E, Poves E, Espinosa L, Barrio J, Torres MÁ, Cuatrecasas M, Elizalde I, Bujanda L, Garmendia M, Ferrández Á, Muñoz G, Andreu V, Paules MJ, Lario S, Ramírez MJ, Gisbert JP. Incomplete type of intestinal metaplasia has the highest risk to progress to gastric cancer: results of the Spanish follow-up multicenter study. J Gastroenterol Hepatol. 2016;31(5):953–8.

36. Tarnawski AS, Ahluwalia A, Jones MK. Angiogenesis in gastric mucosa: an important component of gastric erosion and ulcer healing and its impairment in aging. J Gastroenterol Hepatol. 2014;29(Suppl 4):112–23.

37. Carmeliet P, Jain RK. Principles and mechanisms of vessel normalization for cancer and other angiogenic diseases. Nat Rev Drug Discov. 2011; 10(6):417–27.

38. Spina D, Vindigni C, Presenti L, Schürfeld K, Stumpo M, Tosi P. Cell proliferation, cell death, E-cadherin, metalloproteinase expression and angiogenesis in gastric cancer precursors and early cancer of the intestinal type. Int J Oncol. 2001;18(6):1251–8.

39. Walshe TE, D'Amore PA. The role of hypoxia in vascular injury and repair. Annu Rev Physiol. 2008;3:615–43.

40. Lentsch AB, Ward PA. Regulation of inflammatory vascular damage. J Pathol. 2000;190(3):343–8.

41. Colgan SP, Campbell EL, Kominsky DJ. Hypoxia and mucosal inflammation. Annu Rev Pathol. 2016;11:77–100.

42. Whiteford JR, De Rossi G, Woodfin A. Mutually supportive mechanisms of inflammation and vascular remodeling. Int Rev Cell Mol Biol. 2016; 326:201–78.

43. Li HW, Pan HF, Zhao ZM, Shi YF, Yan Y, Yuan YM, Zeng JH, Lin ZY, Zhao JY. Effect of Weipixiao on plasma tumor necrosis factor alpha and interleukin-4 expression in rats with gastric precancerous lesions. J Guangzhou Univ Tradit Chin Med. 2015;32(2):271–4.

44. Span PN, Bussink J. Biology of hypoxia. Semin Nucl Med. 2015;45(2):101–9.

45. Pan HF, Zhao ZM, Ren JL, Shi YF. Effect of Weipixiao on gastric epithelial intestinal metaplasia in chronic atrophic gastritis rats. Tradit Chin Drug Res Clin Pharmacol. 2012;23(1):55–7.

46. Pan HF, Ren JL, Zhao ZM, Liu J. Effect of Weipixiao on cell generation cycle distribution and apoptosis-related gene expression in gastric mucosal epithelial cells of gastric precancerous lesion rats with spleen-deficiency chronic atrophic gastritis. J Guangzhou Univ Tradit Chin Med. 2010;27(5):488–91.

47. Gao Y, Deng J, Yu XF, Yang DL, Gong QH, Huang XN. Ginsenoside Rg1 inhibits vascular intimal hyperplasia in balloon-injured rat carotid artery by down-regulation of extracellular signal-regulated kinase 2. J Ethnopharmacol. 2011;138(2):472–8.

48. Leung KW, Cheung LW, Pon YL, Wong RN, Mak NK, Fan TP, Au SC, Tombran-Tink J, Wong AS. Ginsenoside Rb1 inhibits tube-like structure formation of endothelial cells by regulating pigment epithelium-derived factor through the oestrogen beta receptor. Br J Pharmacol. 2007; 152(2):207–15.

49. Wang C, Duan H, He L. Inhibitory effect of atractylenolide I on angiogenesis in chronic inflammation in vivo and in vitro. Eur J Pharmacol. 2009;612(1–3):143–52.

50. Wang SG, Xu Y, Chen JD, Yang CH, Chen XH. Astragaloside IV stimulates angiogenesis and increases nitric oxide accumulation via JAK2/STAT3 and ERK1/2 pathway. Molecules. 2013;18(10):12809–19.

51. Wang S, Chen J, Fu Y, Chen X. Promotion of astragaloside IV for EA-hy926 cell proliferation and angiogenic activity via ERK1/2 pathway. J Nanosci Nanotechnol. 2015;15(6):4239–44.

52. Zhang S, Tang D, Zang W, Yin G, Dai J, Sun YU, Yang Z, Hoffman RM, Guo X. Synergistic inhibitory effect of traditional Chinese medicine astragaloside IV and curcumin on tumor growth and angiogenesis in an orthotopic nude-mouse model of human hepatocellular carcinoma. Anticancer Res. 2017;37(2):465–73.

16

Effective antioxidant, antimicrobial and anticancer activities of essential oils of horticultural aromatic crops in northern Egypt

Hosam O. Elansary[1,2,3]* (ID), Samir A. M. Abdelgaleil[4], Eman A. Mahmoud[5], Kowiyou Yessoufou[3], Khalid Elhindi[1] and Salah El-Hendawy[1]

Abstract

Background: Identifying ornamental plants as new natural antioxidant and antimicrobial sources is always of great importance for the ornamental and horticultural industries.

Methods: The antimicrobial activities of leaves and fruits peel essential oils of twelve ornamental and horticultural crops were determined by screening against wide spectrum of fungi and bacteria, and their respective in vitro antioxidant capacity was evaluated. Furthermore, the anticancer activities against several cancer cells, and one normal human cell line (HEK-293) were examined.

Results: *Origanum vulgare* L. essential oil showed the best antioxidant, antibacterial and anticancer activities compared to screened crops by means of the DPPH and linoleic acid assays for antioxidants, MIC and MBC values for antibacterial activities and IC_{50} for antiproliferative activities. Such important activities in *O. vulgare* was attributed to high pulegone ratio (77.45%) as revealed by the GC/MS assay. *Rosmarinus officinallis* L. essential oil showed the highest antifungal activities by means of lowest MIC and MFC values which might be attributed to 1, 8-cineole (19.60%), camphor (17.01%) and α-pinene (15.12%).

Conclusion: We suggest that oxygenated monoterpenes (i.e. linalool, terpinen-4-ol and pulegone) and monoterpene hydrocarbons play an important role in the essential oil antioxidant, antibacterial, antifungal and anticancer activities of diverse Egyptian ornamental and horticultural crops. Some species showed bioactivities similar to standards compounds and might be suitable for pharmaceutical and food industries.

Keywords: Antioxidants, Ornamental plants, Essential oils, Chemical composition

Background

In an attempt to preserve human health and avoid food losses in the face of global growing food insecurity, synthetic preservatives were introduced in the food industries [1, 2]. Unfortunately, some of these preservatives were reported to cause undesirable health side effects to humans [1, 2]. For example, lipid peroxidation in stored food may lead to rancidity and reduction of food quality [3–5].

The consumption of spoiled food can cause a wide spectrum of human diseases. Furthermore, the development of resistant microorganisms to synthetic preservatives is another threat facing the continuous use of these chemicals.

Consequently, renewed interest has been placed on the discovery and use of natural bioactive resources in medicinal plants to control diseases, food spoilage microorganisms and oxidation [6–11]. Such medicinal plants include ornamental and horticultural crops that contain essential oils that are bioactive against the development of certain microorganisms [12–15]. The essential oils with high content of phenolics are recognized as strong

* Correspondence: helansary@ksu.edu.sa; hosammail2003@yahoo.com
[1]Plant production Department, College of Food and Agriculture Sciences, King Saud University, P.O. Box 2460, Riyadh 11451, Saudi Arabia
[2]Floriculture, Ornamental Horticulture and Garden Design Department, Faculty of Agriculture (El-Shatby), Alexandria University, Alexandria, Egypt
Full list of author information is available at the end of the article

antioxidants [16–20] and have antimicrobial activities against different types of microorganisms [21–27].

Essential oils might be used as anticancer agents as found before in *Pinus koraiensis* against HCT116 colorectal cancer cells [28], *Myracrodruon urundeuva* against HeLa, HEK-293, and Vero E6 cells [29] and Yemeni medicinal plants against A-427, 5637 and MCF-7 cancer cells [30]. Such activities might be attributed to major essential oil constitutes including cineol, capillin and others [31, 32]. There are dozens of unstudied medicinal horticultural crops in Egypt with certain traditional uses such as skin, face and hair treatments [33] and urological, gastrointestinal, respiratory, neurological, cardiological and immunological diseases control [34]. This great diversity of alternative medicine application of essential oils and leaf extracts might be of pharmaceutical importance that need to be explored.

The study investigated the antioxidant and antimicrobial activities of essential oils obtained from important horticultural and economic ornamental medicinal plants. We also associate the main components of the essential oil with specific antioxidant and antimicrobial properties found to explore novel crop additive values.

Methods
Plant materials
The leaves or fruit peels of twelve plant species were collected from Alexandria, Behera and Matrouh in northern Egypt in the spring and summer of 2016. The leaves were obtained from mature non flowering herbal plants of *Rosmarinus officinalis* L., *Artemisia judaica* L., *A. monosperma*, *Origanum vulgare* L. and *Pelargonium graveolens* L'Her. Also the mature leaves of ornamental non trees of *Rosmarinus officinalis Callistemon viminalis* G. Don, *Cupressus macrocarpa* Gordon , *Schinus molle* L., and *Thuja occidentalis* L. The fruit peels were obtained from mature fruits of *Citrus aurantifolia* Swingle, *C. limon* (L.) and *C. paradisi*. The plant samples were collected during the months of April to August, 2016. Plants were identified by Prof. Samir Abdelgaleil and Assoc. Prof. Hosam Elansary. Specimens were vouchered in Department of Pesticide Chemistry and Technology, Alexandria University.

Essential oils analysis
The leaves were dried for five days (26 ± 1 °C) while the fruit peels were used fresh. The essential oils were obtained by hydrodistillation in a Clevenger-type apparatus for 1 h. Gas chromatography/mass spectrometry (Hewlett Packard 5890) apparatus detected the the essential oil constitutes after dilution in diethyl ether. Gas chromatography column properties and injection conditions matches those described [3]. Oil compositions were identified by comparing retention time and indices of

identified constitutes to n-alkanes (C_{10}–C_{36}, Sigma-Aldrich, Cairo) subjected to the same conditions. NIST Ver. 2.0 and Wiley libraries were used as well for the identificaton of the compounds.

Microorganisms and cell cultures
The antimicrobial activities were investigated against fungi and bacteria. Fungi included *Aspergillus flavus* (ATCC 9643), *A. ochraceus* (ATCC 12066), *A. niger* (ATCC 6275), *Penicillium ochrochloron* (ATCC 48663), *P. funiculosum* (ATCC 56755), and *Candida albicans* (ATCC 12066)). Bacteria included *Bacillus cereus* (ATCC 14579), *Micrococcus flavus* (ATCC 10240), *Listeria monocytogenes* (clinical isolate), *Staphylococcus aureus* (ATCC 6538), *Pseudomonas aeruginosa* (ATCC 27853), *Dickeya solani* (DS 0432–1) and *Escherichia coli* (ATCC 35210),. The first four bacteria are Gram-positive while the last three are Gram-negative. The microorganisms are either of economic importance for the agricultural industry (e.g. *L. monocytogenes*, *D. solani* and *S. aureus*) or affect human health mainly such as *C. albicans*. Fungi and bacteria were obtained from Alexandria University. Cell cultures including breast adenocarcinoma (MCF-7), cervical adenocarcinoma (HeLa), T-cell lymphoblast (Jurkat), colon adenocarcinoma (HT-29) and urinary bladder carcinoma (T24) were purchased from American Type Culture Collection.

Antioxidants
The antioxidant activity of the essential oils was estimated using the DPPH [35] and the β-carotene-linoleic acid methods [35]. Positive control (BHT) and negative control were treated as samples and a calibration curve was obtained. The amount of the samples that inhibited 50% of each antioxidant solution (IC_{50}) were considered as the antioxidant activities and experiments were repeated twice.

Antifungal activity assay
The antifungal activities of the essential oils were estimated using the microdilution method [36]. The minimum inhibitory concentration (MIC) was the lowest concentration inhibiting the fungal growth using a binocular. The minimum fungicidal concentration (MFC) was estimated by serial sub-cultivations (0.1–4.0 mg/mL). The MFC was determined as the concentration causing no visible growth and killing 99.5% of the original inoculum. Fluconazole (FLZ) and ketoconazole (KLZ) were used as positive control and experiments were repeated twice.

Antibacterial activity assay
The antibacterial activities were determined by the micro-dilution method [36]. To determine the minimum

inhibitory (MIC) and minimum bactericidal (MBC) concentrations the MIC was considered as the lowest concentrations causing no growth using the binocular. The MBC was quantified using serial sub-cultivation of each bacterium (0.1–2.0 mg/mL) into 100 μL of TSB and incubated for one day. MBC was the lowest concentration showed no growth and killed 99.5% of the original inoculum. Experiments were performed twice and negative control (5% DMSO) as well as positive (streptomycin and ampicillin, 0.01–10 mg/mL) were used.

Antiproliferative activity assay

Essential oils antiproliferative activities against MCF-7, HeLa, Jurkat, HT-29,T24 and HEK-293 followed the MTT method [37] with modifications. Five doses of leaf extracts were used to reach a final concentration of 50, 100, 200, 300, and 400 μg/mL culture media. Negative controls and positive (vinblastine sulfate and taxol) were used.

Furthermore, IC_{50} values were obtained by plotting percentage of cell viability against extract concentration and expressed in μg/ml.

Results
Essential oils GC-MS analyses

The essential oils percentage and analyses (Table 1) showed that each species has its own chemical fingerprint. The major oil constitutes (%) were β –thujone (49.83) and chrysanthenone (10.88) in A. judaica In A. monosperma, capillene (36.86) was the major compound while 1,8-cineole (71.77) was the major in C. viminalis. The limonene (40.19) and β-pinene (19.65) were the major compounds in C. aurantifolia. In C. lemon, limonene (56.30) and β-pinene (8.81) were also the major compounds while in C. paradisi limonene (74.29) and linalool (4.61) were the main compounds. Terpinen-4-ol (20.29) and sabinene (18.67) were the major compounds in C. macrocarpawhile pulegone (77.45) and menthone (4.86) were majors in O. vulgare. β-citronellol (35.92) and geraniol (11.66) were major in P. graveolenswhile 1,8-cineole (19.60), camphor (17.01) and α-pinene (15.12) were major in R. officinallis. α-phellandrene (29.87) and β-phellandrene (21.08) were the major compounds in S. mollewhile α-pinene (35.49) and δ-3-carene (25.42) were the major in T. occidentalis.

The results of chemical analysis indicated that components including limonene, α-pinene were found in more than one species, while others were species specific. Essential oils major constitutes could be divided into three groups including oxygenated monoterpenes (i.e. linalool and pulegone); monoterpene hydrocarbons (i.e. limonene and sabinene) and sesquiterpene hydrocarbons (i.e., σ-cadinene and σ-selinene).

Antioxidant activities

The essential oil of O. vulgare showed significantly the highest antioxidant activities with IC_{50} values of 2.8 and 1.1 mg/L in the DPPH and linoleic acid assays, respectively compared to other essential oils (Table 2). The oils of A. judaica, A. monosperma and C. viminalis followed O. vulgare oil in their antioxidant activities and their IC_{50} values ranged between 4.7–5.3 and 2.7–3.3 mg/L in the DPPH and linoleic acid assays, respectively. The oil of S. molle showed the lowest antioxidant activity among all essential oils examined in the study. In addition, the oils of C. limon, C. macrocarpa, P. graveolens and R. officinallis showed no significant differences regarding their antioxidant activities.

Antifungal activities

The activities of the essential oils were expressed as MIC (Table 3) and MFC (Table 4). In general, all examined oils showed antifungal activities against A. flavus, A. ochraceus, A. niger, P. funiculosum, P. ochrochloron and C. albicans. The MIC and MFC values varied between 0.16– 1.31 and 0.33–> 4 mg/mL, respectively. The oils of R. officinallis, O. vulgare, C. macrocarpa and C. aurantifolia showed the lowest MIC values compared to other plants species. The oil of R. officinallis showed the highest antifungal activities among studied essential oils by means of lowest values of MIC and MFC against the six fungi. The most resistant fungi were C. albicans, P. funiculosum and A. niger showing the highest MIC and MFC values. The essential oils of R. officinallis and O. vulgare revealed comparable activities to commercial reagents.

The antibacterial activities

There were large differences regarding essential oils antibacterial activities by means of MIC (Table 5) and MBC (Table 6). The oils of O. vulgare, C. macrocarpa and C. paradisi showed the highest antibacterial activities with MIC values ranged between 0.11–0.76 mg/mL against examined bacteria. O. vulgare, C. macrocarpa and C. paradise were the three most active essential oils, the MBC was in the range of 0.21 to 1.59. The most resistant bacterium in this case of D. solani and L. monocytogenes. In general, the highest MIC values were recorded for the essential oils of A. monosperma, C. lemon, R. officinallis and S. molle. Most essential oils showed slightly higher MIC values compared to antibiotics, however, O. vulgare showed comparable values to antibiotics in some cases. The antibacterial activities were higher than antibiotics.

Anticancer activities

There were variations in essential oils anticancer activities against selected cancer cell lines as shown in Table 7. The inhibition (expressed as IC_{50}) of different

Table 1 Major constituents of essential oils extracted from twelve Egyptian plant species

Plant name Oil yield (% F.W., v/w)	Major components (%, RI[a])
Artemisia judaica (0.2)	β –Thujone (49.83,1100), Chrysanthenone (10.88,1125), α- Thujone (8.21,1116), 1,8-Cineole (4.91,1034), L-Camphor (3.0,1192), Artemisia alcohol (2.20,1083)
Artemisia monosperma (0.8)	Capillene (36.86,1446), capillin (14.68,1572), γ-Terpinene (12.46,1047), β-Pinene (7.85,964), cis-Ocimene (3.26,1043), Terpinen-4-ol (2.59,1192)
Callistemon viminalis (0.5)	1,8-Cineole (71.77,1034), α-Pinene (11.47,946), Terpinen-4-ol (3.18,1192), Octadecanoic acid (3.08,2172), 1-Phellandrene (1.30,1054)
Citrus aurantifolia (0.75)	Limonene (40.19,1029), β-Pinene (19.65,964), α-Citral (8.14,1240), γ-Terpinene (6.34,1047), α-Terpineol (3.71,1185), Terpinen-4-ol (2.62,1192)
Citrus limon (0.2)	Limonene (56.30,1029), β-Pinene (8.81,964), γ-Terpinene (6.42,1047), α-Citral (4.96,1240), β-Citral (3.83,1216), α-Terpineol (3.38,1185)
Citrus paradisi (0.12)	Limonene (74.29,1029), Linalool (4.61,1117), Linalool oxide (4.18,1088), β-Citral (2.66,1216), α-Fenchol (1.99,1168), Nootkatone (1.78,1800)
Cupressus macrocarpa (0.45)	Terpinen-4-ol (20.29,1192), Sabinene (18.67,974), β-Citronellol (13.01,1225), γ-Terpinene (7.59,1047), Camphor (6.66,1139), α-Terpinene (4.50,1018)
Origanum vulgare (0.5)	Pulegone (77.45, 1237), Menthone (4.86, 1152), cis-Isopulegone (2.22, 1161), Piperitenone (2.13, 1253), Limonene (1.08, 1029), Myrcene (0.66,984)
Pelargonium graveolens (0.09)	β-Citronellol (35.92,1225), Geraniol (11.66,1233), Citronellylformate (11.40,1275), Linalool (9.63,1117), (+)-Isomenthone (6.36,1164), σ-Selinene (5.52,1484)
Rosmarinus officinalis (0.33)	1,8-Cineole (19.60,1034), Camphor (17.01,1139), α-Pinene (15.12,946), Verbenone (9.55,1204), Borneol (8.17,1188), Linalool (5.32,1117)
Schinus molle (0.88)	α-Phellandrene (29.87,1005), β-Phellandrene (21.08,1031), Elemol (13.00,1547), τ-Muurolol (5.35,1641), γ-Eudesmol (4.48,1629), σ-Cadinene (3.99,1524)
Thuja occidentalis (0.25)	α-Pinene (35.49,946), δ-3-Carene (25.42,1004), α-Cedrol (9.05,1585), α-Terpinolene (6.76,1092), Limonene (4.91,1029), Myrcene (2.77,984)

[a]Retention indices related to a homologous series of n-alkanes (C_{10}–C_{36}, Sigma-Aldrich, Cairo) analyzed in the same conditions and computer matching with the NIST mass spectral search program Ver. 2.0 and Wiley libraries

types of cancer cells proliferation ranged between 8.1 and ʼ300 μg/ml. The highest antiproliferation activities were found in O. vulgare, Citrus sp. and A. monosperma against MCF-7, HeLa, Jurkat, HT-29 and T24 cancer cells. The lowest antiproliferative activities were found in the essential oils of P. graveolens. No inhibition activity was found in any oil against HEK-293 (kidney epithelial).

Discussion

Essential oils showed high variation in term of composition even among closely related species (i.e. species of the same genera), which is in agreement with previous reports on several plants [39–41]. All essential oils examined showed antioxidant capacities; however, O. vulgare showed the highest antioxidant activities. This might be attributed to specific essential oil such as the pulegone (77.45%). The pulegone is a known compound found in the family Lamiaceae and has been associated with high antioxidant activities [42–44]. Although

previous studies reported that pulegone is the major oil component of O. vulgare [44], environmental conditions of the plant may alter the chemical composition of the oil [41, 43] leading to the variation of chemical composition that we found among closely related species. Similarly, many other species showed high antioxidant activities (e.g. A. judaica, A. monosperma and C. viminalis). cajor components and their synergetic effects. β α. Specifically, we found a high ratio of β –thujone (49.83%) and α-thujone (8.21%) in A. Judaica, supporting the previous report in Artemisia sieberi Besser in Italy and Iran [45]. The essential oil ratio found in Italy and Iran [45] is slightly higher than that found in our study. However, A. monosperma showed high ratios of α-pinene and terpinen-4-ol which are known to have noticeable antioxidant activities [46]. The high antioxidant activities that we found in relation with the presence of β–thujone may indicate that this compound may play a major role in the antioxidant activities of different Artemisia species.

Table 2 Antioxidant activity of essential oils using the corresponding concentrations measured by DPPH and β-carotene-linoleic acid methods[a]

Essential oil	IC$_{50}$ (mg/L)	
	DPPH radical scavenging	β-Carotene-linoleic acid
Artemisia judaica	4.7 ± 0.1b	2.7 ± 0.1b
Artemisia monosperma	5.3 ± 0.3c[b]	3.3 ± 0.1cd
Callistemon viminalis	5.2 ± 0.1c	3.2 ± 0.1c
Citrus aurantifolia	7.2 ± 0.3e	5.6 ± 0.3f
Citrus limon	6.1 ± 0.3d	4.2 ± 0.1e
Cupressus macrocarpa	6.1 ± 0.1d	4.2 ± 0.3e
Origanum vulgare	2.8 ± 0.3a	1.1 ± 0.1a
Pelargonium graveolens	6.2 ± 0.1d	4.1 ± 0.3e
Rosmarinus officinalis	6.0 ± 0.1d	4.2 ± 0.2e
Schinus molle	8.9 ± 0.1f	6.6 ± 0.3 g
Thuja occidentalis	5.6 ± 0.3 cd	3.6 ± 0.4d
Butylated hydroxytoluene (BHT)	2.9 ± 0.1a	2.6 ± 0.2b

[a]Values are expressed as means ± SD
[b]Means followed by different letters within a column indicate significant differences between treatments based on LSD test ($P \leq 0.05$)

The essential oil in *R. officinallis* showed the highest antifungal activities by means of lowest MIC and MFC values which might be attributed to 1,8-cineole (19.60%), camphor (17.01%) and α-pinene (15.12%) as the major oil constituents as previously reported [47]. It was reported that 1,8-cineole, terpinen-4-ol and other compounds showed strong in-vitro antifungal activities against some plant pathogenic fungi including *Fusarium cerealis, Aspergillus tubingensis* and *A. carbonarius*

[48]. In the current study, we report strong antifungal activities of the 1,8-cineole-rich *R. officinallis* against plant and human pathogenic fungi including *A. flavus, A. ochraceus, A. niger, P. funiculosum, P. ochrochloron* and *C. albicans*. The oil of *O. vulgare* followed *R. officinallis* in term of level of antifungal activities, and such interesting bioactivities of the essential oil might be attributed to the presence of pulegone (77.45%) and the menthone (4.86%).

The essential oil in *C. macrocarpa* showed high antifungal activities compared to other species, which is attributed to the presence of essential antifungal compounds including terpinen-4-ol (20.29%), sabinene (18.67%), γ-terpinene (7.59%) and α-terpinene (4.50%) in agreement with previous investigations on other plants [46]. High ratios of limonene (40.19%) and β-pinene (19.65%) were found in *C. aurantifolia*, confirming previous report [40].

In the current study, we document the highest antibacterial activity for the *O. vulgare* essential oil by means of MIC and MBC values compared to other species, potentially because of the high pulegone ratio. Previous investigations reported strong antibacterial activities of essential oils of the pulegone-rich *Mentha longifolia* L. and pulegone-rich *O. vulgare* against different bacteria such as *Pantoea agglumerans* and human pathogenic *Acinetobacter baumannii*, respectively [43, 44]. The high antifungal as well as antibacterial activities of pulegone rich essential oils suggest that this compound might have a wide spectrum of antifungal and antibacterial activities. The oils of *C. macrocarpa* and *C. paradise* followed *O. vulgare* in their level of antibacterial activities, which might be attributed to terpinen-4-ol and

Table 3 Minimum inhibitory concentration (MIC) of essential oils on fungal strains

Essential oil	MIC (mg/mL)					
	A. flavus	A. ochraceus	A. niger	P. funiculosum	P. ochrochloron	C. albicans
Artemisia judaica	0.31 ± 0.01	0.38 ± 0.02	0.31 ± 0.01	2.95 ± 0.11	0.41 ± 0.03	0.72 ± 0.03
Artemisia monosperma	0.22 ± 0.03	0.29 ± 0.01	0.27 ± 0.03	0.71 ± 0.03	0.33 ± 0.01	0.72 ± 0.11
Callistemon viminals	0.25 ± 0.03	0.43 ± 0.01	0.51 ± 0.03	0.96 ± 0.07	0.52 ± 0.05	0.63 ± 0.03
Citrus aurantifolia	0.18 ± 0.01	0.19 ± 0.01	0.27 ± 0.01	1.31 ± 0.11	0.41 ± 0.03	0.35 ± 0.01
Citrus limon	0.33 ± 0.01	0.29 ± 0.01	0.57 ± 0.03	3.55 ± 0.21	0.57 ± 0.03	0.39 ± 0.03
Citrus paradisi	0.38 ± 0.01	0.52 ± 0.03	0.81 ± 0.03	1.35 ± 0.09	0.42 ± 0.01	0.81 ± 0.05
Cupressus macrocarpa	0.17 ± 0.01	0.20 ± 0.01	0.26 ± 0.02	0.25 ± 0.02	0.28 ± 0.01	0.72 ± 0.05
Origanum vulgare	0.16 ± 0.01	0.18 ± 0.02	0.22 ± 0.01	0.25 ± 0.01	0.33 ± 0.01	0.26 ± 0.01
Pelargonium graveolens	0.23 ± 0.01	0.45 ± 0.05	0.39 ± 0.01	0.52 ± 0.01	0.21 ± 0.01	0.83 ± 0.05
Rosmarinus officinalis	0.15 ± 0.01	0.27 ± 0.01	0.17 ± 0.01	0.23 ± 0.01	0.21 ± 0.03	0.22 ± 0.01
Schinus molle	0.27 ± 0.01	0.31 ± 0.01	0.61 ± 0.05	0.43 ± 0.01	0.47 ± 0.01	0.97 ± 0.09
Thuja occidentalis	0.27 ± 0.01	0.41 ± 0.05	0.45 ± 0.03	0.51 ± 0.03	0.19 ± 0.01	1.21 ± 0.07
Fuconazole	0.14 ± 0.01	0.19 ± 0.01	0.16 ± 0.01	0.11 ± 0.01	0.20 ± 0.01	0.11 ± 0.01
Ketoconazole	0.21 ± 0.01	0.20 ± 0.01	0.12 ± 0.01	2.00 ± 0.09	0.20 ± 0.01	0.21 ± 0.01

Table 4 Minimum fungicidal concentration (MFC) of essential oils on fungal strains

Essential oil	MFC (mg/mL)					
	A. flavus	A. ochraceus	A. niger	P. funiculosum	P. ochrochloron	Candida albicans
Artemisia judaica	0.77 ± 0.03	0.63 ± 0.03	0.85 ± 0.03	> 4	0.95 ± 0.05	1.86 ± 0.09
Artemisia monosperma	0.46 ± 0.01	0.61 ± 0.02	0.87 ± 0.05	1.81 ± 0.10	0.61 ± 0.03	1.63 ± 0.13
Callistemon viminalis	0.63 ± 0.05	0.95 ± 0.05	1.13 ± 0.08	> 2	0.95 ± 0.03	1.1 ± 0.05
Citrus aurantifolia	0.39 ± 0.03	0.41 ± 0.02	0.56 ± 0.02	> 2	0.83 ± 0.03	0.71 ± 0.03
Citrus limon	0.74 ± 0.05	0.76 ± 0.04	1.43 ± 0.07	> 4	1.41 ± 0.08	0.91 ± 0.05
Citrus paradisi	0.76 ± 0.03	> 2	> 2	3.91 ± 0.17	0.93 ± 0.05	1.59 ± 0.07
Cupressus macrocarpa	0.37 ± 0.03	0.48 ± 0.03	0.49 ± 0.03	0.73 ± 0.03	0.68 ± 0.03	1.53 ± 0.15
Origanum vulgare	0.35 ± 0.01	0.47 ± 0.03	0.47 ± 0.03	0.61 ± 0.01	0.71 ± 0.02	0.63 ± 0.03
Pelargonium graveolens	0.47 ± 0.01	1.21 ± 0.09	0.83 ± 0.01	1.19 ± 0.08	0.49 ± 0.03	1.92 ± 0.10
Rosmarinus officinalis	0.33 ± 0.01	0.59 ± 0.03	0.38 ± 0.03	0.57 ± 0.03	0.47 ± 0.03	0.49 ± 0.05
Schinus molle	0.67 ± 0.07	0.67 ± 0.07	1.38 ± 0.09	1.12 ± 0.06	0.89 ± 0.05	2.3 ± 0.11
Thuja occidentalis	0.63 ± 0.03	0.96 ± 0.12	1.75 ± 0.11	1.11 ± 0.09	0.52 ± 0.02	2.51 ± 0.11
Fuconazole	0.20 ± 0.03	0.32 ± 0.01	0.27 ± 0.01	0.24 ± 0.01	0.31 ± 0.01	0.20 ± 0.01
Ketoconazole	0.39 ± 0.03	0.40 ± 0.01	0.19 ± 0.01	3.75 ± 0.07	0.40 ± 0.03	0.41 ± 0.03

sabinene in *C. macrocarpa* as well as limonene and linalool in *C. paradise*. A strong antibacterial activity of five different terpenoids was reported [49] against *Campylobacter* spp. In addition, it was previously reported that the monoterpene terpinen-4-ol enhanced the antibacterial performance of *Melaleuca alternifolia* essential oils against *S. aureus* and *E. coli* [50]. In the same trend, limonene is the major component of citrus essential oils in most species and was proven to have specific bacterial inactivation mechanism in *E. coli* and others [51] thus justifying the noticeable antibacterial activities of *C. paradisi*. However, other species studied here (*C. limon* and *C. aurantifolia*) showed slightly lower antibacterial activities which could be partially explained by lower ratios of limonene and synergetic effects with other oil constituents such as the linalool in *C. paradisi*. Some essential oils in *R. officinallis* and *O. vulgare* showed comparable antibacterial and antifungal activities to antibiotics in some cases, which may indicate that these essential oils might be useful sources of natural products

Table 5 Minimum inhibitory concentrations (MIC) of essential oils on bacterial strains

Essential oil	MIC (mg/mL)						
	B. cereus	D. solani	E. coli	L. monocytogenes	M. flavus	P. aeruginosa	S. aureus
Artemisia judaica	0.35 ± 0.01	0.39 ± 0.01	0.45 ± 0.01	0.31 ± 0.01	0.23 ± 0.03	0.16 ± 0.01	0.27 ± 0.01
Artemisia monosperma	0.43 ± 0.01	0.40 ± 0.01	0.58 ± 0.03	0.52 ± 0.01	0.31 ± 0.01	0.52 ± 0.01	0.38 ± 0.00
Callistemon viminals	0.37 ± 0.01	0.31 ± 0.01	0.49 ± 0.01	0.33 ± 0.01	0.31 ± 0.03	0.39 ± 0.01	0.41 ± 0.01
Citrus aurantifolia	0.23 ± 0.01	0.49 ± 0.01	0.21 ± 0.01	0.31 ± 0.01	0.27 ± 0.03	0.21 ± 0.01	0.25 ± 0.01
Citrus limon	0.53 ± 0.01	0.49 ± 0.01	0.27 ± 0.01	0.43 ± 0.01	0.83 ± 0.07	0.21 ± 0.01	0.43 ± 0.01
Citrus paradisi	0.15 ± 0.01	0.27 ± 0.01	0.21 ± 0.01	0.20 ± 0.01	0.13 ± 0.03	0.15 ± 0.01	0.17 ± 0.01
Cupressus macrocarpa	0.19 ± 0.01	0.29 ± 0.01	0.26 ± 0.01	0.21 ± 0.01	0.13 ± 0.03	0.19 ± 0.01	0.24 ± 0.01
Origanum vulgare	0.11 ± 0.01	0.76 ± 0.01	0.25 ± 0.01	0.40 ± 0.01	0.21 ± 0.03	0.15 ± 0.01	0.28 ± 0.01
Pelargonium graveolens	0.25 ± 0.01	0.27 ± 0.01	0.19 ± 0.01	0.25 ± 0.02	0.15 ± 0.01	0.21 ± 0.01	0.20 ± 0.01
Rosmarinus officinalis	0.40 ± 0.01	0.89 ± 0.01	0.43 ± 0.01	0.52 ± 0.01	0.25 ± 0.03	0.22 ± 0.01	0.69 ± 0.01
Schinus molle	0.29 ± 0.01	0.63 ± 0.01	0.72 ± 0.01	0.71 ± 0.03	0.42 ± 0.03	0.51 ± 0.01	0.37 ± 0.01
Thuja occidentalis	0.33 ± 0.03	0.41 ± 0.03	0.26 ± 0.01	0.31 ± 0.01	0.20 ± 0.01	0.41 ± 0.01	0.25 ± 0.01
Streptomycin	0.07 ± 0.01	0.21 ± 0.01	0.09 ± 0.01	0.18 ± 0.01	0.9 ± 0.01	0.07 ± 0.01	0.21 ± 0.01
Ampicillin	0.10 ± 0.01	0.30 ± 0.01	0.24 ± 0.01	0.18 ± 0.01	0.11 ± 0.01	0.12 ± 0.01	0.11 ± 0.01

Table 6 Minimum bactericidal concentration (MBC) of essential oils on bacterial strains

Essential oil	MBC (mg/mL)						
	B. cereus	D. solani	E. coli	L. monocytogenes	M. flavus	P. aeruginosa	S. aureus
Artemisia judaica	0.63 ± 0.03	1.13 ± 0.01	0.93 ± 0.05	0.72 ± 0.01	0.53 ± 0.03	0.31 ± 0.03	0.53 ± 0.03
Artemisia monosperma	0.89 ± 0.03	0.84 ± 0.05	1.31 ± 0.09	1.23 ± 0.09	0.71 ± 0.03	1.96 ± 0.01	0.65 ± 0.03
Callistemon viminals	0.67 ± 0.01	0.75 ± 0.01	0.91 ± 0.07	0.73 ± 0.05	0.76 ± 0.01	1.13 ± 0.09	0.96 ± 0.03
Citrus aurantifolia	0.49 ± 0.03	0.81 ± 0.03	0.47 ± 0.03	0.63 ± 0.07	0.94 ± 0.01	0.61 ± 0.01	0.53 ± 0.00
Citrus limon	1.31 ± 0.01	0.81 ± 0.01	0.49 ± 0.03	0.93 ± 0.07	> 2	0.40 ± 0.03	0.93 ± 0.05
Citrus paradisi	0.37 ± 0.01	0.61 ± 0.01	0.43 ± 0.03	0.83 ± 0.03	0.25 ± 0.01	0.31 ± 0.01	0.63 ± 0.03
Cupressus macrocarpa	0.38 ± 0.01	0.63 ± 0.01	0.51 ± 0.03	0.57 ± 0.03	0.27 ± 0.01	0.53 ± 0.03	0.47 ± 0.03
Origanum vulgare	0.21 ± 0.01	1.59 ± 0.01	0.58 ± 0.03	0.83 ± 0.03	0.42 ± 0.01	0.34 ± 0.03	0.67 ± 0.03
Pelargonium graveolens	0.59 ± 0.03	0.67 ± 0.03	0.83 ± 0.03	0.46 ± 0.03	0.33 ± 0.01	0.43 ± 0.03	0.51 ± 0.03
Rosmarinus officinalis	0.91 ± 0.01	1.81 ± 0.01	0.82 ± 0.03	1.15 ± 0.07	0.71 ± 0.01	0.93 ± 0.01	1.73 ± 0.03
Schinus molle	0.83 ± 0.01	1.57 ± 0.01	1.78 ± 0.03	> 2	0.98 ± 0.01	1.13 ± 0.01	0.89 ± 0.03
Thuja occidentalis	0.79 ± 0.05	0.83 ± 0.01	0.71 ± 0.03	0.97 ± 0.05	0.53 ± 0.01	0.94 ± 0.01	0.53 ± 0.03
Streptomycin	0.14 ± 0.01	0.40 ± 0.02	0.40 ± 0.01	0.35 ± 0.01	0.19 ± 0.01	0.15 ± 0.01	0.41 ± 0.03
Ampicillin	0.18 ± 0.01	0.55 ± 0.01	0.41 ± 0.03	0.30 ± 0.01	0.18 ± 0.01	0.25 ± 0.01	0.19 ± 0.03

for commercial applications in the pharmaceutical and food industries.

Several studies indicated that Gram-positive bacteria are less resistant than negative ones against natural products such as essential oils [52]. This resistance had been attributed to the additional outer membrane (this is likely the case in our study) and that most resistant bacterium was *D. solani*. Finally, the essential oils compositions and percentages obtained from this study are comparable to studies on geranium [53], citrus [54], *C. viminalis* [55], *R. officinallis* [47], *Artimisia* [45], and *O. vulgare* [44]. However, the essential oils composition of the current collection of horticultural crops differed in some cases from those reported in the literature for *S. molle* (mainly composed of pinene [56], *T. occidentalis* (mainly composed of thujone and fenchone [57] and *O. vulgare* (mainly composed of pulegone). Interestingly, other report on *S. molle* found that the essential oil might be composed of cubenol (27.1%) and caryophyllene oxide (15.3%) [58]. Indeed, a great diversity is known in essential oil plants due to environmental as well as genetic factors.

Few species showed promising anticancer activities against the proliferation of cancer cells. The main effect of the essential oils is attributed to main constitutes such as the capillin in *A. monosperama*, limonene in the

Table 7 In vitro antiproliferative activity [IC$_{50}$ (µg/ml)] of twelve aromatic plants essential oils on cancer cell lines

	MCF-7	HeLa	Jurkat	HT-29	T24	HEK-293
Artemisia judaica	28.51 ± 1.1	54.13 ± 1.5	63.71 ± 1.6	73.01 ± 2.1	171.13 ± 1.8	>300
Artemisia monosperma	15.15 ± 1.1	9.1 ± 0.1	11.0 ± 0.5	10.1 ± 0.5	119.0 ± 2.5	>300
Callistemon viminals	25.15 ± 0.3	18.75 ± 1.5	53.10 ± 3.5	10.51 ± 1.0	166.15 ± 2.8	>300
Citrus aurantifolia	11.11 ± 0.3	58.75 ± 1.5	17.10 ± 1.5	230.84 ± 4.1	>300	>300
Citrus limon	9.52 ± 1.6	51.04 ± 1.2	15.34 ± 1.2	231.91 ± 5.1	216.7 ± 4.1	>300
Citrus paradisi	8.1 ± 1.5	46.15 ± 1.8	14.52 ± 1.9	220 ± 5.3	113.6 ± 5.1	>400
Cupressus macrocarpa	25.4 ± 2.6	24.16 ± 1.6	30.54 ± 3.4	124.8 ± 5.2	>300	>300
Origanum vulgare	8.11 ± 1.0	13.41 ± 1.1	27.05 ± 2.1	12.18 ± 1.4	105.5 ± 2.3	>300
Pelargonium graveolens	61.0 ± 1.5	51.24 ± 3.1	178.5 ± 2.8	195.33 ± 5.4	270.13 ± 7.1	>300
Rosmarinus officinalis	36.5 ± 2.1	27.25 ± 1.5	73.11 ± 2.9	18.17 ± 2.0	118.31 ± 2.8	>300
Schinus molle	41.33 ± 2.1	119.5 ± 2.6	14.85 ± 1.7	18.35 ± 1.3	>300	>300
Thuja occidentalis	57.35 ± 2.3	22.5 ± 1.7	95.52 ± 1.3	125.5 ± 3.9	>300	>300
Vinblastine sulfate	–	2.5 ± 0.08	0.1 ± 0.05	21.4 ± 1.5	63.31 ± 1.7	51.5 ± 2.1
Taxol	0.08 ± 0.005	–	–	–	–	–

Table 8 Common names and edible parts of twelve ornamental and horticultural Egyptian plant species

Plant name	Common name	Edible/economic parts	Common uses
Artemisia judaica	Judean wormwood	Leaves and flowers	Spice, soft drink and cosmetic uses [37]
Artemisia monosperma	Delile	Leaves and flowers	Spice, soft drink and cosmetic uses [37]
Callistemon viminalis	weeping bottlebrush	Leaves and flowers	Ornamental and source of antioxidants, antifungal and antibacterial products [47]
Citrus aurantifolia	Key lime	Fruits and leaves	The fruits are eaten and the essential oils are extracted from the fruit coat. The leaves are used for medicinal puposes [46, 58]
Citrus limon	lemon	Fruits and leaves	The fruits are eaten and the essential oils are extracted from the fruit coat. The leaves are used for medicinal puposes [46, 58]
Citrus paradisi	grapefruit	Fruits and leaves	The fruits are eaten and the essential oils are extracted from the fruit coat. The leaves are used for medicinal puposes [46, 58]
Cupressus macrocarpa	Monterey cypress	Stem, leaves and cones	Ornamental and source of antioxidants, antifungal and antibacterial products [38]
Origanum vulgare	wild marjoram	Leaves and flowers	Spice, soft drink and cosmetic uses [25]
Pelargonium graveolens	Geranium	Leaves and flowers	Spice, soft drink and cosmetic uses [45]
Rosmarinus officinalis	Rosemary	Leaves and flowers	Spice, soft drink and cosmetic uses [25]
Schinus molle	American pepper	Leaves, flowers and fruits	Ornamental and source of antioxidants, antifungal and antibacterial products [48]
Thuja occidentalis	northern white-cedar	Stem, leaves and cones	Ornamental and source of antioxidants, antifungal and antibacterial products [49]

Citrus sp. and pulegone in *O. vulgare*. In agreement with our results in *Artemisia judaica* oil (mainly composed of thujone), Torres et al. [59] reported that the thujone enriched fraction has potential anticancer activities. The use of capillin (1–10 uM), isolated from *A. monosperama, inhibited* cell proliferation of HT29, MIA PaCa-2 and HEp-2 [32]. Several recent studies investigated the anticancer activities of several compounds. Murata et al. [31] found that 1, 8-cineole (the main component of *Callistemon viminals*) suppress the proliferation of colon cancer cells by inducing apoptosis (see Miller et al. [60] for in-depth review). On one hand, Shapira et al. [61] found that Terpinen-4-ol inhibited different cancer cells and Shehab and Abu-Gharbieh, [62] suggested that the essential oil of *Micromeria Fruticosa* L. (58.5% pulegone) has antitumor activities against Human Colon Cancer and MCF7 with IC$_{50}$ at 10 and 12.7 µg/Ml, respectively. Fayed [63] on the other hand reported that geranium essential oil (29.90% citronellol) had the highest anticancer activity with the LC$_{50}$ values of 62.50 µg/ml in NB4 cell line and 86.5 µg/ml in HL-60 cell line whereas Lin et al. [64] reported that α-Phellandrene found in *Schinus molle* influenced cell cycle and apoptosis in murine leukemia WEHI-3 cells. Chen et al. [65, 66] found that α-pinene has antitumor activities through inducing cell cycle arrest.

We aimed to highlight the biological activities in ornamental and horticultural aromatic plants against pathogenic microbes in the Mediterranean region. We demonstrated their antioxidant activities by two different methods and their promising role as natural antioxidant resources. One of the important factors influencing the decision of the farmer to grow specific horticultural crop is the availability of different ways of marketing such as the use of the whole crop as a fresh crop or the use of the essential oil for the pharmaceutical industries (Table 8). Here the bioactivity that we found for these crops is an added value that may encourage farmers to grow these crops and increase the marketing possibilities of their end crops. On the medical level, the pharmaceutical values of those medical crops are promising for pathogenic diseases and human cancer control.

Conclusion

O. vulgare had the best antioxidant and antibacterial activities with a high and unique pulegone ratio (77.45%). The essential oil of *R. officinallis* essential oil showed the highest antifungal activities by means of lowest MIC and MFC values which might be attributed to 1,8-cineole, camphor and α-pinene. The essential oils of *O. vulgare*, *Citrus* sp. and *A. monosperma* showed the highest antiproliferation activities against different cancer cells. Oxygenated monoterpenes (i.e. linalool and pulegone) as well as monoterpene hydrocarbons including pinenes plays a pivotal role in the antioxidant, antibacterial, antifungal and anticancer activities of the essential oils of different horticultural aromatic plants. Some species showed antioxidant and antimicrobial activities comparable to standard compounds, which may indicate that these crops are valuable resources of natural compounds useful for pharmaceutical and food industries.

Acknowledgments

The authors would like to extend their sincere appreciation to the Deanship of Scientific Research at King Saud University, Saudi Arabia through research group No (RG 1436-020). The Faculty of Agriculture, Alexandria University (2016-2017) supported the current research.

Funding

The study was funded by the deanship of Scientific Research at King Saud University through research group No (RG 1436–020).

Authors' contributions

HOE, SAMA and EAM designed and performed the experiments. All authors contributed in validating, writing and approving the final version of the manuscript.

Competing interests

The authors declare that they have no competing interests.

Author details

[1]Plant production Department, College of Food and Agriculture Sciences, King Saud University, P.O. Box 2460, Riyadh 11451, Saudi Arabia. [2]Floriculture, Ornamental Horticulture and Garden Design Department, Faculty of Agriculture (El-Shatby), Alexandria University, Alexandria, Egypt. [3]Department of Geography, Environmental Management and Energy Studies, University of Johannesburg, Auckland Park Kingsway Campus (APK) campus 2006, South Africa. [4]Department of Pesticide Chemistry and Technology, Faculty of Agriculture, Alexandria University, ElShatby, Alexandria 21545, Egypt. [5]Department of Food Industries, Damietta University, Damietta, Egypt.

References

1. Misra G, Pavlostathis SG. Biodegradation kinetics of monoterpenes in liquid and soil- slurry systems. Appl Microbiol Biotechnol. 1997;47:572–7.
2. Tripathi P, Singh V, Naik S. Immune response to Leishmania: paradox rather than paradigm. FEMS Immunol Med Microbiol. 2007;51:229–42.
3. Mau JL, Huang PN, Huang SJ, Chen CC. Antioxidant properties of methanolic extracts from two kinds of Antrodia camphorate mycelia. Food Chem. 2004;86:25–31.
4. Dai J, Zhu L, Yang L, Qiu J. Chemical composition antioxidant and antimicrobial activities of essential oil from Wedelia prostrate. EXCLI J. 2013; 12:479–90.
5. Celiktas OY, Kocabas EEH, Bedir E, Verdar SO, Baser KHC. Antimicrobial activities of methanolic extract and essential oils of Rosmarinus officinalis, depending on location and seasonal variations. Food Chem. 2007;100:553–9.
6. Bajpai KV, Dung NT, Kwon JO, Kang SC. Analysis and the potential application of essential oil and leaf extracts of Silene Americana L. to control food spoilage and foodborne pathogens. J Food Technol. 2008;227:1613–20.
7. Raeisi S, Ojagh SM, Sharifi-Rad M, Sharifi-Rad J, Quek SY. Evaluation of Allium paradoxum (M.B.) G. Don. And Eryngium caucasicum trauve. Extracts on the shelf-life and quality of silver carp (Hypophthalmichthys molitrix) fillets during refrigerated storage. J Food Saf. 2017;37(3):e12321.
8. Sharifi-Rad J, Salehi B, Stojanović-Radić ZZ, Fokou PVT, Sharifi-Rad M, Mahady GB, et al. Medicinal plants used in the treatment of tuberculosis-ethnobotanical and ethnopharmacological approaches. Biotechnol Adv 2017; S0734–9750(17)30077–0.
9. Sharifi-Rad M, Tayeboon GS, Sharifi-Rad J, Iriti M, Varoni EM, Razazi S. Inhibitory activity on type 2 diabetes and hypertension key-enzymes, and antioxidant capacity of Veronica persica phenolic-rich extracts. Cell Mol Biol (Noisy-Le-Grand). 2016;62:80–5.
10. Sharifi-Rad J, Salehi B, Varoni EM, Sharopov F, Yousaf Z, Ayatollahi SA, et al. Plants of the Melaleuca genus as antimicrobial agents: from farm to pharmacy. Phytother Res. 2017;31:1475–94.
11. Elansary HO, Szopa A, Kubica P, Ekiert H, Ali HM, Elshikh MS, et al. Bioactivities of traditional medicinal plants in Alexandria. Evid-Based Complementary Altern Med. 2018;2018:1463579.
12. Politeo O, Jukic M, Milos M. Chemical composition and antioxidant activity of essential oils of twelve spice plants. Croat Chem Acta. 2006; 79:545–52.
13. Adrar N, Oukil N, Bedjou F. Antioxidant and antibacterial activities of Thymus numidicus and Salvia officinalis essential oils alone or in combination. Ind Crop Prod. 2016;88:112–9.
14. Si Said ZB, Haddadi-Guemghar H, Boulekbache-Makhlouf L, Rigou P, Remini H, Adjaoud A, Khoudja NK, Madani K. Essential oil composition, antibacterial and antioxidant activities of hydrodistillated extract of Eucalyptus globulus fruits. Ind Crop and Prod. 2016;89:167–75.
15. Elansary HO, Yessoufou K, Shokralla S, Mahmoud EA, Skalicka-Woźniak K. Enhancing mint and basil oil composition and antibacterial activity using seaweed extracts. Ind Crop Prod. 2016;92:50–6.
16. Sharifi-Rad J, Sureda A, Tenore GC, Daglia M, Sharifi-Rad M, Valussi M, et al. Biological activities of essential oils: from plant Chemoecology to traditional healing systems. Molecules. 2017;22:70.
17. Salem MZM, Elansary HO, Ali HM, El-Settawy AA, Elshikh MS, Abdel-Salam EM, Skalicka-Wozniak K. Bioactivity of essential oils extracted from Cupressus macrocarpa branchlets and Corymbia citriodora leaves grown in Egypt. BMC Complement Altern Med. 2018;18:23.
18. Sermukhamedova O, Wojtanowski KK, Widelski J, Korona-Głowniak I, Elansary HO, Sakipova Z, Malm A, Skalicka-Woźniak K. Metabolic profile of and antimicrobial activity in the aerial part of Leonurus turkestanicus V.I. Krecz. et Kuprian. from Kazakhstan. J AOAC Int. 2017;100:1700–5.
19. Radonic A, Milos M. Chemical composition and in vitro evaluation of antioxidant effect of free volatile compounds from Satureja montana L. Free Radic Res. 2003;37:673–9.
20. Kulisic T, Radonic A, Katalinic V, Milos M. Use of different methods for testing antioxidative activity of oregano essential oil. Food Chem. 2004;85:633–40.
21. Jerbi A, Zehri S, Abdnnabi R, Gharsallah N, Kammoun M. Essential oil composition, free-radical-scavenging and antibacterial effect from stems of Ephedra alata alenda in Tunisia. J Essent Oil Bear Plants. 2016;19: 1503–9.
22. Bhat G, Rassol S, Rehman S, Ganaie M, Qazi PH, Shawl AS. Seasonal variation in chemical composition, antibacterial and antioxidant activities of the essential oil of leaves of Salvia officinalis (sage) from Kashmir, India. J Essent Oil Bearing Plant. 2016;19:1129–40.
23. Sartoratto A, Machado ALM, Delarmelina C, Figueira GM, Dusrte MCT, Rehder VLG. Composition and antimicrobial activity of essential oils from aromatic plants used in Brazil. Braz J Microb. 2004;35:275–80.
24. Sonboli A, Eftekhar F, Yousefzadi M, Kanani MR. Antibacterial activity and chemical composition of the essential oil of Grammosciadium platycarpum Boiss. From Iran. Z Naturforsch. 2005;60:30–4.
25. Soković M, Marin PD, Brkić D, Griensven LJ. Chemical composition and antibacterial activity of essential oils of ten aromatic plants against human pathogenic bacteria. Food. 2007;1:220–6.
26. Celikel N, Kavas G. Antimicrobial properties of some essential oils against some pathogenic microorganisms. Czech J Food Sci. 2008;26:174–81.
27. Jnaid Y, Yacoub R, Al-Biski F. Antioxidant and antimicrobial activities of Origanum vulgare essential oil. Int Food Res J. 2016;23:1706–10.
28. Cho S, Lee E, Kim S, Lee H. Essential oil of Pinus koraiensis inhibits cell proliferation and migration via inhibition of p21-activated kinase 1 pathway in HCT116 colorectal cancer cells. BMC. BMC Complement Altern Med. 2014;14:275.
29. Rebouças de Araújo ID, Coriolano de Aquino N, Guerra ACV, Júnior RF, Araújo RM, Júnior RF, Farias KJS, Fernandes JV, Andrade SV. Chemical

composition and evaluation of the antibacterial and cytotoxic activities of the essential oil from the leaves of Myracrodruon urundeuva. BMC Complement Altern Med. 2017;17:419.

30. Mothana RA, Lindequist U, Gruenert R, Bednarski PJ. Studies of the in vitro anticancer, antimicrobial and antioxidant potentials of selected Yemeni medicinal plants from the island Soqotra. BMC Complement Altern Med. 2009;9:7.

31. Murata S, Shiragami R, Kosugi C, Tezuka T, Yamazaki M, Hirano A, Yoshimura Y, Suzuki M, Shuto K, Ohkohchi N, Koda K. Antitumor effect of 1, 8-cineole against colon cancer. Oncol Rep. 2013;30(6):2647–52.

32. Lee G, Park H-G, Choi M-L, Kim YH, Park YB, Song K-S, Cheong C, Bae Y-S. Falcarindiol, a Polyacetylenic compound isolated from Peucedanum japonicum, Inhibits Mammalian DNA Topoisomerase I. J Microbiol Biotechnol. 2000;10:394–8.

33. Elansary HO, Mahmoud EA, Shokralla S, Yessoufou K. Diversity of plants, traditional knowledge and practices in local cosmetics: a case study from Alexandria, Egypt. Econ Bot. 2015;69:114–26.

34. AbouZid SF, Mohamed AA. Survey on medicinal plants and spices used in Beni-Sueif, upper Egypt. J Ethnobiol Ethnomed. 2011;7:18.

35. Elansary HO, Mahmoud EA. Basil cultivar identification using chemotyping still favored over genotyping using core barcodes and possible resources of antioxidants. J Essent Oil Res. 2015;27:82–7.

36. Espinel-Ingroff A. Comparison of the E-test with the NCCLS M38-P method for antifungal susceptibility testing of common and emerging pathogenic filamentous fungi. J Clini Microbiol. 2001;39:1360–7.

37. Mosmann T. Rapid colorimetric assay for cellular growth and survival: application to proliferation and cytotoxicity assays. Immunol Methods. 1983;65:55–63.

38. Parry J, Su L, Moore J, Cheng Z, Luther M, Rao JN, Wang J-Y, Yu LL. Antiproliferative activities of selected fruit seed flours. J Agric Food Chem. 2006;54:3773–8.

39. Crockett SL. Essential oil and volatile components of the genus Hypericum (Hypericaceae). Nat Prod Commun. 2010;5:1493–506.

40. Sharma A, Cannoo DS. Phytochemical composition of essential oils isolated from different species of genus Nepeta of Labiatae family: a review. Pharmacophore. 2013;4:181–211.

41. Elansary HO. Basil morphological and physiological performance under trinexapac-ethyl foliar sprays and prolonged irrigation intervals. Acta Physiol Plant. 2015;37:1–13.

42. Mkaddem M, Bouajila J, Ennajar M, Lebrhi A, Mathieu F, Romdhane M. Chemical composition and antimicrobial and antioxidant activities of Mentha (longifolia L. and viridis) essential oils. J Food Sci. 2009;74:358–63.

43. Elansary HO, Ashmawy NA. Essential oils of mint between benefits and hazards. J Essent Oil Bearing Plant. 2013;16:429–38.

44. Saghi H, Bahador A, Khaledi A, Kachoei RA, Dastjerdi AF, Esmaeili D. Antibacterial effects of Origanum vulgare essence against multidrug-resistant Acinetobacter baumannii isolated from selected hospitals of Tehran. Iran Avicenna J Clin Microb Infec. 2015;2:e22982.

45. Mahmoubi M, Valian M, Kazempour N. Chemical composition, antioxidant and antimicrobial activity of Artemisia sieberi oils from different parts of Iran and France. J Essent Oil Res. 2015;27:140–7.

46. Elansary HO, Salem MZM, Ashmawy NA, Yacout M. Chemical composition, antimicrobial and antioxidant activities of Lantana camara, Cupressus sempervirens and Syzygium cumini leaves oils from Egypt. J Agric Sci. 2012;4:144–52.

47. Takayama C, de-Faria FM, de Almeida ACA, Dunder RJ, Manzo LP, Socca EAR, Batista LM, Salvador MJ, Souza-Brito ARM, Luiz-Ferreira A. Chemical composition of Rosmarinus officinalis essential oil and antioxidant action against gastric damage induced by absolute ethanol in the rat. Asian Pac J Trop Biomed. 2016;6:677–81.

48. Morcia C, Malnati M, Terzi V. In vitro antifungal activity of terpinen-4-ol, eugenol, carvone, 1,8-cineole (eucalyptol) and thymol against mycotoxigenic plant pathogens. Food Addit Contam Part A Chem Anal Control Expo Risk Assess. 2012;29:415–22.

49. Kurekci C, Padmanabha J, Bishop-Hurley SL, Hassan E, Al Jassim RA, McSweeney CS. Antimicrobial activity of essential oils and five terpenoid compounds against Campylobacter jejuni in pure and mixed culture experiments. Int J Food Microbiol. 2013;166:450–7.

50. Hammer KA, Carson CF, Riley TV. Effects of Melaleuca alternifolia (tea tree) essential oil and the major monoterpene component terpinen-4-ol on the development of single- and multistep antibiotic resistance and antimicrobial susceptibility. Antimicrob Agents Chemother. 2012;56:909–15.

51. Espina L, Gelaw TK, de Lamo-Castellví S, Pagán R, García-Gonzalo D. Mechanism of bacterial inactivation by (+)-limonene and its potential use in food preservation combined processes. PLoS One. 2013;8:e56769.

52. Aelenei P, Miron A, Trifan A, Bujor A, Gille E, Aprotosoaie AC. Essential oils and their components as modulators of antibiotic activity against gram-negative bacteria. Medicines. 2016;3:1–34.

53. Sharopov FS, Zhang H, Setzer WN. Composition of geranium (Pelargonium graveolens) essential oil from Tajikistan. American J Essen Oils Nat Prod. 2014;2:13–6.

54. Dejnane D. Chemical profile, antibacterial and antioxidant activity of Algerian citrus essential oils and their application in Sardina pilchardus. Foods. 2015;4:208–28.

55. Salem MZM, El-Hefny M, Nasser R, Ali HM, El-Shanhorey NA, Elansary HO. Medicinal and biological values of Callistemon viminalis extracts: history, current situation and prospects. Asian Pacific J Trop Med. 2017;10:229–37.

56. Diaz C, Quesada S, Brenes O, Aguilar G, Ciccio JF. Chemical composition of Schinus molle essential oil and its cytotoxic activity on tumour cell lines. Nat Prod Res. 2008;22:1521–34.

57. Svajdlenka E, Mártonfi P, Tomasko I, Grancai D, Nagy M. Essential oil compostion of Thuja occidentalis L. samples from Slovakia. J Essn Oil Res. 1998;11:532–6.

58. Cavalcanti AS, Alves MS, Paulo da Silva LC, Sanches MN, Chaves DSA, Alves de Souza MA. Volatiles composition and extraction kinetics from Schinus terebinthifolius and Schinus molle leaves and fruit. Rev Bras Farm. 2015;25: 356–62.

59. Torres A, Vargas Y, Uribe D, Carrasco C, Torres C, Rocha R, Oyarzún C, San Martín R, Quezada C. Pro-apoptotic and anti-angiogenic properties of the α/β-thujone fraction from Thuja occidentalis on glioblastoma cells. J Neuro-Oncol. 2016;128:9–19.

60. Miller JA, Thompson PA, Hakim IA, Chow HS, Thomson CA. D-limonene: a bioactive food component from citrus and evidence for a potential role in breast cancer prevention and treatment. Oncol Rev. 2011;5:31–42.

61. Shapira S, Pleban S, Kazanov D, Tirosh P, Arber N. Terpinen-4-ol: a novel and promising therapeutic agent for human gastrointestinal cancers. PLoS One. 2016;11:e0156540.

62. Shehab NG, Abu-Gharbieh E. Constituents and biological activity of the essential oil and the aqueous extract of Micromeria fruticosa (L.) Druce subsp. serpyllifolia. Pak J Pharm Sci. 2012;25:687–92.

63. Fayed SA. Antioxidant and anticancer activities of Citrus reticulate (Petitgrain mandarin) and Pelargonium graveolens (Geranium) essential oils. Res J Agri Biol Sci. 2009;5:740–7.

64. Lin JJ, Yu CC, Lu KW, Chang SJ, Yu FS, Liao CL, Lin JG. Chung JG.α-Phellandrene alters expression of genes associated with DNA damage, cell cycle, and apoptosis in murine leukemia WEHI-3 cells. Anticancer Res. 2014; 34:4161–80.

65. Chen W, Liu Y, Li M, Mao J, Zhang L, Huang R, Jin X, Ye L. Anti-tumor effect of α-pinene on human hepatoma cell lines through inducing G2/M cell cycle arrest. J Pharmacol Sci. 2015;127:332–8.

66. Bourgou S, Rahali FZ, Ourghemmi I, Tounsi S. Changes of peel essential oil composition of four Tunisian Citrus during fruit maturation. Scientific World J. 2012;2012:528593.

Use of biologically-based complementary medicine in breast and gynecological cancer patients during systemic therapy

Loisa Drozdoff, Evelyn Klein, Marion Kiechle and Daniela Paepke* ⓘD

Abstract

Background: Biologically-based complementary medicines (BB-CAM) including herbs and nutritional supplements are frequently taken by breast- and gynecological cancer patients undergoing systemic therapy. The aim of this study was to analyze the use of these natural CAM methods under systemic therapy.

Methods: From September 2014 to December 2014 and February 2017 to May 2017 all patients ($n= 717$) undergoing systemic therapy at the day care unit, Department of Gynecology and Obstetrics, Technical University Munich, Germany, with breast- and/or gynecological cancer were included in this survey.
The self-administered 8-item questionnaire was developed to obtain information on complementary medication intake during systemic therapy.

Results: Among 448 respondents 74.1% reported to use complementary medication simultaneous to their systemic therapy. The most frequently applied methods during therapy were vitamins and minerals supplements (72.3%), medicinal teas (46.7%), phytotherapy (30.1%), and mistletoe (25.3%).
The analysis showed that various patients-, disease- and therapy characteristics like receiving chemotherapy ($p= 0.002$), and younger age (younger than 60 years; $p=0.017$) are significantly associated with BB-CAM use.

Conclusions: Our data suggest that female cancer patients undergoing systemic therapy frequently use BB-CAM medicine. Therefore, it is indispensable to implement counseling and evidence-based complementary treatments into clinical routine of cancer centers. A counseling service for integrative medicine concepts and an outpatient program (ZIGG) was therefore implemented in our cancer center in 2013. Further research on the CAM intake of cancer patients is needed in order to verify drug interactions and implement specific guidelines for integrative medication concepts.

Background

Herbal medicine, nutritional supplements, acupuncture and many more therapies, also known as complementary and alternative medicines (CAM), have become increasingly popular and a common self-medication tool [1–5].

Furthermore, several studies have shown a great prevalence of CAM therapies in cancer patients [1–17]. The interpretation and identification of reliable data on the prevalence of complementary therapy methods is still difficult, as a consensus on the definition and terminology of CAM is still missing. [18] Ott et al. define *conventional* treatments as accepted and practiced by the mainstream medical community, *complementary* therapies as used in addition to conventional treatments, and *alternative* treatments as being used instead of conventional treatments. The best of conventional and complementary therapies are combined in integrated treatments [19].

But not only the diversity of the terminology of CAM is problematic when interpreting current literature, also the heterogeneity of considered therapies or medications makes data analysis challenging. Complementary therapy methods include a wide range of approaches and products, with some authors including only herbal medications, while others also include dietary supplements and mind-body practices. This is one reason for the enormous variability of CAM use in literature among cancer patients. This is the reason why we chose the specialized term of BB-CAM.

The prevalence of cancer patients using CAM differs from 50 to 70% in Germany, 45–49% in Australia, and

* Correspondence: Daniela.Paepke@mri.tum.de
Department of Gynecology and Obstetrics, University Hospital rechts der Isar, Technical University Munich, Ismaninger Str. 22, 81675 Munich, Germany

up to 95% in the USA [7, 9, 15–17]. A European survey conducted by Molassiotis A. et al., demonstrated that the use of CAM in cancer patients in the EU is approximately 36%. Interestingly, the percentage can be up to 90% in subgroups of cancer patients [11]. Looking at characteristics for CAM users, the data shows that female sex, young age, higher educational level and a non-metastatic disease is more often associated with CAM use [20, 21] In summary, terminology, definition and also the therapy phase is relevant for a systematic analysis of complementary health approaches in cancer patients.

The National Center for Complementary and Integrative Health (NCCIH) classified CAM treatments into two subgroups: natural products (biologically–based complementary and alternative medicine, BB-CAM), which includes dietary supplements, e.g. herbs, vitamins, minerals and probiotics, or mind and body practices, e.g. yoga, acupuncture, relaxing techniques, meditation and others. Some complementary methods such as homeopathy, Ayurveda medicine or traditional Chinese medicine do not fit into either of these two complementary health approaches [22].

The aim of the present study was to systematically analyze the use of biologically-based complementary medication (BB-CAM), such as herbs, dietary supplements and homeopathy in breast and gynecological cancer patients during systemic therapy. Here, we aimed to assess detailed information about a subgroup of BB-CAM and a special patients' cohort to increase missing evidence about this elaborate topic of CAM.

Methods

A cross-sectional descriptive survey was used to collect data about BB-CAM treatments with a questionnaire based on the categorical classification of different BB-CAM methods. The questionnaire was designed after research of actual data on BB-CAM and in consideration of studies and publications on questionnaire design as well as on CAM especially in gynecological oncology. The result was a self-administered 8-item questionnaire. We added the survey as an Additional file 1. Initially, the questionnaire was examined by professional physicians and researchers. Afterwards, it was pre-tested in a pilot project involving 10 selected cancer patients to prove comprehensibility, in particular understanding of specific terms like globules or homoeopathic potencies. It was known that some of the selected patients were users and some non-users of BB-CAM. Finally, we designed a revised 8-item questionnaire which was approved by the Ethics Committee of the Technical University of Munich (TUM) with the project number 412/14.

We calculated the number of participants that was needed to estimate the prevalence of BB-CAM with a 95% confidence interval and a confidence level of 5.0%. The sample size calculation was based on an estimated annual population of approximately 720 patients attending the chemotherapy unit within two different 3-month-periods. On the basis of these considerations and an expected 50% prevalence of BB-CAM use, we extrapolated that 245 participants are required. With an expected response rate of 60% we had to include at least 408 patients to take part in our survey. From September 2014 to December 2014, and again from February 2017 to May 2017, the questionnaire was handed out to all patients undergoing systemic therapy at the day care unit of the Department of Gynecology and Obstetrics, University Hospital rechts der Isar, Technical University of Munich (TUM), Munich, Germany. Two different survey periods were chosen in order to identify differences in the prevalence of BB-CAM during these two periods, as CAM therapies in general have become more popular. Additionally, two different time points of questioning were chosen to account for a potential increase of attendance of our ZIGG, which is rather unique for our Interdisciplinary Breast and Gynecological Cancer Center since its implementation in 2013.

Participation was voluntary and non-anonymous. Patients were eligible if they received any anticancer treatment at present, were older than 18 years, spoke German, and were physically and mentally able to complete the questionnaire.

The patients recorded conventional co-medications and complementary medications. Routinely prescribed supportive medication, such as vitamin D or calcium supplements were excluded from the analysis. Patients' cancer diagnosis and complete medical history including former and current cancer therapy was documented by the treating physician. Patients were classified as BB-CAM users if they used at least one complementary treatment at present.

Data analysis

Descriptive statistics such as mean, standard deviation, median, absolute and relative frequencies were used to describe the distribution of the socio demographic and illness or treatment related characteristics of patients. Hypothesis testing on differences between BB-CAM users and non-users was performed with two-sample t tests and chi-square tests. The relation of patients' age and therapy characteristics to BB-CAM use was analyzed by multivariable logistic regression. Only completely filled-out questionnaires were analyzed. All analyses were conducted with IBM® SPSS® Statistics for Windows, Version 24 (IBM Corp., Armonk, N.Y., USA). Statistical analysis was done in cooperation with the Institute of Medical Informatics, Statistics and Epidemiology, TU Munich.

Results

Four hundred forty-eight (62.5%) of 717 patients participated and completed the survey. After analyzing different time periods separately, we noticed just negligible differences and decided to collect the data and perform calculation of all patients collectively.

With respect to demographics, the cohorts mean age was 62.2 ± 12.4 years. With the exception of one man, all patients were women.

The vast majority of the 362 patients (80.8%) suffered from breast cancer as the primary cancer site.

More than one-third of the patients (171/448; 38.2%) had an early stage cancer and the majority (61.8%) a metastatic and/or recurrent disease, independent of their cancer type. Table 1 shows the distribution of the survey participants´ age and disease characteristics.

62.1% ($n = 278$) of responding patients received CTX, whereas 43.8% ($n = 196$) of the patients were treated with antibodies, 33.5% ($n = 150$) hormone therapy, and 28.8% ($n = 129$) received treatment with bisphosphonates. Various combinations of more than one systemic therapy per patient were possible. The medians of co-medication of users and non-users were nearly similar (2.55 (non-user) vs. 2.51 (user)). The therapy related characteristics of the patients are presented in Table 2.

With respect to prevalence and predictors of BB-CAM use, the majority (74.1%; $n = 332$) of the population surveyed declared that they were currently using BB-CAM during systemic cancer therapy. As far as the different treatment types are concerned, it showed that vitamins and mineral supplements (72.3%; $n = 240$), medicinal teas (46.7%; $n = 155$), homeopathy (34.0%; $n = 113$), phytotherapy (30.1%; $n = 100$), and mistletoe (25.3%; $n = 84$) were frequently used. These findings comparing the use of different treatments are illustrated in Fig. 1.

The category "Other" (13.6%; $n = 45$) included special nutritional supplements in particular. Various combinations of more than one BB-CAM method per patient were also possible.

When evaluating the patients' variables associated with BB-CAM use by applying univariable analysis, we noticed that 79.1% of the patients who were receiving chemotherapy used BB-CAM significantly more often (79,1 vs. 65,9%; $p = 0,002$). In this patient group especially mistletoe was used (24,8 vs. 8,8%; $p = < 0,001$). In contrast, patients receiving endocrine therapy and/or bisphosphonates as a systemic therapy applied significantly fewer complementary methods (endocrine: 66,7 vs. 77,9% $p = 0,011$; bisphosphonates: 67,4 vs. 76,8% $p = 0,041$). Similar results of less intake are seen when comparing the use of mistletoe treatments with endocrine or bisphosphonate medication (8.7% and 10.9%, respectively). Furthermore, significant differences become evident upon analyzing the patients´ age. Here, patients in the age group below or equal to 60 years (79.8 vs. 69.9%; $p = 0.017$) use BB-CAM significant more often than patients older than 60 years.

By analyzing patients' age and therapy characteristics by applying multivariable logistic regression we found that patients older than 60 years had 0.61 lower odds than patients below or equal to 60 years

Table 1 Selected patients- and disease characteristics of the total study cohort with univariable analyses of BB-CAM use

CHARACTERISTICS		ALL PATIENTS		BB-CAM				p^1
				User		Non-user		
		Total Count	% of all patients	Count	% of Total	Count	% of Total	
		448	**100%**	332	74.1%	116	25.9%	
Patients								
Age in years (mean ± SD)		62.2 ± 12.4		61.5 ± 12.5		64.1 ± 12.1		0.378
	≤60 yrs.	193	43.1%	154	79.8%	39	20.2%	*0.017*
	>60 yrs.	255	56.9%	77	30.2%	178	69.8%	
Disease								0.168
Breast-Ca	Early Stage	147	32.8%	114	77.6%	33	22.4%	
	Advanced	201	44.9%	141	70.1%	60	29.9%	
	Recurrence	13	2.9%	9	69.2%	4	30.8%	
Ovarian-Ca	FIGO I-III	23	5.1%	21	91.3%	2	8.7%	
	FIGO IV	15	3.3%	9	60.0%	6	40.0%	
	Recurrence	37	8.3%	30	81.1%	7	18.9%	
Other Gyn-Ca		12	2.7%	8	66.7%	4	33.3%	
Disease state	Early Stage	171	38.2%	135	78.9%	36	21.1%	0.066
	Advanced+ Recurrence	277	61.8%	197	71.1%	80	28.9%	

[1] p values are not adjusted for multiplicity and have to be interpreted to be exploratory

Table 2 Selected therapy characteristics of the total study cohort with univariable analyses of BB-CAM use

CHARACTERISTICS			ALL PATIENTS		BB-CAM				p^1
					User		Non-user		
			Total Count	% of all patients	Count	% of Total	Count	% of Total	
			448	100%	332	74.1%	116	25.9%	
Therapy line									0.053
Breast-Ca	Neoadjuvant		70	15.6%	58	82.9%	12	17.1%	
	Adjuvant		89	19.9%	64	71.9%	25	28.1%	
	Metastasis 1st -line		78	17.4%	45	57.7%	33	42.3%	
	Metastasis 2nd -line		50	11.2%	37	74.0%	13	26.0%	
	Metastasis 3rd -line		20	4.5%	17	85.0%	3	15.0%	
	Metastasis ≥4th -line		53	11.8%	42	79.2%	11	20.8%	
	Recurrence 1st -line		8	1.8%	6	75.0%	2	25.0%	
	Recurrence ≥ 2nd -line		5	1.1%	3	60.0%	2	40.0%	
Ovarian-Ca	Neoadjuvant		1	0.2%	1	100.0%	0	0.0%	
	Adjuvant		37	8.3%	29	78.4%	8	21.6%	
	Recurrent		37	8.3%	30	81.1%	7	18.9%	
Therapy									
Immune modulation			2	0.4%	2	100.0%	0	0.0%	0.402
Chemotherapy			278	62.1%	220	79.1%	58	20.9%	*0.002*
Antibodies			196	43.8%	143	73.0%	53	27.0%	0.625
Endocrine			150	33.5%	100	66.7%	50	33.3%	*0.011*
Bisphosphonates			129	28.8%	87	67.4%	42	32.6%	*0.041*

^1p values are not adjusted for multiplicity and have to be interpreted to be exploratory

(95% CI: 0.39–0.97; $p = 0.038$) and breast cancer patients in metastatic first-line therapy had 0.39 times lower odds than the reference (95% CI: 0.15–0.94). Logistic regression thus suggests that BB-CAM use is significantly unlikely in these patient groups (Table 3). When comparing survey years (2014 vs. 2017), only a negligible difference was seen in the prevalence of BB-CAM use (71.5 vs. 75.2%; $p = 0.409$).

More importantly, there were 82 patients who used BB-CAM (82/332; 24.6%) as they had been participating in a further study design. It is also noteworthy that 23.4% ($n = 105/448$) of the patients surveyed and 31.3% ($n = 104/332$) of the BB-CAM users used the opportunity of consultation for CAM usage in our clinic (ZIGG). A notable increase was seen in the attendance of ZIGG within the survey time. In 2014, 25 patients (18.2%) took part in the integrative medicine counseling service of our clinic. After 3 years, i.e. in 2017, this number increased to 80 patients (25.7%). Despite the increased ZIGG attendance (7.5%) of our patients during the

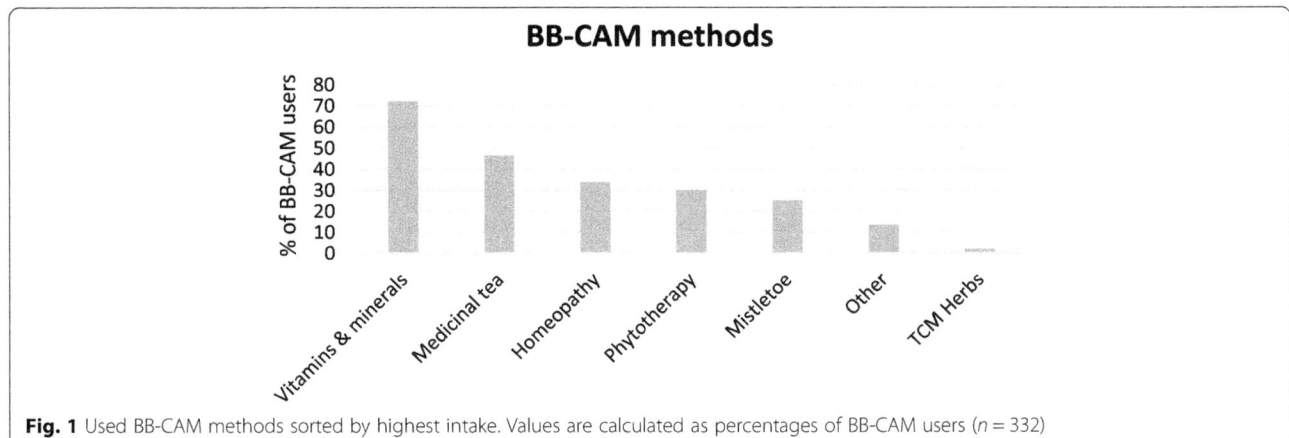

Fig. 1 Used BB-CAM methods sorted by highest intake. Values are calculated as percentages of BB-CAM users ($n = 332$)

Table 3 Bivariate logistic regression model with odds of use of BB-CAM, adjusted for selected patients´ characteristics

CHARACTERISTICS		BB-CAM USE			
		Odds ratio	95% CI		p
			Lower	Upper	
Age (years)					
≤60 yrs.		1.00 (Reference)			
>60 yrs.		.612	.385	.972	*.038*
Therapy					
Bisphosphonates	No medication	1.00 (Reference)			
	Medication	.975	.532	1.787	.934
Antibodies	No medication	1.00 (Reference)			
	Medication	.875	.503	1.521	.635
Endocrine	No medication	1.00 (Reference)			
	Medication	1.018	.547	1.895	.955
Chemotherapy	No medication	1.00 (Reference)			
	Medication	1.576	.879	2.824	.126
Therapy line					.390
Breast-Ca	Neoadjuvant	1.00 (Reference)			
	Adjuvant	.766	.316	1.857	
	Metastasis 1st-line	**.394**	**.159**	**.973**	
	Metastasis 2nd-line	.823	.302	2.242	
	Metastasis 3rd-line	1.649	.384	7.073	
	Metastasis ≥4th-line	.948	.355	2.530	
	Recurrence 1st-line	.892	.149	5.320	
	Recurrence ≥2nd-line	.372	.054	2.544	
Ovarian-Ca	Adjuvant	1.072	.371	3.099	
	Recurrent	1.035	.363	2.955	

two survey periods, the prevalence of BB-CAM usage in the two surveyed cohorts had not changed remarkable.

Discussion

In addition to the growing evidence for the widespread use of CAM, our data suggest a frequent use of biologically based complementary medicine during systemic therapy among patients with breast and gynecological cancer. In our survey population three-quarters (74.1%) of the responding patients reported an ongoing use of BB-CAM. In view of the literature, this is an overall high number. CAM use may have increased in recent years. A study from 1994 [6] suggested that CAM use in gynecological cancer patients in the UK was around 16%, whereas another previous study from 2006 reported a prevalence of 40% among comparable cancer patients in Europe [13]. The group of Horneber et al.

also found an increase in the prevalence of CAM use from an estimated 25% in the 1970s to about 50% in the year 2000 among patients with breast cancer [7]. This information is important for clinicians as it emphasizes that their patients frequently use CAM.

Many studies have tried to characterize a typical profile of a CAM user according to sociodemographic or disease-related data. Young female patients with a higher education suffering from breast cancer are often associated with a frequent use of CAM [8, 17, 20, 21, 23]. However, other studies failed to reveal any significant correlations between gender, cancer diagnosis, age and educational level [9, 12, 24]. Accordingly, our data suggest that CAM use is more popular among patients younger than 60 years.

Furthermore, we investigated that patients in the therapy setting of a first-line metastatic breast cancer therapy were undergoing less BB-CAM treatments than other patients. Nonetheless, our data also show that breast cancer patients in a neoadjuvant therapy setting (82.9% BB-CAM users), or patients in a metastasis third-line therapy (85.0% BB-CAM users), take BB-CAM more commonly than patients during other therapy lines. Divergent data exist concerning the association of therapy lines with CAM use. A study in 2015 reported that receiving adjuvant chemotherapy is associated with frequent CAM use [25], while Fremd et al. showed that patients in further therapy lines of metastatic breast cancer demonstrated increased CAM user rates [20]. Consequently, we could not support or falsify any of the published reports in total. The present study proposes that metastatic breast cancer patients are less willing to use BB-CAM while they are receiving first-line therapy (57.7% of the patients using BB-CAM) compared to patients during advanced therapy lines. This fact may support the observed correlation of Fremd et al. who reported higher rates of CAM user in further metastatic therapy lines.

The by far most commonly used CAM therapies are biologically-based complementary treatments. Wilkinson et al. reported vitamin/mineral supplement as the most frequently used therapy, followed by herbs, chiropractic and massage therapy [17]; in contrast, praying followed by BB-CAM were most often used in a German Comprehensive Cancer Centre [20]. Our findings confirm earlier studies reported in the literature documenting the regular use of BB-CAM [13, 17, 26, 27]. This frequent use is of some concern, as a number of herbs might interact with conventional drugs or produce a variable degree of toxicity. There is an urgent need to evaluate the effects of commonly used remedies and assess their toxicity profile. With our data serving as background, it is important to take into consideration that cancer patients expect the oncologist to be the medical provider of advice and treatment in the context of CAM [28]. In contrast, only 50% of practicing oncologists state to be interested in CAM and 77% rate their level of skills as insufficient [29]. According to recent data, 70% of the patients reported that their oncologist did not take time to discuss CAM treatment options [8]. The information of using BB-CAM is also really important for professionals, especially during an ongoing study design. We could not find any data about this variable in past researches. However, our data confirm that 24.7% of the BB-CAM users had been concomitantly participating in a further study design. This can lead to distortions of the study results and further mistakes in the future treatment of patients. Previous studies showed that information about CAM most frequently came from informal and uncontrolled sources like friends/family and media [30]. In our study cohort almost one third (31.6%) of the BB-CAM users took part a specific counseling program (ZIGG) and therefore were advised professionally.

The integrative consultation program was established at our University Hospital rechts der Isar in 2013 for gynecologic and obstetric patients to create a reliable therapy setting between CAM and conventional drugs. Gynecologists, oncologists and trained nurses work together in an interdisciplinary team to achieve the best comprehensive care for patients. Special skills in phytotherapy, homeopathy, anthroposophical medicine and other CAM treatments contribute to the indispensable know-how of professionals working in such an integrative center. The routine anamnesis should be completed by explicit questions about the use of CAM methods. Good communication skills and an open discussion about CAM issues are the key to protect patients from an inappropriate, unhelpful or even dangerous use of CAM.

One of the study's limitations is that we did not collect more data on patients' sociodemographic aspects and their motivations for using BB-CAM. Studies suggest that patients are looking for different benefits from CAM, for example, to improve the immune system, reduce side effects, and not miss an opportunity for well-being [26, 27]. It would be interesting for future research to analyze patients´ choice of CAM treatment and the contributing factors. Another limitation lies in the study cohort itself. Due to the fact that a structured integrative consultations program exists at the clinic, more patients are becoming aware of integrative therapies and are possibly more likely to use BB-CAMs. Furthermore, we cannot exclude recall bias, because BB-CAM intake was based on self-report.

Conclusion

In comparison to other studies, usage of BB-CAM concomitant with systemic therapy in our department is considered to be common. Although there is a positive trend in using the opportunity of CAM counseling, there are still many patients using BB-CAM without any professional expertise at all. Further research on the safety and efficiency of CAM has to be established to base professional counseling on an extensive evidence of CAM. An implementation of standard operating procedures for CAM counseling in cancer centers and the adjustment of postgraduate medical education will be beneficial for patient management and likely to increase patient satisfaction.

Acknowledgments
We would like to thank all patients who participated in the survey.

Funding
This work was supported by the German Research Foundation (DFG) and the Technical University of Munich (TUM) in the framework of the Open Access Publishing Program.

Authors' contributions
DP conceived of the presented idea, developed the theoretical formalism and designed the study. LD carried out the study, performed the computations and wrote the manuscript with support from EK and DP. MK supervised the project. All authors discussed the results and contributed to the final manuscript. All authors read and approved the final manuscript.

Competing interests
The authors declare that they have no competing interest.

References

1. Eisenberg DM, Davis RB, Ettner SL, Appel S, Wilkey S, Van Rompay M, Kessler RC. Trends in alternative medicine use in the United States, 1990-1997: results of a follow-up national survey. Jama. 1998;280(18):1569–75.
2. Gavin JA, Boon H. CAM in Canada: places, practices, research. Complement Ther Clin Pract. 2005;11(1):21–7.
3. McFarland B, Bigelow D, Zani B, Newsom J, Kaplan M. Complementary and alternative medicine use in Canada and the United States. Am J Public Health. 2002;92(10):1616–8.
4. Xue CC, Zhang AL, Lin V, Da Costa C, Story DF. Complementary and alternative medicine use in Australia: a national population-based survey. J Altern Complement Med. 2007;13(6):643–50.
5. Zollman C, Vickers A. ABC of complementary medicine. Users and practitioners of complementary medicine. BMJ. 1999;319(7213):836–8.
6. Downer SM, Cody MM, McCluskey P, Wilson PD, Arnott SJ, Lister TA, Slevin ML. Pursuit and practice of complementary therapies by cancer patients receiving conventional treatment. BMJ. 1994;309(6947):86–9.
7. Horneber M, Bueschel G, Dennert G, Less D, Ritter E, Zwahlen M. How many cancer patients use complementary and alternative medicine: a systematic review and metaanalysis. Integr Cancer Ther. 2012;11(3):187–203.
8. Huebner J, Muenstedt K, Prott FJ, Stoll C, Micke O, Buentzel J, Muecke R, Senf B. Online survey of patients with breast cancer on complementary and alternative medicine. Breast Care (Basel). 2014;9(1):60–3.
9. Huebner J, Prott FJ, Micke O, Muecke R, Senf B, Dennert G, Muenstedt K. Online survey of cancer patients on complementary and alternative medicine. Oncol Res Treat. 2014;37(6):304–8.
10. Jacobson JS, Verret WJ. Complementary and alternative therapy for breast cancer: the evidence so far. Cancer Pract. 2001;9(6):307–10.
11. Molassiotis A, Fernadez-Ortega P, Pud D, Ozden G, Scott JA, Panteli V, Margulies A, Browall M, Magri M, Selvekerova S, et al. Use of complementary and alternative medicine in cancer patients: a European survey. Ann Oncol. 2005;16(4):655–63.
12. Molassiotis A, Ozden G, Platin N, Scott JA, Pud D, Fernandez-Ortega P, Milovics L, Panteli V, Gudmundsdottir G, Browall M, et al. Complementary and alternative medicine use in patients with head and neck cancers in Europe. Eur J Cancer Care (Engl). 2006;15(1):19–24.
13. Molassiotis A, Scott JA, Kearney N, Pud D, Magri M, Selvekerova S, Bruyns I, Fernadez-Ortega P, Panteli V, Margulies A, et al. Complementary and alternative medicine use in breast cancer patients in Europe. Support Care Cancer. 2006;14(3):260–7.
14. Navo MA, Phan J, Vaughan C, Palmer JL, Michaud L, Jones KL, Bodurka DC, Basen-Engquist K, Hortobagyi GN, Kavanagh JJ, et al. An assessment of the utilization of complementary and alternative medication in women with gynecologic or breast malignancies. J Clin Oncol. 2004;22(4):671–7.
15. Rausch SM, Winegardner F, Kruk KM, Phatak V, Wahner-Roedler DL, Bauer B, Vincent A. Complementary and alternative medicine: use and disclosure in radiation oncology community practice. Support Care Cancer. 2011;19(4):521–9.
16. Smith PJ, Clavarino AM, Long JE, Anstey CM, Steadman KJ. Complementary and alternative medicine use by patients receiving curative-intent chemotherapy. Asia Pac J Clin Oncol. 2016;12(3):265–74.
17. Wilkinson JM, Stevens MJ. Use of complementary and alternative medical therapies (CAM) by patients attending a regional comprehensive cancer care Centre. J Complement Integr Med. 2014;11(2):139–45.
18. Posadzki P, Watson LK, Alotaibi A, Ernst E. Prevalence of use of complementary and alternative medicine (CAM) by patients/consumers in the UK: systematic review of surveys. Clin Med (Lond). 2013;13(2):126–31.
19. Ott MJ. Complementary and alternative therapies in cancer symptom management. Cancer Pract. 2002;10(3):162–6.
20. Fremd C, Hack CC, Schneeweiss A, Rauch G, Wallwiener D, Brucker SY, Taran FA, Hartkopf A, Overkamp F, Tesch H, et al. Use of complementary and integrative medicine among German breast cancer patients: predictors and implications for patient care within the PRAEGNANT study network. Arch Gynecol Obstet. 2017;295(5):1239–45.
21. Judson PL, Abdallah R, Xiong Y, Ebbert J, Lancaster JM. Complementary and alternative medicine use in individuals presenting for Care at a Comprehensive Cancer Center. Integr Cancer Ther. 2017;16(1):96–103.
22. Complementary, Alternative, or Integrative Health: What do these terms mean? [https://nccih.nih.gov/health/integrative-health].
23. Eschiti VS. Lesson from comparison of CAM use by women with female-specific cancers to others: it's time to focus on interaction risks with CAM therapies. Integr Cancer Ther. 2007;6(4):313–44.
24. Zhang Y, Leach MJ, Hall H, Sundberg T, Ward L, Sibbritt D, Adams J. Differences between male and female consumers of complementary and alternative medicine in a national US population: a secondary analysis of 2012 NIHS data. Evid Based Complement Alternat Med. 2015;2015:413173.
25. Strizich G, Gammon MD, Jacobson JS, Wall M, Abrahamson P, Bradshaw PT, Terry MB, Teitelbaum S, Neugut AI, Greenlee H. Latent class analysis suggests four distinct classes of complementary medicine users among women with breast cancer. BMC Complement Altern Med. 2015;15:411.
26. Kessel KA, Lettner S, Kessel C, Bier H, Biedermann T, Friess H, Herrschbach P, Gschwend JE, Meyer B, Peschel C, et al. Use of complementary and alternative medicine (CAM) as part of the oncological treatment: survey about Patients' attitude towards CAM in a university-based oncology Center in Germany. PLoS One. 2016;11(11):e0165801.
27. Lettner S, Kessel KA, Combs SE. Complementary and alternative medicine in radiation oncology : survey of patients' attitudes. Strahlenther Onkol. 2017;193(5):419–25.
28. Munstedt K, Vogt T, Rabanus ME, Hubner J. Wishes and beliefs of cancer patients regarding counseling on integrative medicine. Breast Care (Basel). 2014;9(6):416–20.
29. Trimborn A, Senf B, Muenstedt K, Buentzel J, Micke O, Muecke R, Prott FJ, Wicker S, Huebner J. Attitude of employees of a university clinic to complementary and alternative medicine in oncology. Ann Oncol. 2013;24(10):2641–5.
30. Shen J, Andersen R, Albert PS, Wenger N, Glaspy J, Cole M, Shekelle P. Use of complementary/alternative therapies by women with advanced-stage breast cancer. BMC Complement Altern Med. 2002;2:8.

18

Adenosine and adenosine-5′-monophosphate ingestion ameliorates abnormal glucose metabolism in mice fed a high-fat diet

Ardiansyah[1,2*†] ⓘ, Yuto Inagawa[1†], Takuya Koseki[3], Afifah Zahra Agista[1], Ikuo Ikeda[4], Tomoko Goto[1], Michio Komai[1] and Hitoshi Shirakawa[1,5*]

Abstract

Background: We have previously reported that ingestion of adenosine (ADN) and adenosine-5′-monophosphate (AMP) improves abnormal glucose metabolism in the stroke-prone spontaneously hypertensive rat model of non-obesity-associated insulin resistance. In this study, we investigated the effect of ADN and AMP ingestion on glucose metabolism in mice with high-fat diet-induced obesity.

Methods: Seven-week-old C57BL/6 J mice were administered distilled water (as a control), 10 mg/L ADN, or 13 mg/L AMP via their drinking water for 14 or 25 weeks, during which they were fed a high-fat diet. Oral glucose tolerance test (OGTT) was conducted on 21-week-old mice fasted for 16 h. Insulin tolerance test (ITT) was performed on 22-week-old mice fasted for 3 h. Blood and muscle were collected for further analysis of serum parameters, gene and protein expression levels, respectively.

Results: Glucose metabolism in the ADN and AMP groups was significantly improved compared with the control. OGTT and ITT showed that ADN and AMP groups lower than control group. Furthermore, phosphorylation of AMP-activated protein kinase (AMPK) and mRNA levels of genes involved in lipid oxidation were enhanced in the skeletal muscle of ADN- and AMP-treated mice.

Conclusion: These results indicate that ingestion of ADN or AMP induces activation of AMPK in skeletal muscle and mitigates insulin resistance in mice with high-fat diet-induced diabetes.

Keywords: Adenosine, Adenosine-5′-monophosphate, Glucose metabolism, High-fat diet

Background

The prevalence of obesity has increased because of changing lifestyles, including dietary habits, in both developed and developing countries [1]. Hypertension, diabetes, dyslipidemia, and cardiovascular diseases associated with obesity have been recognized as diseases of worldwide importance [2, 3]. Excessive energy intake causes increased presence of non-esterified fatty acids in the blood and di-acylglycerol and palmitoyl-CoA in the liver and skeletal muscle, followed by heightened oxidative stress [4, 5], factors that are known to induce insulin resistance.

Given that insulin resistance is a major pathogenic event in the occurrence and progression of lifestyle-associated diseases, its alleviation is a key strategy for the prevention of such conditions. Adenosine-5′-monophosphate (AMP)-activated protein kinase (AMPK) has been reported to attenuate insulin resistance, since it enhances lipid oxidation and glucose uptake in the liver and skeletal muscle, in which it regulates the expression of β-oxidation-associated genes. Therefore, much attention is being paid to AMPK as a potential therapeutic target in the treatment of insulin resistance [6, 7].

* Correspondence: ardiansyah@bakrie.ac.id; shirakah@tohoku.ac.jp
†Ardiansyah and Yuto Inagawa contributed equally to this work.
[1]Laboratory of Nutrition, Graduate School of Agricultural Science, Tohoku University, Sendai 980-0845, Japan
Full list of author information is available at the end of the article

Adenosine (ADN) is an endogenous purine nucleoside but also derives from AMP in food via the action of nucleotidase in the small intestine, from which it is absorbed into the body. Cellular ADN levels are regulated by both efflux and influx transporters [8, 9], and this molecule participates in diverse cellular functions, including the inflammatory immune response and lipid metabolism in the liver [10–12].

Various studies have provided evidence to support the role of ADN in health. For example, studies in both rats and humans demonstrated that oral ingestion of ADN in sucrose solutions significantly decreased blood glucose and insulin levels through inhibition of α-glucosidase activity by ADN [13, 14]. ADN has the capacity to attenuate the proliferation of both human and rat glomerular mesangial cells, which are related to hypertension and diabetes [15]. Furthermore, prior research using Sprague–Dawley rats has shown that ADN attenuates high-fat diet-induced increases in blood glucose and insulin, suppresses elevation of plasma corticosterone levels, rectifies altered nutrient transporter expression profiles, and prevents upregulation of TNF-α in the intestine [16]. On the other hand, AMP is well known as a purine nucleotide and participant in ATP metabolism. It has been approved by the FDA as a food additive to block bitter taste or enhance flavor [17, 18]. In addition, the functional properties of AMP have been implicated in thermoregulation of men and induction of hypothermia through ADN receptors [19].

Our group has examined the effect of ADN and AMP administration on the stroke-prone spontaneously hypertensive rat model of non-obesity-induced hypertension and insulin resistance [20, 21]. We found that ingestion of ADN and AMP activates AMPK in skeletal muscle and ameliorates insulin resistance and impaired glucose metabolism. The aim of the present study was to investigate the influence of ADN and AMP ingestion on glucose metabolism in a mouse model of obesity-associated insulin resistance induced by a high-fat diet.

Methods
Animal experiments
Male C57BL/6 J mice (CLEA Japan Inc., Tokyo, Japan) were housed in polycarbonate cages (three mice per cage) under controlled conditions (temperature, 23 ± 3 °C; humidity, $50 \pm 10\%$; 12/12 h light/dark cycle). The mice were sorted by body weight before beginning the study, and those used in experiments were of the same weight. The experimental design of the present study was approved by the Animal Research-Animal Care Committee of Tohoku University. The mouse model of diet-induced obesity has become popular as a tools for understanding high-fat in human and the development of obesity. C57BL/6 J mice as a good model for diet-induced obesity that has correlated closely with human obesity progression [22]. All experiments were conducted in accordance with the guidelines issued by this committee and Japanese legislation (2005). The mice were acclimatized for 7 days with free access to conventional non-purified diet (F-2, Funabashi Farm Co., Ltd., Chiba, Japan) and distilled water. After this period, the 7-week-old mice were administered distilled water (control), ADN, or AMP for 14 or 25 weeks. ADN (Wako Pure Chemical Industries, Osaka, Japan) and AMP (kindly provided by Yamasa Co., Chiba, Japan) were used at 10 and 13 mg/L in distilled water, respectively. All mice received a high-fat diet (HFD32, CLEA Japan Inc.). HFD32 is super-high-fat diet with 32% of crude fat and calorie rate 60% from gross energy (fat kcal %). Food and water intake was recorded every 2 days, and body weight was measured every week during the experimental period. At the end of the experiment, mice were euthanized by decapitation after 6 h of fasting. Blood was collected, and serum was immediately separated by centrifugation and stored at − 20 °C until analysis. Skeletal muscle (the quadriceps femoris muscle) was excised and kept at − 80 °C until needed. The workflow diagram of the experiment is shown in Fig. 1.

Tolerance tests
We subjected mice in the 25-week experimental groups to both oral glucose tolerance tests (OGTT) and insulin tolerance tests (ITT). OGTT were conducted on 21-week-old mice fasted for 16 h. Blood for glucose measurement was collected from the tail vein before (0 min) and 15, 30, 60, and 120 min after administration of glucose at 2.0 g/kg body weight via a gastric tube. Blood glucose levels were measured using a StatStrip Glucose Xpress Meter (Nova Biomedical Co., Waltham, MA, USA).

ITT were performed on 22-week-old mice fasted for 3 h. Blood for glucose measurement was collected from the tail vein before (0 min) and 15, 30, and 60 min after intraperitoneal administration of insulin (Humulin R, Eli Lilly & Co., Indianapolis, IN, USA) at 0.75 U/kg body weight. Blood glucose levels were measured with a StatStrip Glucose Xpress Meter.

Serum parameters
Serum levels of glucose, triglycerides, and non-esterified fatty acids were measured by enzymatic colorimetric methods (Wako Pure Chemical Industries). Serum insulin and adiponectin levels were tested using rat insulin (Morinaga Institute of Biological Science, Inc., Yokohama, Japan) and mouse/rat adiponectin (Otsuka Co., Tokyo, Japan) ELISA kits, respectively. Blood samples were collected, centrifuged at 1870×g for 15 min at 4 °C in a centrifuge (CF7D2; Hitachi Co. Ltd., Tokyo, Japan) and stored at − 80 °C until required for later analyses.

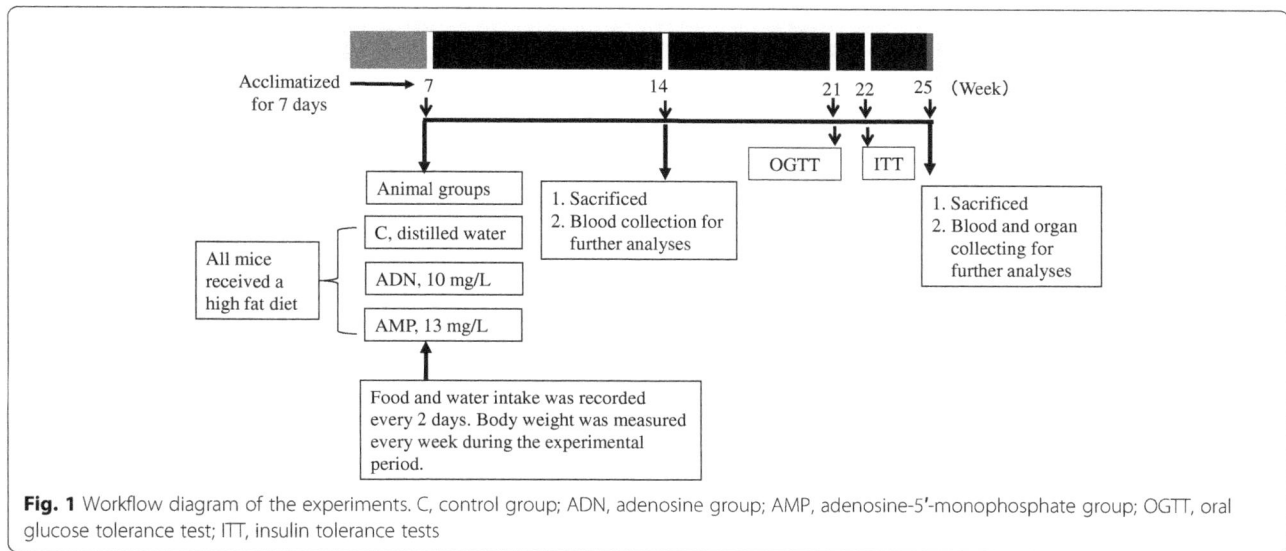

Fig. 1 Workflow diagram of the experiments. C, control group; ADN, adenosine group; AMP, adenosine-5'-monophosphate group; OGTT, oral glucose tolerance test; ITT, insulin tolerance tests

RNA preparation and quantitative RT-PCR

Total RNA was isolated from muscle tissue with the guanidine isothiocyanate-based reagent Isogen (Nippon Gene, Tokyo, Japan), according to the manufacturer's instructions. The isolated RNA was treated with RNase-free DNase (Qiagen, Hilden, Germany) for 10 min at room temperature before being purified using an RNeasy Mini kit (Qiagen). The ratio of absorbance at wavelengths of 260 and 280 nm was measured, and agarose gel electrophoresis was performed for quantitative and qualitative analysis of the isolated RNA. Four micrograms of total RNA was used as a template to synthesize cDNA. The RNA was denatured in the presence of oligo (dT), random primers, and 10 mmol/L dNTP (Amersham Biosciences, Tokyo, Japan) at 65 °C for 5 min. It was then incubated in a 20-μL volume with 50 mmol/L Tris-HCl (pH 8.3) containing 0.1 mol/L DTT, 50 U SuperScript III reverse transcriptase (Invitrogen, Carlsbad, CA, USA), and 20 U RNaseOUT RNase inhibitor (Invitrogen) at 25 °C for 5 min, 50 °C for 60 min, and 70 °C for 15 min. Aliquots of the resulting cDNA were used as templates in subsequent quantitative PCR using an Applied Biosystems (Foster City, CA, USA) 7300 Real-Time PCR System and SYBR Premix Ex Taq (Takara Bio Inc., Kusatsu, Japan) according to the manufacturers' instructions. Relative target gene expression levels were normalized to those of eukaryotic elongation factor-1α1 mRNA [23]. The target sequences were amplified using primers specific to the corresponding cDNA (Additional file 1: Table S1).

Western blot analysis

Skeletal muscle lysate was prepared after removal of adipose tissue by homogenizing the muscle in ice-cold phosphate-buffered saline containing inhibitors of proteinase (Complete Proteinase Inhibitor Cocktail, Roche Applied Science, Mannheim, Germany) and phosphatase (PhosSTOP Phosphatase Inhibitor Cocktail, Roche Applied Science). The lysate was centrifuged at 15,000×g for 30 min for collection of the supernatant, the concentration of protein in which was determined using a protein assay kit (Bio-Rad, Hercules, CA, USA). Twenty micrograms of protein was mixed with SDS gel-loading buffer and resolved by SDS-polyacrylamide gel electrophoresis on 10–20% gels (Wako Pure Chemical Industries). The proteins were subsequently transferred onto a polyvinylidene fluoride membrane (Millipore, Billerica, MA, USA), which was then blocked for 1 h with Tris-buffered saline-Tween 20 (10 mM Tris-HCl at pH 7.4, 150 mM NaCl, and 0.1% Tween 20) containing 5% skim milk or 5% bovine serum albumin (Sigma, St. Louis, MO, USA) and incubated with antibodies against AMPKα2 (Millipore) or phosphorylated AMPKα (Thr172) (Millipore), respectively. The membranes were also probed with an antibody against α-tubulin (Sigma). Protein bands were visualized with Immobilon Western Detection Reagent (Millipore) and an LAS-4000 mini luminescent image analyzer (Fujifilm, Tokyo, Japan). The relative level of each protein was normalized to that of α-tubulin.

Statistical analysis

Data are presented as means ± SEM. Statistical analysis comprised repeated-measures one-way ANOVA followed by the Tukey–Kramer test. A p-value < 0.05 was considered to indicate a significant difference among means.

Results

Body weight and daily ADN and AMP intake

Body weight, body weight gain, and the food efficiency ratio (FER) did not differ among the groups after administration of ADN or AMP for 14 or 25 weeks (Additional file 2: Table S2) when compared with the control group. However, the FER in the ADN group was significantly higher compared with that in the AMP group at 14 weeks. In addition, no differences between the groups were noted in food and water intake and relative organ weights (data not shown). ADN and AMP intake, calculated according to the volume of water consumed, was 25 ± 0.1 and 34 ± 0.3 $\mu g \cdot day^{-1}$, respectively.

Serum parameters

After 6 h of fasting, serum glucose levels at the 14th week of treatment were significantly lower in the ADN group than in the AMP group but did not significantly differ from those in the control group (Fig. 2a). In addition, no differences were noted among the control, ADN, and AMP groups in terms of serum levels of insulin, triacylglycerol, non-esterified fatty acids, and adiponectin (Fig. 2b-e).

OGTT

We performed OGTT at the 14th week of administration. Plasma glucose levels in both the ADN and AMP groups were significantly lower than those in the control group 30 and 60 min after glucose administration (Fig. 3a).

Furthermore, the incremental area under the curve calculated for the ADN and AMP treatments was significantly smaller than that for the control (Fig. 3b). ITT were carried out at the 15th week of treatment. Plasma glucose levels were significantly lower in the ADN group than in the control group 60 min after administration of insulin (Fig. 4).

AMPK phosphorylation and gene expression

We measured levels of phosphorylated and total AMPK α-subunit (AMPKα) protein in skeletal muscle by western blotting to evaluate AMPK activation in this tissue (Fig. 5a, b). The relative quantity of total AMPKα (t-AMPKα) at the 14th week of administration was significantly higher in the AMP group than in the control group (Fig. 5c), and phosphorylated AMPKα (p-AMPKα) levels in the ADN and AMP groups were significantly higher than those in the control group at both week 14 and 25 (Fig. 5d). Moreover, the ratio of p-AMPKα to t-AMPKα was significantly higher in the ADN and AMP groups than in the control group after 14 and 25 weeks of treatment (Fig. 5e). These results suggest that administration of ADN or AMP enhanced AMPK activity in skeletal muscle. mRNA levels of peroxisome proliferator-activated receptor α (Ppara) were significantly increased after

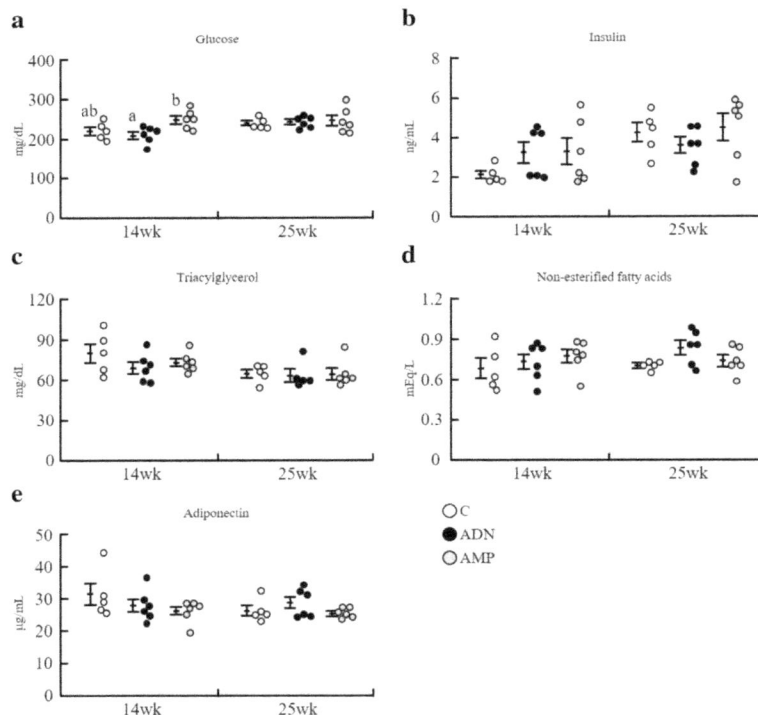

Fig. 2 Serum biochemical parameters of mice with high-fat diet-induced obesity administered ADN or AMP after fasting 6 h. **a** Glucose; (**b**) insulin; (**c**) triacylglycerol; (**d**) non-essential fatty acids; (**e**) adiponectin. Values are means ± SEM, n = 5 or 6. *p < 0.05 versus the control group. Different letters in the same panel represent a significant difference (p < 0.05). C, control group; ADN, adenosine group; AMP, adenosine-5'-monophosphate group

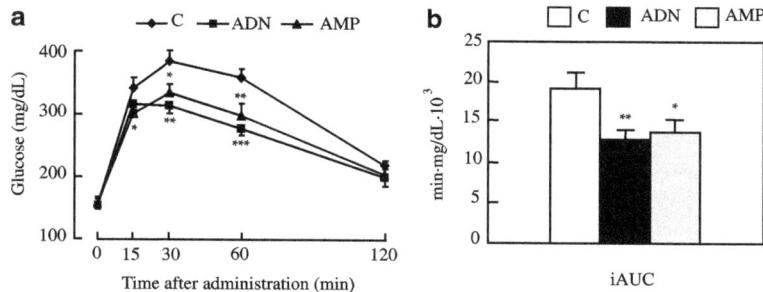

Fig. 3 Oral glucose tolerance tests of mice with high-fat diet-induced obesity administered ADN or AMP. **a** Blood glucose changes; (**b**) incremental areas under the curve (iAUC). Values are means ± SEM, n = 5 or 6. *$p < 0.05$, **$p < 0.01$, ***$p < 0.001$ versus the control group. C, control group; ADN, adenosine group; AMP, adenosine-5'-monophosphate group

14 weeks of ADN or AMP treatment. In addition, those of acyl-CoA synthase (*Acs*), very long chain acyl-CoA dehydrogenase (*Vlcad*), and PPAR gamma coactivator 1α (*Pgc1α*) were significantly higher in the AMP group than in the control group at week 14 (Additional file 3: Table S3). However, no significant differences in the levels of these transcripts were observed between the groups at the 25th week of administration.

Discussion

In our previous work, we investigated the capacity of ADN and AMP to ameliorate metabolic syndrome-related diseases using a stroke-prone spontaneously hypertensive rat model of non-obesity-associated insulin resistance and hypertension-related disorders similar to human essential hypertension [20, 21]. ADN administration reduced blood glucose and insulin levels measured under fasting

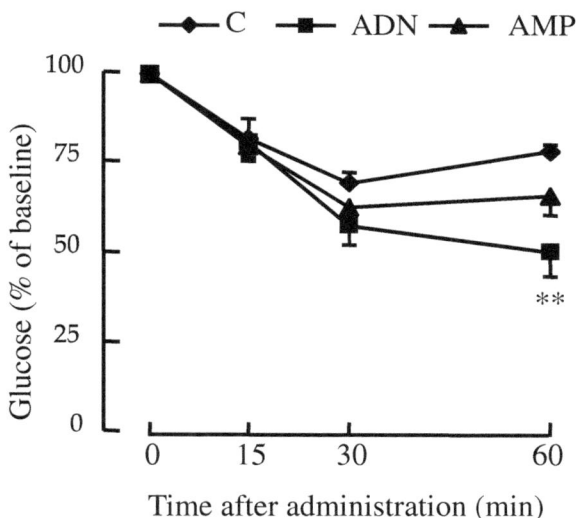

Fig. 4 Changes in blood glucose during insulin tolerance tests of mice with high-fat diet-induced obesity administered ADN or AMP. Values are means ± SEM, $n = 5$ or 6. **$p < 0.01$ versus the control group. C, control group; ADN, adenosine group; AMP, adenosine-5'-monophosphate group

conditions, as well as glucose and insulin tolerance. In addition, we showed for the first time that ingestion of AMP increases plasma adiponectin concentration, upregulates hepatic *Prkaa1* mRNA expression, and elevates levels of p-AMPKα, leading to enhanced expression of genes associated with β-oxidation in the liver.

In the current study, we examined the effect of ADN and AMP administration on glucose metabolism using mice fed a high-fat diet as an animal model of obesity. Human and animal studies have demonstrated that a diet high in fat induces increased lipid accumulation in tissues including adipose tissue and skeletal muscle, followed by insulin resistance [24]. Increased levels of non-esterified fatty acids in the blood and diacylglycerol and palmitoyl-CoA in organs result in activation of c-Jun N-terminal kinase (JNK) and inhibitor of kappa light polypeptide gene enhancer in B-cells, kinase β (IKKβ). Activation of JUN and IKKβ leads to serine phosphorylation of insulin receptor substrate, interfering with insulin signaling via the insulin receptor [25, 26]. We speculate that the effect of ADN and AMP is more pronounced in the early stage of diabetes. Future studies are needed to clarify the detailed mechanism, but ADN and AMP are promising candidates for the prevention of diabetes in both mice and humans.

Even though blood glucose levels in fasted state were not different among the groups (Fig. 1a), tolerance tests revealed that ADN and AMP improved the abnormal glucose tolerance (Fig. 3) and insulin sensitivity (Fig. 4) observed in the mouse model of obesity used in this study. These results indicate that administration of ADN or AMP can mitigate insulin resistance in mice fed a high-fat diet. ADN and AMP treatment may have the ability to reduce blood glucose in postprandial, but not in fasted state.

In this study, we found that oral administration of ADN or AMP can activate AMPK in skeletal muscle (Fig. 5). This is the first in vivo demonstration of AMPK activation by ADN or AMP in the high-fat diet-induced obese mouse model of insulin resistance. AMPK acts as

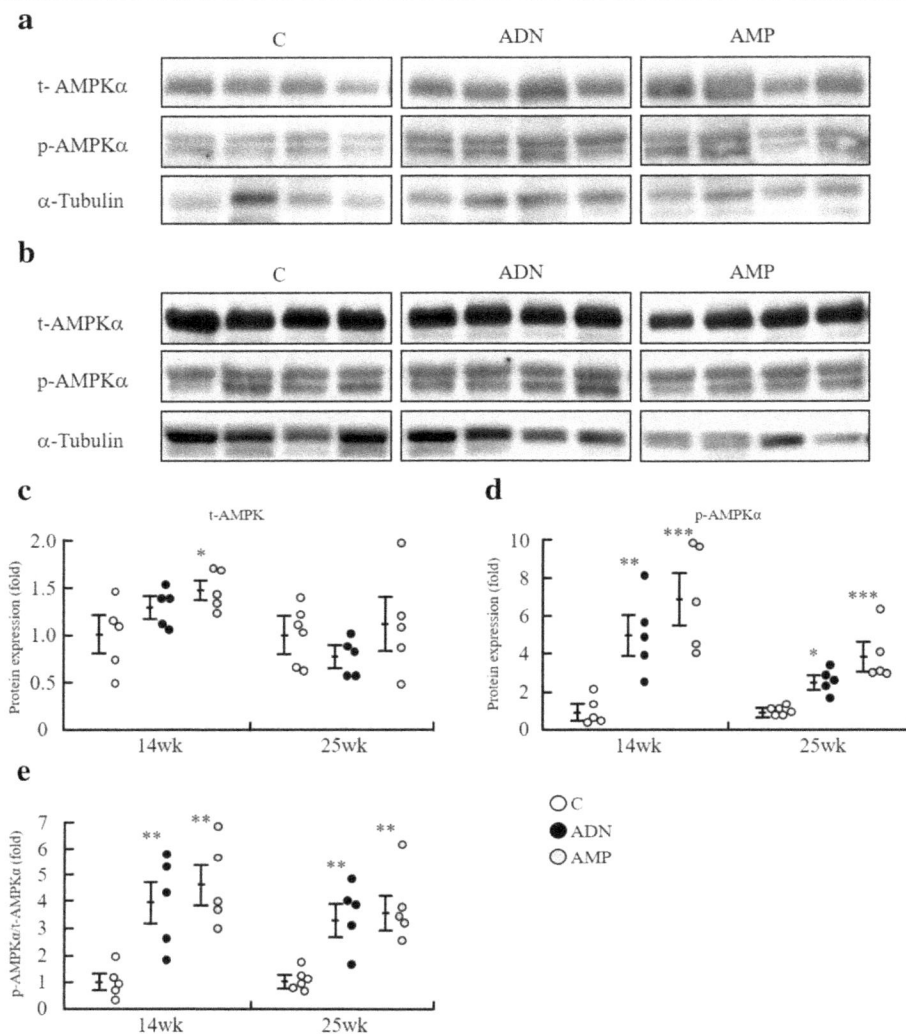

Fig. 5 Representative immunoblot images and quantitative analyses of total AMPKα, phosphorylated AMPKα, and α-tubulin. **a** Western blot images at 14 weeks; (**b**) western blot images at 25 weeks; (**c**) expression of total AMPKα (t-AMPKα); (**d**) expression of phosphorylated AMPKα (p-AMPKα); and (**e**) ratio of t-AMPKα to p-AMPKα. Values are means ± SEM, n = 5 or 6. *$p < 0.05$, **$p < 0.01$, ***$p < 0.001$ versus the control group. C, control group; ADN, adenosine group; AMP, adenosine-5'-monophosphate group

a sensor, and when activated, stimulates mitochondrial biogenesis, energy production, lipid oxidation, and glucose influx, alleviating insulin resistance via activation of sirtuin 1 and PGC1α [27]. AMPK activation in muscle was enhanced after both 14 and 25 weeks of ADN or AMP administration independently of adiponectin. Thus, ADN and AMP may indeed suppress the progression of high-fat diet-induced insulin resistance relatively early in the development of diabetes.

mRNA expression of the gene encoding PPARα, an AMPK target in skeletal muscle, was increased in the AMP and ADN groups after 14 weeks of administration. Furthermore, levels of *Acs* and *Vlcad* mRNA were also higher in the AMP group at this time point (Additional file 3: Table S3). However, these differences were no

longer evident after 25 weeks of treatment, despite continued AMPK activation in the skeletal muscle of ADN- or AMP-treated mice. Thus, although at 14 weeks (Additional file 3: Table S3), activation of AMPK in skeletal muscle stimulated the expression of PPARα and its target genes; it suggests that an adaption had occurred by the 25th week of administration (Additional file 3: Table S3). Skeletal muscle can adapt its metabolic properties in response to a number of physiologic conditions by activation and repression of signaling events that affect the metabolic pathways of several genes related to the oxidation process. The first evidence linking AMPK to the regulation of glucose metabolism in skeletal muscle was provided by treatment with AICAR, an activator of AMPK that enhances fatty acid oxidation [28]. Our results suggest that ADN and AMP contribute to improving the regulation of glucose metabolism through expression of PPARα and its target genes.

Lipid accumulation in the skeletal muscle of obese animals induces abnormal glucose metabolism accompanied by dysregulated insulin signaling and skeletal muscle function. Upregulation of lipid oxidation in skeletal muscle is considered a therapeutic strategy to combat insulin resistance. Unsaturated fatty acids, such as oleic acid, and agonists of PPARα enhance lipid oxidation and are expected to have therapeutic effects in diabetes [29–31]. In our study, administration of ADN or AMP increased the expression of transcripts associated with lipid oxidation in skeletal muscle. As muscle is the major site of ATP production and consumption, enhanced lipid oxidation in skeletal muscle may be involved in the mitigation of abnormal glucose metabolism by ADN and AMP in mice fed a high-fat diet.

Although this study was carefully and well prepared, we were still aware of its limitations. We need to measure locomotor activity of mice. Various studies have shown that in rodent models of obesity locomotor activity is necessary to evaluate. Further studies are needed to evaluate the behavior of mice after administration of ADN and AMP. In addition, further studies are needed to elucidate the complete physiological effect of ADN and AMP to confirm its detailed mechanism of action at the molecular level.

Conclusions

Here, we showed that administration of ADN or AMP to obese mice ameliorates abnormal glucose metabolism induced by a high-fat diet. ADN or AMP treatment also increases the level of activated AMPK in skeletal muscle. Activation of AMPK may upregulate lipid oxidation and attenuates insulin resistance caused by obesity.

Acknowledgments
We are thankful to Yamasa Co. (China, Japan), which kindly provided the AMP used in this study.

Funding
This work was partially supported by the JSPS Core-to-Core Program A (Advanced Research Networks) entitled "Establishment of international agricultural immunology research-core for a quantum improvement in food safety."

Authors' contributions
A and YI performed the experiments and prepared the manuscript. TK, AZA, II, and TG contributed to the design of the experiments and participated in the discussion of the results. MK and HS supervised the entire design of the experiments and drafted the manuscript. All authors read and approved the final manuscript.

Competing interests
The authors declare that they have no competing interest associated with this publication.

Author details
[1]Laboratory of Nutrition, Graduate School of Agricultural Science, Tohoku University, Sendai 980-0845, Japan. [2]Department of Food Science and Technology, Universitas Bakrie, Jakarta 12920, Indonesia. [3]Faculty of Agriculture, Yamagata University, Tsuruoka 997-8555, Japan. [4]Laboratory of Food and Biomolecular Science, Graduate School of Agricultural Science, Tohoku University, Sendai 980-0845, Japan. [5]International Education and Research Center for Food Agricultural Immunology, Graduate School of Agricultural Science, Tohoku University, Sendai 980-0845, Japan.

References
1. Hardus PM, van Vuuren CL, Crawford D, Worsley A. Public health perceptions of the causes and prevention of obesity among primary school children. Int J Obes Relat Metab Disord. 2003;27:1465–71.
2. Haffner S, Taegtmeyer H. Epidemic obesity and the metabolic syndrome. Circulation. 2003;108:1541–5.
3. Sharma AM. The obese patient with diabetes mellitus: from research targets to treatment options. Am J Med. 2006;119:S17–23.
4. Hotamisligil GS. Inflammation and metabolic disorders. Nature. 2006;444: 860–7.
5. Erion DM, Shulman GI. Diacylglycerol-mediated insulin resistance. Nat Med. 2010;16:400–2.
6. Cantó C, Gerhart-Hines Z, Feige JN, Lagouge M, Noriega L, Milne JC, Elliott PJ, Puigserver P, Auwerx J. AMPK regulates energy expenditure by modulating NAD$^+$ metabolism and SIRT1 activity. Nature. 2009;458:1056–60.
7. Yamauchi T, Kamon J, Minokoshi Y, Ito Y, Waki H, Uchida S, Yamashita S, Noda M, Kita S, Ueki K, Eto K, Akanuma Y, Froguel P, Foufelle F, Ferre P, Carling D, Kimura S, Nagai R, Kahn BB, Kadowaki T. Adiponectin stimulates glucose utilization and fatty-acid oxidation by activating AMP-activated protein kinase. Nat Med. 2002;8:1288–95.
8. Zimmermann H. Extracellular metabolism of ATP and other nucleotides. Naunyn Schmiedeberg's Arch Pharmacol. 2000;362:299–309.
9. Duflot S, Riera B, Fernández-Veledo S, Casadó V, Norman RI, Casado FJ, Lluís C, Franco R, Pastor-Anglada M. ATP-sensitive K$^+$ channels regulate the concentrative adenosine transporter CNT2 following activation by A$_1$ adenosine receptors. Mol Cell Biol. 2004;24:2710–9.
10. Hasko G, Linden J, Cronstein B, Pacher P. Adenosine receptors: therapeutic aspects for inflammatory and immune diseases. Nat Rev Drug Discov. 2008; 7:759–70.
11. Dhalla AK, Santikul M, Smith M, Wong MY, Shryock JC, Belardinelli L. Antilipolytic of novel partial A1 adenosine receptor agonist devoid of cardiovascular effects: comparison with nicotinic acid. J Pharmacol Exp Ther. 2007;321:327–33.
12. Dhalla AK, Wong MY, Voshol PJ, Belardinelli L, Reaven GM. A1 adenosine receptor partial agonist lowers plasma FFA and improves insulin resistance induced by high-fat diet in rodents. Am J Physiol Endocrinol Metab. 2007; 292:E1358–63.
13. Fukumori Y, Maeda N, Takeda H, Onodera S, Shiomi N. Serum glucose and insulin response in rats administered with sucrose or starch containing adenosine, inosine or cytosine. Biosci Biotechnol Biochem. 2000;64:237–43.
14. Fukumori Y, Takeda H, Fujisawa T, Ushijima K, Onodera S, Shiomi N. Blood glucose and insulin concentrations are reduced in human administered sucrose with inosine or adenosine. J Nutr. 2000;130:1946–9.
15. Dubey RK, Gillespie DG, Mi Z, Jackson EK. Adenosine inhibit PDGF-induced growth of human glomerular mesangial cells via A2B receptors. Hypertension. 2005;46:628–34.
16. Lee CY. Adenosine protects Sprague Dawley rats from high-fat diet and repeated acute restraint stress-induced intestinal inflammation and altered expression of nutrient transporters. J Anim Physiol Anim Nutr. 2015;99:317–25.
17. Ding M, Yuzo N, Robert FM. Blocking taste receptor activation of gustducin gustatory responses to bitter compounds. Proc Natl Acad Sci U S A. 1999; 96:9903–8.
18. Zhang F, Wang S, Luo Y, Ji X, Nemoto EM. When hypothermia meets hypotension and hyperglycemia: the diverse effects of adenosine 50-monophosphate on cerebral ischemia in rats. J Cereb Blood Flow Metab. 2009;29:1022–34.
19. Swoap SJ, Rathvon M, Gutilla M. AMP does not induce torpor. Am J Physiol Regul Integr Comp Physiol. 2007;293:R468–73.

20. Ardiansyah, Shirakawa H, Shimeno T, Koseki T, Shiono Y, Murayama T, Hatakeyama E, Komai M. Adenosine, an identified active component from the Driselase-treated fraction of rice bran, is effective at improving metabolic syndrome in stroke-prone spontaneously hypertensive rats. J Agric Food Chem. 2009;57:2558–64.

21. Ardiansyah, Shirakawa H, Koseki T, Hiwatashi K, Takahasi S, Akiyama Y, Komai M. Novel effect of adenosine 5'-monophosphate on ameliorating hypertension and the metabolism of lipids and glucose in stroke-prone spontaneously hypertensive rats. J Agric Food Chem. 2011;59:13238–45.

22. Fraulob JC, Ogg-Diamantino R, Fernandes-Santos C, Aguila MB, Mandarim-de-Lacerda CA. A mouse model of metabolic syndrome: insulin resistance, fatty liver and non-alcoholic fatty pancreas disease (NAFPD) in C57BL/6 mice fed a high fat diet. J Clin Biochem Nutr. 2010;46:212–23.

23. Shirakawa H, Ohsaki Y, Minegishi Y, Takumi N, Ohinata K, Furukawa Y, Mizutani T, Komai M. Vitamin K deficiency reduces testosterone production in the testis through down-regulation of the Cyp11a a cholesterol side chain cleavage enzyme in rats. Biochim Biophys Acta. 2006;1760:1482–8.

24. Krssak M, Petersen FK, Dresner A, DiPietro L, Vogel SM, Rothman DL, Roden M, Shulman GI. Intramyocellular lipid concentrations are correlated with insulin sensitivity in humans: a 1H NMR spectroscopy study. Diabetologia. 1999;42:113–6.

25. Gao Z, Hwang D, Bataille F, Lefevre M, York D, Quon MJ, Ye J. Serine phosphorylation of insulin receptor substrate 1 by inhibitor kappa B kinase complex. J Biol Chem. 2002;277:48115–21.

26. Shi H, Kokoeva MV, Inouye K, Tzameli I, Yin H, Flier JS. TLR4 links innate immunity and fatty acid-induced insulin resistance. J Clin Invest. 2006;116: 3015–25.

27. Iwabu M, Yamauchi T, Okada-Iwabu M, Sato K, Nakagawa T, Funata M, Yamaguchi M, Namiki S, Nakayama R, Tabata M, Ogata H, Kubota N, Takamoto I, Hayashi YK, Yamauchi N, Waki H, Fukayama M, Nishino I, Tokuyama K, Ueki K, Oike Y, Ishii S, Hirose K, Shimizu T, Touhara K, Kadowaki T. Adiponectin and AdipoR1 regulate PGC-1alpha and mitochondria by Ca^{2+} and AMPK/SIRT1. Nature. 2010;464:1313–9.

28. Merrill GF, Kurth EJ, Hardie DG, Winder WW. AICA riboside increases AMP-activated protein kinase, fatty acid oxidation, and glucose uptake in rat muscle. Am J Phys. 1997;273:E1107–12.

29. Tsuchiya Y, Hatakeyama H, Emoto N, Wagatsuma F, Matsushita S, Kanzaki M. Palmitate-induced down-regulation of sortilin and impaired GLUT4 trafficking in C2C12 myotubes. J Biol Chem. 2010;285:34371–81.

30. Coll T, Eyre E, Rodríguez-Calvo R, Palomer X, Sánchez RM, Merlos M, Laguna JC, Vázquez-Carrera M. Oleate reverses palmitate-induced insulin resistance and inflammation in skeletal muscle cells. J Biol Chem. 2008;283:11107–16.

31. Coll T, Alvarez-Guardia D, Barroso E, Gómez-Foix AM, Palomer X, Laguna JC, Vázquez-Carrera M. Activation of peroxisome proliferator-activated receptor-δ by GW501516 prevents fatty acid-induced nuclear factor-B activation and insulin resistance in skeletal muscle cells. Endocrinology. 2010;151:1560–9.

19

Complementary and alternative medicine use among persons with multiple chronic conditions

Justice Mbizo[1][*] [ID], Anthony Okafor[2], Melanie A. Sutton[1], Bryan Leyva[3], Leauna M. Stone[1] and Oluwadamilola Olaku[4,5]

Abstract

Background: Although a quarter of Americans are estimated to have multiple chronic conditions, information on the impact of chronic disease dyads and triads on use of complementary and alternative medicine (CAM) is scarce. The purpose of this study is to: 1) estimate the prevalence and odds of CAM use among participants with hypercholesterolemia, hypertension, diabetes, and obesity; and 2) examine the effects of chronic condition dyads and triads on the use of CAM modalities, specifically manipulative and body-based methods, biological treatments, mind-body interventions, energy therapies, and alternative medical systems.

Methods: Data were obtained from the 2012 National Health Interview Survey and the Adult Alternative Medicine supplement. Statistical analyses were restricted to persons with self-reported hypercholesterolemia, hypertension, diabetes, or obesity ($n = 15{,}463$).

Results: Approximately 37.2% of the participants had just one of the four chronic conditions, while 62.4% self-reported multiple comorbidities. CAM use among participants was as follows ($p < 0.001$): hypercholesterolemia (31.5%), hypertension (28.3%), diabetes (25.0%), and obesity (10.8%). All combinations of disease dyads and triads were consistently and significantly associated with the use of mind-body interventions (2–4%, $p < 0.001$). Two sets of three dyads were associated with use of manipulative methods (23–27%, $p < 0.05$) and energy therapies (0.2–0.3%, $p < 0.05$). Use of biological treatments (0.04%, $p < 0.05$) and alternative systems (3%, $p < 0.05$) were each significant for one dyad. One triad was significant for use of manipulative methods (27%, $p < 0.001$).

Conclusions: These findings point to future directions for research and have practical implications for family practitioners treating multimorbid patients.

Keywords: Complementary and alternative medicine, Chronic disease, Comorbidity, Diabetes, Hypercholesterolemia, Hypertension, Integrative medicine, Obesity

Background

The National Center for Complementary and Integrative Health, the federal government's lead agency for scientific research on complementary and alternative medicine (CAM), defines CAM as a category of medicine that includes a variety of treatment approaches that fall outside the realm of conventional medicine. CAM therapies have been grouped into five distinct domains: manipulative and body-based methods, biological treatments, mind-body interventions, energy therapies, and alternative medical systems [1]. Evidence from national studies suggest that approximately one-third of Americans used some form of CAM in the past 12 months [2]. Use of non-conventional medicine in the general population has been increasing in the past decade and contributes substantially to health care spending. In 2007, Americans spent nearly $34 billion in out-of-pocket expenses on CAM, which represented a

* Correspondence: jmbizo@uwf.edu
[1]Department of Public Health, University of West Florida, 11000 University Parkway, Bldg. 38/Room 127, Pensacola, FL 32514, USA
Full list of author information is available at the end of the article

25% increase in spending compared earlier estimates from 1997 trends [3].

A substantial body of research has focused on understanding trends and patterns of CAM use in the general U.S. population [2, 4], as well as among specific patient subgroups. Several studies have examined correlates and predictors of CAM use among patients with specific chronic diseases, including diabetes [5], cancer [6], and cardiovascular disease [7], with evidence suggesting high CAM use among patients with chronic illness. Despite advances in the collective understanding of CAM use among patients with chronic illness, little is known about the utilization of CAM among patients with multiple chronic conditions. Although more than a quarter of Americans are estimated to have multiple co-morbidities, we identified few studies [8] assessing the effect of specific combinations of chronic diseases (dyads and triads) on use of CAM. Notably, none of these studies focused specifically on patients with cardiovascular risk factor combinations such as hypertension, hypercholesterolemia, diabetes, and obesity, all of which are conditions of increasing prevalence and public health significance. Whereas the prevalence of hypertension among adults in the U.S. has remained relatively constant at 30% since 1999 [9–11], the prevalence of diabetes (9–12%), hypercholesterolemia (25–27%), and obesity (31–36%) has been steadily increasing in the past decade [9].

Given the increasing prevalence of these risk factors and their significant contributions to cardiovascular morbidity and mortality in the U.S. [12] and around the world, this is an important gap in the scientific literature. To address this gap, this study sought to: 1) estimate the prevalence and odds of CAM use among participants with major chronic diseases such as hypercholesterolemia, hypertension, diabetes, and obesity; and 2) examine the effects of chronic condition dyads and triads on the use of specific CAM modalities and treatments. We anticipate findings from this study may be useful in generating hypotheses for future research and have practical implications for family physicians and chronic disease self-management specialists.

Methods

Study design and participants

This cross-sectional study consists of men and women ages 18 years and older who responded to the 2012 National Health Interview Survey (NHIS), a nationally-representative surveillance system administered by the Centers for Disease Control and Prevention's National Center for Health Statistics (NCHS). The NHIS serves as "the principal source of information on the health of the civilian non-institutionalized population in the United States." [13] Beginning in 2002, the NCHS added a supplementary module on CAM

utilization that is administered every five years. This study specifically focused on persons with self-reported hypercholesterolemia, hypertension, diabetes, or obesity (n = 15,463). The NHIS survey is a population-based surveillance system administered by the U.S. Centers for Disease Control and Prevention. The survey consists of face-to-face household interviews to obtain data for each respondent selected to complete the NHIS instrument and is administered by NCHS trained interviewers. To ensure a nationally representative data set for the civilian noninstitutionalized population of the United States, a multistage stratified sampling design is used, with interviews conducted in all 50 states and the District of Columbia. Computer-assisted data collection is utilized during each interview to perform data quality checks as responses are made and to ensure the consistency of the questionnaire flow.

The NHIS survey has several components broken down into modules. The Household module provides information on household composition and survey response characteristics. The Family module provides information on participants' relationships and family structure within households. Individual information is contained in the Person and Sample Adult modules. The Person module contains information on individual health status, health care access and utilization, health insurance, basic socio-demographics, income/assets, and family food security. The Sample Adult module contains questions on socio-demographics, health conditions/status, health behaviors, and health care access and utilization administered to randomly selected adults within the family. Finally, the Adult Alternative Medicine module provides information on the adult sample use of non-conventional health care practices. A detailed discussion of the NHIS instrument is described elsewhere [14, 15].

Measures

Overall CAM use was measured by collapsing all reported CAM products into the five domains noted previously: [1] (1) manipulative and body-based methods, including chiropractic/osteopathic approaches and massage therapy; (2) biological treatments, including herbal remedies and special diets; (3) mind-body interventions, including meditation, hypnosis, prayer, and art/music therapy; (4) energy therapies, including biofield and bioelectromagnetic-based therapies, and {5} alternative medical systems, including acupuncture, Ayurvedic medicine, homeopathy, and naturopathy. A composite variable for CAM use was created by combining the domains in which CAM use was present if any one of the five domains was coded as "1", indicating reported CAM use within that domain. The final CAM variable was dichotomized into "0" and "1", where "0" represented absence of CAM use. The independent variables included

Table 1 Characteristics of the study sample and frequency of chronic conditions, national health interview survey, 2012

Characteristics	Overall Sample n(%)	Chronic Condition			
		Hypercholesterolemia n(%)	Hypertension n(%)	Diabetes n(%)	Obesity n(%)
Age Group					
< 35	1241(8.0)	502(39.9)	823(66.6)	137(11.1)	490(39.8)
35–49	2946(18.8)	1658(56.4)	1860(63.1)	516(17.5)	1327(44.9)
50–64	5479(35.5)	3496(63.2)	3966(72.5)	1338(24.0)	2287(41.7)
> 64	5797(37.7)	3833(66.0)	4649(80.2)	1537(26.3)	1523(26.4)
Sex					
Male	6964(44.9)	4322(61.8)	5045(72.5)	1616(22.9)	2503(35.9)
Female	8499(55.1)	5167(60.5)	6253(73.7)	1912(22.3)	3124(36.8)
Race and Ethnicity					
Non-Hispanic White	11,663(75.6)	7423(63.4)	8212(70.5)	2500(21.3)	4186(35.8)
Non-Hispanic Black/African American	2746(17.6)	1377(49.7)	2341(85.6)	762(27.5)	1199(44.2)
Alaska Natives/American Indians	158(1.0)	86(54.1)	122(78.9)	53(33.7)	76(50.8)
Non-Hispanic Other	896(5.8)	603(67.4)	623(69.5)	213(23.3)	166(18.3)
Education Level					
Less than High School	2890(18.5)	1718(59.1)	2291(79.6)	858(29.5)	1062(36.8)
High School Graduate/Some College	8877(57.5)	5358(60.1)	6589(74.3)	2060(22.9)	3445(38.7)
College/Professional Graduate	3696(24.0)	2413(65.2)	2418(65.4)	610(16.7)	1120(30.5)
Marital Status					
Married	8131(52.7)	5219(64.0)	5606(68.9)	1778(21.8)	2996(37.0)
Widowed/Divorced	5114(33.1)	3150(61.2)	4052(79.4)	1293(24.7)	1682(32.7)
Single/Never Married	2218(14.2)	1120(49.9)	1640(74.3)	457(20.5)	949(42.8)
Family Income					
< $20,000	6696(43.2)	3904(58.2)	5322(79.6)	1850(27.2)	2566(38.2)
$20,000–$34,999	2107(13.8)	1312(62.0)	1546(73.4)	460(21.9)	802(38.0)
$35,000–$49,999	2306(14.9)	1448(62.2)	1597(69.4)	473(21.0)	839(36.6)
$50,000–$74,999	3435(22.3)	2256(65.3)	2145(62.5)	544(15.6)	1173(34.2)
$75,000+	919(5.8)	569(61.7)	688(75.4)	201(21.3)	247(26.9)
Health Insurance Coverage					
Yes	13,742(88.8)	8655(62.6)	10,009(73.0)	3198(23.0)	4894(35.7)
No	1721(11.2)	834(48.9)	1289(74.7)	330(19.3)	733(42.2)
Regular Source of Care					
Yes	14,174(91.6)	8836(62.1)	10,389(73.4)	3353(23.4)	5240(37.0)
No	1289(8.4)	653(50.7)	909(70.3)	175(13.5)	387(30.1)
Geographic Region					
Northeast	2554(16.6)	1610(62.4)	1803(70.8)	545(20.9)	878(34.2)
Midwest	3206(20.8)	1981(61.4)	2320(72.2)	694(21.3)	1244(39.0)
South	5962(38.6)	3581(59.9)	4536(76.3)	1478(24.8)	2276(38.4)
West	3741(24.0)	2317(61.9)	2639(70.6)	811(21.4)	1229(32.5)
Hypercholesterolemia					
Yes	9489(61.1)	–	5853(61.8)	2219(23.1)	3390(35.8)
No	5974(38.9)	–	5445(91.1)	1309(21.8)	2237(37.3)

Table 1 Characteristics of the study sample and frequency of chronic conditions, national health interview survey, 2012 *(Continued)*

Characteristics	Overall Sample n(%)	Chronic Condition			
		Hypercholesterolemia n(%)	Hypertension n(%)	Diabetes n(%)	Obesity n(%)
Hypertension					
Yes	11,298(73.2)	5853(51.6)	–	2591(22.7)	4422(39.1)
No	4165(26.8)	3636(87.1)	–	937(22.4)	1205(28.9)
Diabetes					
Yes	3528(22.6)	2219(62.4)	2591(73.4)	–	1722(48.9)
No	11,935(77.4)	7270(60.7)	8707(73.1)	–	3905(32.8)
Body Mass Index					
< 18.5 (Underweight)	782(5.1)	451(57.8)	579(73.5)	178(23.0)	–
18.5–24.9 (Normal)	3618(23.6)	2199(60.2)	2461(68.0)	502(13.9)	–
25.0–29.9 (Overweight)	5436(34.9)	3449(63.2)	3836(70.8)	1126(20.4)	–
30.0+ (Obese)	5627(36.4)	3390(60.1)	4422(78.7)	1722(30.4)	–
Manipulative Methods					
Yes	3778(24.3)	2492(65.7)	2678(71.1)	762(20.2)	1425(38.0)
No	11,685(75.7)	6997(59.6)	8620(73.8)	2766(23.4)	4202(35.9)
Mind-Body Interventions					
Yes	801(5.1)	497(62.0)	518(64.9)	88(11.4)	220(27.7)
No	14,662(94.9)	8992(61.1)	10,780(73.6)	3440(23.2)	5407(36.9)
Biological Treatments					
Yes	42(0.3)	24(58.7)	32(76.2)	7(15.9)	11(27.0)
No	15,421(99.7)	9465(61.1)	11,266(73.2)	3521(22.6)	5616(36.4)
Energy Therapies					
Yes	72(0.5)	49(67.3)	38(51.8)	11(14.5)	29(39.1)
No	15,391(99.5)	9440(61.1)	11,260(73.3)	3517(22.6)	5598(36.4)
Alternative Systems					
Yes	592(3.8)	395(66.9)	394(66.6)	97(16.5)	204(34.8)
No	14,871(96.2)	9094(60.9)	10,904(73.4)	3431(22.8)	5423(36.5)

Note: All frequencies are unweighted; all percentages are weighted

socio-demographic and socio-economic characteristics such as age, sex, race/ethnicity, education, marital status, family income, insurance coverage, having a regular source of care, and region of residence.

Statistical analysis

The analysis consisted of descriptive statistics, bivariate analysis, and multivariate logistic regression. The descriptive analysis included counts, means, standard deviations, and proportions of CAM use. For the bivariate analysis, we performed a Chi-square test of independence to assess the association and significance of each covariate and CAM use. The multivariate logistic regression method, a critical component of the analysis, was used to assess the association between the dichotomous response variable describing CAM use and the predictor variables or covariates [16]. To account for the confounding effect of the covariates in the

multivariate analysis, the adjusted odds ratios (aOR) were calculated. The 95% confidence intervals for the odds ratio were determined and used not only to assess the significance of the covariates but also to determine the magnitude of the effect based on the range of the interval.

All analyses were performed using Stata 15 for Windows (STATA Corp., College Station, Texas). Data from the NHIS Family, Household, Person, Sample Adult, and Adult Alternative Medicine files were merged, and sampling weights were applied to account for the complex probability survey design [13]. Using the multivariate and bivariate analysis previously described, we further stratified the analysis by disease dyads and triads across the five domains of CAM and examined the associations between the different chronic disease dyads and triads with respect to specific CAM modality use. Statistical significance was set at a p-value of less than 0.05.

Table 2 Proportions and odds of CAM use among adults with and without comorbidities

Independent Variables	Overall CAM Use		CAM Use in Patients with 2 or More Chronic Conditions		Adjusted Odds of CAM Use			
					Patients with 1 Chronic Condition		Patients with 2 or More Chronic Conditions	
	n(%)	χ^2, p-value	n(%)	χ^2, p-value	aOR [95% CI]	p-value	aOR [95% CI]	p-value
Age Group		6.69, p < 0.001		14.04, p = 0.003				
< 35 (ref)	349(28.3)		156(26.9)		1.00	–	1.00	–
35–49	887(29.9)		473(27.7)		1.12[0.89,1.39]	0.331	1.04[0.83,1.30]	0.729
50–64	1740(31.6)		1108(31.0)		1.07[0.86,1.32]	0.548	1.21[0.98,1.49]	0.083
> 64	1607(27.6)		1042(27.4)		0.94[0.75,1.18]	0.529	1.10[0.88,1.37]	0.417
Sex		3.28, p = 0.071		2.29, p = 0.130				
Male (ref)	1999(28.7)		1219(28.0)		1.00	–	1.00	–
Female	2584(30.2)		1560(29.4)		1.25[1.11,1.42]	< 0.001	1.29[1.17,1.42]	< 0.001
Race and Ethnicity		79.11, p < 0.001		161.97, p < 0.001				
Non-Hispanic White (ref)	3857(32.9)		2307(32.0)		1.00	–	1.00	–
Non-Hispanic Black/African American	460(16.4)		320(17.2)		0.46[0.37,0.56]	< 0.001	0.52[0.45,0.60]	< 0.001
Alaska Natives/American Indians	39(25.2)		24(22.4)		0.98[0.52,1.85]	0.949	0.64[0.40,1.02]	0.058
Non-Hispanic Other	227(25.6)		128(25.8)		0.61[0.47,0.78]	< 0.001	0.75[0.60,0.94]	0.012
Education Level		111.49, p < 0.001		132.62, p < 0.001				
Less than High School (ref)	533(18.8)		369(19.1)		1.00	–	1.00	–
High School Graduate/Some College	2696(30.0)		1694(29.6)		1.80[1.48,2.19]	< 0.001	1.53[1.34,1.74]	< 0.001
College/Professional Graduate	1354(36.5)		716(35.3)		2.12[1.70,2.65]	< 0.001	1.78[1.51,2.09]	< 0.001
Marital Status		12.49, p < 0.001		16.36, p < 0.001				
Married (ref)	2550(31.2)		1533(30.2)		1.00	–	1.00	–
Widowed/Divorced	1465(28.3)		919(28.0)		1.04[0.90,1.21]	0.589	1.02[0.92,1.15]	0.666
Single/Never Married	568(25.9)		327(24.8)		0.96[0.79,1.16]	0.681	0.92[0.79,1.07]	0.291
Family Income		38.48, p < 0.001		97.68, p < 0.001				
< $20,000 (ref)	1652(24.7)		1097(24.6)		1.00	–	1.00	–
$20,000–$34,999	613(29.0)		367(27.3)		1.12[0.93,1.36]	0.245	0.98[0.85,1.14]	0.838
$35,000–$49,999	801(34.3)		483(34.3)		1.21[1.00,1.46]	0.044	1.30[1.12,1.50]	< 0.001
$50,000–$74,999	1255(36.2)		675(35.1)		1.21[1.01,1.46]	0.040	1.25[1.08,1.44]	0.003
$75,000+	262(28.6)		157(29.1)		1.01[0.78,1.32]	0.931	1.14[0.93,1.41]	0.208
Health Insurance Coverage		4.31, p = 0.039		0.05, p = 0.816				
Yes	4107(29.8)		2489(28.8)		1.05[0.85,1.29]	0.674	0.84[0.71,0.99]	0.041
No (ref)	476(27.2)		290(28.4)		1.00	–	1.00	–
Regular Source of Care		9.36, p = 0.002		7.02, p = 0.008				
Yes	4256(29.9)		2624(29.0)		1.06[0.86,1.31]	0.596	1.09[0.88,1.35]	0.424
No (ref)	327(25.3)		155(24.1)		1.00	–	1.00	–
Geographic Region		33.08, p < 0.001		157.90, p < 0.001				
Northeast (ref)	702(27.3)		389(25.0)		1.00	–	1.00	–
Midwest	1140(35.6)		723(35.8)		1.21[1.00,1.46]	0.046	1.64[1.41,1.90]	< 0.001
South	1441(24.1)		895(23.1)		0.91[0.76,1.08]	0.268	1.03[0.89,1.19]	0.681
West	1300(34.4)		772(34.6)		1.21[1.01,1.45]	0.037	1.61[1.38,1.87]	< 0.001
Hypercholesterolemia		45.22, p < 0.001		13.64, p < 0.001				
Yes	2995(31.5)		2105(29.7)					
No	1588(26.4)		674(25.9)					

Complementary and Alternative Medicine for Health Professionals

Table 2 Proportions and odds of CAM use among adults with and without comorbidities *(Continued)*

Independent Variables	Overall CAM Use		CAM Use in Patients with 2 or More Chronic Conditions		Adjusted Odds of CAM Use			
					Patients with 1 Chronic Condition		Patients with 2 or More Chronic Conditions	
	n(%)	χ^2, p-value	n(%)	χ^2, p-value	aOR [95% CI]	p-value	aOR [95% CI]	p-value
Hypertension		27.19, $p < 0.001$		0.33, $p = 0.566$				
Yes	3210(28.3)		2357(28.6)					
No	1373(32.7)		422(29.4)					
Diabetes		41.12, $p < 0.001$		25.62, $p < 0.001$				
Yes	877(25.0)		814(25.4)					
No	3706(30.8)		1965(30.4)					
Body Mass Index		12.01, $p < 0.001$		22.60, $p < 0.001$				
< 18.5 (Underweight)	158(1.0)		67(19.8)					
18.5–24.9 (Normal)	1092(7.0)		338(25.6)					
25.0–29.9 (Overweight)	1669(10.7)		712(29.6)					
30.0+ (Obese)	1664(10.8)		1662(29.6)					

Note: All frequencies are unweighted; all percentages are weighted

Results

Table 1 presents descriptive statistics and the frequency of the four chronic conditions by covariates. Overall CAM use proportions in general, CAM use in participants with two or more chronic conditions, and a comparison of the adjusted odds of CAM use for those participants with one chronic condition versus two or more conditions are presented in Table 2 Table 3 provides the bivariate proportions for CAM use among disease dyads and triads for the five CAM domains. Finally, Table 5 summarizes statistically significant CAM domain use by disease status, including individual chronic diseases, as well as dyads and triads.

Sample characteristics

As described in Table 1, the sample was predominately White (75.6%), with the Southern region of the U.S. represented approximately twice the proportion of each of the other regions. Approximately 55.1% were female, 52.7% were married, and 73.2% were 50 years of age or older. About 76% had a high school or less education, and about one-quarter had graduated from college. Hypertension was most prevalent (73.2%), followed by hypercholesterolemia (61.1%), obesity (36.4%), and diabetes (22.6%). Approximately 37.2% of the participants had just one of the four chronic conditions, while 62.4% had more than one chronic disease.

Bivariate and multivariate analysis of CAM use
Bivariate analysis

As noted in Fig. 1, overall 29.5% of the sample reported use of CAM of any kind. However, an examination of CAM use by disease status (see Table 2 and Fig. 1) showed lower proportions of participants with hypertension (28.3%), diabetes

(25.0%), or obesity (10.8%) used CAM compared to those without these conditions ($p < 0.001$). Participants with hypercholesterolemia (31.5%) showed higher proportions of CAM use compared to those without this condition ($p < 0.001$). All the covariates except for sex were statistically associated with CAM use ($p < 0.05$). Additional results from the multivariate logistic regression analysis are reported in Table 2 with aORs controlling for potential confounding effects of the covariates in the model (e.g., education, sex, race/ethnicity, insurance status, etc.).

Multivariate analysis: Participants with one chronic condition

After controlling for confounding effects for those with one chronic condition, females were 25% more likely to use CAM than males ($p < 0.001$). Black/African Americans and the Non-Hispanic Other group were 54% and 39% less likely to report CAM use compared to Whites ($p < 0.001$), respectively. Compared to individuals with less than a high school education, high school and college graduates were 80% and 2.12 times more likely to report CAM use, respectively ($p < 0.001$). Participants with incomes in the range $35,000 to $49,999 or $50,000 to $74,999 were each 21% more likely to report CAM use compared to those with incomes less than $20,000 per year ($p < 0.05$). Finally, there was a 21% increased likelihood of using CAM for those participants residing in the Midwest or West, respectively, compared to Northeast residents ($p < 0.05$). For those with one chronic condition, there was no significant relationship in the adjusted odds of CAM use by age, marital status, having health insurance, or having a regular source of care.

Table 3 Utilization of CAM modalities by chronic disease dyads and triads

Disease Combinations	Overall CAM Use (n = 15,463)		CAM Modalities									
			Manipulative Methods (n = 3778)		Biological Treatments (n = 42)		Mind-Body Interventions (n = 801)		Energy Therapies (n = 72)		Alternative Systems (n = 592)	
	(%)	χ^2 value, p-value	(%)	χ^2 value, p-value	(%)	χ^2 value, p-value	(%)	χ^2 value, p-value	(%)	χ^2 value, p-value	(%)	χ^2 value, p-value
Disease Dyads												
ChoBp		0.08, p = 0.773		5.12, p = 0.024		0.03, p = 0.872		30.13, p < 0.001		5.32, p = 0.022		1.02, p = 0.314
Yes	11.2		25.4		0.3		3.9		0.3		3.6	
No	18.3		23.7		0.3		5.9		0.6		4.0	
ChoDiab		6.15, p = 0.014		0.58, p = 0.447		0.25, p = 0.614		29.25, p < 0.001		4.16, p = 0.042		2.83, p = 0.094
Yes	3.8		23.7		0.2		2.6		0.2		3.1	
No	25.7		24.4		0.3		5.6		0.5		3.9	
ChoOb		10.53, p = 0.001		22.79, p < 0.001		1.27, p = 0.261		18.55, p < 0.001		2.64, p = 0.106		1.40, p = 0.238
Yes	6.9		27.4		0.2		3.7		0.7		4.1	
No	22.6		23.5		0.3		5.6		0.4		3.7	
BpDiab		17.18, p < 0.001		4.51, p = 0.035		0.15, p = 0.702		37.98, p < 0.001		4.78, p = 0.030		4.88, p = 0.028
Yes	4.3		22.7		0.2		2.6		0.2		3.0	
No	25.2		24.6		0.3		5.7		0.5		4.0	
BpOb		0.05, p = 0.827		2.61, p = 0.107		1.67, p = 0.197		14.34, p < 0.001		2.68, p = 0.103		3.03, p = 0.083
Yes	8.4		25.1		0.2		4.0		0.3		3.4	
No	21.1		24.0		0.3		5.6		0.5		4.0	
DiabOb		8.55, p = 0.004		2.01, p = 0.157		5.69, p = 0.018		27.74, p < 0.001		1.56, p = 0.212		2.43, p = 0.120
Yes	2.9		22.9		0.04		2.4		0.3		3.1	
No	26.6		24.5		0.3		5.5		0.5		3.9	
Disease Triads												
ChoBpDiab		2.84, p = 0.093		0.04, p = 0.834		0.01, p = 0.933		22.67, p < 0.001		3.74, p = 0.054		1.08, p = 0.299
Yes	3.20		24.1		0.3		2.6		0.2		3.3	
No	26.3		24.3		0.3		5.5		0.5		3.9	
ChoBpOb		5.13, p = 0.024		13.43, p < 0.001		2.68, p = 0.102		14.78, p < 0.001		0.42, p = 0.518		0.02, p = 0.884
Yes	4.9		27.2		0.1		3.6		0.4		3.8	
No	24.6		23.8		0.3		5.4		0.5		3.8	
ChoDiabOb		0.37, p = 0.544		0.28, p = 0.596		2.82, p = 0.094		18.48, p < 0.001		1.30, p = 0.255		0.40, p = 0.528
Yes	2.0		25.0		0.0		2.2		0.2		3.5	
No	27.5		24.3		0.3		5.4		0.5		3.8	
BpDiabOb		4.34, p = 0.038		0.48, p = 0.491		3.89, p = 0.050		18.99, p < 0.001		2.28, p = 0.132		1.04, p = 0.309
Yes	2.3		23.5		0.1		2.5		0.2		3.3	
No	27.2		24.4		0.3		5.4		0.5		3.9	

Note: All percentages are weighted proportions
Disease Dyads: ChoBp = Hypercholesterolemia and Hypertension; ChoDiab = Hypercholesterolemia and Diabetes; ChoOb = Hypercholesterolemia and Obesity; BpDiab = Hypertension and Diabetes; BpOb = Hypertension and Obesity; DiabOb = Diabetes and Obesity
Disease Triads: ChoBpDiab = Hypercholesterolemia and Hypertension and Diabetes; ChoBpOb = Hypercholesterolemia and Hypertension and Obesity; BpDiabOb = Hypertension and Diabetes and Obesity; ChoDiabOb = Hypercholesterolemia and Diabetes and Obesity

Multivariate analysis: Participants with two or more chronic conditions

After adjusting for potential confounders for those with two or more chronic conditions, age, marital status, and having a regular source of care had no statistically significant effect on CAM use. Compared to Non-Hispanic Whites, Black/African Americans were 48% less likely to use CAM ($p < 0.001$), while Non-Hispanic Others were 25% less likely to report CAM use ($p < 0.05$). Those with health insurance and

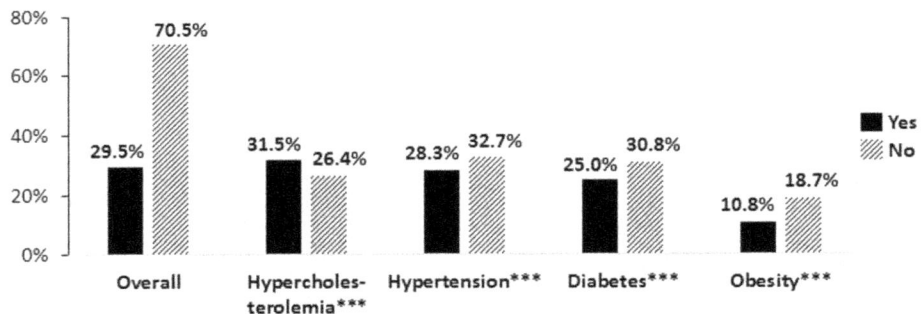

Fig. 1 Overall and Individual Disease-Specific Rates of CAM Use. Overall: [Yes = Used CAM of any kind regardless of disease condition; No = Did not use CAM]; For individual disease conditions: [Yes = Used CAM and had the disease; No = Used CAM but did not have the disease]; Significance levels: *$p < 0.05$, **$p < 0.01$, ***$p < 0.001$

two or more conditions were 16% less likely to report CAM use compared to those without health insurance and two or more conditions ($p < 0.05$). Females were 29% more likely to report CAM use compared to males ($p < 0.001$).

Residents of the Midwest were 64% more likely to report CAM use ($p < 0.001$), while those from the West were 61% more likely to use CAM ($p < 0.001$), compared to those living in the Northeast. Compared to individuals with less than a high school education, high school and college graduates were 53% and 78% significantly more likely to report CAM use, respectively ($p < 0.001$). Finally, compared to participants making less than $20,000, participants with income ranges of $35,000 to $49,999 and $50,000 to $74,999 were 30% ($p < 0.001$) and 25% ($p < 0.01$) more likely to use CAM.

Multivariate analysis: CAM use by disease dyads and triads

Table 3 summarizes the proportions of CAM use by disease dyads and disease triads with respect to overall utilization and the specific CAM domains as operationally defined in this study. Diabetes co-occurring with hypercholesterolemia, hypertension, or obesity was significant for overall CAM use with rates ranging from 2.9 to 4.3% ($p < 0.05$). Those without these comorbidities

using CAM had rates of 25.2% to 26.6%. Similarly, having both hypercholesterolemia and obesity yielded a significantly lower rate (6.9%) of CAM use compared to 22.6% among those using CAM who did not have this disease combination ($p < 0.01$). However, two disease dyads were not significant for CAM use among those with and without the disease combinations (i.e., hypertension and hypercholesterolemia; and hypertension and obesity). However, disease concordance with some of the highest proportions of CAM use (11.2% and 8.4%, respectively) was observed among persons within each of these groups, as noted in Fig. 2.

Across the disease triads, as noted in Table 3, proportions of CAM use ranged from 2.0 to 4.9% for those with these comorbidities. However, as reflected in Fig. 3, with respect to disease triads, only two of the four triads (hypertension and obesity co-occurring with either hypercholesterolemia or diabetes) were significant ($p < 0.05$). Nearly 5% of persons with hypertension, obesity, and hypercholesterolemia reported CAM use compared to 24.6% who used CAM but did not have this disease combination ($p < 0.05$). Similarly, having hypertension, obesity, and diabetes was also significant for CAM use (2.3%) compared to 27.2% who did not have these conditions but used CAM ($p < 0.05$).

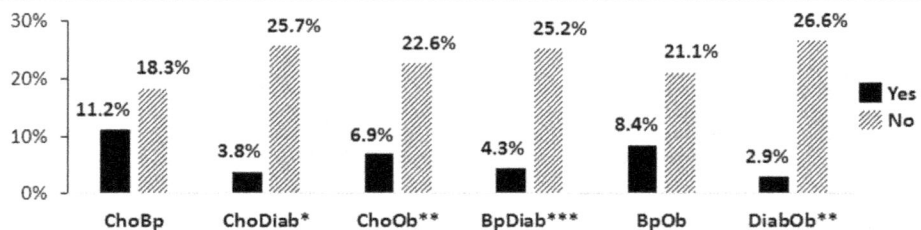

Fig. 2 CAM Use by Disease Dyads. [Yes = Used CAM and had the disease dyad; No = Used CAM but did not have the disease dyad]; Disease Dyads: ChoBp = Hypercholesterolemia and Hypertension; ChoDiab = Hypercholesterolemia and Diabetes; ChoOb = Hypercholesterolemia and Obesity; BpDiab = Hypertension and Diabetes; BpOb = Hypertension and Obesity; DiabOb = Diabetes and Obesity; Significance levels: *$p < 0.05$, **$p < 0.01$, ***$p < 0.001$

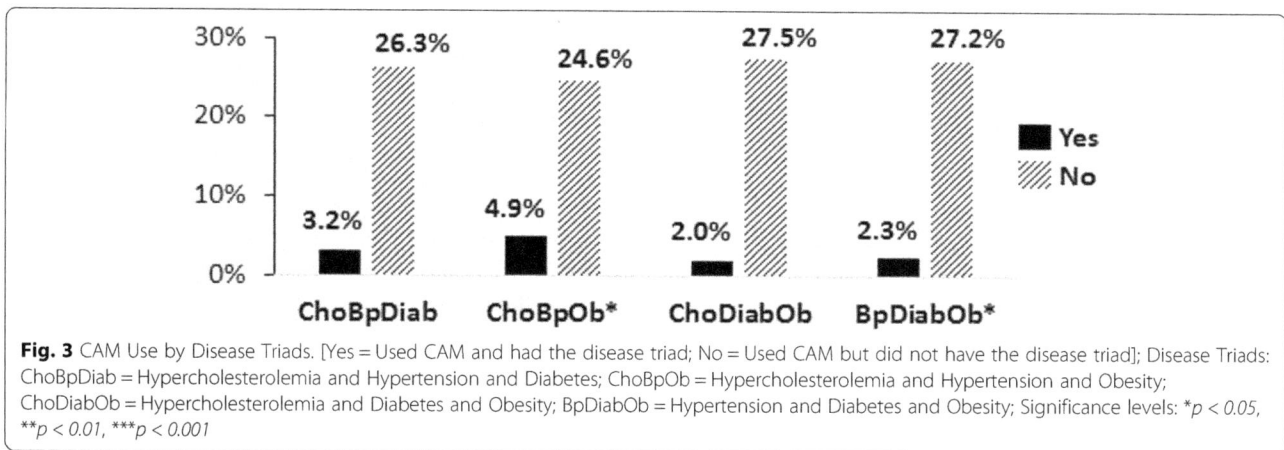

Fig. 3 CAM Use by Disease Triads. [Yes = Used CAM and had the disease triad; No = Used CAM but did not have the disease triad]; Disease Triads: ChoBpDiab = Hypercholesterolemia and Hypertension and Diabetes; ChoBpOb = Hypercholesterolemia and Hypertension and Obesity; ChoDiabOb = Hypercholesterolemia and Diabetes and Obesity; BpDiabOb = Hypertension and Diabetes and Obesity; Significance levels: *$p < 0.05$, **$p < 0.01$, ***$p < 0.001$

After adjusting for potential confounders for those with two or more chronic conditions, for the six dyad combinations (see Table 4), significant results for the adjusted odds ratios were only found for obese diabetic participants, who were 30% less likely to use CAM compared to those without these two chronic conditions (aOR = 0.70; 95% CI:0.55–0.88; $p < 0.01$). For the four disease triad combinations, significantly higher adjusted odds were only found for those participants with a concurrent diagnosis of hypercholesterolemia, diabetes, and obesity, who were 41% more likely to use CAM compared to those without these three chronic conditions (aOR = 1.41; 95% CI:1.02–1.94; $p < 0.05$). Additionally, those with hypercholesterolemia, hypertension, and obesity were 22% more likely to use CAM compared to those without these three comorbidities (aOR = 1.22; 95% CI:1.09–1.36; $p < 0.01$).

Multivariate analysis: CAM domain use by disease status
Across all four individual chronic conditions, manipulative methods had the highest rates of use (22–26%, $p < 0.05$). Alternative medical systems were also used by those with hypertension, hypercholesterolemia, or diabetes (3–4%, $p < 0.01$). For those with hypertension, diabetes, or obesity, approximately 3% to 5% used mind-body interventions ($p < 0.001$). Use of energy therapies (0.3%, $p < 0.001$) was only significant for those with hypertension, while use of biological treatments was not significant for any individual chronic condition. In general, the evidence suggests that there is greater use of manipulative methods, alternative medical systems, and mind-body interventions among participants with these individual chronic conditions. In addition, participants with hypertension utilized the greatest variety of treatments with significant usage across four of the five CAM domains, followed by participants with diabetes significantly utilizing treatments within three of the five CAM domains.

Alternatively, participants with hypercholesterolemia or obesity significantly used CAM treatments within just two of the five CAM domains.

As noted in Table 3, there appears to be higher use of mind-body interventions and manipulative methods among participants with two comorbidities. Whereas mind-body interventions are consistently and statistically associated with all six disease dyads with utilization ranging from 2 to 4% ($p < 0.001$), manipulative methods were significant for three dyads with the highest proportions overall (23–27%, $p < 0.05$). The use of energy therapies was also significant for three of the disease dyads, but with lower proportions (0.2–0.3%, $p < 0.05$). The use of alternative medical systems was significant for just one disease dyad (3%, $p < 0.05$), as was the use of biological treatments (0.04%, $p < 0.05$). In the dyad participant populations, those with hypertension and diabetes utilized the greatest variety of treatments with significant usage across four of the five CAM domains, followed by participants with hypertension and hypercholesterolemia significantly utilizing treatments within three of the five CAM domains. Alternatively, participants with hypercholesterolemia and either diabetes or obesity, as well as obese diabetic participants significantly used treatments within two of the five CAM domains. Finally, obese hypertensive participants significantly used treatments within just one CAM domain.

Similar to the findings in the disease dyads, the use of mind-body interventions was significant ($p < 0.001$) across all disease triads with proportions ranging from 2 to 4%. However, the use of manipulative methods was only significant for persons with hypercholesterolemia, hypertension, and obesity ($p < 0.001$), with a large proportion of use (27%) for this group. The use of biological treatments, energy therapies, and alternative medical systems were not significant for any of the disease triads, with use trends all under 4%. In the triad participant populations, those with

Table 4 Odds of CAM use among adults by chronic disease dyads and triads

Disease Combinations	Adjusted Odds of CAM Use	
	aOR [95% CI]	p-value
Disease Dyads		
ChoBp		
No (ref)	1.04[0.95–1.14]	0.351
Yes	1.00	–
ChoDiab		
No (ref)	0.92[0.75–1.11]	0.368
Yes	1.00	–
ChoOb		
No (ref)	1.08[0.96–1.21]	0.210
Yes	1.00	–
BpDiab		
No (ref)	1.06[0.91–1.24]	0.451
Yes	1.00	–
BpOb		
No (ref)	1.05[0.96–1.15]	0.309
Yes	1.00	–
DiabOb		
No (ref)	0.70[0.55–0.88]	0.003
Yes	1.00	–
Disease Triads		
ChoBpDiab		
No (ref)	1.00	–
Yes	1.11[0.94–1.32]	0.210
ChoBpOb		
No (ref)	1.00	–
Yes	1.22[1.09–1.36]	0.001
ChoDiabOb		
No (ref)	1.00	–
Yes	1.41[1.02–1.94]	0.037
BpDiabOb		
No (ref)	1.00	–
Yes	0.83[0.67–1.03]	0.083

Disease Dyads: ChoBp = Hypercholesterolemia and Hypertension; ChoDiab = Hypercholesterolemia and Diabetes; ChoOb = Hypercholesterolemia and Obesity; BpDiab = Hypertension and Diabetes; BpOb = Hypertension and Obesity; DiabOb = Diabetes and Obesity
Disease Triads: ChoBpDiab = Hypercholesterolemia and Hypertension and Diabetes; ChoBpOb = Hypercholesterolemia and Hypertension and Obesity; BpDiabOb = Hypertension and Diabetes and Obesity; ChoDiabOb = Hypercholesterolemia and Diabetes and Obesity

hypertension, hypercholesterolemia, and obesity utilized the greatest variety of treatments with significant usage across two of the five CAM domains, whereas all other triad participants significantly utilized treatments within just one of the five CAM domains.

Discussion

An alternate study based on 2012 NHIS adult respondents with and without mental illness and two or more chronic physical conditions (including diabetes, hyperlipidemia, hypertension, and others) [17], similarly found higher patterns of CAM use across manipulative methods (15%) compared to mind-body interventions (6%) or alternative medical systems (4%) for those with physical comorbidities only. Manipulative methods, in particular, may appeal to users that prefer collaborative decision making with a supportive CAM practitioner [18]. Other researchers have documented that such therapeutic relationships can occur irrespective of the CAM treatment efficacy [5].

The observed diminished effect of disease triads on overall use of CAM as well as less use of specific modalities may reflect the fact that when individuals have more than two comorbidities, they are likely to be under strict care and management by a conventional health care provider. As such, these patients are likely to be on pharmaceutical agents or intentionally minimizing use of CAM products. With respect to manipulative methods, it is possible that patients with three chronic conditions are in such a debilitated state that engagement with these methods may not be possible.

Limitations

Before discussing further implications of this study, several limitations must be noted. First, self-reported NHIS data are based on a sample of the population, and thus this study may be affected by sampling error and missing data. Second, CAM use trends may have changed since the publication of NHIS 2012 data set. In addition, the self-reported nature of the survey may have resulted in under-reporting of the various chronic diseases and CAM use. Nonetheless, the cross-sectional nature of the study allowed us to examine associations among sociodemographic factors, disease conditions, and use of a myriad of CAM therapies.

Implications for family practitioners

This study has implications for the management of patients with chronic conditions, especially when these ailments co-exist. In this study, as summarized in Table 5, two CAM modalities (i.e., mind-body interventions and manipulative methods) dominated use patterns of participants with individual chronic conditions, as well as with disease dyads and triads composed of hypercholesterolemia, hypertension, diabetes, and obesity. These modalities have little interference and minimal to no side effects with conventional medicines that may be prescribed for these conditions. Alternatively, for some chronic diseases, alternative medical systems (3 individual disease conditions and 1 dyad), energy therapies (1

Table 5 Statistically Significant CAM Modality Use by Disease Status

MIND-BODY INTERVENTIONS			MANIPULATIVE METHODS		
Hypertension***	ChoBp***	ChoBpDiab***	Hypercholesterolemia***	ChoBp*	ChoBpOb***
Diabetes***	ChoDiab***	ChoBpOb***	Hypertension**	ChoOb***	
Obesity***	ChoOb***	ChoDiabOb***	Diabetes***	BpDiab*	
	BpDiab***	BpDiabOb***	Obesity*		
	BpOb***				
	DiabOb***				
ALTERNATIVE SYSTEMS			ENERGY THERAPIES		
Hypercholesterolemia** Hypertension***	BpDiab*		Hypertension***	ChoBp*	
Diabetes**				ChoDiab*	
				BpDiab*	
BIOLOGICAL TREATMENTS					
	DiabOb*				

Disease Dyads: ChoBp = Hypercholesterolemia and Hypertension; ChoDiab = Hypercholesterolemia and Diabetes; ChoOb = Hypercholesterolemia and Obesity; BpDiab = Hypertension and Diabetes; BpOb = Hypertension and Obesity; DiabOb = Diabetes and Obesity
Disease Triads: ChoBpDiab = Hypercholesterolemia and Hypertension and Diabetes; ChoBpOb = Hypercholesterolemia and Hypertension and Obesity; BpDiabOb = Hypertension and Diabetes and Obesity; ChoDiabOb = Hypercholesterolemia and Diabetes and Obesity
Significance levels: *$p < 0.05$, **$p < 0.01$, ***$p < 0.001$

individual disease condition and 3 dyads), and biological treatments (1 dyad) were also significant choices for some participants.

Conclusions

As integrative medicine becomes commonplace, family practitioners will play a pivotal role in educating patients on the benefits and potential harm of CAM products [19, 20]. This is especially true as more patients require maintenance medications that may increase the risk for multi-drug or herb-drug interactions or nullify the sometimes narrowly windowed therapeutic effects of the pharmaceutical agents indicated for these conditions [7, 21]. Our study provides prevalence data concerning the use of CAM modalities among persons with a variety of chronic condition dyads and triads, and these disease combinations have gone largely understudied in the scientific literature with respect to specific CAM domain usage rates. Patients with multiple comorbidities use various non-conventional approaches, and as such, it is important for health care providers at every level to proactively probe patients on the use of CAM products and or services and to offer personalized information about the possible risks, benefits, and potential implications of using CAM. Indeed, research has consistently shown patients do not always voluntarily divulge information on CAM use to providers [5, 22, 23]. This study focused on four chronic conditions due to their prevalence in the general population. As clinical practice guidelines and life-style recommendations for multimorbid patients continue to be developed to include CAM, future research on these and other comorbidities may contribute to improved health care utilization and patient outcomes.

Authors' contributions
JM and AO designed the study and methodology and executed the data analysis. MAS, LMS, BL, and OO were major contributors in data interpretation and in writing the manuscript. All authors read and approved the final manuscript.

Competing interests
The authors declare that they have no competing interests. The views and opinions expressed in this article are those of the authors and do not necessarily represent the views of the National Institutes of Health or any other government agency.

Author details
[1]Department of Public Health, University of West Florida, 11000 University Parkway, Bldg. 38/Room 127, Pensacola, FL 32514, USA. [2]Department of Mathematics and Statistics, University of West Florida, Pensacola, FL, USA. [3]Warren Alpert Medical School, Brown University, Providence, RI, USA. [4]Office of Cancer Complementary and Alternative Medicine, National Cancer Institute, Bethesda, MD, USA. [5]Kelly Government Solutions, Bethesda, MD, USA.

References
1. Straus SE. Expanding horizons of healthcare: five-year strategic plan, 2001-2005. Bethesda: NIH; 2000. p. 1–47.
2. Clark TC, Black LI, Stussman BJ, et al. Trends in the use of complementary health approaches among adults: United States, 2002-2012. Natl Health Stat Rep. 2015;79:1–16.
3. Nahin RL, Barnes PM, Stussman BJ, Bloom B. Costs of complementary and alternative medicine (CAM) and frequency of visits to CAM practitioners: United States, 2007. Natl Health Stat Rep. 2009;18:1–16.
4. Barnes PM, Bloom B, Nahin RL. Complementary and alternative medicine use among adults and children: United States, 2007. Natl Health Stat Rep. 2008;12:1–24.
5. Warren N, Canaway R, Unantenne N, Manderson L. Taking control: complementary and alternative medicine in diabetes and cardiovascular disease management. Health. 2012;17:323–39.
6. Leong M, Smith TJ, Rowland-Seymour A. Complementary and integrative medicine for older adults in palliative care. Clin Geriatr Med. 2015;31:177–91.
7. Zencirci AD. Complementary therapy use of cardiovascular patients. Intern Med. 2013;3:e113.
8. Anderson JG, Taylor AG. Use of complementary therapies by individuals with or at risk for cardiovascular disease: results of the 2007 National Health Interview Survey. J Cardiovasc Nurs. 2012;27:96–102.
9. Bauer UE, Briss PA, Goodman RA, Bowman BA. Prevention of chronic disease in the 21st century: elimination of the leading preventable causes of premature death and disability in the USA. Lancet. 2014;384:45–52.

10. Go AS, Mozaffarian D, Roger VL, et al. Heart disease and stroke statistics--2014 update: a report from the American Heart Association. Circ. 2013;129:e28–e292.

11. Nwankwo T, Yoon SS, Burt V, Gu Q. Hypertension among adults in the United States: National Health and nutrition examination survey, 2011-2012. NCHS Data Brief. 2013;133:1–8.

12. Ward BW, Schiller JS, Goodman RA. Multiple chronic conditions among US adults: a 2012 update. Prev Chronic Dis. 2014;11:E62.

13. National Center for Health Statistics. National Health Interview Survey. 2012. https://www.cdc.gov/nchs/nhis/nhis_2012_data_release.htm

14. Parsons VL, Moriarity C, Jonas K, et al. Design and estimation for the National Health Interview Survey, 2006-2015. Vital Health Stat. 2014;165:1–53.

15. Su D, Li L. Trends in the use of complementary and alternative medicine in the United States: 2002-2007. J Health Care Poor Underserved. 2011;22:296–310.

16. Agresti A. Asymptotic theory for parametric models. In: Agresti A, editor. Categorical data analysis. 2nd ed. New York: John Wiley & Sons; 2003. p. 576–99.

17. Alwhaibi M, Bhattacharya R, Sambamoorthi U. Type of multimorbidity and complementary and alternative medicine use among adults. Evid Based Complement Alternat Med. 2015;2015:362582.

18. Bishop FL, Yardley L, Lewith GT. A systematic review of beliefs involved in the use of complementary and alternative medicine. J Health Psychol. 2007;12:851–67.

19. Frank R, Stollberg G. Medical acupuncture in Germany: patterns of consumerism among physicians and patients. Sociol Health Illn. 2014;26:351–72.

20. Ventola CL. Current issues regarding complementary and alternative medicine (CAM) in the United States: part 1: the widespread use of CAM and the need for better-informed health care professionals to provide patient counseling. Pharm Ther. 2010;35:461–8.

21. Zhang J, Onakpoya IJ, Posadzki P, Eddouks M. The safety of herbal medicine: from prejudice to evidence. Evid Based Complement Alternat Med. 2015;2015:316706.

22. Robinson A, McGrail MR. Disclosure of CAM use to medical practitioners: a review of qualitative and quantitative studies. Complement Ther Med. 2004;12:90–8.

23. Tasaki K, Maskarinec G, Shumay DM, et al. Communication between physicians and cancer patients about complementary and alternative medicine: exploring patients' perspectives. Psychooncology. 2002;11:212–20.

20

Steroidal alkaloids and conessine from the medicinal plant *Holarrhena antidysenterica* restore antibiotic efficacy in a *Galleria mellonella* model of multidrug-resistant *Pseudomonas aeruginosa* infection

Thanyaluck Siriyong[1], Supayang Piyawan Voravuthikunchai[1] and Peter John Coote[2]* 🆔

Abstract

Background: This study aimed to evaluate the efficacy of combinations of steroidal alkaloids and conessine from the Thai medicinal plant *Holarrhena antidysenterica* with antibiotics against *Pseudomonas aeruginosa* strains possessing different efflux-pump-mediated multidrug-resistant (MDR) phenotypes in a *Galleria mellonella* infection model.

Methods: *P. aeruginosa* strains with defined mutations that result in the overexpression of the MexAB-OprM, MexCD-OprJ and MexEF-OprN efflux pumps, and a strain with all three of these pumps deleted, were used. In vitro, the effect of combinations of steroidal alkaloids and conessine with antibiotics was compared with antibiotic treatment alone via MIC determination and time-kill assays. Efficacy of combinations of the steroidal alkaloids and conessine with levofloxacin were compared with monotherapies against infections in *G. mellonella* larvae by measuring larval mortality and bacterial burden.

Results: Combination therapies of conessine or steroidal alkaloids with levofloxacin enhanced bacterial inhibition in vitro and restored antibiotic efficacy in vivo compared to the constituent monotherapies. Neither conessine nor the steroidal alkaloids induced any detectable toxicity in *G. mellonella* larvae. The enhanced efficacy of the combination treatments was most pronounced with conessine and correlated with reduced larval burden of infecting *P. aeruginosa*. Notably, the enhanced efficacy of conessine/levofloxacin combinations was only detected in the parent strain and strains that overexpressed the MexAB-OprM or MexEF-OprN efflux systems.

Conclusions: Steroidal alkaloids from *Holarrhena antidysenterica*, and particularly the principal active ingredient conessine, restored levofloxacin efficacy against resistant *P. aeruginosa* strains possessing efflux-mediated MDR phenotypes. The compounds should be investigated further as a potential novel therapy.

Keywords: Conessine, Efflux pump inhibitor, *Galleria mellonella*, *Holarrhena antidysenterica*, Mex efflux systems

Background

Global emergence of multidrug-resistant (MDR) *Pseudomonas aeruginosa* is now a growing threat to antibiotic therapy. Chromosomally encoded antibiotic efflux mechanisms greatly contribute to antibiotic resistance in this organism, in particular, the multidrug efflux pumps of the resistance-nodulation-division (RND) superfamily such as MexAB-OprM, MexCD-OprJ, MexEF-OprN, and MexXY-OprM [1, 2]. Clinical isolates of *P. aeruginosa* are often identified with mutations in regulatory genes that result in the over-expression of these RND efflux pumps and confer a MDR phenotype [1, 3]. The MDR phenotype occurs due to the broad and overlapping range of antibiotic substrates that the RND pumps efflux, particularly MexAB-OprM [3]. Thus, multidrug efflux pumps represent potential targets for the development of novel treatment regimens for MDR *P. aeruginosa*.

* Correspondence: pjc5@st-andrews.ac.uk
[2]Biomedical Sciences Research Complex, School of Biology, University of St Andrews, The North Haugh, St Andrews, Fife, UK
Full list of author information is available at the end of the article

The use of efflux pump inhibitors (EPIs) as adjuncts in combination therapies with existing antibiotics is a potential strategy for preventing efflux-mediated resistance and restoring antibiotic efficacy [4]. Many synthetic compounds such as phenylalanine-arginine β-naphthylamide (PAβN), carbonyl cyanide m-chlorophenylhydrazone (CCCP), quinoline derivatives, and 1-(1-naphthylmethyl)-piperazine (NMP) display efflux pump inhibitory activity however none have yet been developed for clinical application [5, 6]. Some existing drugs have also been found to possess efflux-pump inhibitory properties and could be repurposed as resistance modifying agents when administered in combination with antibiotics. Examples include trimethoprim and the selective serotonin reuptake inhibitor sertraline [5, 7, 8].

Currently, a number of naturally-occurring compounds with possible EPI activity including berberine [9], curcumin [10, 11], and p-coumaric acid [12] are being actively researched for potential future application [13, 14]. Extracts made from the stem bark of the plant Holarrhena antidysenterica (Linn) Wallich belonging to the family Apocynaceae, are used in Thai and Ayurvedic traditional medicine to treat amoebic dysentery and diarrhoea [15, 16]. Steroidal alkaloids present within the extracts possess antibacterial, anti-diarrhoeal and astringent properties [15, 16]. Previous studies indicated that H. antidysenterica extract, and the principal active ingredient alone (the steroidal alkaloid conessine [16]), were able to restore the inhibitory activity of novobiocin and rifampicin against extensively drug-resistant Acinetobacter baumannii in vitro [17–19]. Exposure to either H. antidysenterica extract, or conessine alone, at concentrations that did not result in increased membrane disruption, resulted in accumulation of the fluorescent dye Pyronin Y suggesting that both treatments may have EPI-like properties [19]. Moreover, exposure to conessine restored the MICs of antibiotics against a P. aeruginosa strain over-expressing MexAB-OprM to values comparable with the wild-type parent and conessine induced the accumulation of Hoechst 33342 in cells over-expressing the same efflux pump [20].

Previous work has employed Galleria mellonella larvae to demonstrate enhanced efficacy of putative EPIs in combination with antibiotics versus infections by MDR strains of P. aeruginosa that over-express various RND efflux pumps [10, 21]. The aim of this study was to evaluate the efficacy of combinations of antibiotics with either H. antidysenterica extracts, or the steroidal alkaloid conessine, using a G. mellonella infection model to determine if these combinations were toxic, or could treat successfully, infections with P. aeruginosa strains possessing an efflux-pump dependent MDR phenotype due to over-expression of either MexAB-OprM, MexCD-OprJ or MexEF-OprN.

Methods
Bacteria and growth media
P. aeruginosa strains PAM1020 (PAO1 prototroph, wild-type); PAM1032 (nalB), MexAB-OprM overexpressed; PAM1033 (nfxB), MexCD-OprJ overexpressed; PAM1034 (nfxC), MexEF-OprN overexpressed; and PAM1626 (Δmex), MexAB-OprM, MexCD-OprJ and MexEF-OprN deletion, were a generous gift from Dr. Olga Lomovskaya, Rempex Pharmaceuticals, USA [22]. The strains were grown to mid-log phase in Mueller–Hinton broth (MHB; Merck, Darmstadt, Germany) at 37 °C with shaking (at 200 rpm) to prepare inocula for antibiotic susceptibility testing in vitro and efficacy testing in vivo.

Chemicals and G. mellonella larvae
Conessine and the antibiotics ceftazidime, piperacillin, meropenem, amikacin, and levofloxacin were purchased from Sigma–Aldrich Ltd. (Dorset, UK). Stock solutions of antibiotics were prepared in sterile deionized water. Conessine was made in 70% Tween 80 (Sigma–Aldrich Ltd., Dorset, UK) and 30% ethanol. Sub-stocks of all antibiotics and conessine used in experiments were dissolved in sterile deionized water. G. mellonella larvae were obtained from UK Waxworms Ltd. (Sheffield, UK). Stock solutions of steroidal alkaloids from H. antidysenterica bark extract were prepared in 100% ethanol as previously described [15]. Briefly, fresh barks were washed with distilled water and dried at 60 °C overnight. Finely powdered bark (4 kg) was macerated with 95% ethanol (1:2 w/v) to obtain an alcohol extract, evaporated to dryness, and then suspended in methanol. The suspension was adjusted to pH = 3.2 by addition of HCl (2 M). The solution was basified to pH = 9 with NaOH (2 M) and then extracted with chloroform (0.4 L × 5) to obtain the total alkaloids (25.63 g). Sub-stocks used in experiments were made in sterile deionized water.

Antibiotic susceptibility testing
MICs of antibiotics (ceftazidime, piperacillin, meropenem, amikacin, and levofloxacin), conessine, or steroidal alkaloids against each of the P. aeruginosa strains were determined in 96-well microplates as previously described [23]. Briefly, doubling dilutions of each antibiotic, conessine or steroidal alkaloids were prepared in MHB and subsequently inoculated with 1.0×10^6 cfu/mL of P. aeruginosa. The effect of conessine or steroidal alkaloids in combination with each antibiotic was measured by first preparing 96-well plates with doubling dilutions of each antibiotic in MHB as described above. Following this, single concentrations of either steroidal extracts (1024 mg/L) or conessine ($MIC_{0.5}$–32 mg/L or $MIC_{0.25}$–16 mg/L) were added to each well prior to inoculation with P. aeruginosa as before. Microplates were incubated at 37 °C and the MIC was defined as the

concentration(s) present in the first optically clear well after 24 h. Each experiment was performed at least twice. Fractional inhibitory concentration index (FICI) = (MIC$_{drug + steroidal\ alkaloids\ or\ conessine}$/MIC$_{steroidal\ alkaloids\ or\ conessine}$) + (MIC$_{drug + steroidal\ alkaloids\ or\ conessine}$/MIC$_{antibiotic}$) were calculated for each combination and synergy was defined as FICI ≤0.5 [24].

Determination of *P. aeruginosa* viability

P. aeruginosa viability was assessed after 24 h exposure to levofloxacin (0.125, 1, 2 mg/L), conessine (32 mg/L), or steroidal alkaloids (1024 mg/L), and combinations of levofloxacin with conessine or steroidal alkaloids. Aliquots of tested compounds were added to 96-well microplate wells containing MHB, while identical volumes of sterile water were added to control wells. Microplates were inoculated with 1.0×10^6 cfu/mL of *P. aeruginosa* and the plates were incubated at 37 °C for 24 h. Subsequently, viable bacteria were determined by serial dilution in MHB and plating on nutrient agar (NA; Merck, Darmstadt, Germany). Plates were incubated at 37 °C for 24 h prior to counting colonies. Each treatment was replicated in quadruplicate and a mean value was calculated. Synergy was defined as a ≥ 2-log$_{10}$ decrease in colony count at 24 h by the combination therapies compared with the most effective single treatments, as well as a ≥ 2-log$_{10}$ decrease in colony count compared with the starting inoculum [25].

G. mellonella model of *P. aeruginosa* infection

G. mellonella at their final instar larval stage were kept at room temperature in darkness. Larvae weighing within the range of 250 to 350 mg were selected for each experiment to ensure consistency in subsequent drug administrations and were used within 1 week of receipt.

Efficacy of conessine or steroidal alkaloids in combination with levofloxacin versus *G. mellonella* larvae infected with the *P. aeruginosa* strains was carried out exactly as described previously [21, 23, 26]. Briefly, groups of 15 larvae were infected with an inoculum of 2.5×10^3 cfu/mL of *P. aeruginosa* cells. Treatments with three doses of conessine or steroidal alkaloids, levofloxacin, and combinations of these compounds were administered 2, 4, and 6 h post-infection. Levofloxacin doses of 1 and 0.05 mg/kg were used for *P. aeruginosa* PAM1020 and PAM1626 respectively and a dose of 5 mg/kg of levofloxacin was utilized for PAM1032, PAM1033 and PAM1034 [21]. Conessine was administered at 50 mg/kg and steroidal alkaloids at 50, 100 and 200 mg/kg in all tested strains. The experiments were repeated in triplicate using larvae from different batches and the data from these replicate experiments were pooled to give *n* = 45. Survival data were plotted using the Kaplan–Meier method [27] and comparisons made between groups using the log-rank test [28]. In all comparisons with the negative control it was the uninfected control (rather than the unmanipulated control) that was used. Holm's correction was applied to account for multiple comparisons in all tests and $P ≤ 0.05$ was considered significant [29].

G. mellonella haemolymph burden

Larval burden of five randomly selected caterpillars from each treatment group was measured at 24 h intervals exactly as described previously [10, 21, 26]. Groups of 30 larvae were infected with 2.5×10^3 cfu/mL of *P. aeruginosa*. Conessine (50 mg/kg) or steroidal alkaloids (50, 100 or 200 mg/kg), levofloxacin (1 or 5 mg/kg), and the combinations were administered at 2, 4, and 6 h post-infection. Larvae were incubated in Petri dishes at 37 °C. The detection limit for this assay was 100 cfu/mL of larval homogenate.

Results

H. antidysenterica steroidal alkaloids and conessine increase the susceptibility of *P. aeruginosa* to antibiotics in vitro

Alone, the steroidal alkaloids had no inhibitory action and the MIC for the parent strain and the strains overexpressing each of the efflux systems was > 1024 mg/L. However, deletion of all three efflux systems (PAM1626) did induce some sensitivity as the MIC for this strain was 256 mg/L. In contrast, the MIC for conessine was identical for all of the strains tested: 64 mg/L, suggesting that conessine is not a substrate for the MexAB-OprM, MexCD-OprJ, and MexEF-OprN efflux pumps.

The susceptibility of the *P. aeruginosa* strains to a group of anti-pseudomonal antibiotics alone or in the presence of steroidal alkaloids (128 or 1024 mg/L) or conessine (32 mg/L) is shown in Table 1. In this study, steroidal alkaloids extract at 1024 mg/L contained approximately 37 mg/L conessine content [19]. The strain overexpressing the MexAB-OprM efflux pump (PAM1032) was more resistant to ceftazidime, piperacillin, meropenem and levofloxacin in comparison to the parent strain (PAM1020). In contrast, the strains overexpressing the MexCD-OprJ (PAM1033) and MexEF-OprN (PAM1034) efflux systems displayed resistance to levofloxacin only. Deletion of all three efflux systems (PAM1626) resulted in increased susceptibility to all of the antibiotics compared to the parent strain. These results are in accordance with published reports on the substrate specificity of these efflux pumps [1, 21].

Generally, but with some exceptions, combination of the steroidal alkaloids or conessine with the antibiotics resulted in minor reductions of the MICs of the antibiotics versus each of the *P. aeruginosa* strains tested (Table 1). However, this enhancement of antibiotic inhibition was not synergistic as none of the calculated FICI values for each of the drug combinations was ≤0.5 (Table 1).

Further study of the inhibitory action of the steroidal alkaloids or conessine in combination with levofloxacin

Table 1 MICs of five antibiotics alone and in the presence of *Holarrhena antidysenterica* steroidal alkaloids or conessine against *P. aeruginosa* PAM1020, 1032, 1033, 1034 and 1626

Strain	Drug	Drug MIC (mg/L) with			FIC index[b]	
		Alone	Steroidal alkaloids[a]	Conessine[a]	Drug + Steroidal alkaloids	Drug + Conessine
PAM1020	CAZ	1	0.5	1	1.50	1.50
	PIP	2	1	2	1.50	1.50
	MEM	0.5	0.5	0.25	2.00	1.00
	LVX	0.5	0.5	0.25	2.00	1.00
	AMK	1	0.5	0.5	1.50	1.00
PAM1032	CAZ	4	2	2	1.50	1.00
	PIP	16	16	8	2.00	1.00
	MEM	4	4	2	2.00	1.00
	LVX	2	1	1	1.50	1.00
	AMK	1	0.5	0.5	1.50	1.00
PAM1033	CAZ	1	0.5	1	1.50	1.50
	PIP	2	1	2	1.50	1.50
	MEM	0.5	0.25	0.5	1.50	1.50
	LVX	4	4	4	2.00	1.50
	AMK	0.5	0.25	0.5	1.50	1.50
PAM1034	CAZ	1	1	0.5	2.00	1.00
	PIP	1	0.5	0.03125	1.50	0.53
	MEM	0.5	0.5	0.125	2.00	0.75
	LVX	4	2	0.25	1.50	0.56
	AMK	0.5	0.25	0.5	1.50	1.50
PAM1626	CAZ	0.5	0.5	0.25	1.50	1.00
	PIP	0.5	0.25	0.5	1.00	1.50
	MEM	0.0625	0.0625	0.0625	1.50	1.50
	LVX	0.03125	0.00781	0.00391	0.75	0.63
	AMK	0.5	0.25	0.25	1.00	1.00

CAZ ceftazidime, *PIP* piperacillin, *MEM* meropenem, *LVX* levofloxacin, *AMK* amikacin

[a]The concentration of steroidal alkaloids or conessine added to each well reflected the previously characterized MICs and were selected to be lower than the MIC for each strain: PAM1020, 1032, 1033, and 1034: Steroidal alkaloids (1024 mg/L), Conessine (32 mg/L); PAM1626: Steroidal alkaloids (128 mg/L), Conessine (32 mg/L)

[b]Fractional inhibitory concentration index (FIC index) where synergistic ($\leq$ 0.5), non- synergistic (> 0.5 - $\leq$ 4.0), and antagonistic (> 4.0). For the strains where the steroidal alkaloids did not have a measurable MIC, the highest value tested (1024 mg/L) was used in the FICI calculation to provide a conservative estimate of the FICI value

was carried out because the fluoroquinolones are known substrates for all three of the overexpressed efflux systems studied in this work [1]. Furthermore, in a recent study that employed the same strains, levofloxacin in combination with unrelated, putative EPIs generated optimal results [21].

The effect of exposure to levofloxacin alone at MIC$_{0.5}$, or combinations of levofloxacin with steroidal alkaloids or conessine, on the viability of the *P. aeruginosa* strains was measured using an in vitro 24 h time-kill assay (Table 2). The *P. aeruginosa* strain overexpressing the MexCD-OprJ efflux system (PAM1033) and the triple deletion strain (PAM1626) were omitted because the levofloxacin MIC of PAM1033 was unchanged by exposure to either the

alkaloids or conessine, and PAM1626 is already hypersensitive to levofloxacin (Table 1).

Combination of levofloxacin with either the steroidal alkaloids or conessine did enhance killing of the *P. aeruginosa* strains overexpressing MexAB-OprM and MexEF-OprN compared to the single drug treatments. The greatest enhancement of killing occurred with combinations of levofloxacin and conessine. However, similar to the findings shown in Table 1, the enhanced killing due to the combination treatments was not sufficiently potent to be termed synergistic.

In summary, combination of *H. antidysenterica* steroidal alkaloids and conessine with antibiotics resulted in enhanced inhibition in vitro of *P. aeruginosa* strains

Table 2 Effect of conessine and steroidal alkaloids in combination with levofloxacin on the viability of *P. aeruginosa* PAM1020, PAM1032 and PAM1034

	Strain	Agent (s)	Concentration (mg/L)	Log CFU/ml			
				Inoculum	Untreated control	Treatment (±SD)	Log reduction
Single treatment at MIC$_{0.5}$[a]	PAM1020	Conessine	32			9.47 ± 0.03	0.27
		Alkaloids	1024	5.16 ± 0.06	9.74 ± 0.06	8.76 ± 0.01	0.98
		LVX	0.125			8.91 ± 0.02	0.83
	PAM1032	Conessine	32			9.42 ± 0.01	0.45
		Alkaloids	1024	5.44 ± 0.08	9.87 ± 0.14	8.82 ± 0.06	1.05
		LVX	1			8.19 ± 0.68	1.68
	PAM1034	Conessine	32			9.54 ± 0.09	0.13
		Alkaloids	1024	5.64 ± 0.21	9.67 ± 0.02	8.88 ± 0.23	0.79
		LVX	2			8.18 ± 0.10	1.49
Combinations at MIC$_{0.5}$	PAM1020	Conessine + LVX	32 + 0.125	5.16 ± 0.06	9.74 ± 0.06	9.25 ± 0.03	0.49
		Alkaloids + LVX	1024 + 0.125			8.12 ± 0.16	1.62
	PAM1032	Conessine + LVX	32 + 1	5.44 ± 0.08	9.87 ± 0.14	**5.35 ± 0.43**	**4.52**
		Alkaloids + LVX	1024 + 1			**7.70 ± 0.13**	**2.17**
	PAM1034	Conessine + LVX	32 + 2	5.64 ± 0.21	9.67 ± 0.02	**5.54 ± 0.09**	**4.13**
		Alkaloids + LVX	1024 + 2			**6.85 ± 0.67**	**2.82**

[a]A MIC was not detectable for the steroidal alkaloids so the highest concentration tested was used in this assay
Viability was determined in 96-well microplates after 24 h exposure to the antibiotics in MHB at 37 °C. Data shown is the mean and standard deviation from quadruple experiments. Highlighted treatments are those that resulted in ≥2 log$_{10}$ reduction compared to untreated controls

that over-express different efflux-pump systems that can confer a MDR phenotype.

Combination treatments of levofloxacin with *H. antidysenterica* steroidal alkaloids, or conessine, show enhanced efficacy compared to the component monotherapies versus *G. mellonella* larvae infected with MDR strains of *P. aeruginosa*

The efficacy of antibiotic combinations with steroidal alkaloids or conessine were investigated in vivo using the *G. mellonella* infection model. Initially, larvae were injected with triple doses (at 2, 4 and 6 h intervals after the start of the experiment) of the steroidal alkaloids (up to 200 mg/kg) or conessine (up to 50 mg/kg) alone to determine if either were toxic and neither had any detrimental effect on the larvae after 96 h incubation at 37 °C (Additional file 1).

Preliminary studies showed that combinations of the steroidal alkaloids or conessine with the antibiotic levofloxacin gave the best results so these were investigated further in detail. Appropriate strain specific dosing regimens of levofloxacin, steroidal alkaloids and conessine were determined that provided little, or no, therapeutic benefit to larvae infected with the *P. aeruginosa* strains when administered as monotherapies (Additional file 2). Thus, any enhanced efficacy induced upon administration of combinations of the antibiotics with the steroidal alkaloids or conessine could be readily observed.

The effect of triple doses (2, 4 and 6 h post-infection (p.i)) of levofloxacin in combination with steroidal alkaloids

on the survival and bacterial burden of *G. mellonella* larvae infected with *P. aeruginosa* PAM1032 and PAM1034 is shown in Fig. 1. Treatment with triple doses of steroidal alkaloids alone (50, 100 or 200 mg/kg) had no therapeutic benefit on all of the strains tested (Fig. 1a and b). Death of the infected larvae correlated with the recovery of high numbers of *P. aeruginosa* PAM1032 or PAM1034 from within the larvae after just 24 h (Fig. 1c and d respectively). Similarly, a triple dose of levofloxacin (5 mg/kg) resulted in only a minor increase in survival of infected larvae compared to infected larvae treated with PBS (Fig. 1a and b) and the rapid growth of both *P. aeruginosa* strains within the larvae was not significantly reduced (Fig. 1c and d).

Notably, treatment with the same triple doses of the steroidal alkaloids in combination with 5 mg/kg of levofloxacin resulted in significantly enhanced survival compared to triple doses of the monotherapies ($P < 0.05$). Enhanced survival after combination therapy was most pronounced with PAM1032 infections but was also evident with PAM1034 to a lesser extent (Fig. 1a and b). Furthermore, combination therapy completely prevented the rapid proliferation of bacteria within the larvae reflected by large reductions in bacterial burden compared to that seen with the monotherapies over the duration of the experiment (Fig. 1c and d). The enhanced efficacy of levofloxacin occurred in a dose-dependent fashion increasing as the co-administered dose of the steroidal alkaloids increased. Significantly enhanced efficacy was only observed with the strains overexpressing

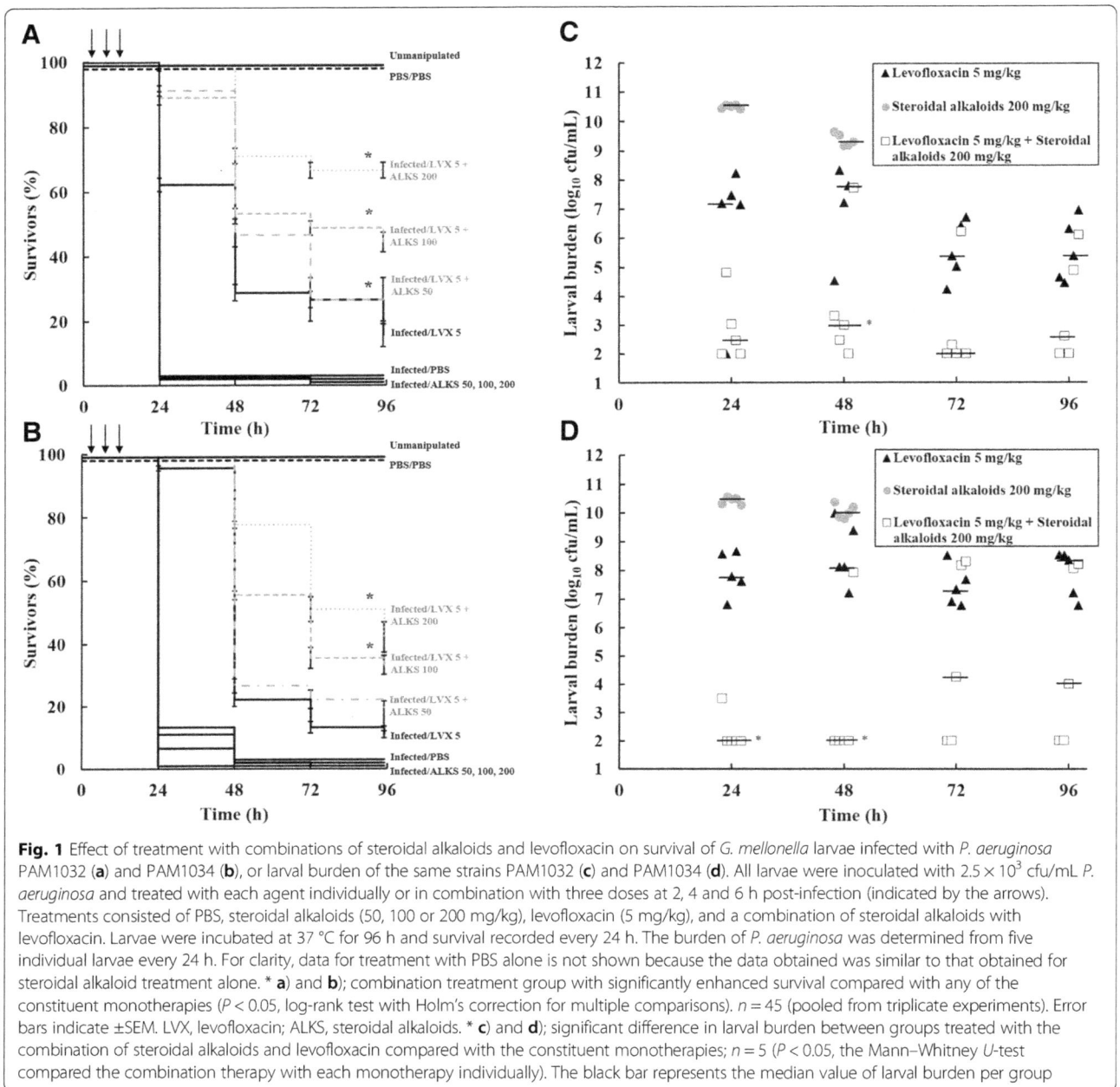

Fig. 1 Effect of treatment with combinations of steroidal alkaloids and levofloxacin on survival of *G. mellonella* larvae infected with *P. aeruginosa* PAM1032 (**a**) and PAM1034 (**b**), or larval burden of the same strains PAM1032 (**c**) and PAM1034 (**d**). All larvae were inoculated with 2.5 × 10³ cfu/mL *P. aeruginosa* and treated with each agent individually or in combination with three doses at 2, 4 and 6 h post-infection (indicated by the arrows). Treatments consisted of PBS, steroidal alkaloids (50, 100 or 200 mg/kg), levofloxacin (5 mg/kg), and a combination of steroidal alkaloids with levofloxacin. Larvae were incubated at 37 °C for 96 h and survival recorded every 24 h. The burden of *P. aeruginosa* was determined from five individual larvae every 24 h. For clarity, data for treatment with PBS alone is not shown because the data obtained was similar to that obtained for steroidal alkaloid treatment alone. * **a**) and **b**); combination treatment group with significantly enhanced survival compared with any of the constituent monotherapies (*P* < 0.05, log-rank test with Holm's correction for multiple comparisons). *n* = 45 (pooled from triplicate experiments). Error bars indicate ±SEM. LVX, levofloxacin; ALKS, steroidal alkaloids. * **c**) and **d**); significant difference in larval burden between groups treated with the combination of steroidal alkaloids and levofloxacin compared with the constituent monotherapies; *n* = 5 (*P* < 0.05, the Mann–Whitney *U*-test compared the combination therapy with each monotherapy individually). The black bar represents the median value of larval burden per group

MexAB-OprM (PAM1032) and MexEF-OprN (PAM1034). A small enhancement (*P* < 0.05) in survival was observed in the parent strain (PAM1020) but only at the highest dose of steroidal alkaloids administered (Additional file 3a). No enhancement in survival after combination therapy was observed in the strain overexpressing MexCD-OprJ (PAM1033) or the strain with the three efflux-pump systems deleted (PAM1626) (Additional file 3b and c respectively).

Similar studies were carried out with combinations of conessine with levofloxacin rather than the steroidal

alkaloids (Fig. 2). Treatment with a triple dose of conessine (50 mg/kg) alone had no therapeutic effect on larvae infected with all of the *P. aeruginosa* strains tested and did not prevent the rapid increase in bacterial burden of the inoculated *P. aeruginosa* strains that occurred after the first 24 h p.i (Fig. 2). Similarly, strain-specific, triple doses of levofloxacin alone were administered that resulted in only a small increase in survival of infected larvae compared to those treated with PBS: PAM1020–1 mg/kg (Fig. 2a) and PAM1032 or PAM1034 5 mg/kg (Fig. 2b and c, respectively). Correlating with larval survival, these

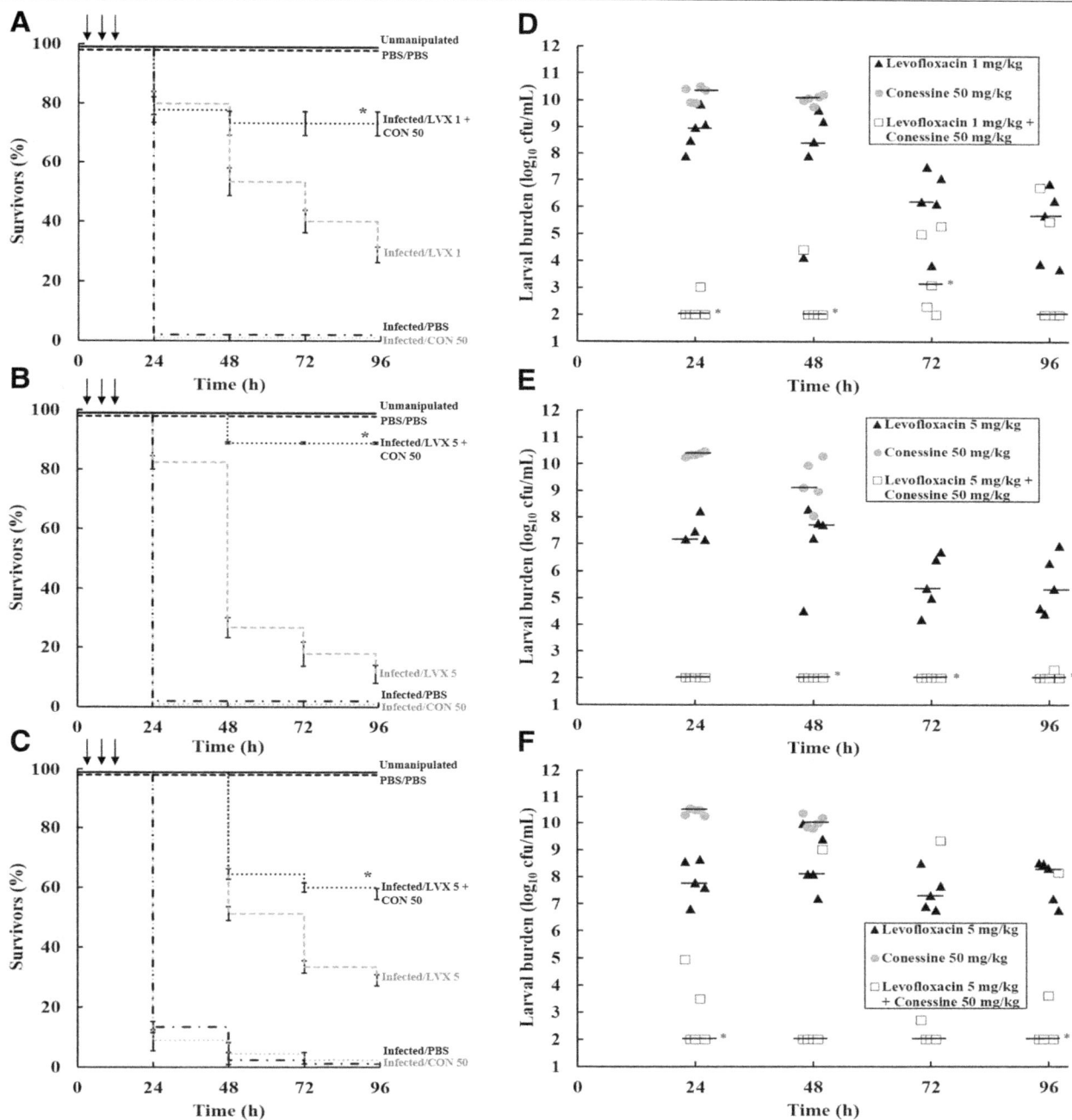

Fig. 2 Effect of treatment with combinations of conessine and levofloxacin on survival of *G. mellonella* larvae infected with *P. aeruginosa* PAM1020 (**a**), PAM1032 (**b**) and PAM1034 (**c**), or larval burden of the same strains PAM1020 (**d**), PAM1032 (**e**) and PAM1034 (**f**). All larvae were inoculated with 2.5×10^3 cfu/mL *P. aeruginosa* and treated with each agent individually or in combination with three doses at 2, 4 and 6 h post-infection (indicated by the arrows). Treatments consisted of PBS, conessine (50 mg/kg), levofloxacin (1 or 5 mg/kg, indicated on graph), and a combination of conessine with levofloxacin. Larvae were incubated at 37 °C for 96 h and survival recorded every 24 h. The burden of *P. aeruginosa* was determined from five individual larvae every 24 h. For clarity, data for treatment with PBS alone is not shown because the data obtained was similar to that obtained for conessine treatment alone. ***a), **b**) and **c**); combination treatment group with significantly enhanced survival compared with any of the constituent monotherapies ($P < 0.05$, log-rank test with Holm's correction for multiple comparisons). $n = 45$ (pooled from triplicate experiments). Error bars indicate ±SEM. LVX, levofloxacin; CON, conessine. * **d**), **e**) and **f**); significant difference in larval burden between groups treated with the combination of conessine and levofloxacin compared with the constituent monotherapies; $n = 5$ ($P < 0.05$, the Mann–Whitney *U*-test compared the combination therapy with each monotherapy individually). The black bar represents the median value of larval burden per group

doses of levofloxacin resulted in only a minor reduction in the bacterial burden within the larvae over the 96 h duration of the experiment (Fig. 2d, e and f).

Treatment with a triple dose of a combination of conessine (50 mg/kg) with the same, strain-specific levofloxacin doses mentioned previously, resulted in significantly enhanced survival compared to triple doses of the monotherapies ($P < 0.05$). Enhanced efficacy was most notable versus the *P. aeruginosa* strain overexpressing the MexAB-OprM efflux pump (PAM1032) (Fig. 2b) but the combination therapy also resulted in enhanced survival of the parent strain (PAM1020) (Fig. 2a) and the strain overexpressing MexEF-OprN (PAM1034) (Fig. 2c). As before, the combination treatment resulted in correlative reductions in bacterial burden within infected larvae over the 96 h duration of the experiment with the inhibitory effect on bacterial growth being most notable for PAM1032 (Fig. 2e) but was also evident in larvae infected with either PAM1020 (Fig. 2d) or PAM1034 (Fig. 2f). As shown with the steroidal alkaloids previously, combination therapy of conessine with levofloxacin did not result in enhanced survival of larvae infected with either PAM1033 (overexpressing MexCD-OprJ) or PAM1626 (the strain with the three efflux-pump systems deleted) (Additional file 4a and b respectively).

In summary, combination therapies of conessine or steroidal alkaloids with levofloxacin restored antibiotic efficacy in vivo versus infections with strains of *P. aeruginosa* overexpressing either the MexAB-OprM or MexEF-OprN efflux pumps. These observations were supported by the results obtained in vitro. The enhanced efficacy of the combination treatments was reflected in high levels of larval survival that correlated with reduced larval burden of the infecting pathogens. In some cases the combination treatment completely eradicated detectable bacteria within the larvae with numbers remaining below the level of detection ($\leq 2 \log_{10}$ cfu/mL).

Discussion
Mutations that result in the over-expression of efflux pumps and confer a MDR phenotype on *P. aeruginosa* strains are frequently isolated from infected patients [1, 3]. Thus, the overexpression of efflux pumps such as MexAB-OprM, MexCD-OprJ, MexEF-OprN, and MexXY-OprM render many therapeutic options for serious *P. aeruginosa* infections redundant. As a consequence, many studies have addressed the possibility of co-administering EPIs with antibiotics to restore the clinical efficacy of antibiotics that are otherwise rendered ineffective [4, 5].

A previous study conducted in the corresponding author's lab employed well-characterized *P. aeruginosa* strains (gifted by [22]) that over-express the RND efflux pumps in conjunction with a *G. mellonella* larva infection model [21]. Notably, this demonstrated that infection with strains that overexpress efflux pumps resulted in antibiotic treatment failure in *G. mellonella* larvae, reproducing the treatment outcomes seen

in human patients, and illustrating that this invertebrate model can be employed to identify novel treatments for MDR *P. aeruginosa* infections. Subsequently, the model was used to identify putative EPI/antibiotic combinations that restored antibiotic efficacy versus efflux-pump mediated *P. aeruginosa* infections in vivo [10, 21]. The present work has used the same *P. aeruginosa* strains and presents evidence that combinations of levofloxacin with *H. antidysenterica* extract, and the principal active ingredient alone (the steroidal alkaloid conessine), show no toxicity in vivo but enhanced efficacy in vitro and in vivo and represent a novel treatment option meriting further investigation.

Available evidence suggests that *H. antidysenterica* steroidal crude extract, and conessine may be acting as EPIs [19, 20]. The steroidal extract and the alkaloid conessine have recently been reported to enhance antibiotic activity due to interference with the AdeIJK efflux pump in *A. baumannii* [19] which is functionally equivalent to the MexAB-OprM pump of *P. aeruginosa* [30]. Furthermore, conessine restored antibiotic susceptibility to an otherwise resistant *P. aeruginosa* strain that overexpressed the MexAB-OprM efflux pump [20]. The data reported in the present study does not demonstrate that either the steroidal extracts or conessine are EPIs but is consistent with this hypothesis. For example, both the steroidal extracts and conessine restored the in vivo efficacy of levofloxacin only against the parent strain (where MexAB-OprM is known to be constitutively expressed; [3]) and the strains overexpressing the MexAB-OprM or MexEF-OprN efflux pumps. They had no restorative effect on the strain overexpressing MexCD-OprJ or the strain with all three of the Mex efflux pumps deleted. This specificity for certain Mex efflux systems does imply that compounds within the extract and conessine could be acting as EPIs. Furthermore, the finding that the restorative effect on levofloxacin efficacy was much less potent with the crude extract of steroidal alkaloids compared to the principal active ingredient alone (the steroidal alkaloid conessine; [16]) also suggests that it is conessine that posesses these EPI-like properties. Nonetheless, it also cannot be discounted that the restorative effect of the extract and conessine on levofloxacin efficacy with the strains containing the *nalB* (MexAB-OprM overexpressed) or *nfxC* (MexEF-OprN overexpressed) mutations could be explained by other unknown effects of these mutations that are unconnected with the over-expression of the two Mex efflux pumps.

Irrespective of the precise mode of action, the ability of conessine to restore antibiotic efficacy versus MDR *P. aeruginosa* infections merits further investigation and development for potential clinical application. Precise evaluation of the toxicity of *H. antidysenterica* bark extracts has not been carried out in humans. A study of acute and subacute toxicity of the methanol extract of a related plant, *Holarrhena floribunda*, that also contains conessine and is widely used to treat gastrointestinal disorders in Cameroon, revealed a

LD_{50} of 7 g/kg for female rats, indicating low levels of toxicity [31]. However, conessine alone was found to have an LD_{50} of 28.7 mg/kg after administration to mice intraperitoneally and was also observed to depress the heart and central nervous system [32]. Notably, the dose employed in the present study that elicited the optimal restorative effect on levofloxacin efficacy was higher at 50 mg/kg. Clearly, additional studies are required to identify if either the plant extracts or conessine alone are able to be safely used in human patients. Furthermore, showing that the steroidal extracts and conessine restore antibiotic efficacy in *G. mellonella* larvae does not mean that the same effects would be observed in mammals. Whilst this study has once again revealed the success of the *G. mellonella* infection model as a 'first *in vivo*' test for novel antimicrobial therapies, additional studies will also need to determine if the therapeutic benefit observed here also occurs in more traditional mammalian infection models.

Conclusions

In summary, combination therapies of conessine or steroidal alkaloids with levofloxacin restored the efficacy of the antibiotic in vivo versus infections of *G. mellonella* larvae with strains overexpressing either the MexAB-OprM or MexEF-OprN efflux pumps. No restorative effect was observed on infections with strains overexpressing MexCD-OprJ or the strain with all three of the Mex efflux pumps deleted. The enhanced efficacy of the combination treatments was reflected in high levels of larval survival that correlated with large reductions in larval burden of the infecting pathogens.

Additional files

Additional file 1: Raw data for steroidal alkaloid and conessine toxicity in vivo. (XLS 39 kb)

Additional file 2: Raw data for single treatments in vivo. (XLS 198 kb)

Additional file 3: Effect of treatment with combinations of steroidal alkaloids and levofloxacin on survival of *Galleria mellonella* larvae infected with *Pseudomonas aeruginosa* PAM1020 (a), PAM1033 (b) and PAM1626 (c). All larvae were inoculated with 2.5×10^3 cfu/mL *P. aeruginosa* and treated with each agent individually or in combination with three doses at 2, 4 and 6 h post-infection (indicated by the arrows). Treatments consisted of PBS, steroidal alkaloids (50, 100 or 200 mg/kg), levofloxacin (0.05, 1 or 5 mg/kg), and a combination of steroidal alkaloids with levofloxacin. Larvae were incubated at 37 °C for 96 h and survival recorded every 24 h. * combination treatment group with significantly enhanced survival compared with any of the constituent monotherapies ($P < 0.05$, log-rank test with Holm's correction for multiple comparisons). $n = 30$ (pooled from duplicate experiments). LVX, levofloxacin; ALKS, steroidal alkaloids.

Additional file 4: Effect of treatment with combinations of conessine and levofloxacin on survival of *Galleria mellonella* larvae infected with *Pseudomonas aeruginosa* PAM1033 (a) and PAM1626 (b). All larvae were inoculated with 2.5×10^3 cfu/mL *P. aeruginosa* and treated with each agent individually or in combination with three doses at 2, 4 and 6 h post-infection (indicated by the arrows). Treatments consisted of PBS, conessine (50 mg/kg), levofloxacin (0.05 or 5 mg/kg), and a combination of conessine with levofloxacin. Larvae were incubated at 37oC for 96 h and survival recorded every 24 h. * combination

treatment group with significantly enhanced survival compared with any of the constituent monotherapies ($P < 0.05$, log-rank test with Holm's correction for multiple comparisons). $n = 30$ (pooled from duplicate experiments). LVX, levofloxacin; CON, conessine.

Abbreviations
CCCP: Carbonyl cyanide m-chlorophenylhydrazone; EPI: Efflux pump inhibitor; FICI: Fractional inhibitory concentration index; LD_{50}: 50% Lethal dose; MDR: Multidrug-resistant; MHB: Mueller-Hinton broth; MIC: Minimal inhibitory concentration; NMP: 1-(1-Naphthylmethyl)-piperazine; PAβN: Phenylalanyl arginyl β-naphthylamide; RND: Resistance–nodulation–division

Acknowledgements
Not applicable.

Funding
This work was supported by the Thailand Research Fund through the Royal Golden Jubilee Ph.D. Program (Grant No. PHD/0041/2556) co-funded by the Newton Fund of the British Council and TRF Senior Research Scholar (Grant No. RTA 5880005).

Authors' contributions
TS designed and performed experiments, analyzed data, prepared figures and tables, and wrote the first draft of a manuscript. SPV and PJC supervised parts of the experimental work and revised the manuscript. All authors read and approved the final manuscript.

Competing interests
The authors declare that they have no competing interests.

Author details
[1]Department of Microbiology, Faculty of Science and Natural Product Research Center of Excellence, Prince of Songkla University, Songkhla, Thailand. [2]Biomedical Sciences Research Complex, School of Biology, University of St Andrews, The North Haugh, St Andrews, Fife, UK.

References
1. Lister PD, Wolter DJ, Hanson ND. Antibacterial-resistant *Pseudomonas aeruginosa*: clinical impact and complex regulation of chromosomally encoded resistance mechanisms. Clin Microbiol Rev. 2009;22:582–610.
2. Piddock LJ. Clinically relevant chromosomally encoded multidrug resistance efflux pumps in bacteria. Clin Microbiol Rev. 2006;19:382–402.
3. Poole K. *Pseudomonas Aeruginosa*: Resistance to the Max. Front Microbiol. 2011;2:65.
4. Tegos GP, Haynes M, Strouse JJ, Khan MM, Bologa CG, Oprea TI, et al. Microbial efflux pump inhibition: tactics and strategies. Curr Pharm Des. 2011;17:1291–302.
5. Bohnert JA, Kern WV. Antimicrobial drug efflux pump inhibitors. In: Li XZ, et al., editors. Efflux-Mediated Antimicrobial Resistance in Bacteria. Switzerland: Springer International Publishing; 2016. p. 755–95.
6. Sun J, Deng Z, Yan A. Bacterial multidrug efflux pumps: mechanisms, physiology and pharmacological exploitations. Biochem Biophys Res Commun. 2014;453:254–67.
7. Bohnert JA, Szymaniak-Vits M, Schuster S, Kern WV. Efflux inhibition by selective serotonin reuptake inhibitors in *Escherichia coli*. J Antimicrob Chemother. 2011;66:2057–60.
8. Piddock LJV, Garvey MI, Rahman MM, Gibbons S. Natural and synthetic compounds such as trimethoprim behave as inhibitors of efflux in gram-negative bacteria. J Antimicrob Chemother. 2010;65:1215–23.
9. Morita Y, Nakashima K, Nishino K, Kotani K, Tomida J, Inoue M, et al. Berberine is a novel type efflux inhibitor which attenuates the MexXY-mediated aminoglycoside resistance in *Pseudomonas aeruginosa*. Front Microbiol. 2016;7:1223.

10. E B, PJ C. Enhancement of antibiotic efficacy against multi-drug resistant *Pseudomonas aeruginosa* infections via combination with curcumin and 1-(1-Naphthylmethyl)-piperazine. J Antimicrob Agents. 2016;2:116.

11. Negi N, Prakash P, Gupta ML, Mohapatra TM. Possible role of curcumin as an efflux pump inhibitor in multidrug resistant clinical isolates of *Pseudomonas aeruginosa*. J Clin Diagn Res. 2014;8:DC04-7.

12. Choudhury D, Talukdar AD, Chetia P, Bhattacharjee A, Choudhury MD. Screening of natural products and derivatives for the identification of RND efflux pump inhibitors. Comb Chem High Throughput Screen. 2016; 19:705-13.

13. Prasch S, Bucar F. Plant derived inhibitors of bacterial efflux pumps: an update. Phytochem Rev. 2015;14:961-74.

14. Stavri M, Piddock LJV, Gibbons S. Bacterial efflux pump inhibitors from natural sources. J Antimicrob Chemother. 2007;59:1247-60.

15. Chakraborty A, Brantner AH. Antibacterial steroid alkaloids from the stem bark of *Holarrhena pubescens*. J Ethnopharmacol. 1999;68:339-44.

16. Kumar N, Singh B, Bhandari P, Gupta AP, Kaul VK. Steroidal alkaloids from *Holarrhena antidysenterica* (L.) WALL. Chem Pharm Bull. 2007;55:912-4.

17. Chusri S, Siriyong T, Na-Phatthalung P, Voravuthikunchai SP. Synergistic effects of ethnomedicinal plants of Apocynaceae family and antibiotics against clinical isolates of *Acinetobacter baumannii*. Asian Pac J Trop Med. 2014;7:456-61.

18. Phatthalung PN, Chusri S, Voravuthikunchai SP. Thai ethnomedicinal plants as resistant modifying agents for combating *Acinetobacter baumannii* infections. BMC Complement Altern Med. 2012;12:56.

19. Siriyong T, Chusri S, Srimanote P, Tipmanee V, Voravuthikunchai SP. *Holarrhena antidysenterica* extract and its steroidal alkaloid, conessine, as resistance-modifying agents against extensively drug-resistant *Acinetobacter baumannii*. Microb Drug Resist. 2016;22:273-82.

20. Siriyong T, Srimanote P, Chusri S, Yingyongnarongkul B, Suaisom C, Tipmanee V, et al. Conessine as a novel inhibitor of multidrug efflux pump systems in *Pseudomonas aeruginosa*. BMC Complement Altern Med. 2017;17:405.

21. Adamson DH, Krikstopaityte V, Coote PJ. Enhanced efficacy of putative efflux pump inhibitor/antibiotic combination treatments versus MDR strains of *Pseudomonas aeruginosa* in a *Galleria mellonella in vivo* infection model. J Antimicrob Chemother. 2015;70:2271-8.

22. Lomovskaya O, Lee A, Hoshino K, Ishida H, Mistry A, Warren MS, et al. Use of a genetic approach to evaluate the consequences of inhibition of efflux pumps in *Pseudomonas aeruginosa*. Antimicrob Agents Chemother. 1999;43:1340-6.

23. Hill L, Veli N, Coote PJ. Evaluation of *Galleria mellonella* larvae for measuring the efficacy and pharmacokinetics of antibiotic therapies against *Pseudomonas aeruginosa* infection. Int J Antimicrob Agents. 2014; 43:254-61.

24. Eliopoulous G, Moellering R. Antimicrobial combinations. In: Lorian V, editor. Antibiotics in Laboratory Medicine 3. Baltimore: Williams and Wilkins; 1996. p. 330-96.

25. White RL, Burgess DS, Manduru M, Bosso JA. Comparison of three different *in vitro* methods of detecting synergy: time-kill, checkerboard, and E test. Antimicrob Agents Chemother. 1996;40:1914-8.

26. Krezdorn J, Adams S, Coote PJ. A *Galleria mellonella* infection model reveals double and triple antibiotic combination therapies with enhanced efficacy versus a multidrug-resistant strain of *Pseudomonas aeruginosa*. J Med Microbiol. 2014;63:945-55.

27. Bland JM, Altman DG. Survival probabilities (the Kaplan-Meier method). Brit Med J. 1998;317:1572.

28. Bland JM. The logrank test. Brit Med J. 2004;328:1073.

29. Holm S. A simple sequentially rejective multiple test procedure. Scand J Stat. 1979;6:65-70.

30. Damier-Piolle L, Magnet S, Bremont S, Lambert T, Courvalin P. AdeIJK, a resistance-nodulation-cell division pump effluxing multiple antibiotics in *Acinetobacter baumannii*. Antimicrob Agents Chemother. 2008;52:557-62.

31. Bogne KP, Penlap BV, Mbofung CM, Etoa F-X. Acute and subacute toxicity of the methanol extract from *Holarrhena floribunda* G. Don (Apocynaceae). Europ. J Exp Biol. 2012;2:1284-8.

32. Stephenson RP. The pharmacological properties of conessine, isoconessine and neoconessine. Brit J Pharmacol. 1948;3:237-45.

21

Integrative oncology and complementary medicine cancer services in Australia

Caroline A. Smith[1]* (iD), Jennifer Hunter[1,2], Geoff P. Delaney[4,5,6], Jane M. Ussher[3], Kate Templeman[1], Suzanne Grant[1] and Eleanor Oyston[7]

Abstract

Background: Individuals living with and beyond a cancer diagnosis are increasingly using complementary therapies and medicines (CM) to enhance the effectiveness of cancer treatment, manage treatment-related side effects, improve quality-of-life, and promote self-efficacy. In response to the increasing use and demand for CM by cancer patients, interest in the implementation of Integrative Oncology (IO) services that provide CM alongside conventional cancer care in Australia and abroad has developed. The extent that cancer services in Australia are integrating CM is uncertain. Thus, the aim of this study was to identify IO services in Australia and explore barriers and facilitators to IO service provision.

Methods: A national, cross-sectional survey of healthcare organisations was conducted in 2016. Organisations in the public and private sectors, including not-for-profit organisations that provided cancer care in hospital or community setting, were included.

Results: A response rate of 93.2% was achieved ($n = 275/295$). Seventy-one organisations (25.8%) across all states/territories, except the Northern Territory, offered IO albeit in a limited amount by many. Most common IO services included massage, psychological-wellbeing, and movement modalities in hospital outpatient or inpatient settings. There were only a few instances where biological-based complementary medicine (CM) therapies were prescribed. Funding was often mixed, including patient contributions, philanthropy, funding by the organisation, and volunteer practitioners.

Of the 204 non-IO providers, 80.9% had never provided any IO service. Overwhelmingly, the most common barrier to IO was a lack of funding, followed by uncertainty about patient demand, choice of services, and establishing such services. Less-common barriers were a lack of evidence, and support from oncologists or management. More funding, education and training, and building the evidence-base for CM were the most commonly suggested solutions.

Conclusion: IO is increasingly being provided in Australia, although service provision remains limited or non-existent in many areas. Mismatches appear to exist between low IO service provision, CM evidence, and high CM use by cancer patients. Greater strategic planning and policy guidance is indicated to ensure the appropriate provision of, and equitable access to IO services for all Australian cancer survivors.

Keywords: Cancer, Supportive care, Complementary medicine, Integrative oncology, Integrative medicine

* Correspondence: caroline.smith@westernsydney.edu.au
[1]NICM Health Research Institute, Western Sydney University, Westmead campus, Locked Bag 1797, Penrith, NSW 2751, Australia
Full list of author information is available at the end of the article

Background

Individuals living with and beyond a cancer diagnosis (hereafter referred to as cancer survivors) in Australia, are increasingly using complementary medicine (CM) [1] and some cancer services are providing integrative oncology (IO) services [2, 3]. Integrative oncology (IO) is described as: *"a patient-centred, evidence-informed field of cancer care that utilizes mind and body practices, natural products, and/or lifestyle modifications alongside conventional cancer treatments. IO aims to optimize health, quality of life, across the cancer care continuum and to empower people to prevent cancer and become active participants before, during, and beyond cancer treatment"* [4].

The prevalence of CM use by cancer survivors in Australia has risen from 22% in 1996 [5], to 65% in 2008 [6], with an estimated period prevalence rate between 1985 and 2009 of 43% (95% CI: 19–67%) [1]. The most commonly used CM interventions include biological-based therapies (such as nutritional supplements, special diet and foods, and traditional herbal medicines) followed by non-biologically-based therapies (such as prayer/spiritual practices, meditation/imagery, massage, yoga, acupuncture, Tai Chi/Qigong, and relaxation) [6]. CM is mostly used by cancer survivors as an adjuvant rather than an alternative to their conventional cancer treatment. Reasons for use include desire to augment the effectiveness of treatment, manage treatment-related side effects, improve quality-of-life, and promote self-efficacy [7, 8].

Whilst the research reporting CM use and the experiences of cancer survivors in Australia continues to grow [9–13], little is known about its integration with other cancer services. Only two studies have explored this issue, and the results from both surveys were limited by small sample sizes, restricted inclusion criteria, and suboptimal response rates [2, 3]. Questions remain about the current provision of IO services, the types of CM therapies that are being integrated, the healthcare settings in which they are provided, how they are funded, and key determinants influencing the provision of such services.

Methods

The aim of this study was to examine current IO service provision in Australia and explore barriers and facilitators to service delivery. A cross-sectional survey of Australian healthcare organisations with cancer services was conducted throughout 2016. The sample was obtained through extensive search strategies to identify all cancer services from both the public and private sectors, including not-for-profit organisations that provided cancer care in either a hospital or community setting. A short-list of potentially eligible organisations was generated from searching public and private hospital databases and organisations that were located in community settings [14–16]. To ensure potential services were not missed,

volunteers from each State who were familiar with the cancer services in their region were given specific instructions for conducting Internet searches on Google and Bing search engines. In addition, further services and sites were identified through conversations with industry experts from peak organisations (e.g. Cancer Nurses Society of Australia, Clinical Oncology Society of Australia, Cancer Council Australia), cancer care networks (e.g. Integrated Cancer Services Managers Group), collaborative groups (e.g. Complementary and Integrative Therapies Group, Western Australian Clinical Oncology Group), and managers and survey participants who provided information about affiliated sites, and/or other locations.

Excluded from the survey were small businesses with specialist consultation rooms only; palliative care services and hospices that were not part of an organisation with cancer services; and organisations that only provided information, support groups, counselling or ad-hoc retreats for cancer survivors. For those services meeting the eligibility criteria, the research officer made contact with organisation volunteers and presented an invitation to participate. Each participating organisation nominated an appropriate staff member to answer the survey. Written, informed consent was obtained from each respondent.

A 52-item questionnaire was designed and pilot tested Additional file 1). Content and questions were based on a NSW survey instrument of CM practices and policies in cancer services [3] and a Scottish scoping study of OM services [17] The online and paper versions of the questionnaire were pilot-tested with staff working in a local cancer service that provided IO and modified accordingly. On-line or paper versions of the questionnaire were available. The online version was administered through SurveyMonkey [18]. Most questions included an option for an open-ended response or comments.

The following broad definitions were provided at the beginning of the questionnaire and are jointly referred to hereafter as IO:

- CM – acupuncture, aromatherapy, chiropractic, herbs and supplements, massage, meditation, music or art therapy, naturopathy, osteopathy, Reiki, relaxation, Tai Chi, therapeutic touch, yoga.
- integrative medicine (IM) – healthcare practitioners who combine evidence-based conventional medicine with CM.

A more comprehensive list of CM services was used when inquiring about service provision for different CM categories (see supplementary material).

Every survey was checked to ensure that there was only one response per organisation and that respondents had not inadvertently selected an incorrect response to the skip question about CM service provision. If either occurred, relevant respondents were contacted and asked to amend their responses. In instances where more than one staff answered the survey, the responses from the most senior person were kept. Those respondents who reported that their cancer service was in the planning stages of delivering a CM service were recontacted before closing date to determine if this prior status was still valid.

Descriptive statistics detailing the counts and percentages was the primary statistical method used. Statistical analysis was undertaken using SPSS V24 [19]. Questions requiring inferential statistical analysis were determined a priori using Chi-squared and Fishers exact tests. Statistical significance set at $p < 0.05$. Qualitative data from the open questions were independently coded for content into descriptive categories by authors CS and JH, and analysed using conventional content analysis [20]. Many of the questions were compulsory, and as such, provided a 'don't know' option. Missing data included unanswered questions. A map of the distribution of IO services was generated using The software use for mapping in this project was ArcGis [21].

Results

A total of 366 healthcare organisations were identified, from which 295 met the inclusion/exclusion criteria. The response rate was 93.2%, with 275 of the eligible organisations participating in the study. Response rates in the Northern Territory and the Australian Capital Territory were significantly lower than other states, at 66.7%

and 75.0% respectively (Fisher's exact, $p < 0.05$). There were no incomplete surveys.

Most of the 275 respondents (55.6%, $n = 153$) reported dual roles in the organisation as both a healthcare professional and administrator/manager. For the remaining, 73 (26.5%) reported their role as a healthcare professional only, and 49 (17.8%) were an administrator/manager only. Of the healthcare professionals, 60.2% ($n = 136$) had a nursing background, and only a few were an oncologist/haematologist (3.1%, $n = 7$).

Integrative oncology service provision

Seventy-one organisations (25.8%) stated they offered some type of IO service (Table 1). The median duration of service provision was 6 years, ranging from 2 months to 42 years. Some respondents reported incremental service development, reflecting changes in attitudes towards IO, pressure to provide evidence-informed therapies, and responsiveness to patient needs.

All states, except the Northern Territory, offered IO (Fig. 1). No significant differences between the states were observed (Fisher's exact, $p = 0.10$). Significant differences, however, were observed between the ownership and the likelihood of providing IO (Fisher's exact, $p < .001$). IO providers were most likely to be owned by a not-for-profit organisation (46.5%) or were government owned (38.0%), and least likely to be owned by a for-profit organisation (15.5%). In comparison, most non-IO providers were government owned (53.4%), followed by for-profit organisations (32.8%), and not-for-profit companies (13.7%).

IO services were mostly provided in hospital inpatient or outpatient settings (Table 2). In general, the most notable

Table 1 Location and ownership of integrative oncology providers and non-providers

Healthcare organisations with specialised cancer services $n = 275$	IO providers		Non-IO providers		Total	
	n	%	n	%	n	%
Location						
Australian Capital Territory	1	0.4	2	0.7	3	1.1
New South Wales	25	9.1	57	20.7	82	29.8
Northern Territory	0	0.0	2	0.7	2	0.7
Queensland	9	3.3	58	21.1	67	24.4
South Australia	6	2.2	22	8.0	28	10.2
Tasmania	2	0.7	5	1.8	7	2.5
Western Australia	11	4.0	17	6.2	28	10.2
Victoria	17	6.2	41	14.9	58	21.1
Ownership*						
Government	27	9.8	109	39.6	136	49.5
For-profit company	11	4.0	67	24.4	78	28.4
Not-for-profit company	33	12.0	28	10.2	61	22.2
Total	71	25.8	204	74.2	275	100.0

* X^2 (2) = 33.6, $p < 0.001$

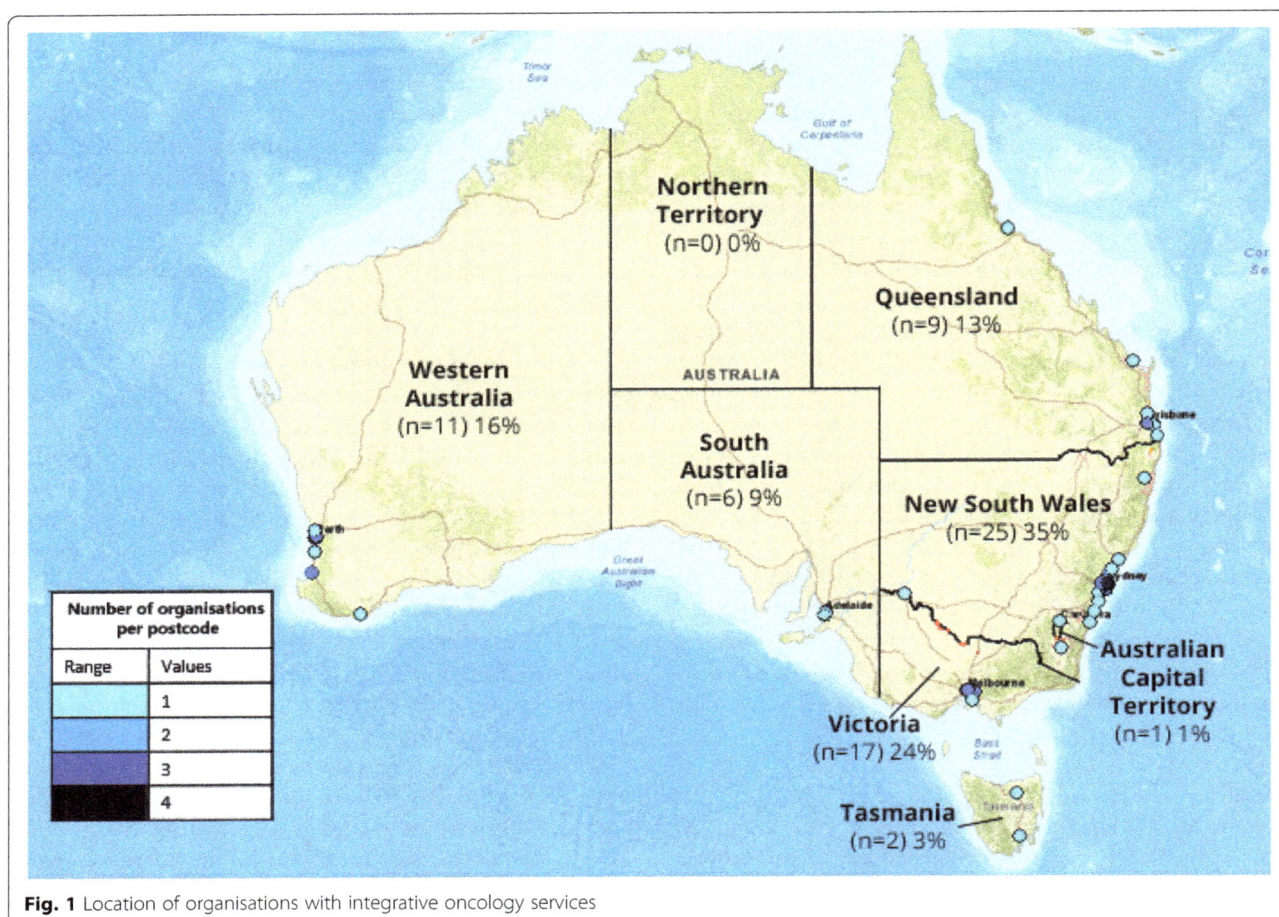

Fig. 1 Location of organisations with integrative oncology services

difference between the settings in which IO was provided compared to cancer services was that only 4.2% (n = 3/71) of the IO services were provided to patients at home or in residential care compared to 27.6% (n = 76/275) for all cancer services. Twenty-five organisations provided some or all of their IO services in a dedicated centre.

Of the organisations offering IO services the most common IO services were massage (76.1%, n = 54/71), psychological wellbeing services (71.8%, n = 51/71), and movement modalities (39.4%, n = 28/71) (Table 3). The

median number of the different categories of IO services (Table 3) was two; 19 organisations provided only one category, and 10 organisations provided four or more. Practitioners generally worked on a part-time basis.

A wide range of massage, touch, and body realignment therapies were offered, with oncology massage (defined as massage provided by a certified oncology massage therapist) being the most prevalent (55.6%, n = 30/54). Osteopathy and chiropractic services were not provided by any of the cancer services. The most commonly provided psychological

Table 2 Settings where cancer services are provided

Setting[b]	IO providers IO services[a]		IO providers all cancer services		Non-IO providers all cancer services		All providers (total)	
	n	%	n	%	n	%	n	%
Hospital inpatient	37	13.5	54	19.6	120	43.6	174	63.3
Hospital outpatient / clinic	56	20.4	64	23.3	187	68.0	251	91.3
(Dedicated IO centre)	(25	9.1)						
Community centre / facility	14	5.1	22	8.0	54	19.6	76	27.6
Home / residential care visits	3	1.1	23	8.4	53	19.3	76	27.6
Total	71	25.8	71	25.8	204	74.2	275	100.0

[a]IO services are a sub set of all cancer services [b] more than one response allowed

Table 3 Integrative oncology (IO) service provision

Service category	Number of organisations		Number of practitioners / organisation		Hours available per week / organisation	
	n	%	Median	range	Median	range
Massage, Touch, or Body Alignment Therapies	54	76.1	2.5	1 to 27	12	2 to 65
Psychological Wellbeing Services	51	71.8	2	1 to 10	7	0.5 to 72
Movement Modalities *(non-CM physiotherapy & exercise physiology excluded)*	28	39.4	2	1 to 20	3	1 to 20
Integrative Medicine *(consultation or advice)*	13	18.3	1	1 to 4	40	24 to 46
Acupuncture *(either medical or Chinese)*	9	12.7	1	1 to 3	6	2 to 24
Other *(naturopath, nutritionist not a dietitian service)*	3	4.2	1	1 to 3	16	6 to 60

Total number of organisations providing IO services n = 71

wellbeing services were art therapy, meditation, music therapy, and relaxation. Yoga and Tai Chi were the most frequently reported movement modalities. Ten services reported offering movement modalities delivered by either a physiotherapist (*n* = 7) or exercise physiologist (n = 3); however, nine of these were not included in the final count as the modality was not classified as a CM. Less frequently provided was acupuncture (*n* = 9).

Aside from Western naturopathy, no other holistic traditional healing practices, specifically Chinese herbal medicine, Ayurveda medicine or Indigenous Australian healing practices, were offered. Overwhelmingly, biological-based CM therapies (e.g. herbs, vitamins or minerals) were not provided. There were only four cancer services where such therapies could have been formally prescribed by either an IM doctor or CM practitioner. Formal IM advice from a pharmacist about CM products was available at nine services.

Qualifications of practitioners
Twenty of the 71 organisations with IO services (28.2%) indicated they had practitioners with dual qualifications (defined as practitioners who held both qualifications as a biomedical trained practitioner and complementary medicine practitioner); however, a similar number (*n* = 21, 29.6%) did not know the answer to this question. Several examples were given that included a nurse certified in oncology massage and another who was also a naturopath; a medical practitioner with acupuncture qualifications; and an occupational therapist who trained as a music therapist.

Integration of practitioners
Most of the cancer services that provided IO held multidisciplinary team meetings or case conferences (83.1%, *n* = 58) from which just under half (*n* = 28) invited the IO practitioners to participate. Almost an equal number (*n* = 27) indicated that these practitioners were not invited, and four respondents did not know the answer to this question.

Funding of services
Funding resources were mixed. Organisations used a variety of sources: patient contributions (49.2%, *n* = 35), philanthropic contributions (47.9%, n = 34), funding by the organisation (47.8%, n = 34), and volunteer practitioners (42.2%, *n* = 30). Patient contributions were defined as 'any combination of out-of-pocket costs or rebates from either private health insurance or Medicare'. IM services were the only category of service (Table 3) where none of the IO providers funded the service with philanthropic contributions nor through the help of volunteer practitioners. Not-for-profit organisations were significantly more likely to engage volunteer practitioners (X^2 (2) = 8.9, $p < 0.05$). No significant differences were found between the ownership of the organisation and the likelihood of the IO services being funded by the other three sources.

Organisations not providing IO
Of the 204 non-IO providers, 80.9% (*n* = 165) had never provided IO services, 7.8% (n = 16) previously provided IO services, and 5.8% (*n* = 12) were planning to provide IO services. Eleven (5.4%) of the non-IO providers commented that the cancer service actively provided information and/or referred patients to nearby IO or CM services. Multiple reasons, including qualitative comments, were given for why the cancer services did not provide IO and barriers to providing IO (Table 4).

Integrative oncology barriers and facilitators
Nearly two-thirds (123/188) of respondents identified insufficient funding as the most common reason their organisation did not provide IO services. Similarly, the most common solutions suggested were to address funding dilemmas and establish sustainable business models. How IO services should be funded was more contentious. Some called for *"Medicare funding to support the use of appropriate complementary medicine."* Others suggested higher rebates from private health insurers. Philanthropy, *"fundraising"* or finding practitioners *"that want to volunteer"* were also proposed. A few respondents from the private health sector considered it was

Table 4 Barriers to providing Integrative oncology (IO) services and potential solutions

Barriers (n = 204)	Number	Percent	Potential Solutions (n = 130)	Number	Percent
Lack of funding	123	60.3	Funding	59	45.4
Low patient demand / awareness	65	31.9	Staff education / training	30	23.1
Unsure about which IO services to provide	64	31.4	Build the evidence-base	18	13.8
Unsure how to set up an IO service	55	27.1	Help with developing a business model	8	6.2
Lack of support or interest from oncologists	51	25.0	Determine clinical governance	7	5.4
Organisational policy does not allow IO	38	18.6	Change organisational attitudes / culture	7	5.4
Not enough evidence	22	10.8	Ensure sufficient demand for service	5	3.8
Management does not want IO services	16	7.8	Policy support	4	3.1
Other Comments:			More space to provide services	3	2.3
Inadequate resources e.g. time, staff, space	17	8.3			
No champion or organisational interest	8	3.9			
Unsure of patient demand	7	3.4			
Difficulty recruiting CM practitioners	6	2.9			
Patient affordability / high out-of-pocket costs	2	1			

Only non-IO providers were asked these questions. More than one response was allowed

the responsibility of the public service to provide IO services. This view, however, was not always shared by those in the public health sector who, for example, stated that *"given the number of competing demands for resources within a public hospital"*, accessing IO *"would need to be patient/consumer-driven"* and patients could *"seek this if they wish to"* in the community. Other respondents highlighted the challenges with providing affordable, equitable services for their population base.

"We are currently trying to develop integrative therapies in the centre. Sustainability and cost will always be a factor. We are in a demographically struggling area." (Administrator/ Manager and Healthcare professional)

Funding issues were intertwined with other challenges, such as providing value in healthcare and prioritising essential services. For some, IO was considered a non-essential service that would require external funding and evidence to justify its provision.

"We are too busy complying with accreditation and providing the best possible known treatment services to our patients. I feel we are here to heal people not be airy fairy, there are plenty of places for that. I also feel these complementary treatments belittle what we are trying to achieve. But if they were paid by the Health Funds as inpatient services at great reward I would reconsider this." (Administrator/Manager)

"Difficult, government authorities do not recognise complementary therapies as being essential in

supporting cancer patients through cancer treatment and beyond. Grants are great but when the funding runs out the service has to cease in most cases." (Administrator/Manager and Healthcare professional)

"If evidence supports better outcomes for patients when they receive complementary therapy, a business case could be made to include their services" (Healthcare professional)

Although only a few respondents (10.8%, n = 22/204) considered inadequate evidence as a barrier to providing IO services, building a stronger evidence base (13.8%, n = 18/130) and educating staff about existing evidence (23.1%, n = 30/130) were more commonly suggested as potential solutions (31.3%, n = 64/130). For some, establishing an evidence base was paramount.

"Until there is adequate evidence to support significant objective benefit the other barriers are irrelevant. Oncologist support will only come with evidence." (Healthcare professional)

In addition to more research investigating efficacy and cost-effectiveness, respondents also identified uncertainty about patient needs for IO (31.9%, n = 65/204). These individuals discussed the importance of obtaining more information about patient demand and needs (2.9%, n = 6/130).

"Research as to what the patients would like us to consider and how we would fund it." (Administrator/ Manager and Healthcare professional)

Discussion

The cross-sectional survey of CM services within healthcare organisations was the largest and most comprehensive of its kind to have been conducted in Australia [2, 3] identifying 295 healthcare organisations with cancer services. Although the provision of IO by these services appears to have doubled over the past 6 years, albeit in a limited capacity by many cancer services, most of the 275 surveyed organisations (74.2%) were yet to provide any type IO service. For the 71 organisations that did, IO services were largely provided in hospital inpatient or outpatient settings, including those with a dedicated IO centre. Access, however, was often limited by availability with services being offered for a limited number of hours per week. Services relied heavily on funding from patients and philanthropy, and the generosity of volunteer CM practitioners.

Challenges with funding IO services, coupled with the need for more guidance on how to establish these services, were considered the greatest obstacles reported by non-IO providers. Insufficient evidence of safety and efficacy, and a lack of support or interest from oncologists or senior management, were other important barriers. These findings are consistent with other research, including a recently published small study of IO organisations in Australia [22], suggesting that barriers to providing IO include challenges with determining an appropriate service model and revenue structure; concerns with clinical governance and legal issues, such as regulations and credentialing; a lack of education about CM; and inadequate evidence about safety and effectiveness of CM [23–27]. Many of these challenges are not unique to IO, and to some extent, reflect the challenges with providing supportive cancer care more generally [28–31], and translating evidence into practice when evidence is established and recommended in clinical guidelines [32]. Indeed, delivering value-based healthcare, along with evidence for effectiveness and cost-effectiveness, places what patients value at the centre of healthcare decision making [33].

Notwithstanding these challenges, the provision of IO services in 2016 are substantially higher at 25.8% (30.5% for New South Wales) compared to earlier estimates of 8.9% for Australia in 2014 [2] (19% for New South Wales in 2009) [3]. Different sampling frames and definitions of IO service provision may explain some of the observed differences. The 2009 New South Wales survey only inquired about CM services for inpatients that were provided by practitioners who were not employees of the hospital [3]. Similarly, the 2014 national survey used only one hospital database to identify organisations with an oncology department, no community-based organisations were included, and it was unclear if inpatient services were included [2]. If community-based organisations and

inpatient CM services were excluded from the current analysis, 2016 estimates would remain substantially higher at 20.4% ($n = 56$). Coupled with a six-year mean duration of operation, and a further 12 (4%) organisations that were planning to provide IO, results from the 2016 survey demonstrate substantial ongoing growth of IO service provision in Australia.

Despite this apparent growth, Australian IO service provision appears similar to some comparable countries. In 2009, the estimated number of National Health Service cancer treatment centres in the United Kingdom providing IO ranged from 2.2 per 1 million population in England to 5.0 in Northern Ireland [34]. The comparison rate for Australia is estimated at 2.9 healthcare organisations with an IO service per 1 million population (2016 total population in Australia 24.4million) [35]. A 2013 mapping survey of oncology centres and hospitals in Europe identified 47 of the 99 responding cancer centres provided IO [36]. Response bias, however, may have resulted in an overestimate. Rates for the US, Canada, and New Zealand are yet to be reported, although most of the National Cancer Institute designated comprehensive cancer centres in the US purportedly provide IO [37, 38].

Non-biological IO services were mostly provided by cancer services; massage/touch therapies and psychological wellbeing services were the most common followed by movement modalities. Aside from much lower rates of IM consultations/advice and acupuncture, the types of IO services that were provided mostly align with international IO services [34, 37], evidence-based clinical guidelines for breast cancer and lung cancer [32, 39], and the CM therapies commonly used by cancer survivors in Australia [6]. The low rates of acupuncture services, however, were somewhat surprising. Whilst the quality of the evidence for effectiveness is variable clinical practice guidelines conclude there is moderate certainty that the net benefit from treatment is small [32, 39]. In Australia, credentialing of acupuncturists should be relatively straightforward as all acupuncturists (be they medical doctors or Chinese medicine practitioners) are statutorily regulated through the Australian Health Practitioner Regulation Agency.

Perhaps the largest mismatch was the high rates of biological-based therapies used by cancer survivors (e.g. herbs and nutritional supplements, and consultations with traditional medicine practitioners) [6, 9–11] compared to the negligible provision of biological-based IO services. Botanicals and supplements continue to be controversial due to concerns over safety, especially regarding interactions with pharmaceuticals and contraindications [40]. Decision making in this context is complex. Oncologists consistently identify a lack of knowledge and education as major barriers to discussing CM use with their patients

[41–43]. An analysis of over 2000 IO consultations in a comprehensive cancer centre in the US found the most common reasons why cancer survivors sought an IO consultation with a medical doctor was to pursue a holistic integrative approach (34%), and/or to obtain expert advice on CM product use (34%) and nutrition (21%) [38]. Cancer survivors may, therefore, benefit from building positive therapeutic alliances with medical doctors and pharmacists who have specific IO training to guide the safe and effective use of CM products [38]. Little is known about the IO capacity of medical practitioners who work in cancer care in Australia. In Canada almost 70% of 100 health care providers surveyed reported that they felt unprepared to monitor cancer patients' CM use, and fewer than 9% of participants reported being capable of searching for credible evidence-based information on CM and cancer [44]. In a survey of 176 Australian health care providers caring for patients with haematological cancer patients, 91% supported the use of mind/body therapies and 41% the use of natural products, only 19% felt they could advise patients, and 77% wanted to learn more [45, 46].

Limitations of this study include the under-representation of specialist oncologists and haematologists completing the survey. This may have biased the results that found insufficient evidence was much less important than financial and logistical barriers to providing IO. Although the acceptance of CM by Australian oncologists appears to be increasing [47], more information is needed about their views on providing IO services. It is also possible that the question enquiring whether the organisation provided IO services was answered incorrectly with some crossover regarding what was considered a non-IO service. For some respondents, CM services that were provided within existing conventional allied health services (with no additional CM practitioners) were considered non-IO, whereas others thought this was inclusive of IO. For example, physiotherapy was often associated with movement modalities. To mitigate this risk, clarification was provided to all participants during data collection, survey responses were carefully reviewed, and relevant participants were contacted to clarify their responses. Lower response rates in Northern Territory and the Australian Capital Territory limit the generalisability to these states. Despite these limitations, however, the high overall response rate and coverage of the targeted sample supports the validity and generalisability of the findings.

Conclusion

In summary, healthcare organisations across Australia are increasingly providing IO services. Service provision, however, appears to remain limited or non-existent in many areas. Healthcare organisations signalled a need for more funding, and assistance with clinical governance and business models. Building and translating the evidence of CM and developing clinical guidelines is, therefore, suggested to inform the decisions made by clinicians, patients, and policy makers. Greater top-down strategic planning and policy guidance is indicated to ensure the appropriate provision of, and equitable access to, IO services for all cancer survivors living across Australia.

Acknowledgements

The authors acknowledge and thank the Oncology Massage Ltd. volunteers for their assistance with Internet searches to identify eligible healthcare organisations.

Funding

This project was funded through a 2016 Research Partnerships Program, Western Sydney University. Partner funding was obtained from Oncology Massage Ltd., a registered charity that provides training to massage practitioners in Australia and internationally; and from South West Sydney Local Health District.
Additional support was provided by NICM and THRI, University of Western Sydney.
The funding bodies had no role in the design of the study and collection, analysis, and interpretation of data and in writing the manuscript section.

Authors' contributions

All authors read and approved the final manuscript. CS, JH, GdL and JU conceptualised the design of the study. CS, JH and JH assumed overall responsibility for project management. CS and JH analysed the data. KT and SG were responsible for data collection. EO contributed to data collection. All authors read and approved the final manuscript.

Competing interests

Author's JH, CS, KT and SG are academic researchers at NICM. As a medical research institute, NICM receives research grants and donations from foundations, universities, government agencies, individuals and industry. Sponsors and donors provide untied funding for work to advance the vision and mission of NICM. The project that is the subject of this article was not undertaken as part of a contractual relationship with any donor or sponsor. Author EO is the Founder of Oncology Massage Ltd., a not-for-profit company and registered charity in Australia that provides education, training and advocacy for oncology massage. Authors GPD and JU have no competing interests to declare.

Author details

[1]NICM Health Research Institute, Western Sydney University, Westmead campus, Locked Bag 1797, Penrith, NSW 2751, Australia. [2]Menzies Centre for Health Policy, School of Public Health, Sydney Medical School, The University of Sydney, Sydney, NSW, Australia. [3]Translational Health Research Institute, School of Medicine, Western Sydney University, Campbelltown, NSW, Australia. [4]South-Western Sydney Clinical School, Faculty of Medicine, University of New South Wales, Kensington, NSW, Australia. [5]Cancer Services, South Western Sydney Local Health District, Liverpool, NSW, Australia. [6]Ingham Institute of Applied Medical Research, Liverpool, NSW, Australia. [7]Oncology Massage Limited, PO Box 109, Deakin West, ACT 2600, Australia.

References

1. Horneber M, Bueschel G, Dennert G, Less D, Ritter E, Zwahlen M. How many cancer patients use complementary and alternative medicine: a systematic review and meta-analysis. Integr Cancer Ther. 2012;11(3):187–203.
2. Lim E, Vardy JL, Oh B, Dhillon HM. Integration of complementary and alternative medicine into cancer-specific supportive care programs in Australia: a scoping study. Asia Pac J Clin Oncol. 2017;13(1):6–12.
3. Raszeja V, Jordens CFC, Kerridge IH. Survey of practices and polices relating to the use of complementary and alternatives medicines and therapies in New South Wales cancer services. Intern Med J. 2013;43:84–8.
4. Witt CM, Balneaves LG, Cardoso MJ, Cohen L, Greenlee H, Johnstone P, Kücük Ö, Mailman J, Mao JJ. A comprehensive definition for integrative oncology. Natl Cancer Inst Monogr. 2017;52:229-38.
5. Begbie SD, Kerestes ZL, Bell DR. Patterns of alternative medicine use by cancer patients. Med J Aust. 1996;165(10):545.

6. Oh B, Butow P, Mullan B, Beale P, Pavlakis N, Rosenthal D, Clarke S. The use and perceived benefits resulting from the use of complementary and alternative medicine by cancer patients in Australia. Asia Pac J Clin Oncol. 2010;6(4):342–9.

7. Bell RM. A review of complementary and alternative medicine practices among cancer survivors. Clin J Oncol Nurs. 2010;14(3):365–70.

8. Anmichai T, Grossman M, Richard M. Lung cancer patients' beliefs about complementary and alternative medicine in the promotion of their wellness. Eur J Oncol Nurs. 2012;16:520–7.

9. Hunter D, Marinakis C, Salisbury R, Cray A, Oates R. Complementary therapy use in metropolitan and regional Australian radiotherapy centres; do patients report effective outcomes? Support Care Cancer. 2016;24(4):1803–11.

10. Sullivan A, Gilbar P, Curtain C. Complementary and alternative medicine use in Cancer patients in rural Australia. Integr Cancer Ther. 2015;14(4):350–8.

11. Adams J, Valery PC, Sibbritt D, Bernardes CM, Broom A, Garvey G. Use of traditional indigenous medicine and complementary medicine among indigenous Cancer patients in Queensland, Australia. Integr Cancer Ther. 2015;14(4):359–65.

12. Wilkinson JM, Stevens MJ. Use of complementary and alternative medical therapies (CAM) by patients attending a regional comprehensive cancer care Centre. J Complement Integr Med. 2014;11(2):139–45.

13. Klafke N, Eliott JA, Olver IN, Wittert GA. The role of complementary and alternative medicine (CAM) routines and rituals in men with cancer and their significant others (SOs): a qualitative investigation. Support Care Cancer. 2014;22(5):1319–31.

14. YZnet-Communications. Australian health directory. Available from: http://www.healthdirectory.com.au 2016

15. Australian hospitals and aged care directory 2014. Doonan: ATA Professional Service; 2013.

16. AIHW. My Hospitals: Australian Institute of Health and Welfare. Australian Government.

17. IRIS, Iris Cancer Partnership: Scottish scoping survey of massage services for people living with cancer. 2014.

18. SuveyMonkey Inc. San Mateo: Available from: www.surveymonkey.com. Accessed June 2015.

19. SPSS Statistics for Windows, Version 24.0.

20. Hsieh HF, Shannon SE. Three approaches to qualitative content analysis. Qual Health Res. 2005;15(9):1277–88.

21. ESRI. ArcGIS Desktop: Release 10. Redlands: Environmental Systems Research Institute; 2011.

22. Lim E, Vardy JL, Oh B, Dhillon HM. Mixed methods study to investigate models of Australian integrative oncology. J Alt Comp Med. 2017;23(12):980–8.

23. Scott C. The Dr Dorothea Sandars and Irene lee Churchill fellowship to study the integration of complementary and supportive therapies with conventional medical care for people with cancer – USA, UK. Australia: The Winston Churchill Memorial Trust of Australia; 2012.

24. Kerridge IH, McPhee JR. Ethical and legal issues at the interface of complementary and conventional medicine. Med J Aust. 2004;181(3):164–6.

25. Robotin MC, Penman AG. Integrating complementary therapies into mainstream cancer care: which way forward? Med J Aust. 2006;185(7):377–9.

26. Stub T, Quandt SA, Arcury TA, Sandberg JC, Kristoffersen AE, Musial F, Salamonsen A. Perception of risk and communication among conventional and complementary health care providers involving cancer patients' use of complementary therapies: a literature review. BMC Complement Alt Med. 2016;16:353.

27. Braun L, Harris J, Katris P, Cain M, Dhillon H, Koczwara B, Olver I, Robotin M. Clinical oncology Society of Australia position statement on the use of complementary and alternative medicine by cancer patients. Asia Pac J Clin Oncol. 2014;10(4):289–96.

28. Carey M, Lambert S, Smits R, Paul C, Sanson-Fisher R, Clinton-McHarg T, et al. Support Cancer Care. 2012;20(2):207–19.

29. Currow DC, Allingham S, Bird S, Yates P, Lewis J, Dawber J, Eagar K. Referral patterns and proximity to palliative care inpatient services by level of socio-economic disadvantage. A national study using spatial analysis. BMC Health Serv Res. 2012;12:424.

30. Brennan M, Gormally JF, Butow P, Boyle FM, Spillane AJ. Survivorship care plans in cancer: a systematic review of care plan outcomes. Br J Cancer. 2014;111:1899–908.

31. Fox P, Boyce A. Cancer health inequality persists in regional and remote Australia. Med J Aust. 2014;8:445–6.

32. Greenlee H, Balneaves LG, Carlson LE, Cohen M, Deng G, Hershman D, Mumber M, Perlmutter J, Seely D, Sen A, et al. Clinical practice guidelines on the use of integrative therapies as supportive care in patients treated for breast cancer. J Nat Cancer Inst. 2014;50:346–58.

33. Gentry S, Badrinath P. Defining health in the era of value-based care: lessons from England of relevance to other health systems. Cureus. 2017;9(3):e1079.

34. Egan B, Gage H, Hood J, McDowell C, Maguire G, Storey L. Availability of complementary and alternative medicine for people with cancer in the British National Health Service: results of a national survey. Complement Ther Clin Pract. 2012;18(2):75–80.

35. ABS. In: Statistics ABo, editor. Australian Demographic Statistics, Dec 2016 (released 27/06/2017). Canberra; 2017.

36. Rossi E, Vita A, Baccetti S, Stefano MD, Voller F, Zanobini A. Complementary and alternative medicine for cancer patients: results of the EPAAC survey on integrative oncology centres in Europe. Support Care Cancer. 2015;23(6):1795–806.

37. Seely DM, Weeks LC, Young S. A systematic review of integrative oncology programs. Curr Oncol. 2012;19(6):e436–61.

38. Lopez G, McQuade J, Cohen L. Integrative oncology physician consultations at a comprehensive cancer center: analysis of demographic, clinical and patient reported outcomes. J Cancer. 2017;8(3):395–402.

39. Deng GE, Rausch SM, Jones LW, Gulati A, Kumar NB, Greenlee H, Pietanza MC, Cassileth BR. Complementary therapies and integrative medicine in lung cancer: diagnosis and management of lung cancer, 3rd ed: American College of Chest Physicians evidence-based clinical practice guidelines. Chest. 2013;143(Suppl):e420S-36S.

40. Alsanad SM, Williamson EM, Howard RL. Cancer patients at risk of herb/food supplement–drug interactions: a systematic review. Phytother Res. 2014;28(12):1749–55.

41. Lee RT, Barbo A, Lopez G, Melhem-Bertrandt A, Lin H, Olopade OI, Curlin FA. National survey of US oncologists' knowledge, attitudes, and practice patterns regarding herb and supplement use by patients with cancer. J Clin Oncol. 2014;32(36):4095–101.

42. Davis EL, Oh B, Butow PN, Mullan BA, Clarke S. Cancer patient disclosure and patient-doctor communication of complementary and alternative medicine use: a systematic review. Oncologist. 2012;17(11):1475–81.

43. Chang KH, Brodie R, Choong MA, Sweeney KJ, Kerin MJ. Complementary and alternative medicine use in oncology: a questionnaire survey of patients and health care professionals. BMC Cancer. 2011;11:196.

44. King N, Balneaves LG, Levin GT, Nguyen T, Nation JG, Card C, et al. Surveys of cancer patients and cancer health care providers regarding complementary therapy use, communication, and information needs. Integr Cancer Ther. 2015;14(6):515–24.

45. King T, Grant S, Taylor S, Houteas K, Barnett C, White K. A CAM do Approach: the attitudes, use and disclosure of the use of complementary and alternative medicine (CAM) in those with myeloma. Clin Lymphoma Myeloma Leuk. 2015;15:e317–8.

46. Newell S, Sanson-Fisher RW. Australian oncologists' self-reported knowledge and attitudes about non-traditional therapies used by cancer patients. Med J Aust. 2000;172(3):110–3.

47. Burnett L, Dhillon H, Vardy J. Knowledge and attitudes of oncologists about complementary and alternative therapies used by cancer patients. AJC. 2013;12(4):229-38.

22

A Lanosteryl triterpene from *Protorhus longifolia* augments insulin signaling in type 1 diabetic rats

Sihle Ephraim Mabhida[1*], Rabia Johnson[2,3], Musawenkosi Ndlovu[1], Nonhlakanipho Felicia Sangweni[1], Johan Louw[2], Andrew Opoku[1] and Rebamang Anthony Mosa[1]

Abstract

Background: A substantial literature supports antidiabetic properties of the lanosteryl triterpene (methyl-3β-hydroxylanosta-9,24-dien-21-oate, RA-3) isolated from *Protorhus longifolia* stem bark. However, the molecular mechanism(s) associated with the antihyperglycemic properties of the triterpene remained to be explored. The current study aimed at investigating the molecular mechanism(s) through which RA-3 improves insulin signaling in streptozotocin-induced type 1 diabetic rats.

Methods: The type 1 diabetic rats were treated daily with a single oral dose of RA-3 (100 mg/kg) for 28 days. The rats were then sacrificed, and blood, skeletal muscle and pancreases were collected for biochemical, protein expression and histological analysis, respectively.

Results: Persistently high blood glucose levels in the diabetic control rats significantly increased expression of IRS-1^{Ser307} while the expression of p-Akt ^{Ser473}, p-GSK-3β ^{Ser9}, GLUT 4 and GLUT 2 were decreased. However, enhanced muscle insulin sensitivity, which was indicated by a decrease in the expression of IRS-1^{ser307} with a concomitant increase in the p-Akt^{Ser473}, p-GSK-3β ^{Ser9}, GLUT 4 and GLUT 2 expression were observed in the diabetic rats treated with RA-3. The triterpene-treated animals also showed an improved pancreatic β-cells morphology, along with increased C-peptide levels. An increase in the levels of serum antioxidants such as catalase, superoxide dismutase, and reduced glutathione was noted in the rats treated with the triterpene, while their serum levels of interleukin-6 and malondialdehyde were reduced.

Conclusions: It is apparent that RA-3 is able to improve the insulin signaling in type 1 diabetic rats. Its beta (β)-cells protecting mechanism could be attributed to its ability to alleviate inflammation and oxidative stress in the cells.

Keywords: Hyperglycemia, Glucose transporter 4, Oxidative stress, Type 1 diabetes and lanosteryl triterpene

Background

Type 1 diabetes mellitus (T1DM) is a multifactorial disease that is characterized by insulin deficiency due to destruction of the insulin producing pancreatic beta (β)-cells. To date, the exact causes of T1DM remain unknown. However, its onset is linked to an autoimmune attack on the body's own pancreatic β-cells as a result of environmental stimuli on genetically predisposed individuals. T1DM which is common amongst young children and adults, accounts for 5–10% of diabetes cases world-wide [1, 2]. According to the latest statistical report from the Center of Disease Control and Prevention (CDC, 2017), T1DM affects 80,000 children annually and this number is expected to increase by 1.4% each year [3]. Due to early onset and longer duration of the disease, affected individuals are at increased risk of developing cardiac failure at a young age [4]. This does not only place a financial burden on individual households, but also on the countries' health system budgets.

* Correspondence: sihlemabhida@gmail.com
[1]Department of Biochemistry and Microbiology, University of Zululand, Private Bag X1001, KwaDlangezwa 3886, South Africa
Full list of author information is available at the end of the article

Insulin secretion and action are crucial in maintaining glucose homeostasis, which is mediated through translocation of glucose transporters (GLUTs). Skeletal muscle is responsible for 75% of insulin-mediated glucose disposal [5] through activation of the phosphatidylinositol 3-kinase (PI3-K)/protein kinase B (2) (Akt2) pathway and subsequent translocation of GLUT 4 to the plasma membrane [6]. Persistent hyperglycemia or glucotoxicity observed in diabetic patients, as a result of insulin signaling impairment, is the underlying cause of various diabetic complications. This impairment is known to be concomitant to oxidative stress and an augmented pro-inflammatory response [7].

Though regular intravenous insulin injection is used to manage T1DM, this management strategy neither cures nor prevents onset of diabetes-induced complications. Thus, more effective treatment regimens are required in a quest to prevent, delay or more effectively treat the disease. Therefore, there is a growing interest in plant-derived bioactive compounds as potential candidates in the development of drug formulations with multiple targets to combat diabetes and its associated complications.

Various in vitro and in vivo studies have shown that triterpenes, a diverse group of natural compounds, have the ability to inhibit intestinal glucose absorption [8–10] and supress raised blood glucose levels through increased insulin secretion and cellular glucose uptake in peripheral tissues [11, 12]. A lanosteryl triterpene (RA-3, Fig. 1) isolated from Protorhus longifolia (Benrh.) Engl. (Anacardiaceae) stem bark has been reported to possess hypoglycemic properties, which are also associated with stimulation of cellular glucose uptake [13] and improved glucose tolerance [14, 15]. However, the molecular mechanism(s) associated with these antidiabetic properties of the compound remained to be elucidated. Therefore, this study was

set out to explore the molecular mechanism(s) through which RA-3 exerts its hypoglycemic effect. Its effect on peripheral insulin signaling in skeletal muscle of STZ-induced type 1 diabetic rats was investigated in this study.

Methods
Extraction and isolation of RA-3
Fresh stem bark of *Protorhus longifolia* (specimen voucher number RA01UZ) was collected from KwaHlabisa, KwaZulu-Natal (KZN), South Africa. The plant was verified by Dr. N.R. Ntuli from the Botany Department, University of Zululand, South Africa. The plant material was then air-dried and ground to powder. The targeted lanosteryl triterpene, RA-3 (Fig. 1), was extracted and isolated from the chloroform extract of *P. longifolia* using chromatographic techniques as previously reported [13, 16]. Spectroscopic (IR, NMR) data analysis was used to confirm the chemical structure of the compound.

Induction of type 1 diabetes
Approval for use of laboratory animals (*Rattus norvegicus*) and experimental procedures was granted by the University of Zululand research ethics committee (ethical clearance number: UZREC 171110–030 PGM 2016/329). Male *Sprague-Dawley* rats ($n = 20$, 150–200 g) were obtained from the Biochemistry and Microbiology Department, University of Zululand. The animals were maintained under standard conditions (12-h light/dark cycle, relative humidity, ~ 50%, and temperature, 23–25 °C). Before commencement of experimental procedures, rats were acclimatized for five days with free access to water and pelleted rat feed, ad libitum. T1DM was induced by giving the rats a single intraperitoneal injection of streptozotocin (STZ) solution (60 mg/kg). Five days after the STZ injection, blood samples were obtained by tail prick for blood glucose measurement. The

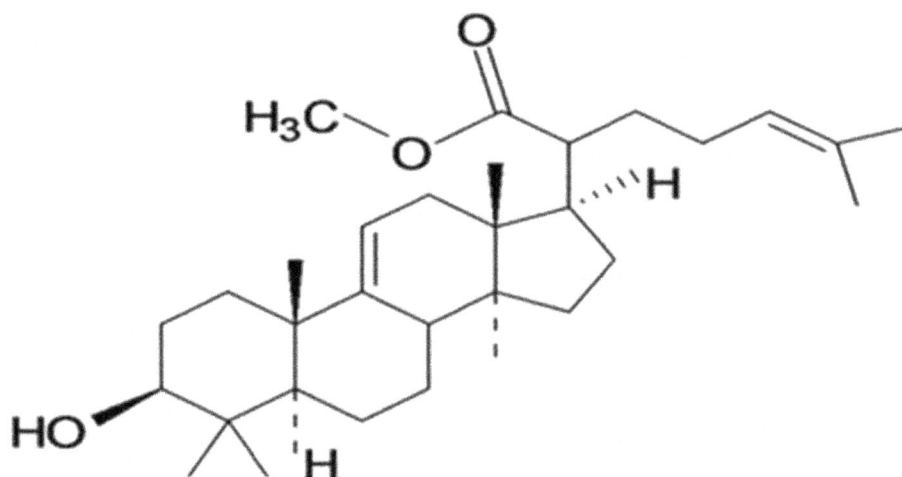

Fig. 1 Chemical structure of lanosteryl triterpene (RA-3)

fasting blood glucose level was measured with ACCU TREND PLUS® glucometer (Roche Diagnostics, Mannheim, Germany). The rats with the fasting blood glucose levels higher than or equal to 11 mmol/L were considered diabetic and they were used in the study.

Preparation of RA-3 solution
RA-3 was dissolved in Tween 20 (2%) to prepare a working solution of 100 mg/kg body weight of the rat. The prepared dosage was based on previous studies performed in our laboratory [14, 16].

Treatment of diabetic animals with RA-3
STZ-induced diabetic rats were randomly divided into three groups with each group consisting of five animals ($n = 5$). The animals were then orally administered with the drugs or carrier solvent as follows: (I) diabetic control group was given Tween 20 (2% diluted with distilled water); (II) diabetic animals treated with RA-3 (100 mg/kg); and (III) diabetic animals treated with metformin (100 mg/kg). The normal control group (IV) was given an equivalent volume of distilled water. The animals received an oral single dose of the RA-3 and metformin (standard antidiabetic drug) daily for 28 days. Fasting blood glucose levels of the rats were measured at seven days intervals using the ACCUTREND PLUS® glucometer (Roche Diagnostics, Mannheim, Germany) for the full duration of the experimental period. Upon completion of the experiment, the animals were fasted overnight, and then placed in an induction chamber were it was anesthetized by inhalation (2% isoflurane mixed with 98% Oxygen).The loss of sensation was further confirmed by the pedal withdrawal reflex before any procedure was performed. Blood from the animals was collected by cardiac puncture for serum analysis. Thereafter, the pancreas, liver and skeletal muscles were harvested for histology and western blot analysis, respectively.

Biochemical analysis of serum antioxidants, malondialdehyde, interleukin-6 and C-peptide levels
Blood samples were centrifuged (Eppendorf® MiniSpin® 5454 Micro centrifuge, Merck) at 4 °C for 10 min at 1200 rpm. Serum was then collected into fresh tubes and stored at – 80 °C until required. The serum levels of catalase (CAT), superoxide dismutase (SOD), reduced glutathione (GSH) and malondialdehyde (MDA) were measured using commercially available assay kits from Sigma-Aldrich (St. Louis, MO, USA). An enzyme-linked immunosorbent assay (ELISA) kit obtained from Sigma-Aldrich Co. Ltd. (Steinheim, Germany) was used to measure the serum interleukin-6 (IL-6) level. Standard clinical laboratory (Global Clinical & Viral Laboratory, Richards Bay, SA) procedures were followed to measure the serum level of C-peptide.

Hematoxylin and eosin stain of pancreas
The excised pancreatic tissues were fixed in neutral buffered formalin (10%) until they were required for histological analysis. The formalin fixed tissues were routinely processed by a Leica TP 1020 automated processor (Leica Biosystems, Buffalo Grove, IL, USA) and embedded in paraffin wax. Tissues were sectioned and attached to aminopropyltriethoxysilane coated glass slides, after which they were stained with hematoxylin and eosin [15]. Examination of the slides was performed by an independent Pathologist without prior knowledge of the experimental groups (Vet Diagnostix Laboratories, Pietermaritzburg, South Africa).

Western blot analysis
To investigate effect of RA-3 on some known proteins involved in insulin signaling pathway, immunoblots against IRS-1^{ser307}, p- Akt^{Ser473}, p- GSK-3β^{Ser9}, GLUT 4 and GLUT 2 were performed. Snap frozen skeletal muscle and liver tissues (100 mg each) were separately lysed in lysis buffer (Pierce Biotechnologies, Rockford, CA, USA) using a tissue lyser. Thereafter, the samples were centrifuged (Eppendorf® MiniSpin® 5454 Micro centrifuge, Merck) at 4 °C for 20 min at 12,000 rpm. Supernatant was collected and stored at – 20 °C until required. Protein (30 μg) was mixed with an equal volume of 2× Laemmli sample buffer (Biorad) before it was denatured at 95 °C. The denatured protein samples (30 μg) were loaded on a 12% SDS-polyacrylamide gel (Bio-Rad, Hercules, CA, USA) and transferred to a polyvinylidene fluoride (PVDF) membrane (Bio-Rad, Hercules, CA, USA) [17] and membranes containing the proteins of interest were then incubated at 4 °C for 16 h with the following primary antibodies: anti- IRS-1^{Ser307} (1:500), phospo-Akt^{Ser473} (1:1000), phospho-GSK-3β^{Ser9} (1:1000) (Cell signaling, Danvers, MA, USA), anti-GLUT 4 (1:1000) (Sigma-Aldrich Chemical Co., St. Louis, MO, USA) and GLUT 2 (1:500) (Sigma-Aldrich Chemical Co., St. Louis, MO, USA). Membranes were then washed and incubated with the appropriate horseradish peroxidase conjugated secondary antibody at room temperature for 90 min. All proteins were normalized to a loading control (β-Actin) (1:500) (Santa Cruz Biotechnology, Dallas, TX, USA). Chemidoc-XRS imager and Quantity One software (Bio-Rad Laboratories, Hercules, CA, USA) were used to detect and quantify the proteins. Image J software was used to quantify the signal intensity of the bands.

Data analysis
Data were analyzed using GraphPad Prism software (version 5.03). Experiments were performed in triplicates and data were expressed as mean ± SEM. Statistical differences between groups was determine by One-way analysis of variance (ANOVA), followed by Tukey post-hoc test.

Table 1 Results of the effect of RA-3 on fasting blood glucose levels of the STZ-induced type 1 diabetic rats

Group	Baseline (mmol/L)	Blood glucose levels Day 28 (mmol/L)	ΔBlood glucose levels (%)
Non-diabetic control	4.2 ± 0.22	4.3 ± 0.04	
Diabetic control	14.0 ± 0.58****	27.0 ± 1.14****	
Diabetic + RA-3	13.3 ± 0.58****	4.4 ± 0.44####	67
Diabetic + metformin	13.8 ± 0.40****	4.3 ± 0.44####	69

Results are expressed as the mean ± SEM, $n = 5$. **** $p \leq 0.0001$ versus non-diabetic control, #### $p \leq 0.0001$ versus diabetic control

The values were considered statistically significant where $p \leq 0.05$.

Results

Fasting blood glucose levels of the STZ-induced diabetic rats

Table 1 shows the results of the effect of RA-3 on the fasting blood glucose levels of the STZ-induced diabetic rats following the experimental period of 28 days. Persistently higher fasting plasma glucose levels were observed in the diabetic control rats. However, treatment of the diabetic rats with RA-3 significantly lowered the blood glucose levels by 67%. The observed effect was similar and comparable to the metformin treated group (69%), which served as the positive control group.

Serum antioxidants and C-peptide levels

The effect of RA-3 on serum antioxidants and C-peptide levels in the STZ-induced diabetic animals are presented in Table 2. The STZ-induced type 1 diabetic rats showed a significant decrease in GSH (4.31 ± 0.150, $p \leq 0.001$), SOD (29 ± 0.040, $p \leq 0.01$), CAT (0.05 ± 0.006, $p \leq 0.05$) and C-peptide levels (0.5 ± 0.220, $p \leq 0.0001$) when compared to the normal control group. Treatment of the animals with either RA-3 or metformin was able to significantly increase the serum glutathione (6.05 ± 0.130, $p \leq 0.05$), superoxide dismutase (55 ± 0.011, $p \leq 0.05$) catalase (0.10 ± 0.004, $p \leq 0.05$) and C-peptide (0.8 ± 1.020, $p \leq 0.0001$) levels when compared to their diabetic control counterparts.

Serum MDA and IL-6

The effect of RA-3 on the serum MDA and IL-6 levels are presented in Fig. 2. The STZ-induced type 1 diabetic rats showed a significant increase of serum MDA (270 ± 13.4%, $p \leq 0.0001$) and IL-6 (153 ± 2.70%) when compared to the normal control group. After 28 days of treatment, a decreased in the levels of serum MDA (121 ± 12.5%, $p \leq 0.0001$) and IL-6 (135 ± 10.9%) was observed in the RA-3 treated group as compared to the diabetic control group. This was consistent with the observed increase in antioxidant levels in the RA-3 treated group. A similar and comparable effect was also observed in the metformin treated group. However, the effect of either RA-3 or metformin to reduce IL-6 levels was not significant.

Effect of RA-3 on the morphology of β-cells of the STZ-induced diabetic rats

Histological evaluation of the pancreatic sections from the different experimental groups was performed. The results of the histology are shown in Fig. 3. The pancreas of the normal rats (Fig. 3a) showed normal islet morphology. Whereas the pancreatic tissues from the untreated diabetic group (Fig. 3b) confirmed shrinkage of the islets. However, treatment of the diabetic animals with RA-3 as well as metformin appeared to preserve islet size as shown in Fig. 3c and d, respectively.

Western blot analysis

IRS-1^{ser307}, p-Akt, p-GSK-3β, GLUT 4 and GLUT 2 are major proteins involved in the insulin-dependent signaling pathway (Fig. 4). The results revealed that high blood glucose levels in the untreated diabetic rats significantly increased the expression of IRS-1^{Ser307} (183 ± 4.06%, $p \leq 0.0001$), while decreasing expression of p-Akt^{Ser473} (41 ± 0.91%, $p \leq 0.0001$) and p-GSK-3β ^{Ser9} (10 ± 2.71%, $p \leq 0.0001$) as compared to the non-diabetic group. The observed effects of high blood glucose levels were reversed following the 28 days treatment of the diabetic rats with RA-3 (96 ± 2.61%, $p \leq 0.0001$; 109 ± 3.14%, $p \leq 0.0001$ and 94 ± 3.67%, $p \leq 0.0001$, respectively) when compared to the diabetic control group. The observed effects were comparable to the metformin treated group. This study showed that while a decrease in GLUT 4 (30 ± 3.97%, $p \leq 0.0001$) and GLUT 2 (40 ± 1.63%, $p \leq 0.0001$) expression

Table 2 Effect of RA-3 on serum antioxidants and C-peptide levels of the diabetic animals

Group	GSH (nmol/mL)	SOD (Inhibition rate %)	CAT (Units/mL)	C-peptide (µg/L)
Non-diabetic control	7.33 ± 0.010	56 ± 0.005	0.12 ± 0.005	0.8 ± 0.010
Diabetic control	4.31 ± 0.150***	29 ± 0.040**	0.05 ± 0.006*	0.5 ± 0.220****
Diabetic + RA-3	6.05 ± 0.130*#	55 ± 0.011#	0.10 ± 0.004#	0.8 ± 1.020####
Diabetic + metformin	6.40 ± 0.140*#	54 ± 0.012#	0.10 ± 0.006#	0.8 ± 0.410####

Results are expressed as the mean ± SEM, $n = 5$. * $p \leq 0.05$, ** $p \leq 0.01$, *** $p \leq 0.001$, **** $p \leq 0.0001$ versus non-diabetic control, # $p \leq 0.05$, #### $p \leq 0.0001$ versus diabetic control

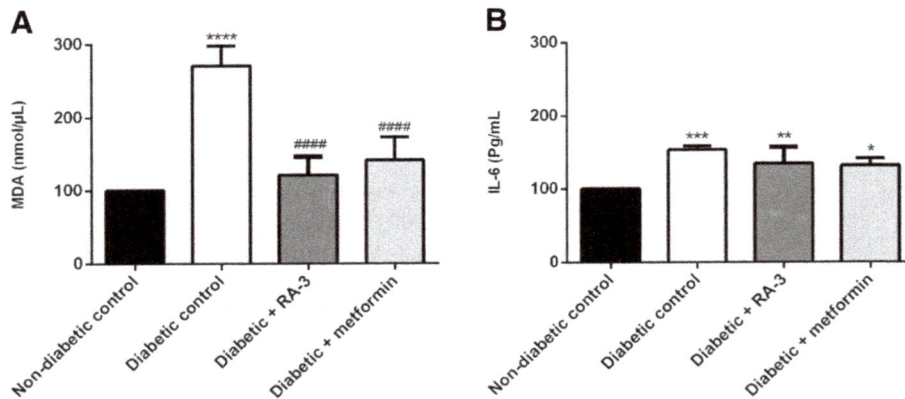

Fig. 2 Effect of RA-3 on serum (**a**) MDA and (**b**) IL-6 levels in STZ-induced type 1 diabetic animals. Results are expressed as the mean ± SEM, $n =$ 5. * $p \leq 0.05$, ** $p \leq 0.01$, *** $p \leq 0.001$, **** $p \leq 0.0001$ vs. non-diabetic control, #### $p \leq 0.0001$ vs. diabetic control

was observed in the diabetic control group, an increased expression ($80 \pm 8.16\%$, $p \leq 0.01$) and ($110 \pm 3.14\%$, $p \leq 0.01$) of these proteins was observed in the skeletal muscle and the liver tissues of the diabetic animals that received RA-3 (Fig. 4d and e).

Discussion

Understanding the molecular mechanism that leads to the development and progression of T1DM is an important objective in the management of the disease. Despite the use of

current hypoglycemic drugs and insulin injections to manage the disease, the search for new drugs that can prevent and/or effectively treat the disease is on-going. Previous studies have demonstrated the anti-hyperglycemic property of the lanosteryl triterpene (RA-3). This was evidenced by its ability to stimulate cellular glucose uptake in C2C12 myocytes and 3 T3-1 L adipocytes [13] and then improve glucose tolerance in diabetic rats [14, 15]. However, the molecular mechanism(s) through which RA-3 exerts its hypoglycemic effect remained to be explored and

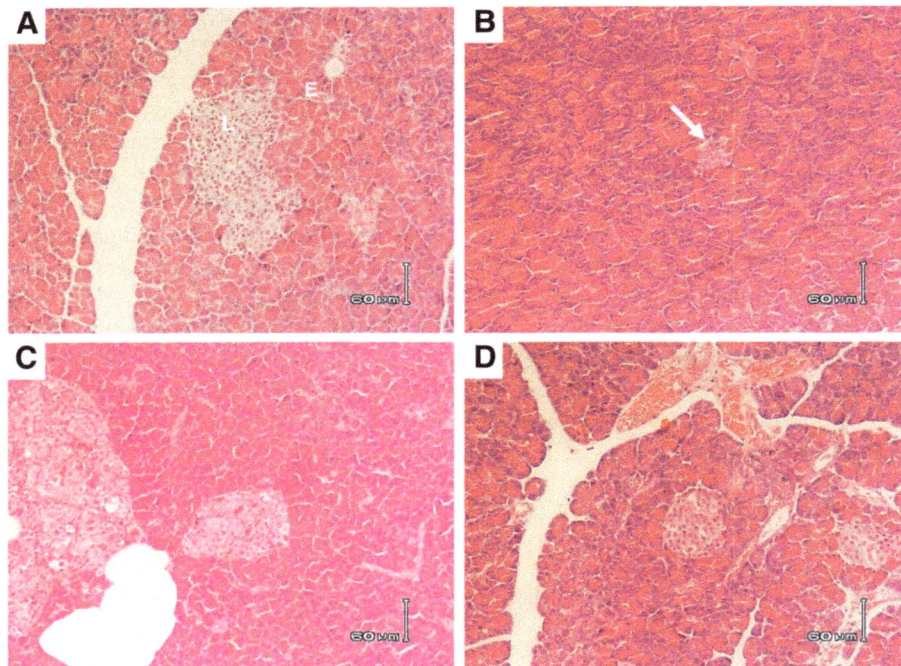

Fig. 3 The effect of RA-3 on pancreatic islet morphology of STZ-induced type 1 diabetic rats. **a** Normal control group, (**b**) Untreated diabetic group, (**c**) RA-3 treated group, and (**d**) Metformin treated group. (L) indicates a normal islet without any histological alterations, (E) exocrine portion of pancreatic tissue and an arrow illustrates STZ-induced shrinkage of islets .NB: For each image the magnification (200X). Bar indicator is 60 μm

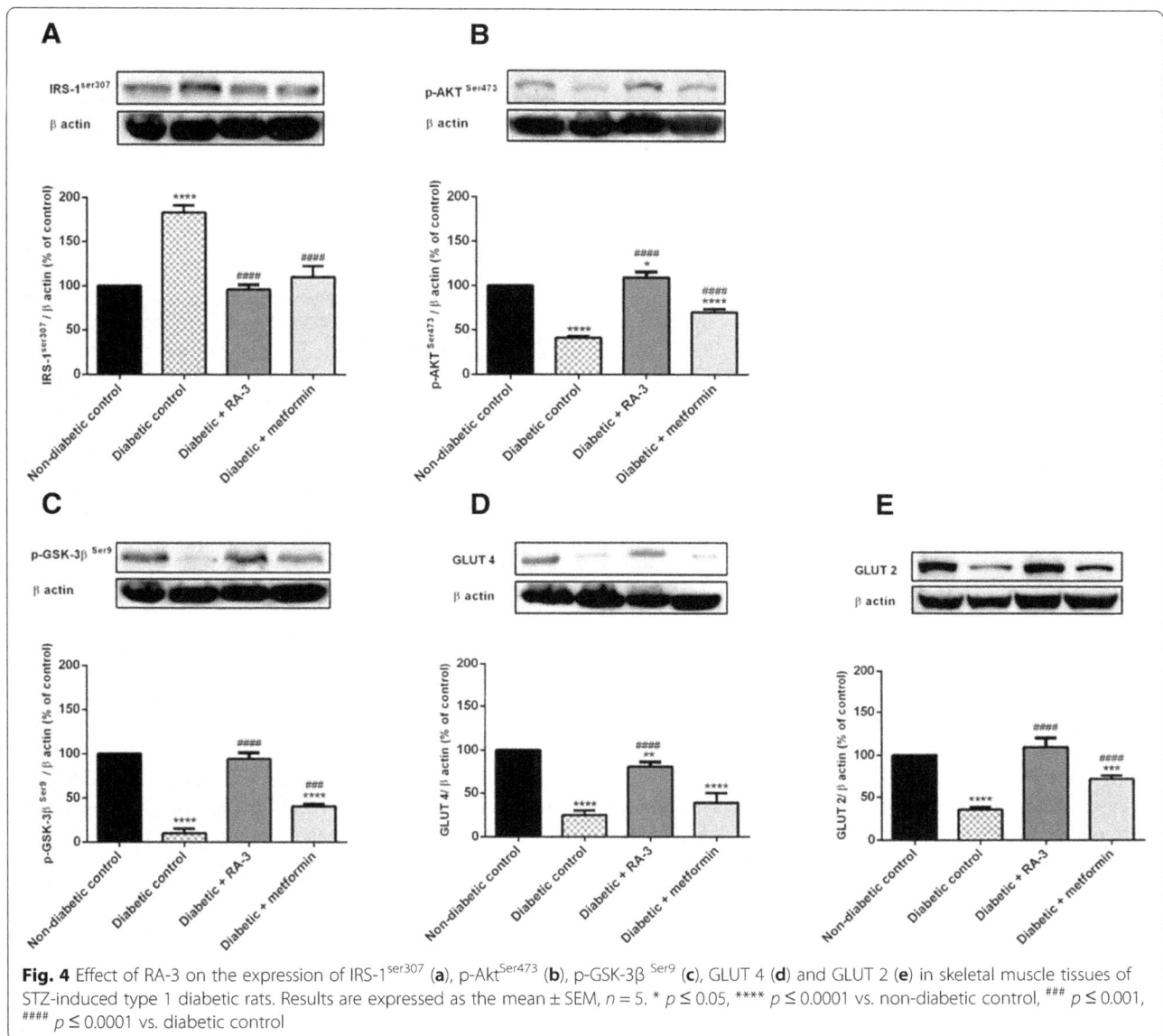

Fig. 4 Effect of RA-3 on the expression of IRS-1^{ser307} (**a**), p-Akt^{Ser473} (**b**), p-GSK-3β ^{Ser9} (**c**), GLUT 4 (**d**) and GLUT 2 (**e**) in skeletal muscle tissues of STZ-induced type 1 diabetic rats. Results are expressed as the mean ± SEM, $n = 5$. * $p \leq 0.05$, **** $p \leq 0.0001$ vs. non-diabetic control, ### $p \leq 0.001$, #### $p \leq 0.0001$ vs. diabetic control

understood. Thus, this study investigated potential of RA-3 to augment insulin signaling in the STZ-induced type 1 diabetic rats.

Insulin stimulates muscle glucose uptake by promoting recruitment of GLUT 4 or GLUT 2 via activation of the phosphatidylinositol 3-kinase (PI3-K) and Akt2 pathway [6]. Under physiological conditions, an increase in the expression of IR-IRS-PI3K-Akt signaling cascade is observed. However, the expression of these proteins is down regulated in the diabetic state. The results from the current study showed that the hypoglycemic effect of RA-3 could partly be linked to its ability to augment insulin signalling (Fig. 5). This is indicated by the observed decrease in IRS-1^{Ser307} expression and increase in p-Akt and p-GSK-3β expression, which was well correlated with the increased expression of GLUT 4 and GLUT 2 in the RA-3

treated group. Increased expression of GLUT 4 and GLUT 2 expression was further supported by the lower blood glucose levels in the RA-3 treated diabetic animals. A pentacyclic triterpene, oleanolic acid, has also been reported to enhance the insulin signaling pathway in the skeletal muscle of STZ-induced diabetic rats [18]. High expression of p-Akt activates translocation of GLUT 4 and thus increases glucose uptake by the cell. p-Akt also further phosphorylates GSK-3β, promoting the glucose storage as glycogen. The ability of RA-3 to increase the expression of p-GSK-3β shows potential of this compound to control glucose homeostasis. These results further support the previous report in which RA-3 inhibited glucose-6-phosphatase and increased hepatic glycogen storage in the STZ-induced diabetic rats [14].

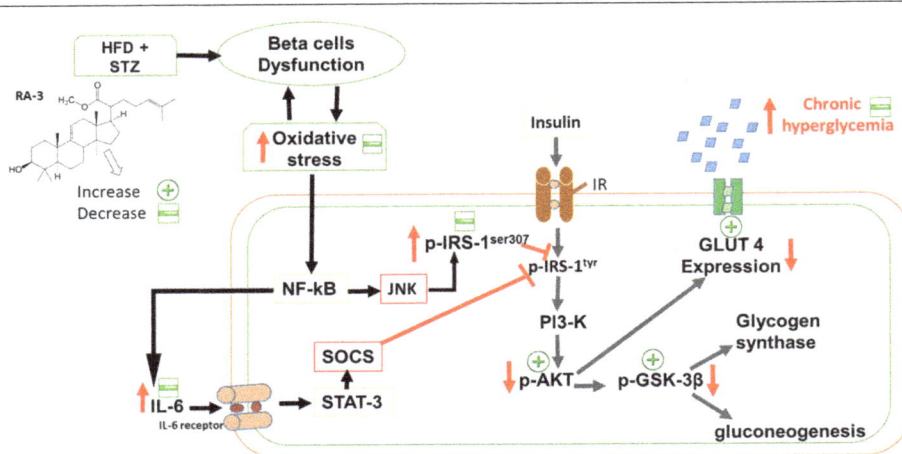

Fig. 5 Overview of insulin regulation of major metabolic responses in the cells. Under physiological conditions, insulin binds to its receptor (IR) to enhance positive tyrosine IRS-1 phosphorylation, promoting the activation of PI3-K which in turn phosphorylates and activates p-Akt. High expression of p-Akt activates translocation of glucose transporter 4 and thus increasing glucose uptake by the cell. p-Akt also further phosphorylates GSK-3β, promoting the glucose storage as glycogen. Under pathophysiological conditions, oxidative stress and pro-inflammatory cytokines such as IL-6 enhance negative phosphorylation of IRS-1 serine (307), causing insulin resistance. Activated NF-κB activates serine/threonine kinases (JNK) which phosphorylates IRS-1 and also works via other pathways such as SOCS expression to inhibit the insulin signaling pathway

Effective antidiabetic therapeutics should also possess pancreatic β-cells protective properties in order to maintain their production of insulin. RA-3 also showed potential to improve morphology of the pancreatic β-cells of the diabetic rats. The potential β-cells protective effect of the triterpene could be attributed to its ability to increase tissue antioxidant status which was evidenced by increases in GSH, CAT and SOD serum levels in the RA-3 treated group. The decrease in serum MDA levels, a marker of lipid peroxidation, and IL-6 further supported the antioxidant protective potential of the compound. The observed increase in serum C-peptide levels, a reliable indicator of well-functioning pancreatic β-cells [19], further supported the potential β-cells protective effect of the triterpene. The ability of the lanosteryl triterpene to improve pancreatic β-cells morphology and thus increase serum C-peptide levels has recently been demonstrated in type 2 diabetic rats [15]. Furthermore, since oxidative stress and pro-inflammatory cytokines such as IL-6 are implicated in the insulin signaling impairment and β-cells dysfunction [20], the antioxidant and anti-inflammatory effects mediated by RA-3 further support its β-cells protective effect and stimulation of cellular glucose uptake.

Conclusions

The present study provides evidence that the anti-hyperglycaemic activity of RA-3 could be linked to its ability to protect pancreatic β-cells and improve insulin signaling in skeletal muscles of the diabetic rats. This is indicated by increased expression of proteins involved in insulin signaling and eventual increased expression of

GLUT 4 in the muscle of the diabetic animals treated with RA-3. The lanosteryl triterpene also reduced oxidative stress and inflammation which are important mediators of cellular insulin resistance, pancreatic β-cells dysfunction and tissue damage in the diabetic animals. Thus, future research directions, which are also important in addressing limitations of the present study, involve immunohistochemistry of the skeletal muscle to confirm the effect of the triterpene on the insulin signalling in skeletal muscle, unravelling molecular mechanisms through which RA-3 improves the pancreatic islets size and quantification of the number of islet cells in the diabetic rats. Furthermore, the consistent similar results exhibited by RA-3 and metformin, a standard antidiabetic drug, suggests a need to evaluate the antidiabetic effects of a combination of the two drugs.

Abbreviations
Akt2: protein kinase B (2); GLUT 4: Glucose transporter 4; GLUTs: Glucose transporters; GSK-3β: Glycogen synthase kinase 3 beta; IL-6: Interleukin-6; IR: Insulin receptor; IRS-1: Insulin receptor substrate 1; PI3-K: Phosphatidylinositol 3-kinase; RA-3: Methyl-3β-hydroxylanosta-9,24-dien-21-oate; STZ: Streptozotocin; T1DM: Type 1 diabetes mellitus

Acknowledgements
The authors are indebted to Zanka Yuroukova for her expertise in histopathological analysis of the pancreatic tissue, the University of Zululand Research Committee (UZRC) for funding this work and South African National Research Foundation (NRF) for sponsorship awarded to M.S.E.

Funding
This work was financially supported by the University of Zululand Research Committee (UZRC), South African National Research Foundation (SA-NRF) and South African Medical Research Council's Biomedical Research and Innovation Platform.

Authors' contributions

MRA and OA conceived and designed the experiments; MSE and SNF performed the experiments; MRA, JR and JL experimental design and interpretation of western blot analysis; MSE and NM analysed the data; OA, MSE, JR and MRA wrote the manuscript. All authors have read and approved the manuscript.

Competing interests

"The authors declare that they have no competing interests."

Author details

[1]Department of Biochemistry and Microbiology, University of Zululand, Private Bag X1001, KwaDlangezwa 3886, South Africa. [2]Biomedical Research and Innovation Platform (BRIP), South African Medical Research Council, Tygerberg 7505, South Africa. [3]Division of Medical Physiology, Faculty of Medicine and Health Sciences, Stellenbosch University, Tygerberg 7505, South Africa.

References

1. World health Organization (WHO). World health statistics 2017. Available online: http://apps.who.int/iris/bitstream/10665/44844/1/9789241564441_eng.pdf?ua=1 (accessed on 29 May 2017).

2. Wherrett D, Huot C, Mitchell B, Pacaud D. Type 1 diabetes in children and adolescents. Can J Diabetes. 2013;37:153–62.

3. Centers for Disease Control and Prevention. National diabetes statistics report, 2017. Atlanta, GA: Centers for Disease Control and Prevention, US Department of Health and Human Services; 2017.

4. International Diabetes Federation (IDF). IDF Diabetes Atlas, 7th ed. Available online: http://www.diabetesatlas.org/ (accessed on 29 May 2017).

5. Wei Y, Chen K, Whaley-Connell AT, Stump CS, Ibdah JA, Sowers JR. Skeletal muscle insulin resistance: role of inflammatory cytokines and reactive oxygen species. Am J Phys Regul Integr Comp Phys. 2008;294(3):673–80.

6. Li X, Wang F, Xu M, Howles P, Tso P. ApoA-IV improves insulin sensitivity and glucose uptake in mouse adipocytes via PI3K-Akt signaling. Sci Rep. 2017;7:216–26.

7. Solinas G, Becattini B. JNK at the crossroad of obesity, insulin resistance, and cell stress response. Molecular Metabolism. 2017;6(2):174.

8. Hou W, Li Y, Zhang Q, Wei X, Peng A, Chen L, Wei Y. Triterpene acids isolated from *Lagerstroemia speciosa* leaves as α-glucosidase inhibitors. Phytother Res. 2009;23(5):614–8.

9. Musabayane CT, Tufts MA, Mapanga RF. Synergistic antihyperglycemic effects between plant-derived oleanolic acid and insulin in streptozotocin-induced diabetic rats. Ren Fail. 2010;32(7):832–9.

10. Khathi A, Serumula MR, Myburg RB, Van Heerden FR, Musabayane CT. Effects of Syzygium aromaticum-derived triterpenes on postprandial blood glucose in streptozotocin-induced diabetic rats following carbohydrate challenge. PLoS One. 2013;8(11):81632.

11. Lee MS, Thuong PT. Stimulation of glucose uptake by triterpenoids from *Weigela subsessilis*. Phytother Res. 2010;24(1):49–53.

12. Castellano JM, Guinda A, Delgado T, Rada M, Cayuela JA. Biochemical basis of the antidiabetic activity of oleanolic acid and related pentacyclic triterpenes. Diabetes. 2013;62(6):1791–9.

13. Mosa RA, Naidoo JJ, Nkomo FS, Mazibuko SE, Muller CJF, Opoku AR. In vitro anti-hyperlipidemic potential of triterpenes from stem bark of *Protorhus longifolia*. Planta Med. 2014;80:1685–91.

14. Mosa RA, Cele ND, Mabhida SE, Shabalala SC, Penduka D, Opoku AR. In vivo antihyperglycemic activity of a lanosteryl triterpene from *Protorhus longifolia*. Molecules. 2015;20:13374–83.

15. Mabhida SE, Mosa RA, Penduka D, Osunsanmi FO, Dludla PV, Djarova TG, Opoku AR. A lanosteryl triterpene from *Protorhus longifolia* improves glucose tolerance and pancreatic beta cell ultrastructure in type 2 diabetic rats. Molecules. 2017;22(8):1252.

16. Machaba KE, Cobongela SZZ, Mosa RA, Lawal AO, Djarova TG, Opoku AR. In vivo anti-hyperlipidemic activity of the triterpene from the stem bark of *Protorhus longifolia* (Benrh) Engl. Lipids Health Dis. 2014;13:131.

17. Johnson R, Shabalala S, Louw J, Kappo AP, Muller CJF. Aspalathin reverts doxorubicin-induced cardiotoxicity through increased autophagy and decreased expression of p53/mTOR/p62 signaling. Molecules. 2017;22(10):1589.

18. Mukundwa A, Mukaratirwa S, Masola B. Effects of oleanolic acid on the insulin signaling pathway in skeletal muscle of streptozotocin-induced diabetic male Sprague-Dawley rats. J Diabetes. 2016;8(1):98–108.

19. Leighton E, Sainsbury CA, Jones GC. A practical review of C-peptide testing in diabetes. Diabetes Therapy. 2017;5:1–13.

20. Elmarakby AA, Sullivan JC. Relationship between oxidative stress and inflammatory cytokines in diabetic nephropathy. Cardiovasc Ther. 2012;30:49–59.

23

The actual conditions of traditional Japanese Kampo education in all the pharmacy schools in Japan

Yoshinobu Nakada[1][*] [ID] and Makoto Arai[1,2]

Abstract

Background: To investigate the present status of Kampo education, which has still not been elucidated, after the introduction of the new core national curriculum of 2015 into nationwide pharmacy education, in all 74 pharmacy schools in Japan.

Methods: A postal questionnaire survey was conducted from August 2015 to January 2016. The completed questionnaires were returned by mail. Web-based syllabi were also investigated to ascertain the detailed lecture curricula in each school. Descriptive analyses were conducted without statistics.

Results: A total of 74 questionnaires were collected (response rate, 100%). In 2015, the numbers of clinical Kampo classes as required subjects during the 6 years of regular pharmacy school education ranged from 0 to 36 (median, 13; mean, 11.8 ± 7.6). Of the 74 schools, 49 schools (66%) provided Kampo education from a clinical standpoint. Pharmacists employed in pharmacies and physicians taught most of these classes. The major problems to be solved first are: selecting and retaining teachers to teach clinical Kampo medicine (43 of 74 schools, 58%), preparing standard textbooks (37 schools, 50%), and improving the environment for practical Kampo training (30 schools, 41%).

Conclusions: Curricula for teaching Kampo medicine significantly differ at each of the 74 Japanese pharmacy schools. In addition to selecting teachers who can adequately teach clinical Kampo medicine, improving training environments, and nationwide standardization of the curricula and textbooks are critical.

Keywords: Core curriculum, Education, Kampo medicine, Pharmacy school, Questionnaire survey

Background

Japanese traditional medicine (Kampo medicine) was uniquely developed, especially in the Edo period (1603–1868), after having been introduced from China centuries prior to that [1, 2]. It was the primary medicine until the end of the Edo period. Western medicine, however, gradually took over during the Meiji period (1868–1912) and has continued as the primary form of medicine in Japan until the present day. The large factor of this change was that the national licensing examination for physicians only asked questions related to Western medicine. Under this long slump in Kampo medicine, Kampo theories (especially those in herbal medicine) were only handed down by a very few pharmacists and physicians in their own offices. Finally, the situation in clinical sites gradually began to change due to the listing of Kampo medicines in the national health insurance program in 1967. Over the subsequent years, Kampo therapy has become increasingly popular among Japanese people [3–5]. Moreover, 70 to 90% of Japanese

* Correspondence: yoshinobu_nakada@tsc.u-tokai.ac.jp
[1]Department of Kampo Medicine, Tokai University School of Medicine, Isehara, Kanagawa, Japan
Full list of author information is available at the end of the article

physicians regularly prescribe Kampo medicine in their medical practices according to clinical evidence and reports of mechanisms of action and/or by following guidelines from modern Western medicine [6–8]. The education of Kampo medicine, however, was still largely inadequate until the early days of the twenty-first century.

The curricula in Japanese pharmacy schools changed significantly in 2006, when they extended their 4-year program to 6 years and increased their clinical medicine classes. Since then, Kampo medicine education has been definitely incorporated into the curricula of all the pharmacy schools. Furthermore, in 2015 the newly revised core curriculum has been added, in which concepts, education of uses, side effects, adverse events, and interactions with Western medicines of Kampo medicine have been emphasized. In addition, topics on the way to catch patients' patterns, systematic classifications of Kampo formulae, Kampo medicines in contemporary medicine, management of Kampo drugs in pharmacies, and education for patients have all been newly added, which are namely educational points from the clinical side, compared with the prior curriculum which emphasized education of crude drugs, active ingredients of crude drugs, and drug efficacy evaluations. Traditionally, however, pharmacists have been able to sell Kampo medicines in their drugstores without prescriptions. One hundred forty-eight kinds of Kampo formulae are currently approved by the Japanese national health insurance system. If patients are treated within these Kampo medicines and want to use the national health insurance, they have to ask their physicians and get a prescription. On the other hand, if patients opt not use the insurance, they can go directly to pharmacies or hospitals providing treatment which is not covered by the national health insurance. Namely, pharmacists can sell Kampo medicine directly, over-the-counter (OTC), and Kampo formulae of crude drugs to their customers in their pharmacies, even though the Japanese national health insurance does not cover it. Moreover, pharmacists have the right to ask physicians (indeed, they have the professional responsibility to ask), if they notice any mistakes, or points of concern, in any prescriptions they handle. Therefore, it is imperative that pharmacists have standard and adequate knowledge of Kampo medicine. E.g., especially the mineralocorticoid action of Glycyrrhiza containing glycyrrhizin and its interactions with diuretics, and the sympathomimetic effect of the Ephedra herb containing ephedrine are some of the crude drugs which physicians and pharmacists should remember. Similarly, they have to know their contraindications and they have to identify the excess overlapping of crude drugs among multiple Kampo prescriptions from multiple hospitals [9]).

Interestingly, it was not until 2001, for the first time in Japanese medical schools, that the national guidelines on medical education core curriculum approved the education of Japanese traditional medicine. Since then, however, among all the 80 Japanese university medical schools, an increasing number of them have integrated Kampo medicine into their curricula [1]. According to our previous study [10], which shows the outcomes of a questionnaire survey of all the Japanese medical schools in 2011, 98% of them conducted at least one Kampo medicine class, and 81% taught Kampo medicine on the basis of the traditional Japanese theory. The most outstanding problems to be solved first discovered from the survey were selecting and retaining teachers to teach Kampo medicine (65%), curricula standardization (63%), and preparation of standardized textbooks (51%). In the pharmacy education in Japan, however, to our knowledge, no such survey has ever been done after introducing the new national core curriculum of 2015. The aims of this study are to elucidate the present conditions of Kampo education in all the Japanese pharmacy schools and, from these data, to put together basic materials to teach Kampo medicine in the near future.

Methods

We conducted a postal questionnaire survey of the present status of Kampo education in all 74 pharmacy schools (17 national and public schools and 57 private schools) in Japan from August 2015 to January 2016. The questionnaires (see the Additional file 1) were distributed by postal mail to the pharmacy directors in every university pharmacy school first and subsequently by them to the teachers who teach Kampo medicine.

There were two main categories of questions. One category was regarding, "The present status of Kampo related education in your pharmacy school," which asked about the number of units offered, the types of classes (lectures and/or workshops), the contents of the education, and its concepts. The other category was, "Opinions regarding Kampo related education," which asked the teachers detailed questions about their opinions of Kampo medicine. The questions were about the present opinions about the number of lectures, the education about crude drugs and their extracts, the basics of Kampo medicine, the clinical uses of Kampo medicine, and the side effects, adverse events, and interactions with Western medicines. Questions were also asked about the necessity of standardized textbooks, the necessary education about the future of Kampo medicine, and any other related problems that have to be solved as soon as possible. In addition to the questionnaire, we referred to Web-based syllabi to investigate the detailed lecture curricula in each school. In the question about the items that should be added to Kampo education, a "circle" answer (indicating an item that should be required in future curricula) was calculated as 1 point, and a "triangle" answer (indicating an item that should be an elective) was calculated as 0.5 points.

To prepare the questionnaires for the present study, we mainly used the semantic differential method, which is often applied in psychological research, to assure their validity [11]. Completed questionnaires were returned by postal mail. To increase the response rate, directors of any schools that did not return responses were asked again for their completed questionnaires by postal mail. We conducted descriptive analysis without statistics to show everyone that this survey accurately reflects the present status of Kampo education in the pharmacy schools throughout Japan. All the responders gave written informed consent to participate in this study.

This survey was approved by the Institutional Review Board for Clinical Research of Tokai University School of Medicine and conformed to the principles of the Helsinki Declaration. The survey was also approved by the Medical and Pharmaceutical Society for WAKAN-YAKU, the official Japanese scientific organization dealing with Japanese traditional medicine.

Results
Study population
A total of 74 questionnaires were collected, meaning that responses were obtained from every pharmacy school in Japan (response rate, 100%).

Percentages of graduates becoming clinical pharmacists after graduating from Japanese pharmacy schools
Seventy-three pharmacy schools (99%) answered this question. After graduating from Japanese pharmacy schools, the percentages of graduates becoming clinical pharmacists were as follows. Twenty-five schools (34%) answered more than 90%. In 16 schools (22%) it was from 70 to 90%, 11 schools (15%) was from 50 to 70%, 10 schools (14%) was from 30 to 50%, 6 schools (8%) was from 10 to 30%, and 5 schools (7%) was less than 10% (median, 70–90%) (Table 1).

Table 1 Percentages of graduates becoming clinical pharmacists after graduating from Japanese pharmacy schools

Proportions	Schools
≥90%	25 (34%)
70 to 90%	16 (22%)
50 to 70%	11 (15%)
30 to 50%	10 (14%)
10 to 30%	6 (8%)
< 10%	5 (7%)
Total	73

Present status of Kampo related education in Japanese pharmacy schools
The length of 1 class (lecture or workshop) ranged from 60 to 105 min, with a median of 90 min, for which 71 schools answered (96%). Most schools (60 schools, 85%) offered 90 min per unit. The class lengths per unit offered at other schools were: 60 min (1 school), 70 min (5 schools), 75 min (1 school), 80 min (3 schools), and 105 min (1 school).

The number of clinical Kampo classes, except for pharmacognosy, pharmaceutical botany, natural products chemistry, complementary and alternative medicine other than Kampo medicine (e.g., acupuncture, acupressure, and qigong), and practical training, as required subjects during the 6 years of pharmacy schools ranged from 0 to 36 classes with a mean of 11.8 ± 7.6 classes and a median of 13 classes in 2015. These data were extracted in detail from Web-based syllabi and by referring to the questionnaires collected from 74 schools (Fig. 1). In addition, 51 schools (69%) offered clusters of consecutive Kampo classes (lectures and/or workshops). On the contrary, however, 5 schools (7%) had no clinical Kampo classes as required subjects, which means that pharmacy students in those schools had no opportunities to receive any clinical Kampo education. One of those 5 schools was in a transitional period of developing its curriculum, so that there were no required clinical Kampo medicine classes in 2015.

Regarding the concepts in Kampo related education, 72 schools (97%) were teaching Japanese traditional medicine. While 19 schools (26%) were teaching traditional Chinese medicine (TCM), 25 schools (34%) were teaching Western evidence-based medicine (EBM), 64 schools (86%) were teaching pharmacognosy and/or pharmaceutical botany, and only 1 school was teaching the general history of medicine (multiple responses) (Fig. 2).

Forty-nine schools (66%, of all 74 schools) provided Kampo education from a clinical standpoint. These classes were taught most by pharmacists employed in pharmacies and physicians. Thirty-one schools (63%) selected part-time teachers from among those pharmacists employed in pharmacies and physicians and these teachers taught all the classes (lectures and/or workshops) on Kampo related education in 7 of these schools. Physicians taught Kampo medicine in 24 schools (49%). In addition to these specialists, lectures were given by TCM specialists (in 3 schools, 6%), a medical representative (in 1 school), a teacher other than a pharmacist or a physician (in 2 schools), and educational video lectures (in 2 schools) (multiple responses) (Fig. 3). Finally, some Kampo related classes were offered in "hands-on" practical training (in 10 of 66 schools, 15%).

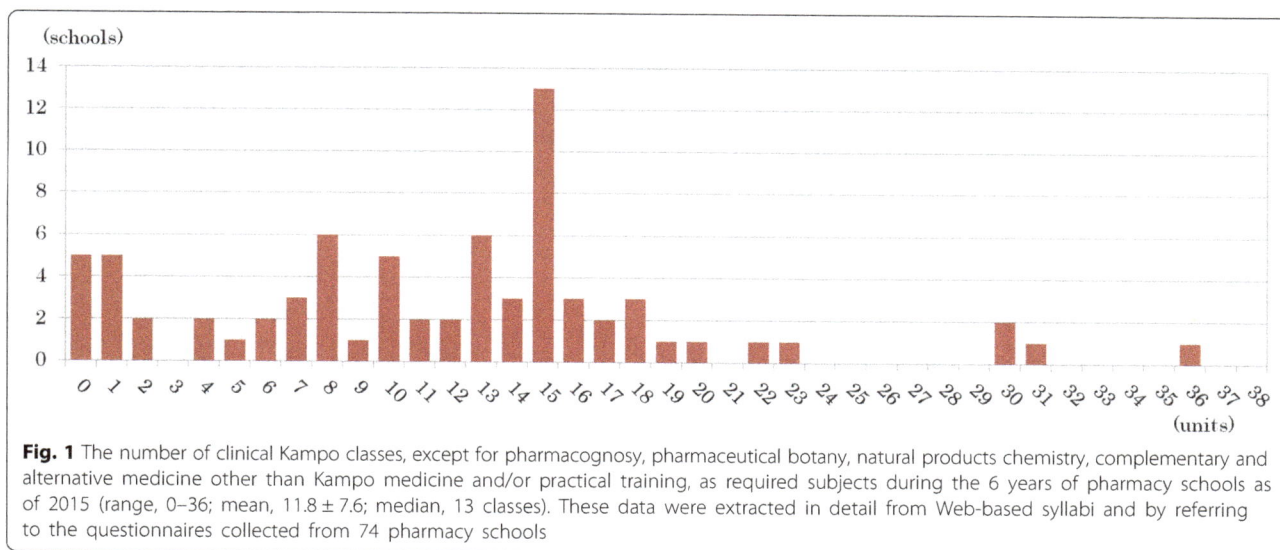

Fig. 1 The number of clinical Kampo classes, except for pharmacognosy, pharmaceutical botany, natural products chemistry, complementary and alternative medicine other than Kampo medicine and/or practical training, as required subjects during the 6 years of pharmacy schools as of 2015 (range, 0–36; mean, 11.8 ± 7.6; median, 13 classes). These data were extracted in detail from Web-based syllabi and by referring to the questionnaires collected from 74 pharmacy schools

Opinions regarding the present Kampo related education

Forty-one of 72 schools (57%) answered that the number of lectures in the curricula was reasonable; however, 29 schools (40%) noted a shortage of lectures (Fig. 4a).

Education about Kampo-related crude drugs and their extracts (Fig. 4b) and about the basics of Kampo medicine (features, technical terms, and core concepts, among others) (Fig. 4c) were reported as being adequate in 46 and 44 schools of 73 and 74 schools (63 and 59%), respectively. The education of clinical applications (diagnostic methods, how to "catch" [i.e., correctly diagnose] the patterns of the "Sho" [the patient's symptoms at a given moment], standardized prescription processes, and the roles of Kampo medicine in contemporary medicine, among others) (Fig. 4d) were reported as being adequate in 32 of 73 schools (44%) but not in 41 schools (56%). Finally, regarding the education of the points to be

emphasized in Kampo medicine (side effects, adverse events, and drug interactions, among others), 53 of 74 schools (72%) answered that they were adequate (Fig. 4e).

Opinions on the future of Kampo related education

About pre-training of Kampo medicine (i.e., at the undergraduate level), 16 of 74 schools (22%) answered that it should be a required subject, and 53 (71%) thought that it ought to remain an elective subject. However, 5 schools (7%) indicated that it was needless.

Fifty-two of 73 schools (71%) answered that nationwide standardized textbooks were necessary, and 21 schools (29%) answered that standardized textbooks were "especially" necessary. No schools indicated that they were, "Unnecessary."

The answers of the items that should be added to Kampo education, except for the items that have already

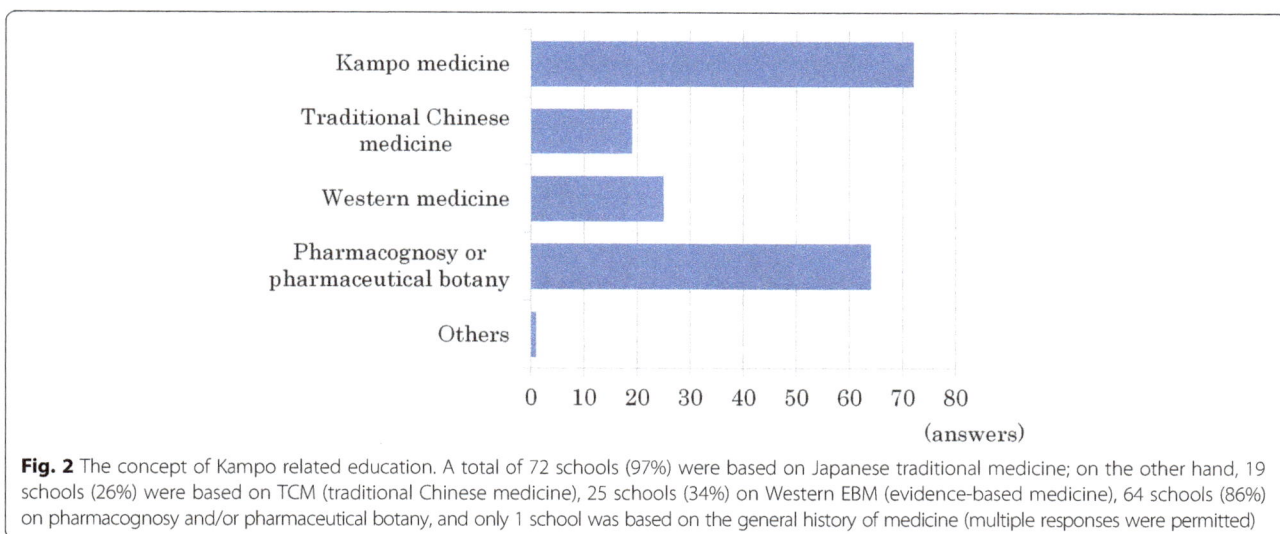

Fig. 2 The concept of Kampo related education. A total of 72 schools (97%) were based on Japanese traditional medicine; on the other hand, 19 schools (26%) were based on TCM (traditional Chinese medicine), 25 schools (34%) on Western EBM (evidence-based medicine), 64 schools (86%) on pharmacognosy and/or pharmaceutical botany, and only 1 school was based on the general history of medicine (multiple responses were permitted)

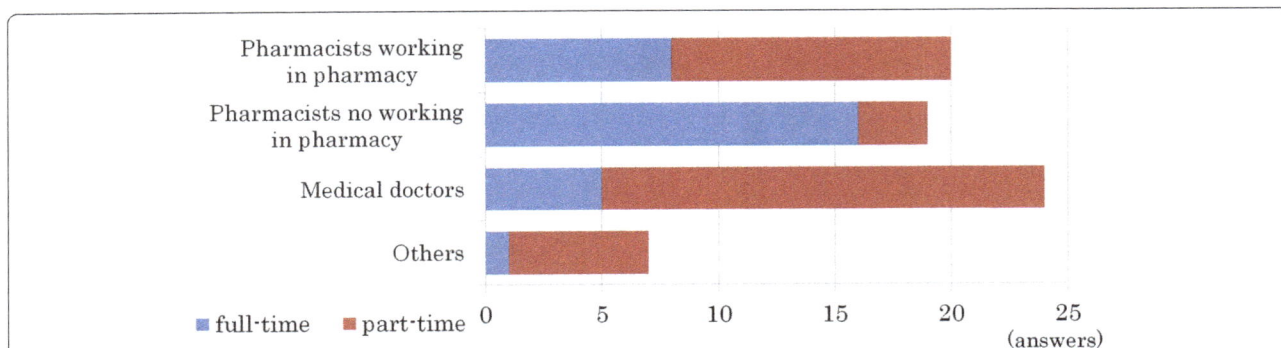

Fig. 3 Teachers' qualifications, of those who taught clinical-based medicine in the pharmacy schools answered by 49 schools (66%). These classes were mostly taught by pharmacists employed in pharmacies and physicians. Thirty-one schools (63%) recruited part-time teachers from among pharmacists employed in pharmacies and physicians. Physicians were recruited in 24 schools (49%)

been listed in the new 2015 core curriculum, are given below (multiple responses, from 74 schools). The most common answer was Case studies (61%), followed by EBM in Kampo medicine (51%), Kampo medicine dispensing training (42%), and Observation of medical treatment (35%). These data suggest that many pharmacy schools are interested in improving their clinical Kampo education. "Others" (5%) consisted of crude drug resources, composition of crude drugs and their extracts in Kampo formulae, traditional medicines around the world, and research methods (1 answer each) (Fig. 5).

The problems with Kampo related education

Selecting and retaining adequate teachers to teach clinical Kampo medicine was the most critical problem (43 of 74 schools, 58%), followed by preparation of standard textbooks (37 schools, 50%) and improvement of the environment for practical training (30 schools, 41%). Among others were, "There was a change in teachers' individual approval of Kampo medicine" (Fig. 6).

Discussion

We reported on the present status of Kampo medicine education in all 74 pharmacy schools in Japan and the related problems that should be solved as soon as possible as revealed by data acquired from a postal questionnaire survey. We found significant differences in the Kampo medicine curricula among the schools, including the number and length of classes (be they lectures and/ or workshops), and the actual contents of the education, among other important issues. Clinical-based Kampo education was largely provided by part-time teachers, who were usually pharmacists employed in pharmacies or physicians. More than half of the schools answered that the education for the clinical use of Kampo medicine was insufficient. As for future outlooks, 93% of the schools answered that pre-training (i.e., at the undergraduate level) in some form of Kampo medicine was

necessary, and more than half wanted to incorporate case studies and EBM into Kampo related medical education as required subjects. Finally, "Selecting and retaining teachers to teach clinical Kampo medicine" and "Preparation of standard textbooks" were selected by more than half of the schools as critical problems.

As we previously pointed out, Kampo therapy has become increasingly popular among Japanese people [3–5]. And moreover, 70 to 90% of Japanese physicians regularly prescribe Kampo medicine in their medical practice. [6–8] Concurrently, more extensive scientific evidence of Kampo formulae has been accumulated [12, 13], and their quality and safety have been maintained at higher levels with the progress of Kampo extract formulae [14] resulting in their more substantial integration into Western medicine [15, 16]. In most cases of patients being prescribed Kampo drugs, patients benefited from Kampo medicine when it was used in combination with Western medicine (when they simultaneously received biomedical drugs) [17].

However, there are some points that should be noted when pharmacists sell Kampo medicines. Firstly, when patients buy OTC Kampo medicines, pharmacists must consult with them to help avoid any side effects, adverse events, and/or interactions with any other medications they may be taking. Secondly, pharmacists have the right and the professional responsibility to ask physicians about any uncertainties on the prescriptions. Therefore, pharmacists working in pharmacies have to have general knowledge about the use and any major drawbacks of Kampo medicine.

However, the present survey showed that standardization of Kampo education in pharmacy schools was a long way off and that a few schools provided no clinical Kampo education at all. Presently, many pharmacists, who want to learn more about Kampo medicine, find Kampo education programs themselves, often after getting their national pharmacist license. Similarly, as reported by Arai, et al. [10],

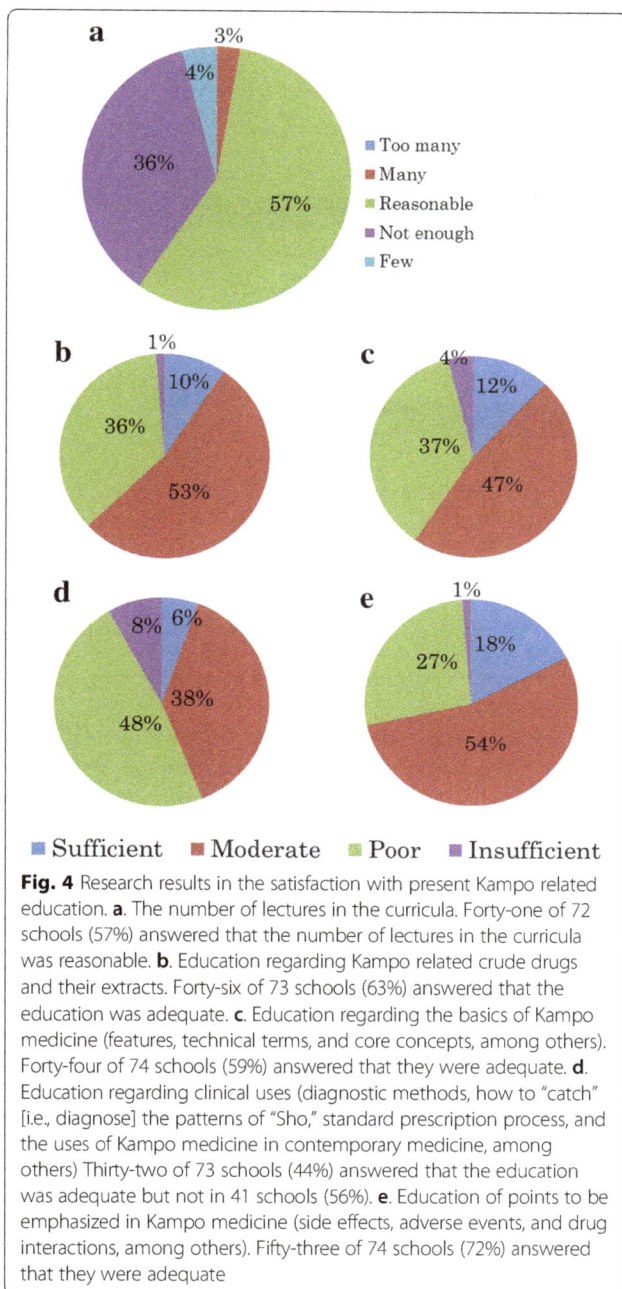

Fig. 4 Research results in the satisfaction with present Kampo related education. **a**. The number of lectures in the curricula. Forty-one of 72 schools (57%) answered that the number of lectures in the curricula was reasonable. **b**. Education regarding Kampo related crude drugs and their extracts. Forty-six of 73 schools (63%) answered that the education was adequate. **c**. Education regarding the basics of Kampo medicine (features, technical terms, and core concepts, among others). Forty-four of 74 schools (59%) answered that they were adequate. **d**. Education regarding clinical uses (diagnostic methods, how to "catch" [i.e., diagnose] the patterns of "Sho," standard prescription process, and the uses of Kampo medicine in contemporary medicine, among others) Thirty-two of 73 schools (44%) answered that the education was adequate but not in 41 schools (56%). **e**. Education of points to be emphasized in Kampo medicine (side effects, adverse events, and drug interactions, among others). Fifty-three of 74 schools (72%) answered that they were adequate

pharmacists. On the other hand, 7% of respondents answered that pre-training of Kampo medicine was needless. It is considered that the yearly schedule in each school is very busy. However, Kampo pre-training will help new pharmacists work proficiently with Kampo medicine.

Selecting and retaining teachers is one of the big issues in Kampo medicine education. This was revealed to be the largest problem to be solved as soon as possible in Japanese medical education [1, 10]. The present survey showed that more than half of the pharmacists working in pharmacies and physicians were hired as part-time teachers to teach clinical Kampo medicine. However, the other schools employ pharmacists who do not work in pharmacies or other specialists to teach their clinical Kampo medicine classes. This problem requires an immediate solution because even new pharmacists, who have just gotten their licenses, sell Kampo medicines in their pharmacies on a daily basis. Minimal essential clinical knowledge of Kampo medicine should be obtained before their employment in a pharmacy. Therefore we suppose that Kampo education from a clinical standpoint, which is provided by pharmacists employed in pharmacies and physicians who know the current situation in clinical medicine, is required. Cooperation among schools, e.g., teachers sharing and faculty development [10], could be a solution to the problem of the lack of teachers in Kampo education from a clinical standpoint. Thereby, many pharmacy schools will be able to begin teaching Kampo education from the clinical side.

In Kampo education in some medical schools, to attract students, certain techniques have been used, e.g., actual interviews with patients [18], students receiving acupuncture [19], and students undergoing medical examinations given by classmates (diagnosing each other using the "qi, blood, and fluid" system) [20, 21]. On the other hand, experience with crude drugs and crude drug extracts is offered in pharmacy schools [22]. If pharmacy students learn to use Kampo medicine during their first year of training in hospitals, they will become increasingly more interested in Kampo medicine [23]. According to a questionnaire survey targeting students in Kyushu University of Health and Welfare [24], it was revealed that pharmacy students realized the importance of Kampo medicine in contemporary medical settings. At the same time, they indicated that the study of Kampo medicine increasingly becomes more difficult as they advanced in their school years. Students in their fourth through sixth years of pharmacy school wanted to study clinical Kampo medicine through case studies and learn about drug interactions between Kampo and Western medicines. They indicated that they wanted to learn how to provide patients with actual, practical Kampo treatments [24, 25].

Kampo education in medical schools throughout Japan has not been standardized; although, that procedure has begun. To ensure that pharmacists and physicians have the same knowledge about Kampo prescriptions, to help patients and avoid patient confusion, standardization is mandatory. Furthermore, examples of clinical use, including case studies and EBM, should adequately be taught, and preparation of standard textbooks should certainly be a common objective among all the schools. Moreover, standardization of Kampo education and standard textbooks among all the pharmacy schools is essential for the Japanese licensing exam for

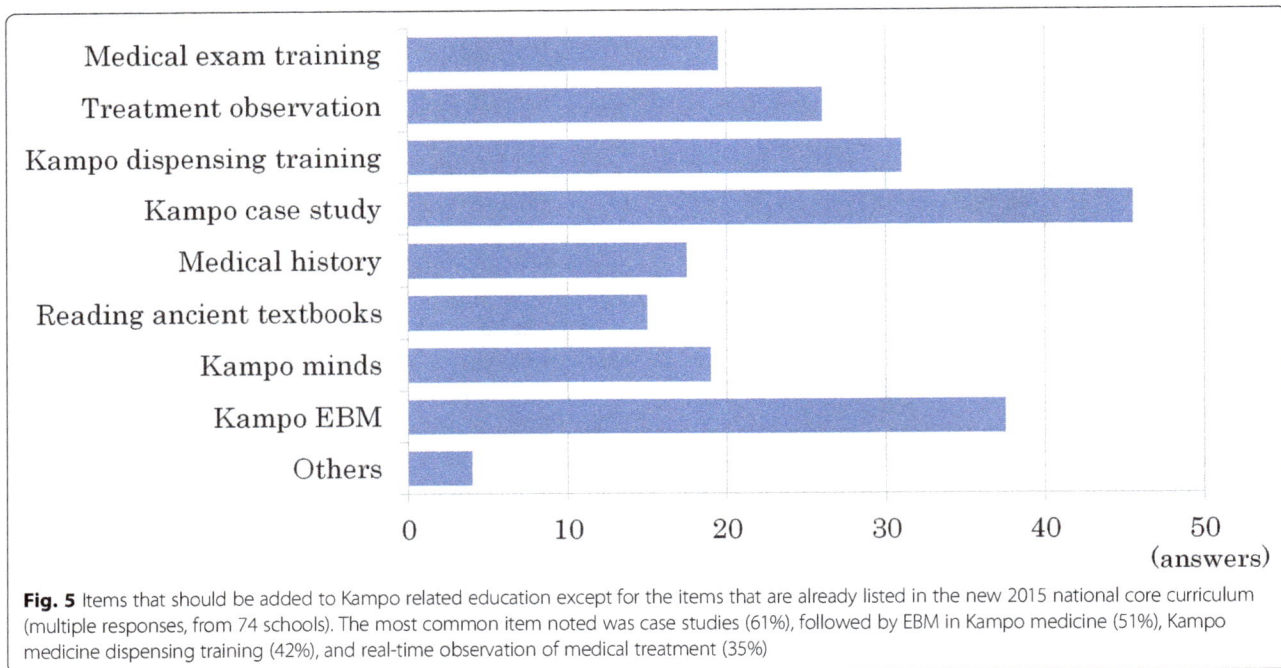

Fig. 5 Items that should be added to Kampo related education except for the items that are already listed in the new 2015 national core curriculum (multiple responses, from 74 schools). The most common item noted was case studies (61%), followed by EBM in Kampo medicine (51%), Kampo medicine dispensing training (42%), and real-time observation of medical treatment (35%)

Finally, according to a fact-finding survey of Japanese undergraduate education in Sino-Japanese traditional medicine for pharmacy students published in 2002, 10 of 46 pharmacy schools (21%) provided no Kampo education at all, and only 3 schools offered Kampo education as a required subject [26]. In comparison, according to the present survey, although there are more than a few problems remaining to be solved (e.g., selecting adequate teachers and preparing standard textbooks), Kampo medicine education in Japanese pharmacy schools is improving exponentially on a nationwide basis. Many graduates from pharmacy schools choose to work in pharmacies, therefore, Kampo clinical knowledge in contemporary medicine is essential not only for patients' safety but also for a positive mindset and motivation of pharmacy students and new

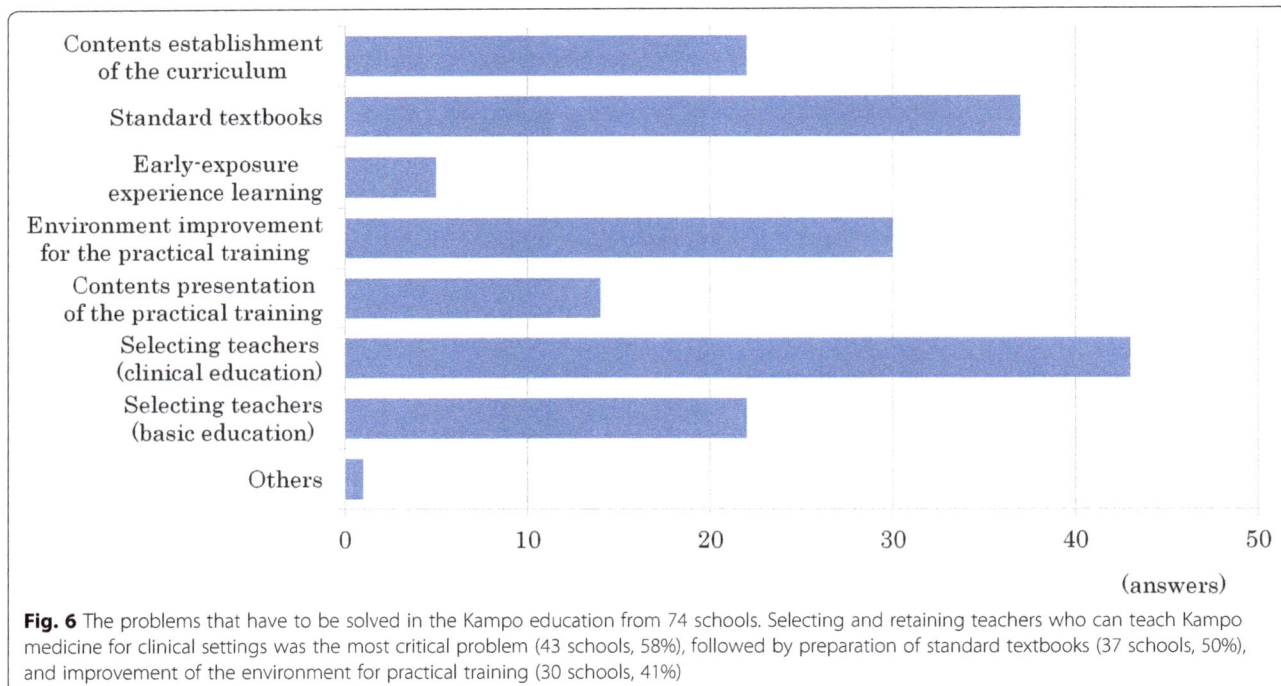

Fig. 6 The problems that have to be solved in the Kampo education from 74 schools. Selecting and retaining teachers who can teach Kampo medicine for clinical settings was the most critical problem (43 schools, 58%), followed by preparation of standard textbooks (37 schools, 50%), and improvement of the environment for practical training (30 schools, 41%)

pharmacists to keep studying and learning about Kampo medicine.

This survey was carried out just after the commencement of the new core curriculum. Therefore, the Kampo educational program at each school may be under revision. Further survey is warranted to elucidate the mature status of Kampo education in pharmacy schools teaching the 2015 core curriculum.

Conclusion

The educational curricula of Kampo medicine significantly differ nationwide among Japanese pharmacy schools. To solve this problem, in addition to selecting and retaining teachers who can adequately teach clinical Kampo medicine, the preparation of standard textbooks and curricula standardization is especially warranted, and among the many other related problems that must be solved immediately, to ensure that the best Kampo education possible is provided in pharmacy schools throughout Japan.

Acknowledgements
We thank Keiko Matsukawa for collecting and analyzing the data. We also thank Robert E. Brandt, Founder, CEO, and CME, of MedEd Japan, Suginami, Tokyo, for helpful advice on the English language in the preparation, editing, and formatting of this manuscript.
A part of these data was presented at a symposium of the 33rd Annual Meeting of the Medical and Pharmaceutical Society for WAKAN-YAKU (2016, Tokyo, Japan).

Funding
We received postage for this study from the Medical and Pharmaceutical Society for WAKAN-YAKU, the official Japanese scientific organization dealing with Japanese traditional medicine.

Authors' contributions
YN wrote the manuscript and MA conceived the study. Both authors participated in the data collection, data analysis, and interpretation of the data, carefully revised the manuscript, and read and approved the final manuscript.

Competing interests
The Department of Kampo Medicine, Tokai University School of Medicine, received a grant from Tsumura, a Japanese manufacturer of Kampo medicine; however, the authors declare that they have no competing interests.

Author details
[1]Department of Kampo Medicine, Tokai University School of Medicine, Isehara, Kanagawa, Japan. [2]Medical and Pharmaceutical Society for WAKAN-YAKU, Kanagawa, Japan.

References
1. Motoo Y, Seki T, Tsutani K. Traditional Japanese medicine, Kampo: its history and current status. Chin J Integr Med. 2011;17:85–7.
2. Yu F, Takahashi T, Moriya J, Kawaura K, Yamakawa J, Kusaka K, et al. Traditional Chinese medicine and kampo: a review from the distant past for the future. J Int Med Res. 2006;34:231–9.
3. Yamashita H, Tsukayama H, Sugishita C. Popularity of complementary and alternative medicine in Japan: a telephone survey. Complement Ther Med. 2002;10:84–93.
4. Hori S, Mihaylov I, Vasconcelos JC, McCoubrie M. Patterns of complementary and alternative medicine use amongst outpatients in Tokyo, Japan. BMC Complement Altern Med. 2008;8:14. https://doi.org/10.1186/1472-6882-8-14.
5. Togo T, Urata S, Sawazaki K, Sakuraba H, Ishida T, Yokoyama K. Demand for CAM practice at hospitals in Japan: a population survey in Mie prefecture. Evid Based Complement Alternat Med. 2011. https://doi.org/10.1093/ecam/neq049.
6. Oka T. The role of Kampo (Japanese traditional herbal) medicine in psychosomatic medicine practice in Japan. Int Congr Ser. 2006;1287:304–8.
7. Terasawa K. Evidence-based reconstruction of Kampo medicine: part-III-how should Kampo be evaluated? Evid Based Complement Alternat Med. 2004;1:219–22. https://doi.org/10.1093/ecam/neh046.
8. Muramatsu S, Aihara M, Shimizu I, Arai M, Kajii E. Current status of Kampo medicine in community health care. Gen Med. 2012;13:37–45.
9. Textbook of Traditional Japanese Medicine. Part 1: Kampo. Health and Labour Sciences Research Grant. http://kampotextbook.sakura.ne.jp/pdf/Part1_Kampo_Textbook_of_Traditional_Japanese_Medicine_en.pdf. Accessed 5 Nov 2018.
10. Arai M, Katai S, Muramatsu S, Namiki T, Hanawa T, Izumi S. Current status of Kampo medicine curricula in all Japanese medical schools. BMC Complement Altern Med. 2012;12:207–13.
11. Osgood CE. Studies on the generality of affective meaning systems. Am Psychol. 1962;17:10–28.
12. Evidence reports of Kampo treatment. 2013. 402 RCT. http://www.jsom.or.jp/medical/ebm/ere/pdf/EKATE2013.pdf. Accessed 5 Nov 2018.
13. Motoo Y, Arai I, Hyodo I, Tsutani K. Current status of Kampo (Japanese herbal) medicines in Japanese clinical practice guidelines. Complement Ther Med. 2009;17:147–54.
14. Nishimura K, Plotnikoff GA, Watanabe K. Kampo medicine as an integrative medicine in Japan. JMAJ. 2009;52:147–9.
15. Fuyuno I. Japan: will the sun set on Kampo? Nature. 2011;480:S96. https://doi.org/10.1038/480S96a.
16. Watanabe K, Matsuura K, Gao P, Hottenbacher L, Tokunaga H, Nishimura K, et al. Traditional Japanese Kampo medicine: clinical research between modernity and traditional medicine-the state of research and methodological suggestions for the future. Evid Based Complement Alternat Med. 2011. https://doi.org/10.1093/ecam/neq067.
17. Katayama K, Yoshino T, Munakata K, Yamaguchi R, Imoto S, Miyano S, et al. Prescription of Kampo drugs in the Japanese health care insurance program. Evid Based Complement Alternat Med. 2013. https://doi.org/10.1155/2013/576973.
18. Takayama S, Ishii S, Takahashi F, Saito N, Arita R, Kaneko S, et al. Questionnaire-based development of an educational program of traditional Japanese Kampo medicine. Tohoku J Exp Med. 2016;240:123–30.
19. Takashi M, Nakada Y, Arai K, Arai M. Educational importance of acupuncture and moxibustion: a survey at the Tokai University School of Medicine Japan. Tokai J Exp Clin Med. 2016;41:76–80.
20. Arai M, Arai K, Hioki C, Takashi M, Matsumoto K, Honda M, et al. Evaluation of medical students using the "qi, blood, and fluid" system of Kampo medicine. Tokai J Exp Clin Med. 2013;38:37–41.
21. Arai M, Arai K, Hioki C, Takashi M, Honda M. Evaluation of Kampo education with a focus on the selected core concepts. Tokai J Exp Clin Med. 2013;38:12–20.
22. Kobayashi Y. Kampo medicine in the new model Core curriculum of pharmaceutical education. Yakugaku Zasshi. 2016;136:423–32 (in Japanese).
23. Matsuda H. Approach to teaching Kampo medicine at Kyoto Pharmaceutical University. Yakugaku Zasshi. 2016;136:405–9 (in Japanese).
24. Atsumi T, Uehara N, Kawasaki R, Ohtsuka I, Kakiuchi N. Attitudes of pharmacy students at Kyushu University of health and welfare toward Kampo medicine from a questionnaire survey conducted in 2012. Kampo Med. 2015;66:155–64 (in Japanese).
25. Kim S, Matsumoto T, Kiyohara H, Hayasaki T, Muranishi A, Hanawa T, et al. Evaluation of Kampo medical education by pharmaceutical students. J Trad Med. 2004;21:241–9 (in Japanese).
26. Shoji N. A fact-finding survey of Japanese undergraduate education in Sino-Japanese traditional medicine for pharmacy students. J Trad Med. 2002;19:1–6 (in Japanese).

24

'Trying to put a square peg into a round hole': a qualitative study of healthcare professionals' views of integrating complementary medicine into primary care for musculoskeletal and mental health comorbidity

Deborah Sharp[1], Ava Lorenc[1][*] [iD], Gene Feder[1], Paul Little[2], Sandra Hollinghurst[1], Stewart Mercer[3] and Hugh MacPherson[4]

Abstract

Background: Comorbidity of musculoskeletal (MSK) and mental health (MH) problems is common but challenging to treat using conventional approaches. Integration of conventional with complementary approaches (CAM) might help address this challenge. Integration can aim to transform biomedicine into a new health paradigm or to selectively incorporate CAM in addition to conventional care. This study explored professionals' experiences and views of CAM for comorbid patients and the potential for integration into UK primary care.

Methods: We ran focus groups with GPs and CAM practitioners at three sites across England and focus groups and interviews with healthcare commissioners. Topics included experience of co-morbid MSK-MH and CAM/integration, evidence, knowledge and barriers to integration. Sampling was purposive. A framework analysis used frequency, specificity, intensity of data, and disconfirming evidence.

Results: We recruited 36 CAM practitioners (4 focus groups), 20 GPs (3 focus groups) and 8 commissioners (1 focus group, 5 interviews).

GPs described challenges treating MSK-MH comorbidity and agreed CAM might have a role. Exercise- or self-care-based CAMs were most acceptable to GPs. CAM practitioners were generally pro-integration.

A prominent theme was different understandings of health between CAM and general practitioners, which was likely to impede integration. Another concern was that integration might fundamentally change the care provided by both professional groups. For CAM practitioners, NHS structural barriers were a major issue. For GPs, their lack of CAM knowledge and the pressures on general practice were barriers to integration, and some felt integrating CAM was beyond their capabilities. Facilitators of integration were evidence of effectiveness and cost effectiveness (particularly for CAM practitioners). Governance was the least important barrier for all groups.

There was little consensus on the ideal integration model, particularly in terms of financing. Commissioners suggested CAM could be part of social prescribing.

(Continued on next page)

* Correspondence: ava.lorenc@bristol.ac.uk
[1]Centre for Academic Primary Care, School of Social and Community Medicine, University of Bristol, Canynge Hall, 39 Whatley Road, Bristol BS8 2PS, UK
Full list of author information is available at the end of the article

(Continued from previous page)

Conclusions: CAM has the potential to help the NHS in treating the burden of MSK-MH comorbidity. Given the challenges of integration, selective incorporation using traditional referral from primary care to CAM may be the most feasible model. However, cost implications would need to be addressed, possibly through models such as social prescribing or an extension of integrated personal commissioning.

Keywords: Primary care, Complementary medicine, Integrated medicine, Qualitative, NHS, Musculoskeletal, Mental health, Comorbidity

Background

Mental health (MH) and musculoskeletal (MSK) conditions create a huge burden for patients, society and healthcare services. Globally, low back pain is the leading cause of disability [1], and in the UK MSKs account for 30% of GP consultations [2] and 30.8 million working days lost annually [3]. Mental ill health is the single largest cause of disability in the UK [4], uses more than 11% of the NHS (National Health Service) budget [5] and costs the UK economy £70–£100 billion/year [4]. Comorbidity of MH and MSK conditions is common - MH problems (anxiety or depression) are 4 times more common in those with persistent pain than in those without [6, 7] and MSK and MH conditions co-occur in 3% of working age (16–64 years) people in England [8]. People with low back pain are significantly more likely to have depression, anxiety and sleep disorders, and to be prescribed medication for these conditions, than those without [9]. Comorbidity is particularly concerning to GPs [10] and poorly addressed by current guidelines, evidence and practice [11], representing an 'effectiveness gap' (where available treatments are sub-optimally effective), which complementary and alternative medicine (CAM) may be able to fill [11–13]. CAM is commonly used by those with comorbid MH and MSK conditions [14, 15].

Although most commonly accessed privately in the UK, CAM can be integrated with conventional (NHS) care. Wiese and colleagues [16] describe three models of integration: 1) pluralism, a patient-based model, where the patient chooses which approach to use, in a 'supermarket' approach [17]; 2) selective incorporation, or integrated medicine, the co-optation of CAM by biomedicine, with CAM as an add-on, provided by trained conventional practitioners or CAM practitioners (on-site or off-site and funded by the NHS/patient/charity; and 3) integrative medicine or transformative integration, which aims to merge biomedicine into a new health paradigm incorporating a holistic approach and providing optimum treatment from any tradition [17–19]. This paper focusses on the second model. Compared to the consumerist approach of the first model, integrated and integrative medicine can promote continuity of care, address safety concerns, and reduce professional power

struggles [20]. The third model, transformative integration, may still be a utopian ideal [19], whereas selective incorporation is preferred by biomedical staff [16]. In primary care, selectively incorporated CAM is more commonly delivered by CAM practitioners than conventional practitioners [21, 22]. Selective incorporation, where patients are referred from conventional healthcare to an off-site CAM practitioner, is similar to social prescribing, a system enabling primary care clinicians to refer patients to a broad range of community services, for example an exercise class or gardening club [23].

Many of the defining values of CAM are now considered part of mainstream care. These include patient-centred care and a holistic approach [24, 25], and emphasis on self-management and prevention, which are prominent goals in current UK health service policy planning [26, 27]. Person- and community-centred approaches to health and wellbeing have a key role in these plans, which can include CAM [28]. Primary care may be the area of the NHS where CAM would fit most comfortably, due to both primary care and CAM having a holistic outlook, emphasis on self-care and strong therapeutic relationships.

Primary healthcare professionals, including GPs, tend to be most positive about CAM for chronic self-limiting conditions or those with limited treatment options e.g. musculoskeletal [29] or chronic pain [29–31]. Other 'effectiveness gaps' include depression, anxiety and stress [13].There is very little research on CAM for comorbid MSK-MH. The sparse qualitative research with GPs and CAM practitioners about integration of CAM into publicly funded health care is rarely health condition-specific, and rarely addresses commissioning issues. Doctors' views on CAM in general vary widely, from enthusiastic to sceptical, with sceptical or uncertain the dominant view [32], although one survey found that only 6% of primary care professionals were against integration of CAM [29]. Attitudes vary depending on the specific CAM approach – a survey of general practitioners (GPs) found that nearly 60% support acupuncture provision on the NHS [33]. Healthcare practitioners' views on CAM are mainly based on professional rather than personal factors [34], in particular the limited evidence base [30, 32], although referral is often determined by patient preference [29, 35].

However, there are challenges to transformative integration and selective incorporation. Based on previous studies of generic integrative services, mainly from the point of view of conventional and CAM clinicians, these can include: preserving the epistemological stance of CAM, as conventional medicine tends to dominate [12, 19, 20]; differing 'corporate cultures' [36, 37]; professional conflicts; conventional practitioners' lack of knowledge regarding CAM [38]; a lack of communication and collaboration between the two groups [37]; a limited evidence base for many CAM; and lack of time in NHS settings [31, 39]. Integration can also give rise to issues around regulation of quality and safety, and duty of care. This particularly applies to a referral model, given UK General Medical Council advice that GPs delegating care must be satisfied with the safety and quality of care, and the practitioner's knowledge, skills and experience [40].

Integrated medicine may help to address comorbid MSK and MH conditions, but there is a lack of research specific to this clinical area. This study therefore sought to explore healthcare professionals' views and experiences to identify the feasibility of integrating CAM for comorbid MH and MSK into UK National Health Service (NHS) primary care.

Methods

We have followed COREQ guidelines in reporting this study [41].

This study explored the views and experiences of GPs, CAM practitioners and healthcare commissioners. This included their views of CAM and any experiences of CAM provision in an integrated fashion in NHS primary care settings; and their views on the potential for and challenges of integrating CAM into primary care, particularly for comorbid MSK and MH conditions.

For GPs and CAM practitioners, focus groups were conducted at three sites across England (A, B, C). A is a fairly large city in the south of England. B and C are moderately sized cities, B in the North and C in the South of England. For commissioners, a combination of focus groups and telephone interviews were conducted, as participants were located throughout England.

CAM practitioners were recruited through a variety of routes including the Complementary and Natural Healthcare Council (CNHC) mailing list and Facebook group, professional organisation online registers (CNHC, British Acupuncture Council, General Osteopathic Council, British Chiropractic Association, UK Tai chi union), Google searches, NHS hospital pain clinics using CAM, and NHS physiotherapy services. GPs were recruited by local CLRNs (Clinical Local Research Networks). Commissioners were recruited via an NHS management fellow at Bristol University, the project steering group, and

commissioners of integrated medicine services in the UK. All potential participants were contacted by email, with telephone follow-up.

Sampling was purposive. For CAM practitioners, the criteria were type of CAM and NHS experience/training. For GPs they were practice location (urban/rural), practice socioeconomic characteristics, gender, ethnic background, attitudes to and experiences of CAM (as self-reported by potential participants in an email). We aimed to include commissioners with experience of commissioning CAM, particularly for MSK and MH, as well as in a variety of geographical locations. We did not collect data on reasons for non-response.

GP/CAM focus groups lasted 90 min and were held on university premises. Two researchers attended each focus group, one (AL) to lead the group and ask the questions, the other noting who spoke and non-verbal communication. AL is a senior research associate with experience of conducting interviews and focus groups, including a PhD using qualitative methods. Participants were offered payment for their time, for themselves or their employer. They were aware that the researcher was pro-CAM. The researcher aimed to maintain an objective stance regarding CAM during the interviews. Participants were assigned codes to ensure confidentiality. Topic guides were developed for the study (see Additional file 1). For CAM practitioners, questions focussed on experience in the NHS, experience treating patients with MSK and MH comorbidity, the evidence base for their therapy, relationships with GPs and barriers to integrating CAM into NHS primary care. GPs were asked about their experience of treating patients with comorbid MSK and MH, their knowledge and experience of CAM (in particular, referring their patients to CAM practitioners), and barriers to integrating CAM into NHS primary care.

Commissioners' focus groups and interviews lasted between 15 and 60 min and were conducted by one researcher (AL). Interviews were either face–to-face, via telephone or video link. The choice between interview or focus group was based on participant preference and availability. Commissioners were offered payment for their time. The topic guide was developed for the study (see Additional file 1) and included questions about definitions and beliefs regarding CAM, experience of commissioning CAM, factors in commissioning decisions, experience of MSK and MH services, barriers to integration of CAM, and thoughts about what evidence might persuade them to commission a CAM service.

Digital audio recordings were transcribed verbatim by a professional company, with non-verbal communication added from our notes. Based on content analysis, a framework was used for all data analysis [42, 43]. Framework analysis is highly structured and systematic, providing a clear map of how analysis and interpretation were performed [42]. It facilitates constant reference back to the original data, to remain grounded [42], but is also structured around pre-set aims and objectives, allowing the answering of specific research questions in the participants' language, in concordance with the abductive stance taken [44]. It consists of five key stages: familiarisation, identifying a framework, indexing, charting and mapping/interpreting [43]. The first four are mainly data management strategies, to order, sort, synthesise and condense the raw data, the bulk of interpretation takes place in the final mapping stage [43]. Data analysis was facilitated using Microsoft Excel and NVivo (computer assisted qualitative data analysis software developed to facilitate systematic and clear analysis) [45]. Familiarisation came through reading the transcripts. A framework of codes was developed from the data, with some a priori themes from the topic guides. Indexing involved comprehensively labelling all the data using the final framework, marking quotations (sentences, paragraphs) which belonged to a code. Charting was performed using the Framework function in NVivo, which uses a matrix, where each row was a participant and each column a code. A summary of the data was entered into each cell in the framework, using quotations as much as possible, with some synthesis and abstraction to make meaning clear [46] but using participant's words and terms, to stay grounded in the data [42]. The final stage of mapping and interpreting was done in Microsoft Excel. Each column was interrogated for themes. At all stages the 'strength' of data was considered, which was based on the following criteria:

- Frequency (number of people) and extensiveness (length) of comments, not as absolute data but to provide an indication of importance [42].
- Specificity: quotes relating to a personal experience were considered more important than hypothetical references [47].
- Intensity or depth of feeling, for example, are the words positive, negative, middling [48]. Internal consistency (changes in individual's views) was also considered [48].
- Disconfirming evidence [49] and negative/deviant cases [50] either proposed alternative explanations, reinforced normative theories by providing unusual examples, explained individual variation from the norm, or refined theories

The study was approved by the University of Bristol Faculty of Medicine and Dentistry Research Ethics Committee (FREC) on 3rd July 2015, reference 21,603. Assurance was provided by the relevant NHS organisations for each of the sites.

Results

Of the 55 CAM practitioners invited, 36 took part in 4 focus groups (65% response rate), two in Site A, one in Site B and one in Site C. Table 1 provides their details. Five practiced tai chi, four acupuncture, and three practiced each of yoga, mindfulness, hypnotherapy, osteopathy, massage. Two practiced nutritional therapy and two chiropractic, one practised homeopathy and one herbal medicine. Participants worked in a variety of settings: most were private but fourteen were located in the NHS, including GP practices, psychological therapy and pain clinics. Seven were NHS professionals (GP, consultant, nurse, occupational therapist, physiotherapist). Eleven were statutorily regulated (NHS professionals, osteopaths or chiropractors) and 21 voluntarily regulated (voluntarily registered with a regulatory body).

Fifty-five GPs expressed an interest in participating, seven of whom subsequently declined and 28 could not attend due to timing. The final sample was predominantly based on GPs' availability, although purposive sampling criteria were met. Twenty GPs (see Table 2) participated, in three focus groups, ten in Site A, six in Site B and four in Site C. Most stated their views as neutral or in favour of CAM, three were 'sceptical'. Four practised CAM.

Of 30 commissioners invited, eight took part, most of whom were also GPs (Table 3). Six worked in CCGs (clinical commissioning group – NHS bodies responsible for commissioning local services), one in an integrated personal commissioning (a scheme using personal health budgets for patients/carers) demonstration site and one for the voluntary sector. One focus group was conducted with three participants; the others' views were obtained through telephone interviews.

The key themes arising from the data were: what is CAM; the role of CAM; feasibility of integrated medicine in the NHS; barriers to integration; GP education; regulation; and models of integration.

What is CAM?

CAM was a difficult term for many GPs as it covers a wide range of interventions. Three GPs mentioned the 'huge' range of CAM and grouping this diverse range of treatments as 'CAM', was seen as 'unhelpful'.

> "I really, really struggle with this umbrella term of complementary and alternative medicine, because I see a huge spectrum" (GP A9)

Two described a spectrum of CAM based on effectiveness and safety, with chiropractic and osteopathy at one end and "mumbo jumbo", e.g. homeopathy and reiki at the other. Some therapies – Pilates, yoga, tai chi, mindfulness and acupuncture – were not necessarily

Table 1 Participants in CAM practitioner focus groups

Code[a]	CAM	Clinical setting	Statutorily regulated?	Voluntarily regulated?	NHS professional?	Practices in NHS?	Is your practice integrated into NHS?
A1.1	Mindfulness	Improving access to psychological therapies (IAPT), occupational therapy, pain clinic	YES	YES	YES	YES	YES
A1.2	Yoga	Private	NO	YES	NO	NO	NO
A1.3	Holistic massage, reiki	Private	NO	NO	NO	NO	NO
A1.4	Mindfulness	IAPT	NO	YES	NO	YES	YES
A1.5	Osteopathy	Private, in GP practice	YES	NO	NO	YES	NO
A1.6	Osteopathy	Private, in GP practice	YES	NO	NO	YES	NO
A1.7	Manipulation, Bach flowers, homeopathy, acupressure	General practice	YES	YES	YES	YES	YES
A1.8	Pilates, yoga	Private	Missing data				
A1.9	Massage, yoga (individual)	Private	NO	YES	NO	NO	NO
A2.1	Tai chi, qigong	Private; chronic patients	NO	NO	NO	NO	NO
A2.10	Homeopathy, Director of integrative medicine centre	Community interest company; NHS	NO	YES	YES	YES	YES
A2.2	Physiotherapy, adapted tai chi, Pilates	NHS rheumatology	YES	NO	YES	YES	YES
A2.3	Hypnotherapy	Private clinic with a physiotherapist	NO	YES	NO	NO	NO
A2.4	Massage, reiki	Private osteopathy clinic attached to a GP surgery	NO	YES	NO	YES	Yes
A2.5	Acupuncture	Low cost clinic	NO	YES	NO	NO	NO
A2.6	Acupuncture, meditation	Cancer centre, multi-bed clinic, community interest company	NO	YES	NO	NO	YES
A2.7	Tai chi	Private	NO	NO	NO	NO	NO
A2.8	Pain management	NHS pain clinic	YES	NO	YES	YES	YES
A2.9	Alexander technique, medical acupuncture	Nurse, NHS pain clinic	YES	YES	YES	YES	YES
B1	Tai chi	Private; collaboration with NHS	YES	YES	NO	YES (PREVIOUS)	SOMETIMES
B2	Mindfulness	Charitable; previously local educational authority	YES	NO	NO	NO	NO
B3	Mindfulness	Former GP; private	NO	YES	NO (retired GP)	NO	NO
B4	Microsystems Acupuncture	Private; charitable	NO	YES	NO	YES	NO
B5	Medical herbalist, nutritional therapist	Private	NO	YES	NO	NO	NO
B6	Tai chi	Primary and secondary care and community mental health	NO	NO	NO	NO	YES
B7	Yoga therapy	Private	NO	YES	NO	NO	NO
B8	Craniosacral, acupuncture, Kampo herbs	Private	NO	YES	NO	NO	NO
C1	Chiropractic	Private	YES	NO	NO	NO	NO
C2	Tai Chi and qigong	Private	NO	YES	NO	NO	NO
C3	Hypnotherapy	Private	Missing data				
C4	Chiropractic	Private	YES	NO	NO	NO	NO
C5	Yoga	Hospital; private	NO	YES	NO	NO	NO
C6	Physio	NHS Hospital	YES	N/A	YES	YES	YES

Table 1 Participants in CAM practitioner focus groups *(Continued)*

Code[a]	CAM	Clinical setting	Statutorily regulated?	Voluntarily regulated?	NHS professional?	Practices in NHS?	Is your practice integrated into NHS?
C7	Acupuncture, Chinese herbal medicine	Private	NO	YES	NO	NO	NO
C8	Hypnotherapy	Private; volunteer	NO	YES	NO	YES	NO
C9	Osteopathy, Heart Math, Alexander technique	Homeless health care; private	Missing data			YES	Missing data

[a]As two focus groups were conducted at Site A these are coded A1 and A2

considered to be complementary, and exercise-based CAM – Pilates, tai chi, yoga – seemed to be more acceptable to GPs. Some were also more positive about CAM which 'foster' self-management.

> "...nothing weird or wonderful there at all [acupuncture, tai chi, yoga], those are all things that are part of our everyday...I wouldn't even particularly class any of those as complementary medicines" (GP A6)

> "Self-care is so important. Teach someone to look after their sleep and not be so concerned about it, or to increase their core stability by using something for themselves, is much better than perhaps referring them to the homoeopathist and

Table 2 Participants in GP focus groups

Code	Attitude to CAM[a]	CAM practitioner?	Deprivation in practice area (as reported by the GP)	Ethnicity	Practice location
A1	Neutral	No	Average	White	Semi-rural
A2	In favour	No	Deprived	Mixed race (Asian/ Caucasian)	Urban
A3	Neutral but open	Yes, anthroposophic medicine	Mixed	Non-White	Urban
A4	In favour	Yes, acupuncture (British Medical Acupuncture Society, BMAS)	Deprived	White	Urban
A5	In favour	Previously (acupuncture, homeopathy)	Average	White	Semi-rural/ suburban
A6	Opposed to NHS funded CAM	No	Fairly deprived	White	Urban
A7	Mixed (depends on therapy)	Yes, acupuncture (BMAS)	Not deprived	White	Urban
A8	In favour	No	Not deprived	White	Semi urban
A9	Mixed (depends on therapy, payment etc)	No	Some deprivation	White	Urban
A10	In favour	No	Students	White	Urban
B1	Previously sceptical, becoming more open	No (acupuncture provided at surgery)	Deprived	White	Rural
B2	Neutral	No	Data missing	White	Locum
B3	Sceptical	No	Locum	White	Variety
B4	Open-minded but depends on the evidence	No (acupuncture provided at surgery)	Lower deprivation	Non-White	Suburban
B5	Data missing	No	Mixed	White	Data missing
B6	Data missing	Yes, acupuncture	Data missing	Data missing	Data missing
C1	Neutral	No	Affluent	White	Rural/urban
C2	In favour (if evidence-based)	No	Pockets of deprivation	White	Semi-rural
C4	Sceptical/neutral	No	Deprived	White	Urban
C5	Sceptical (but open to persuasion)	No	Mixed	White	Urban

[a]This is the respondent's response to asking in an email "We are hoping that the focus groups comprise people with a diversity of opinion - would you say in general you are in favour of CAM, opposed to CAM or simply neutral?"

Table 3 Participants in commissioner focus groups/interviews

Code	Commissioning body/employer	Clinician?	Location in UK	Focus group or interview
1	CCG[a]	Former GP	South West	Focus group
2	CCG	GP	London	Telephone interview
3	CCG (pharmacy services)	GP	South West	Focus group
4	Integrated personal commissioning	No	South West	Telephone interview
5	CCG	GP	North	Telephone interview
6	CCG	GP	London	Focus group
7	CCG (self-care lead)	GP	South West	Telephone interview
8	Voluntary sector - social prescribing	No	North	Telephone interview

[a]Clinical commissioning group

they lay out their store of symptoms again" (GP B5)

The most common criteria used to define CAM were its 'philosophical approach' and its lack of an evidence base. Six GPs talked about CAM as being treatments with a philosophy they perhaps did not accept or understand. For four GPs, the lack of evidence defined CAM, although another felt this did not distinguish it from conventional care. For commissioners, CAM was defined as treatment outside the mainstream.

"I suppose it's [CAM] almost defined by what is in conventional, it's the other things that are not considered conventional" (commissioner 7)

"I would say that anything that doesn't have a solid evidence base would come under the principles of complementary medicine" (GP A6)

GPs discussed two particular areas of overlap between CAM and conventional medicine: exercise (e.g. tai chi) and social support (e.g. personal health budgets). For commissioners, CAM overlapped considerably with broader approaches such as social prescribing and holistic care.

A role for CAM in primary care and MSK-MH comorbidity
All three groups felt that CAM had a role in the provision of primary care services, although GPs were the least enthusiastic and saw CAM's role as limited. CAM practitioners were generally pro-integration.
Unsurprisingly, CAM practitioners were very positive about CAM, citing evidence for its effectiveness, and believed it to be commonly used and demanded by patients. The commissioners were generally positive about CAM, although this may reflect potential selection bias towards pro-CAM commissioners.

"I am very pro a more holistic approach" (commissioner 2)

GPs and CAM practitioners both saw MSK-MH comorbidity commonly in their practice. For GPs, common examples were fibromyalgia, "frequent attenders"/"heart sink patients", overweight, back/chronic pain with anxiety/MH issues, and osteoarthritis. Many CAM practitioners gave examples of comorbidity and how CAM (in their opinion) could help treat it.

"I think most of the patients in general practice have more than one thing going on, so most patients with, you know, anxiety or depression have something else going on. Not all, but most, most I would say. Particularly perhaps when they get into their sort of 30s or 40s or whatever" (GP B2)

"there's definitely an inter-connectedness, particularly with back pain and erm, mental health issues" (GP A9)

"I was just thinking I would love to see someone with just one problem. I was trying to think when was the last time? - I actually can't remember" (CAM C6)

GPs and CAM practitioners both identified challenges in treating comorbidity, mainly NHS service issues, for example waiting lists for physiotherapy or pain clinics. CAM practitioners felt conventional treatment was often of limited benefit. Commissioners also recognised these challenges (although comorbidity per se did not tend to influence their decisions).

"I just feel that the services that we have to use on these people, such as the pain clinic and MATS [Musculoskeletal Assessment Triage Service] are often not meeting their needs" (GP A10)

"[Patients say] "Oh, well the GP just dishes out painkillers", and it doesn't solve the roots of their issue, their problem. So they'll come to me. They say "I want a more holistic approach""(CAM A2.2)

There was some agreement across all three groups that CAM had a role in treating MSK-MH comorbidity, given the limited conventional treatment options or availability. Some GPs felt that something extra, possibly CAM, was needed to offer these patients. CAM practitioners explained that CAM can treat comorbidity using a holistic approach.

"those chronic pain patients who, we all know who they are in our practice, we all dread them popping up on our list, and we need something else to work with them, because more and more evidence says that actually up titrating opiates, has lots of implications, it isn't good for our prescribing, it has lots of side effects for them. So we need something else to reach for, instead of our prescription pads, for these group of patients [chronic pain]. And I think that's sort of the other side of it, that almost makes it a little bit exciting in the sense that it's [integrative medicine] a new area that we could maybe tap into and get some real benefits" (GP B1)

Is integrated medicine feasible in NHS primary care?

A number of GPs highlighted concerns that integrating CAM into NHS primary care would present challenges and might not be feasible. Although many of these concerns were only raised by a few GPs, the repeated emergence of the message across several themes justifies its inclusion as a key issue.

First, CAM was seen by a small number of GPs to be addressing much broader problems than those which primary care should be treating, described by two GPs as 'first world problems' – issues around wellbeing, preventative care, dis-ease. Similarly, some GPs saw CAM as a form of self-care overlapping with social support and exercise. This view of CAM contrasted with the GP's primary role in treating disease.

"the extended, sort of, integration of integrated medicine is that there will be all of these services potentially who we could then refer into. And you're creating the burden of dis-ease rather than disease, and then you're increasing our burden" (GP A6)

Second, a small number of GPs, contemplating integrated medicine becoming part of their practice, thought it would involve fundamental changes to the GP consultation and communication i.e. becoming more patient-centred and 'meaningful'. This was challenging, given the limitations and pressures of UK primary care (bureaucracy, overwork, time constraints).

"There's lots of competing priorities though in terms of GP time, so where do you put complementary medicine as a priority?" (GP B4)

Barriers to integration – The brick wall between CAM and NHS care

A central message, occurring across several themes (mostly from CAM practitioners), was the idea that CAM and conventional medicine have significant conceptual differences which are barriers to integration. The language used strengthens these data. CAM practitioners regarded CAM as holistic, promoting self-care and behavioural change, while conventional care was described as reductionist, paternalistic and passive. They perceived the conceptual differences between the "two worlds" of "mainstream medicine" and CAM as a barrier to integration.

"[CAM is] a completely different concept of really how the world is" (CAM A1.9)

"the Western approach is very much more reductionist, ooking for diagnosis. Whereas I think there's a completely different approach from complementary therapies which is looking at a holistic and outward perspective. So there's quite a lot of adjustments to be made which I think an NHS approach can't cater for" (CAM C9)

Many CAM practitioners were concerned that attempts to overcome these differences would 'secularise', reduce and standardise CAM, and reduce the techniques practitioners could use, diminishing its value and holistic nature and reducing benefits. A few GPs concurred with this view, demonstrated by their concerns about feasibility of true integration in primary care.

"If you secularised qigong totally, if you strip it from all its, in a sense its spiritual value...if you take away the underlying principles in a sense, if you take away the theory and the philosophy... you leave it with a shell...just a form of exercise, a callisthenic, a dynamic movement exercise, a meditation without meditation" (CAM A2.1)

"there seems to be a sort of slight debate going on as to whether you could really, sort of, provide the range of services an osteopath would do privately within the NHS setting... a bit like trying to put a square peg into a round hole and whether or not you lose what, you know, what we think osteopathy is good for, or the good points" (CAM A1.6)

"I think the danger about being integrated into the Health Service if, if, if it stays as it is, is we'll just be very limited as to what we can do" (CAM C4)

CAM practitioners saw CAM being used in the NHS more out of desperation - when conventional care fails or cannot offer anything more - than for its ability to prevent ill-health and promote wellness. They thought true and worthwhile integrative medicine would require a major change to conventional medical thinking, a view which some GPs also expressed. The only constructive suggestion for overcoming the gap between the 'two worlds' was through the planned changes in the NHS 'Five Year Forward View (a policy document describing a new shared vision for the future of the NHS and new models of care which aimed to reduce health disparities and improve care).

For CAM practitioners, structural barriers such as NHS guidelines and bureaucracy were very challenging. Their emotional language emphasised the importance of this theme. Commissioners agreed that guidelines were very influential in their decisions. For GPs, key structural barriers were lack of time and competing priorities in GP consultations.

"...the therapists round here all have something to give, but at the moment we all just seem to be bashing our heads to a large extent against a large brick wall and hopefully this [project] is a chink in the wall" (CAM C8)

"[We] don't have time during a GP consultation to give advice on CAM, you tend to move on to things which are more relevant to you as a GP, which you feel more confident about and which you have more knowledge about or can do something about" (GP B2)

Evidence of effectiveness appeared more important to CAM practitioners than GPs or commissioners. For CAM practitioners, evidence was the most important facilitator of integration and generating and implementing evidence was the biggest barrier.

"...that's one of the things that's incredibly difficult to get anything in to the NHS, it relies on evidence base. And, you know, whether it's complementary or an orthodox approach, it's got to have evidence base" (CAM C6)

For commissioners, the main factor influencing their commissioning decisions was evidence of cost-saving or affordability, and the current cold financial climate posed the biggest challenge to commissioning. Restrictive funding models were also seen as challenging, especially in

general practice. CAM practitioners also recognised the importance of evidence of cost-saving which was 'the only way' to obtain NHS funding for CAM.

"...even drugs that come into us with really good evidence, um, we're having to say, "where can you find the money to pay for this new treatment"" (commissioner 3)

"...everything has to be either cost neutral or saving money. That's the kind of mantra, so it's quite a difficult climate to suggest new services" (commissioner 7)

GP knowledge

For GPs, a clear theme was the need to improve their knowledge and education about CAM, which commissioners and CAM practitioners agreed with. Lack of dialogue between the two professions was a related issue. The importance of GPs' lack of knowledge and understanding of CAM reflects concerns that integration would extend the role of the GP beyond their current abilities or comfort zone.

"I would say my big barrier is my current understanding. I think it comes back to at the end of the day of my actual knowledge of what's available and what's proven erm, and locally what's sort of available" (GP B1)

"...there's a lack of education, formal education about complementary medicine at all, in GP training. We often just pick it up as we go along" (GP B4)

"So I think if you can even get [medical] students before they're qualified to know what's out there [CAM], know what the evidence base is, know who is regulated, know the training and the hoops that people have to jump through, I think it will be really helpful. I think the CCGs yes, but it's too late, because you've got to get the GPs with that knowledge earlier" (CAM C6)

Governance of CAM

Regulation of CAM practitioners was not a major issue for participants although some CAM practitioners felt that greater regulation of practitioners, and improved NHS awareness of regulation, were important. GPs did not mention regulation as a major factor, but that may be due to lack of awareness of the issues.

"I don't see the chance of [hypnotherapy] getting integrated into NHS and NHS funded practice as long as there is a lack of regulation" (CAM A2.3)

"it's giving confidence to the, to the GPs if they are referring to a CAM then if you are CNHC [Complementary and Natural Healthcare Council] registered, then there is a lot of, um, ground to that" (CAM C5)

Commissioners' views varied on whether regulation of CAM practitioners would influence their decisions.

"...if it's mainstream, those are fairly standard, for example, you know, a doctor or a nurse or a therapist for example, but when it comes to some of the alternative or complementary therapies then I don't think always the systems are necessarily quite as rigorous" (commissioner 5)

"[Regulation] is something really that I do not want...imposed on all these other people [CAM practitioners]...The regulation in the health service is an unmitigated disaster now and is costing the system a fortune with...no evidence that it improves quality" (commissioner 6)

Models of integration

CAM practitioners, GPs and commissioners all felt that CAM might address some limitations of NHS provision for patients with MSK-MH comorbidity. For example, where waiting times for NHS treatment were long or the course of treatment/consultations too short; where lifestyle change or an active approach could reduce secondary care burden; where additional treatment options were needed; or to create a more holistic service.

"People, at the moment, are frustrated because they're, they're going to doctors and they're being like, sometimes given just an option of pain relief or physio, but there's a waiting list which is too long for them" (CAM A2.2)

CAM practitioners varied in their views as to whether paying for CAM can improve commitment, adherence, and its perceived value, and that co-payment by patients, on a sliding scale depending on ability to pay, might be the best model. This was also seen as a way of raising awareness of the cost of healthcare, including NHS care, which is often not clear to patients.

"I would see that you would have perhaps council paying a third, NHS paying a third, and it would be

wonderful if the patient paid a third to show a commitment. Would be a nice vision. Would help with the cost saving [laughs]." (CAM A1.2)

Commissioners suggested models for integrating CAM into NHS services. The most promising appeared to be integrated personal commissioning budgets (a scheme using personal health budgets for patients/carers to take more control over their health, and to integrate health, social care and voluntary services) and social prescribing, although the available data have limited generalisability and these models are wider than just CAM. Signposting to CAM (mentioning it without formally referring patients) was also mentioned. Alternatives to NHS-funding were suggested, including charity-funding, voluntary practitioners and public-sector funding. Other considerations included improving communication between CAM and NHS practitioners (which was reported as poor by GPs), and providing CAM through a social enterprise.

Discussion
Summary of findings

GPs, CAM practitioners and commissioners agreed that CAM may be useful to address the limitations of NHS care for the prevalent issue of MSK-MH comorbidity, which include availability and limited effective treatments. Exercise- or self-care-based CAMs were the most acceptable to GPs.

Although they agreed that MSK-MH comorbidity is prevalent and burdensome and needs a new approach, the three groups' views on the barriers to using CAM within the NHS varied. A central message regarding integration was the different understandings of health between CAM and conventional medicine, which were likely to impede integration. CAM practitioners and GPs were concerned about integration fundamentally changing the care they provide, and both groups agreed that GPs' lack of education, knowledge, and understanding regarding CAM was a barrier to integration. For CAM practitioners, NHS structural barriers were a major hurdle. For GPs, lack of time and resources and current pressures were important issues, causing them to feel integration of CAM was beyond their capability. GPs emphasised that integrated medicine would have to relieve their burden rather than add to it. In terms of facilitating integration, evidence was more important to CAM practitioners than GPs and certainly than commissioners, who were more focussed on cost saving. Governance was not a major issue.

Various models of integration were discussed, with little consensus. GPs and commissioners saw an overlap of CAM with social support and exercise and current UK policy regarding self-care and patient activation.

Integration could therefore be seen as one facet of social prescribing and holistic GP care.

Comparison with previous literature

A systematic review has confirmed that GPs see comorbidity as challenging to treat [51]. Our results support previous findings that GPs see MSK pain as an effectiveness gap suitable for an integrated/integrative approach [12, 13, 29, 30], and suggest this also applies to MSK-MH comorbidity. GPs' preference for exercise- or self-care- based CAM aligns with UK healthcare guidelines for low back pain (NICE guideline NG59), depression (NICE guideline CG91) and anxiety (NICE guideline CG113).

Our findings confirm previously identified challenges of integration that are recognised by UK healthcare professionals and may apply to MSK-MH comorbidity. These include: different 'world-views' in understanding health/health care [16, 37, 52]; concerns about secularising CAM when integrating [12, 19, 20] or having to fundamentally change conventional care [16]; NHS bureaucracy (for CAM practitioners) [31, 53]; GPs' lack of knowledge and need for education in CAM [54–56]; and lack of time in NHS settings [31, 39]. GPs' concern that integration of CAM was beyond their current capacity appears to be a new finding and is discussed under Implications below. Although we focussed on an integrated (selective incorporation) model in our topic guides, the challenges raised by participants, particularly those regarding the conceptual differences between CAM and biomedicine, are more pertinent to a transformative model of integration –described by GP A6 as "the extended...integration of integrated medicine". They confirm the view that transformative integration may be a 'utopian ideal' [19].

The concern about 'trying to put a square peg into a round hole' - the 'secularisation' of CAM - is raised by Hollenberg & Muzzin, as 'colonisation' of CAM [57]. Wiese and colleagues found that incompatibility between the ethos of science and CAM mean integration often involves 'co-optation' of CAM, and biomedical domination. There are examples of such secularisation in mindfulness-based approaches and herbal medicine [58, 59].

Poor GP knowledge implies education is needed about CAM – in the UK GPs are keen [29] and in the USA, CAM is often part of the medical curriculum [60]. Inter-professional education is an option [61].

The relatively low importance commissioners gave to evidence is interesting, but confirms findings from conventional medicine [62]. That CAM practitioners believe evidence is important has been reported before [63, 64]. However, CAM practitioners may lack research training [65], and have concerns about the appropriateness of traditional research methodology in CAM [66, 67].

Commissioners' emphasis on cost-saving evidence reflects an emphasis on prioritisation of health service funding [68] and more economic evidence is needed for CAM [69].

Implications

In our study, all three groups of healthcare professionals believed that an integrated approach using certain CAM may be worth pursuing to address limitations of conventional approaches in treating MSK-MH comorbidity, but they had different concerns about how an integrated approach might be implemented.

Findings highlight the burden that GPs are carrying in the UK – their workload has substantially increased [70, 71], a significant proportion of which is MSK and MH conditions [72, 73]. This 'crisis' creates reluctance to even contemplate anything new, e.g. integrated medicine, even if potentially beneficial. GPs and commissioners both felt successful integrated medicine would need to relieve NHS pressures, by reducing GP burden and costs. Integrating CAM may relieve GP workload for patients with limited treatment options [37]. Our study confirms 2003 findings that GPs and commissioners see integration of CAM as potentially helping to meet NHS targets [68]. Current policy drivers include the self-care and patient activation components of the NHS England Five Year Forward View [25, 28], in which primary care is central [26]. This aligns with "expansionism"- which favours the inclusion of alternative approaches [26, 74] e.g. social prescribing and holistic care. Conversely, some GPs' concerns about integration reflect "reductionists'" arguments for GPs to reduce their duties to focus on the "genuinely vulnerable and sick" [75]. This is in line with the 2004 General Practitioner contract which has resulted in GPs practicing a more biomedical model of health and illness [76].

In terms of an integration model, transformative models are unlikely to be successful due to severe restrictions on NHS spending and concerns that these models would necessitate secularisation of CAM or fundamentally changing conventional care [77]. Instead, selective incorporation using referral from NHS primary care, as in social prescribing, may help the NHS address the needs of comorbid patients. Social prescribing is increasingly popular, with a national social prescribing network [78], and funding for social prescribing schemes/interventions from the UK Department of Health [79]. Regulatory implications - GPs would need to be sure of CAM practitioners' regulation, quality and safety - may necessitate CAM practitioners becoming allied health practitioners, facilitated by the Professional Standards Authority's CAM registers [80]. This referral model would require GP education and referral protocols/guidelines [20, 56], and has cost implications, as CAM is almost always patient-funded or part-funded [81, 82]. Co-payment by patients/NHS may be an option, but has equity implications and would need to consider ability to pay, particularly as MSK-MH comorbid patients tend to be of lower socioeconomic status [83, 84]. The King's Fund recently rejected the controversial issue of patients paying for NHS treatment [85]. Another funding option is public health funding, given the overlap between integrative medicine, preventative medicine and public health [86].

For anyone attempting to integrate CAM into a conventional health system we suggest: identifying the evidence for effectiveness and cost-effectiveness; careful consideration of terminology; working with practitioners to develop a CAM approach which respects the philosophies of both conventional medicine and CAM; considering exercise- or self-care-based CAM; including education for GPs; and linking to relevant conventional health policies/strategic priorities e.g. in the UK the Five Year Forward View [56].

There is a need for more evidence of effectiveness and particularly cost-effectiveness of CAM; MSK-MH comorbidity is a fertile area for research. Exercise- and self-care-based CAM may be the best approaches to evaluate as they appear to be most acceptable to GPs.

Strengths and limitations

We were successful in recruiting a large number of practitioners, however we did not aim for data saturation so a larger sample may provide new themes or understandings. Purposive sampling captured the views of a wide range of individuals, and we met all the criteria in our sampling frame, despite GPs' limited availability. However, the professionals who took part were likely to have a more pro-CAM stance than average, which may mean our results are skewed towards the positive aspects of an integrated approach. The researcher's pro-CAM stance may have biased responses although we made efforts to emphasise that we were interested in a range of views and remaining grounded in the objective data from the literature review phase. Commissioners were very difficult to recruit, due to lack of a central organising body or mailing list, and busy schedules. For the large part, we relied on personal contacts, giving a skewed sample with mainly positive experiences regarding commissioning CAM. Their limited availability to attend a focus group necessitated more one-on-one interviews, which may have influenced the findings. More research with commissioners would be very valuable.

Conclusions

GPs, commissioners, and CAM practitioners felt that integration of CAM may offer a useful solution to the challenges faced by the NHS in treating MSK-MH comorbid patients. However, integration of CAM into NHS care/settings for these patients is limited by structural barriers, philosophical differences and concerns about changing both types of care fundamentally. Selective incorporation using referral from NHS primary care into CAM services may be a feasible model of integration, although cost implications would need to be addressed, possibly through models such as social prescribing or co-payment. Regulatory issues would also need to be addressed, including raising GPs' awareness of CAM registers.

Acknowledgements
We are very grateful to the participants in the study. We would also like to thank Mwenza Blell and Kate Morton for their assistance in running the focus groups.

Funding
The report is based on independent research commissioned and funded by the NIHR Policy Research Programme (The Effectiveness And Cost Effectiveness Of Complementary And Alternative Medicine (CAM) For Multimorbid Patients With Mental Health And Musculoskeletal Problems In Primary Care In The UK: A Scoping Study). The views expressed in the publication are those of the author(s) and not necessarily those of the NHS, the NIHR, the Department of Health, 'arms' length bodies or other government departments.

Authors' contributions
DS, GF, PL, SH, SM, AL and HM collaboratively developed the topic guides and helped provide sources of participants. AL organised recruitment for, conducted and analysed the focus groups, and drafted the paper. HM assisted in running one set of focus groups. DS, GF, PL, SH, SM, AL and HM revised the draft paper and read and approved the final version.

Competing interests
The authors declare that they have no competing interests.

Author details
[1]Centre for Academic Primary Care, School of Social and Community Medicine, University of Bristol, Canynge Hall, 39 Whatley Road, Bristol BS8 2PS, UK. [2]Primary Medical Care, Faculty of Medicine, University of Southampton, Aldermoor Close, Southampton SO16 5ST, UK. [3]General Practice and Primary Care, Institute for Health and Wellbeing, University of Glasgow, 1 Horseletthill Road, Glasgow G12 9LX, UK. [4]Department of Health Sciences, University of York, Heslington, York YO10 5DD, UK.

References
1. Hartvigsen J, Hancock MJ, Kongsted A, Louw Q, Ferreira ML, Genevay S, Hoy D, Karppinen J, Pransky G, Sieper J, et al. What low back pain is and why we need to pay attention. Lancet. https://doi.org/10.1016/S0140-6736(18)30480-X [e-pub ahead of print].
2. Department of Health: The Musculoskeletal Services Framework: A joint responsibility: doing it differently. In.; 2006.
3. Office for National Statistics (ONS): Sickness Absence Report. In.; 2016.
4. Davies SC. Annual Report of the Chief Medical Officer 2013, Public Mental Health Priorities: Investing in the Evidence. London: Department of Health; 2014.
5. Knapp M, Lemmi V. The economic case for better mental health. In: Davies S, editor. Annual Report of the Chief Medical Officer 2013, Public Mental Health Priorities: Investing in the Evidence. London: Department of Health; 2014. p. 147–56.
6. Gureje O, Von Korff M, Simon GE, Gater R. Persistent pain and well-being: a World Health Organization study in primary care. Jama. 1998;280(2):147–51.
7. Lepine JP, Briley M. The epidemiology of pain in depression. Hum Psychopharmacol. 2004;19(Suppl 1):S3–7.
8. Department for Work and Pensions, Department of Health: Work, health and disability green paper data pack, supplementary tables; source: table 1n. labour force survey april to june 2016. In.; 2016.
9. Gore M, Sadosky A, Stacey BR, Tai K-S, Leslie D. The burden of chronic low Back pain: clinical comorbidities, treatment patterns, and health care costs in usual care settings. Spine. 2012;37(11):E668–77.
10. NICE: Multimorbidity: clinical assessment and management NICE guideline [NG56]. In.; 2016.
11. Mangin D, Heath I, Jamoulle M. Beyond diagnosis: rising to the multimorbidity challenge. BMJ. 2012;344:e3526.

12. Wye L, Shaw A, Sharp D. Designing a 'NHS friendly' complementary therapy service: a qualitative case study. BMC Health Serv Res. 2008;8(1):173.

13. Fisher P, van Haselen R, Hardy K, Berkovitz S, McCarney R. Effectiveness gaps: a new concept for evaluating health service and research needs applied to complementary and alternative medicine. J Altern Complement Med. 2004; 10(4):627–32.

14. Alwhaibi M, Bhattacharya R, Sambamoorthi U. Type of multimorbidity and complementary and alternative medicine use among adults. Evid Based Complement Alternat Med. 2015;2015. https://doi.org/10.1155/2015/362582.

15. Bystritsky A, Hovav S, Sherbourne C, Stein MB, Rose RD, Campbell-Sills L, Golinelli D, Sullivan G, Craske MG, Roy-Byrne PP. Use of complementary and alternative medicine in a large sample of anxiety patients. Psychosomatics. 2012;53(3):266–72.

16. Wiese M, Oster C, Pincombe J. Understanding the emerging relationship between complementary medicine and mainstream health care: a review of the literature. Health (London). 2010;14(3):326–42.

17. Luff DT, Kate. Models of complementary therapy provision in primary care. In: Medical care research unit. Sheffield: Medical Care Research Unit, University of Sheffield; 1999.

18. Hu X-Y, Lorenc A, Kemper K, Liu J-P, Adams J, Robinson N. Defining integrative medicine in narrative and systematic reviews: a suggested checklist for reporting. Eur J Integr Med. 2015;7(1):76–84.

19. Hollenberg D. Uncharted ground: patterns of professional interaction among complementary/alternative and biomedical practitioners in integrative health care settings. Soc Sci Med. 2006;62(3):731–44.

20. Chung VCH, Ma PHX, Hong LC, Griffiths SM. Organizational determinants of interprofessional collaboration in integrative health care: systematic review of qualitative studies. PLoS One. 2012;7(11):e50022.

21. Wilkinson J, Peters D, Donaldson J: Clinical governance for complementary and alternative medicine in primary care. Final Report to the Department of Health and the King's Fund 2004.

22. Thomas K, Coleman P, Nicholl J. Trends in access to complementary or alternative medicines via primary care in England: 1995–2001 results from a follow-up national survey. Fam Pract. 2003;20(5):575–7.

23. Templeman K, Robinson A. Integrative medicine models in contemporary primary health care. Complement Ther Med. 2011;19(2):84–92.

24. Kemper KJ. APA Presendential address: holistic pediatrics = good medicine. Pediatrics. 2000;105:214–8.

25. Liberating the NHS white paper [https://www.gov.uk/government/publications/liberating-the-nhs-white-paper]. Accessed 15 Oct 2018.

26. Five Year Forward View [https://www.england.nhs.uk/ourwork/futurenhs/nhs-five-year-forward-view-web-version/]. Accessed 15 Oct 2018.

27. Delivering the forward view: NHS planning guidance 2016/17–2020/21 [https://www.england.nhs.uk/ourwork/futurenhs/deliver-forward-view/]. Accessed 15 Oct 2018.

28. At the heart of health: realising the value of people and communities [https://media.nesta.org.uk/documents/at_the_heart_of_health_-_realising_the_value_of_people_and_communities.pdf]. Accessed 15 Oct 2018.

29. van Haselen RA, Reiber U, Nickel I, Jakob A, Fisher PAG. Providing complementary and alternative medicine in primary care: the primary care workers' perspective. Complement Ther Med. 2004;12(1):6–16.

30. Jarvis A, Perry R, Smith D, Terry R, Peters S. General practitioners' beliefs about the clinical utility of complementary and alternative medicine. Prim Health Care Res Dev. 2015;16(03):246–53.

31. Bishop FL, Amos N, Yu H, Lewith GT. Health-care sector and complementary medicine: practitioners' experiences of delivering acupuncture in the public and private sectors. Prim Health Care Res Dev. 2012;13(03):269–78.

32. Maha N, Shaw A. Academic doctors' views of complementary and alternative medicine (CAM) and its role within the NHS: an exploratory qualitative study. BMC Complement Altern Med. 2007;7(1):17.

33. Lipman L, Dale J, MacPherson H. Attitudes of GPs towards the provision of acupuncture on the NHS. Complement Ther Med. 2003;11(2):110–4.

34. Lorenc A, Blair M, Robinson N. Personal and professional influences on practitioners' attitudes to traditional and complementary approaches to health in the UK. J Tradit Chin Med Sci. 2014;1(2):148–55.

35. Brien S, Howells E, Leydon GM, Lewith G. Why GPs refer patients to complementary medicine via the NHS: a qualitative exploration. Prim Health Care Res Dev. 2008;9:205–15.

36. Perard M, Mittring N, Schweiger D, Kummer C, Witt CM. Merging conventional and complementary medicine in a clinic department - a theoretical model and practical recommendations. BMC Complement Altern Med. 2015;15(1):172.

37. Luff D, Thomas KJ. Sustaining complementary therapy provision in primary care: lessons from existing services. Complement Ther Med. 2000;8(3):173–9.

38. Peters D, Chaitow L, Harris G, Morrison S. Integrating complementary therapies in primary care. London: Churchill Livingstone; 2002.

39. Paterson C, Britten N. The patient's experience of holistic care: insights from acupuncture research. Chronic Illn. 2008;4(4):264–77.

40. Good medical practice [http://www.gmc-uk.org/guidance/index.asp]. Accessed 15 Oct 2018.

41. Tong A, Sainsbury P, Craig J. Consolidated criteria for reporting qualitative research (COREQ): a 32-item checklist for interviews and focus groups. Int J Qual Health Care. 2007;19(6):349–57.

42. Ritchie J, Spencer L, O'Connor W. Carrying out qualitative analysis. In: Ritchie J, Lewis J, editors. Qualitative research practice: a guide for social science students and researchers. Edn. London: Sage Publications Ltd.; 2003. p. 219–62.

43. Ritchie J, Spencer L. Qualitative data analysis for applied policy research. In: Bryman A, Burgess R, editors. Analysing qualitative data. London: Routledge; 1993.

44. Pope C, Ziebland S, Mays N. Qualitative research in health care: analysing qualitative data. BMJ. 2000;320:114–6.

45. Spencer L, Ritchie J, O'Connor W. Analysis:practices, principles and processes. In: Ritchie J, Lewis J, editors. Qualitative Research Practice. London: Sage Publications Ltd; 2003. p. 200–18.

46. Pope C, Ziebland S, Mays N. Analysing qualitative data. In: Pope C, Mays N, editors. Qualitative Research in Health Care. Volume 3rd Edition. Oxford: BMJ Books; 2006. p. 63–82.

47. Denzin N, Lincoln YS. Collecting and interpreting qualitative materials. London: Sage Publications Ltd; 1998.

48. Rabiee F. Focus-group interview and data analysis. ProcNutrSoc. 2004;63(4): 655–60.

49. Arksey H, Knight P. Interviewing for social scientists: an introductory resource with examples. London: Sage Publications Ltd; 1999.

50. Seale C. The quality of qualitative research. London: Sage Publications Ltd; 1999.

51. Sinnott C, Mc Hugh S, Browne J, Bradley C. GPs' perspectives on the management of patients with multimorbidity: systematic review and synthesis of qualitative research. BMJ Open. 2013;3(9):e003610.

52. Quah SR. Traditional healing systems and the ethos of science. Soc Sci Med. 2003;57(10):1997–2012.

53. Cant S, Watts P, Ruston A. The rise and fall of complementary medicine in National Health Service hospitals in England. Complement Ther Clin Pract. 2012;18(3):135–9.

54. Sewitch MJ, Cepoiu M, Rigillo N, Sproule D. A literature review of health care professional attitudes toward complementary and alternative medicine. Complement Health Pract Rev. 2008;13(3):139–54.

55. Niemtzow RC, Burns SM, Piazza TR, Pock AR, Walter J, Petri R, Hofmann L, Wilson C, Drake D, Calabria K, et al. Integrative medicine in the Department of Defense and the Department of Veterans Affairs: cautious steps forward. J Altern Complement Med. 2016;22(3):171–3.

56. Crane R, Kuyken W. The implementation of mindfulness-based cognitive therapy: learning from the UK health service experience. Mindfulness. 2013; 4(3):246–54.

57. Hollenberg D, Muzzin L. Epistemological challenges to integrative medicine: an anti-colonial perspective on the combination of complementary/alternative medicine with biomedicine. Health Sociol Rev. 2010;19(1):34–56.

58. Secular mindfulness: potential & pitfalls [https://www.bcbsdharma.org/article/secular-mindfulness-potential-pitfalls/]. Accessed 15 Oct 2018.

59. Singer J, Fisher K. The impact of co-option on herbalism: a bifurcation in epistemology and practice. Health Sociol Rev. 2007;16(1):18–26.

60. Kreitzer MJ, Mann D, Lumpkin M. CAM competencies for the health professions. Complement Health Pract Rev. 2008;13(1):63–72.

61. Willison KD. Advancing integrative medicine through interprofessional education. Health Sociol Rev. 2008;17(4):342–52.

62. Wye L, Brangan E, Cameron A, Gabbay J, Klein JH, Pope C. Evidence based policy making and the 'art' of commissioning – how English healthcare commissioners access and use information and academic research in 'real life' decision-making: an empirical qualitative study. BMC Health Serv Res. 2015;15:430.

63. Hall G. Attitudes of chiropractors to evidence-based practice and how this compares to other healthcare professionals: a qualitative study. Clin Chiropr. 2011;14(3):106–11.

64. Kim Y, Cho S-H. A survey of complementary and alternative medicine practitioner's perceptions of evidence-based medicine. Eur J Integr Med. 2014;6(2):211–9.

65. Hadley J, Hassan I, Khan KS. Knowledge and beliefs concerning evidence-based practice amongst complementary and alternative medicine health care practitioners and allied health care professionals: a questionnaire survey. BMC Complement Altern Med. 2008;8(1):45.

66. Hansen K. Attitudes to evidence in acupuncture: an interview study. Med Health Care Philos. 2012;15(3):279–85.

67. Barry CA. The role of evidence in alternative medicine: contrasting biomedical and anthropological approaches. Soc Sci Med. 2006;62(11): 2646–57.

68. Thomas KJ, Coleman P, Weatherley-Jones E, Luff D. Developing integrated CAM services in primary care Organisations. Complement Ther Med. 2003; 11(4):261–7.

69. Herman PM, Craig BM, Caspi O. Is complementary and alternative medicine (CAM) cost-effective? A systematic review. BMC Complement Altern Med. 2005;5:11.

70. Dale J, Potter R, Owen K, Parsons N, Realpe A, Leach J. Retaining the general practitioner workforce in England: what matters to GPs? A cross-sectional study. BMC Fam Pract. 2015;16(1):140.

71. Neher JO, Borkan JM, Wilkinson MJ, Reis S, Hermoni D, Hobbs FD. Doctor-patient discussions of alternative medicine for back pain. Scand J Prim Health Care. 2001;19(4):237–40.

72. The Musculoskeletal Services Framework: A joint responsibility: doing it differently [http://webarchive.nationalarchives.gov.uk/20130107105354/http:/www.dh.gov.uk/prod_consum_dh/groups/dh_digitalassets/@dh/@en/documents/digitalasset/dh_4138412.pdf]. Accessed 15 Oct 2018.

73. No Health Without Mental Health: A cross-government mental health outcomes strategy for people of all ages [https://www.gov.uk/government/uploads/system/uploads/attachment_data/file/213761/dh_124058.pdf]. Accessed 15 Oct 2018.

74. Nearly two million patients to receive person-centred support to manage their own care [https://www.england.nhs.uk/2016/04/person-centred-support/]. Accessed 15 Oct 2018.

75. GPs shun homeopathy as prescriptions halve [http://www.pulsetoday.co.uk/gps-shun-homeopathy-as-prescriptions-halve/10984426.article#.VadIrq3bKM8]. Accessed 15 Oct 2018.

76. Checkland K, Harrison S, McDonald R, Grant S, Campbell S, Guthrie B. Biomedicine, holism and general medical practice: responses to the 2004 general practitioner contract. Sociol Health Illn. 2008;30(5):788–803.

77. Wye L. Mainstreaming complementary therapies into primary care: the role of evidence, 'ideal' service design and delivery and alterations in clinical practice. Phd thesis: University of Bristol; 2007.

78. New National Social Prescribing Network Addresses NHS Healthcare Accessibility Issues [https://www.westminster.ac.uk/news-and-events/news/2016/new-national-social-prescribing-network-addresses-nhs-healthcare-accessibility-issues]. Accessed 15 Oct 2018.

79. Matthews-King A. Providers invited to bid for £4m worth of funding for social prescribing schemes. Pulse. 2017. http://www.pulsetoday.co.uk/clinical/prescribing/providers-invited-to-bid-for-4m-worth-of-funding-for-social-prescribing-schemes/20035430.article.

80. Let's Work Together [https://www.professionalstandards.org.uk/what-we-do/accredited-registers/lets-work-together]. Accessed 15 Oct 2018.

81. Bodeker G, Kronenberg F, Public Health A. Agenda for traditional, complementary, and alternative medicine. Am J Public Health. 2002;92(10):1582–91.

82. Sharp D, Lorenc A, Morris R, Feder G, Little P, Hollinghurst S, Mercer SW, MacPherson H. Complementary medicine use, views and experiences – a national survey in England. BJGP Open. 2018; Paper submitted for publication. https://doi.org/10.1016/S0140-6736(12)60240-2.

83. Barnett K, Mercer SW, Norbury M, Watt G, Wyke S, Guthrie B. Epidemiology of multimorbidity and implications for health care, research, and medical education: a cross-sectional study. Lancet. 2012;380(9836):37–43.

84. McLean G, Gunn J, Wyke S, Guthrie B, Watt GCM, Blane DN, Mercer SW. The influence of socioeconomic deprivation on multimorbidity at different ages: a cross-sectional study. Br J Gen Pract. 2014;64(624):e440–7.

85. Barker K: A new settlement for health and social care. In: The King's Fund; 2014.

86. Ali A, Katz DL. Disease prevention and health promotion: how integrative medicine fits. Am J Prev Med. 2015;49(5 Suppl 3):S230–40.

Permissions

All chapters in this book were first published in CAM, by BioMed Central; hereby published with permission under the Creative Commons Attribution License or equivalent. Every chapter published in this book has been scrutinized by our experts. Their significance has been extensively debated. The topics covered herein carry significant findings which will fuel the growth of the discipline. They may even be implemented as practical applications or may be referred to as a beginning point for another development.

The contributors of this book come from diverse backgrounds, making this book a truly international effort. This book will bring forth new frontiers with its revolutionizing research information and detailed analysis of the nascent developments around the world.

We would like to thank all the contributing authors for lending their expertise to make the book truly unique. They have played a crucial role in the development of this book. Without their invaluable contributions this book wouldn't have been possible. They have made vital efforts to compile up to date information on the varied aspects of this subject to make this book a valuable addition to the collection of many professionals and students.

This book was conceptualized with the vision of imparting up-to-date information and advanced data in this field. To ensure the same, a matchless editorial board was set up. Every individual on the board went through rigorous rounds of assessment to prove their worth. After which they invested a large part of their time researching and compiling the most relevant data for our readers.

The editorial board has been involved in producing this book since its inception. They have spent rigorous hours researching and exploring the diverse topics which have resulted in the successful publishing of this book. They have passed on their knowledge of decades through this book. To expedite this challenging task, the publisher supported the team at every step. A small team of assistant editors was also appointed to further simplify the editing procedure and attain best results for the readers.

Apart from the editorial board, the designing team has also invested a significant amount of their time in understanding the subject and creating the most relevant covers. They scrutinized every image to scout for the most suitable representation of the subject and create an appropriate cover for the book.

The publishing team has been an ardent support to the editorial, designing and production team. Their endless efforts to recruit the best for this project, has resulted in the accomplishment of this book. They are a veteran in the field of academics and their pool of knowledge is as vast as their experience in printing. Their expertise and guidance has proved useful at every step. Their uncompromising quality standards have made this book an exceptional effort. Their encouragement from time to time has been an inspiration for everyone.

The publisher and the editorial board hope that this book will prove to be a valuable piece of knowledge for researchers, students, practitioners and scholars across the globe.

List of Contributors

Nurul Elyani Mohamad
Department of Cell and Molecular Biology, Faculty of Biotechnology and Biomolecular Science, Universiti Putra Malaysia, 43400 Serdang, Selangor, Malaysia

Noorjahan Banu Alitheen
Department of Cell and Molecular Biology, Faculty of Biotechnology and Biomolecular Science, Universiti Putra Malaysia, 43400 Serdang, Selangor, Malaysia
Institute of Bioscience, Universiti Putra Malaysia, Serdang, Selangor, Malaysia

Swee Keong Yeap
China-ASEAN College of Marine Sciences, Xiamen University Malaysia, Jalan Sunsuria, Bandar Sunsuria, 43900 Sepang, Selangor, Malaysia

Boon-Kee Beh
Institute of Bioscience, Universiti Putra Malaysia, Serdang, Selangor, Malaysia
Biotechnology Research Centre, Malaysian Agricultural Research and Development Institute (MARDI), 43400 Serdang, Selangor, Malaysia

Shaiful Adzni Sharifuddin and Kamariah Long
Biotechnology Research Centre, Malaysian Agricultural Research and Development Institute (MARDI), 43400 Serdang, Selangor, Malaysia

Huynh Ky
Department of Genetics and Plant Breeding, College of Agriculture and Applied Biology, Cantho University, 3/2 Street, CanTho City, Vietnam

Kian Lam Lim
Faculty of Medicine and Health Sciences, Universiti Tunku Abdul Rahman, Sungai Long Campus, Jalan Sungai Long, Bandar Sungai Long, Cheras, 43000 Kajang, Selangor, Malaysia

Wan Yong Ho
School of Biomedical Sciences, the University of Nottingham Malaysia Campus, Jalan Broga, 43500 Semenyih, Selangor, Malaysia

Emily M. Hagel Campbell, Lynsey R. Miron and Paul D. Thuras
Minneapolis VA Health Care System, One Veterans Drive, Minneapolis, MN 55417, USA

Melvin T. Donaldson
Minneapolis VA Health Care System, One Veterans Drive, Minneapolis, MN 55417, USA
University of Minnesota Medical Scientist Training Program, Minneapolis, MN 55455, USA

Elizabeth S. Goldsmith
Minneapolis VA Health Care System, One Veterans Drive, Minneapolis, MN 55417, USA
Division of Epidemiology and Community Health, University of Minnesota School of Public Health, Minneapolis, MN 55454, USA. 4University of Minnesota Medical School, Minneapolis, MN 55455, USA

Melissa A. Polusny and Erin E. Krebs
Minneapolis VA Health Care System, One Veterans Drive, Minneapolis, MN 55417, USA
University of Minnesota Medical School, Minneapolis, MN 55455, USA

Rich F. MacLehose
Division of Epidemiology and Community Health, University of Minnesota School of Public Health, Minneapolis, MN 55454, USA

Wei-ming He and Wei Sun
Affiliated Hospital of Nanjing University of Chinese Medicine, Nanjing 210029, Jiangsu, China

Jia-qi Yin, Li Ni, Yi Xi, Gui-dong Yin, Guo-yuan Lu and Ming-gang Wei
The First Affiliated Hospital of Soochow University, Suzhou 215006, Jiangsu, China

Xu-dong Cheng
Suzhou Hospital of Traditional Chinese Medicine, Suzhou 215006, Jiangsu, China

Xun Lu
Suzhou Municipal Hospital, Affiliated Hospital of Nanjing Medical University, Suzhou 215006, Jiangsu, China

Jie Sun, Beidong Chen, Yanyang Zhao and Huan Gong
MOH Key Laboratory of Geriatrics, Beijing Hospital, National Center of Gerontology, Beijing, China

Ming Zhang and Ruomei Qi
MOH Key Laboratory of Geriatrics, Beijing Hospital, National Center of Gerontology, Beijing, China
Graduate School of Peking Union Medical College, Chinese Academy of Medical Sciences, Beijing, China

Yun You
Institute of Chinese Materia Medica, China Academy of Chinese Medical Sciences, Beijing, China

Shaohui Wang , Yanlan Hu, Yu Yan and Zhekang Cheng
School of Pharmacy, Minzu University of China, No. 27 Zhongguancun South Street, Haidian District, Beijing 100081, China

Tongxiang Liu
School of Pharmacy, Minzu University of China, Key Laboratory of Ethnomedicine (Minzu University of China), Minority of Education, No. 27 Zhongguancun South Street, Haidian District, Beijing 100081, China

Raissa Tioyem Nzogong, Mathieu Tene and Pierre Tane
Laboratory of Natural Products Chemistry, Department of Chemistry, Faculty of Science, University of Dschang, Dschang, Cameroon

Maurice Ducret Awouafack
Laboratory of Natural Products Chemistry, Department of Chemistry, Faculty of Science, University of Dschang, Dschang, Cameroon
Institute of Natural Medicine, University of Toyama, 2630-Sugitani, Toyama 930-0194, Japan.

Fabrice Sterling Tchantchou Ndjateu
Laboratory of Natural Products Chemistry, Department of Chemistry, Faculty of Science, University of Dschang, Dschang, Cameroon
H.E.J Research Institute of Chemistry, University of Karachi, -75270, Karachi, Pakistan

Steve Endeguele Ekom, Jules-Arnaud Mboutchom Fosso and Jean-de-Dieu Tamokou
Laboratory of Microbiology and Antimicrobial substances, Department of Biochemistry, Faculty of Science, University of Dschang, Dschang, Cameroon

Hiroyuki Morita
Institute of Natural Medicine, University of Toyama, 2630-Sugitani, Toyama 930-0194, Japan

Muhammad Iqbal Choudhary
H.E.J Research Institute of Chemistry, University of Karachi, -75270, Karachi, Pakistan

Yu-Heng Lai
Department of Chemistry, Chinese Culture University, Taipei 11114, Taiwan

Cheng-Pu Sun
Institute of Biomedical Sciences, Academia Sinica, Taipei 11529, Taiwan

Hsiu-Chen Huang
Department of Applied Science, National Tsing Hua University South Campus, Hsinchu 30014, Taiwan

Jui-Chieh Chen
Department of Biochemical Science and Technology, National Chiayi University, Chiayi 60004, Taiwan

Hui-Kang Liu
National Research Institute of Chinese Medicine, Ministry of Health and Welfare, Taipei 11221, Taiwan
Program in Clinical Drug Development of Chinese Herbal Medicine, Taipei Medical University, Taipei 11001, Taiwan

Cheng Huang
Department of Biotechnology and Laboratory Science in Medicine, National Yang-Ming University, No. 155, Sec. 2, Linong St., Beitou District, Taipei 11221, Taiwan
Department of Earth and Life Sciences, University of Taipei, Taipei 11153, Taiwan

Yizhe Cui, Qiuju Wang†, Rui Sun, Li Guo, Mengzhu Wang, Junfeng Jia, Chuang Xu and Rui Wu
College of Animal Science and Veterinary Medicine, Heilongjiang Bayi Agricultural University, 2# Xinyang Road, New Development District, Daqing 163319, Heilongjiang, China

Cyrille Ngoufack Tagousop and David Ngnokam
Research Unit of Environmental and Applied Chemistry, Department of Chemistry, Faculty of Science, University of Dschang, Dschang, Cameroon

Jean-de-Dieu Tamokou and Steve Endeguele Ekom
Research Unit of Microbiology and Antimicrobial Substances, Department of Biochemistry, Faculty of Science, University of Dschang, Dschang, Cameroon.

Laurence Voutquenne-Nazabadioko
Groupe Isolement et Structure, Institut de Chimie Moléculaire de Reims (ICMR), CNRS UMR 7312, Bat. 18 BP.1039, 51687 Reims cedex 2, France

Yuan-Chang Yang, Wing-Ming Chou, Debora Arny Widowati and Chi-Chung Peng
Department of Biotechnology, National Formosa University, Huwei District, Yunlin, Taiwan

I-Ping Lin
Department of Biotechnology, National Formosa University, Huwei District, Yunlin, Taiwan
Department of Research and Development, Challenge Bioproducts Co., Ltd., Yunlin, Taiwan

O. E. Kale and T.O.Ogundare
Department of Pharmacology, Benjamin S. Carson (Snr.) School of Medicine, Babcock University, Ilishan-Remo, Ogun State, PMB, Ikeja 21244, Nigeria

O. B. Akinpelu, A. A. Bakare, F. O. Yusuf, R. Gomba, D. C. Araka, A. C. Okolie, O. Adebawo and O. Odutola
Department of Biochemistry, Benjamin S. Carson (Snr.) School of Medicine, Babcock University, Ilishan-Remo, Ogun State, PMB, Ikeja 21244, Nigeria

Li Gao, Chunhua Jia and Huiwen Huang
Beijing University of Chinese Medicine, No. 11 North 3rd Ring East Road, Chaoyang District, Beijing 100029, China

Seo Hyun Kim, Sang Hee Lee, Won Kyun Im, Young Dong Kim and Sung Ho Jeon
Department of Life Science, Multidisciplinary Genome Institute, Hallym University, Chuncheon, Gangwon 24252, South Korea

Sung Won Lee, Hyun Jung Park and Seokmann Hong
Department of Integrative Bioscience and Biotechnology, Institute of Anticancer Medicine Development, Sejong University, Seoul 05006, South Korea

Kyung Hee Kim and Sang Jae Park
Medience Co.,Ltd., 301, Chuncheon Bioindustry Foundation, Chuncheon, Gangwon 24232,South Korea

Qi Sun, Shiyue Li, Junjun Li, Qiuxia Fu, Zhongyuan Wang, Shan-Shan Liu, Zijie Su, Jiaxing Song and Desheng Lu
Guangdong Key Laboratory for Genome Stability & Disease Prevention, Carson International Cancer Center, Department of Pharmacology, Shenzhen University Health Science Center, Shenzhen 518060, Guangdong, China

Bo Li
Key Laboratory of Systems Bioengineering (Ministry of Education), Tianjin University, Tianjin 300072, China

Jinhao Zeng, Ran Yan, Fengming You, Chuan Zheng, Daoyin Gong and Yi Zhang
Chengdu University of Traditional Chinese Medicine, Chengdu 610075, China

Huafeng Pan, Tiantian Cai and Wei Liu
Guangzhou University of Chinese Medicine, Guangzhou 510405, China

Ziming Zhao
Guangdong Provincial Institute of Chinese Medicine, Guangzhou 510095, China

Longhui Chen
Guangzhou Institutes of Biomedicine and Health, Chinese Academy of Sciences, Guangzhou 510530, China

Khalid Elhindi and Salah El-Hendawy
Plant production Department, College of Food and Agriculture Sciences, King Saud University, Riyadh 11451, Saudi Arabia

Hosam O. Elansary
Plant production Department, College of Food and Agriculture Sciences, King Saud University, Riyadh 11451, Saudi Arabia
Floriculture, Ornamental Horticulture and Garden Design Department, Faculty of Agriculture (El-Shatby), Alexandria University, Alexandria, Egypt
Department of Geography, Environmental Management and Energy Studies, University of Johannesburg, Auckland Park Kingsway Campus (APK) campus 2006, South Africa

Kowiyou Yessoufou
Department of Geography, Environmental Management and Energy Studies, University of Johannesburg, Auckland Park Kingsway Campus (APK) campus 2006, South Africa

Samir A. M. Abdelgaleil
Department of Pesticide Chemistry and Technology, Faculty of Agriculture, Alexandria University, ElShatby, Alexandria 21545, Egypt

Eman A. Mahmoud
Department of Food Industries, Damietta University, Damietta, Egypt

Loisa Drozdoff, Evelyn Klein, Marion Kiechle and Daniela Paepke
Department of Gynecology and Obstetrics, University Hospital rechts der Isar, Technical University Munich, Ismaninger Str. 22, 81675 Munich, Germany

Yuto Inagawa, Afifah Zahra Agista, Tomoko Goto1 and Michio Komai
Laboratory of Nutrition, Graduate School of Agricultural Science, Tohoku University, Sendai 980-0845, Japan

Ardiansyah
Laboratory of Nutrition, Graduate School of Agricultural Science, Tohoku University, Sendai 980-0845, Japan
Department of Food Science and Technology, Universitas Bakrie, Jakarta 12920, Indonesia

Hitoshi Shirakawa
Laboratory of Nutrition, Graduate School of Agricultural Science, Tohoku University, Sendai 980-0845, Japan
International Education and Research Center for Food Agricultural Immunology, Graduate School of Agricultural Science, Tohoku University, Sendai 980-0845, Japan

Takuya Koseki
Faculty of Agriculture, Yamagata University, Tsuruoka 997-8555, Japan

Ikuo Ikeda
Laboratory of Food and Biomolecular Science, Graduate School of Agricultural Science, Tohoku University, Sendai 980-0845, Japan

Justice Mbizo, Melanie A. Sutton and LeaunaM. Stone
Department of Public Health, University of West Florida, 11000 University Parkway, Bldg. 38/Room 127, Pensacola, FL 32514, USA

Anthony Okafor
Department of Mathematics and Statistics, University of West Florida, Pensacola, FL, USA

Bryan Leyva
Warren Alpert Medical School, Brown University, Providence, RI, USA

Oluwadamilola Olaku
Office of Cancer Complementary and Alternative Medicine, National Cancer Institute, Bethesda, MD, USA
Kelly Government Solutions, Bethesda, MD, USA

Thanyaluck Siriyong and Supayang Piyawan Voravuthikunchai
Department of Microbiology, Faculty of Science and Natural Product Research Center of Excellence, Prince of Songkla University, Songkhla, Thailand

Peter John Coote
Biomedical Sciences Research Complex, School of Biology, University of St Andrews, The North Haugh, St Andrews, Fife, UK

Caroline A. Smith, Kate Templeman and Suzanne Grant
NICM Health Research Institute, Western Sydney University, Westmead campus, Locked Bag 1797, Penrith, NSW 2751, Australia

Jennifer Hunter
NICM Health Research Institute, Western Sydney University, Westmead campus, Locked Bag 1797, Penrith, NSW 2751, Australia
Menzies Centre for Health Policy, School of Public Health, Sydney Medical School, The University of Sydney, Sydney, NSW, Australia

Jane M. Ussher
Translational Health Research Institute, School of Medicine, Western Sydney University, Campbelltown, NSW, Australia

Geoff P. Delaney
South-Western Sydney Clinical School, Faculty of Medicine, University of New South Wales, Kensington, NSW, Australia
Cancer Services, South Western Sydney Local Health District, Liverpool, NSW, Australia
Ingham Institute of Applied Medical Research, Liverpool, NSW, Australia

Eleanor Oyston
Oncology Massage Limited, Deakin West, ACT 2600, Australia

Sihle Ephraim Mabhida, Musawenkosi Ndlovu, Nonhlakanipho Felicia Sangweni, Andrew Opoku and Rebamang Anthony Mosa
Department of Biochemistry and Microbiology, University of Zululand, Private Bag X1001, KwaDlangezwa 3886, South Africa

Johan Louw
Biomedical Research and Innovation Platform (BRIP), South African Medical Research Council, Tygerberg 7505, South Africa

Rabia Johnson
Biomedical Research and Innovation Platform (BRIP), South African Medical Research Council, Tygerberg 7505, South Africa
Division of Medical Physiology, Faculty of Medicine and Health Sciences, Stellenbosch University, Tygerberg 7505, South Africa

Yoshinobu Nakada
Department of Kampo Medicine, Tokai University School of Medicine, Isehara, Kanagawa, Japan

Makoto Arai
Department of Kampo Medicine, Tokai University School of Medicine, Isehara, Kanagawa, Japan
Medical and Pharmaceutical Society for WAKAN-YAKU, Kanagawa, Japan

Deborah Sharp, Ava Lorenc , Gene Feder and Sandra Hollinghurst
Centre for Academic Primary Care, School of Social and Community Medicine, University of Bristol, Canynge Hall, 39 Whatley Road, Bristol BS8 2PS, UK

Paul Little
Primary Medical Care, Faculty of Medicine, University of Southampton, Aldermoor Close, Southampton SO16 5ST, UK

Stewart Mercer
General Practice and Primary Care, Institute for Health and Wellbeing, University of Glasgow, 1 Horseletthill Road, Glasgow G12 9LX, UK

Hugh MacPherson
Department of Health Sciences, University of York, Heslington, York YO10 5DD, UK

Index

9 781632 418166